Over 10,000 products reviewed,
including the latest skin-care information.

Don't Go to the Cosmetics Counter Without Me

Completely revised
and updated **4th** *Edition*

An Eye-Opening Guide to
Brand-Name Cosmetics

by

PAULA BEGOUN

Subscribe today to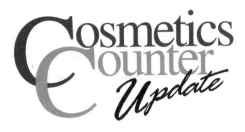

Dear Reader,

Why should you subscribe to my bimonthly newsletter? Because the cosmetics industry is always changing, and as much as I would like to tell you that **Don't Go to the Cosmetics Counter Without Me** provides ALL the product reviews you'll ever need, that simply wouldn't be the truth. There are new products and new cosmetic lines created practically every day, which is the reason I created *Cosmetics Counter Update*.

In each issue of *Cosmetics Counter Update* you'll find:

- **An endless array of the latest product reviews**
- **Full evaluations of new lines**
- **Answers to readers' "Dear Paula" questions**
- **Clear explanations of new research and studies**
- **Critiques of makeup techniques**
- **Hair-care product reviews**

I personally guarantee my newsletter. If you are not 100% satisfied, you will receive an immediate refund. Please give **Cosmetics Counter Update** a try. See if, like many other readers, you notice a money-saving difference in your beauty budget. I look forward to hearing from you!

Warmest regards,

Paula Begoun

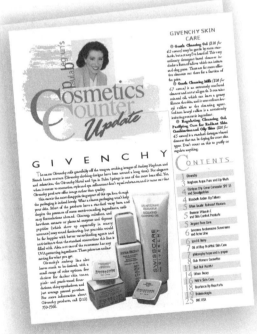

Cosmetics Counter Update:
Beauty and Brains
Finally, a newsletter for women like you!

☐ 1 Year **Cosmetics Counter Update** (US)	$25.00	_____
☐ 1 Year **Cosmetics Counter Update** (Canada)	$35.00	_____
☐ 1 Year **Cosmetics Counter Update** (All Other Countries)	$45.00	_____
☐ E-mail Subscription to **Cosmetics Counter Update**	$12.50	_____

E-mail address _____

☐ One-Time Introductory copy of **Cosmetics Counter Update**	$ 1.00	_____
☐ **The Beauty Bible**	$16.95	_____
☐ **Don't Go to the Cosmetics Counter Without Me**, 4th Edition	$19.95	_____
☐ **Don't Go Shopping for Hair Care Products Without Me**, 2nd Edition	$19.95	_____
☐ Paula's Choice Skin Care brochure	**FREE**	

	If your order totals	Add	
	$00.00–$20.00	$5.00	**All Prices Are Listed in US Funds**
Shipping	$20.01–$40.00	$6.00	
Charges	$40.01–$60.00	$7.00	**Subtotal** _____
	$60.01–$80.00	$8.00	**WA State Residents Add 8.6% Sales Tax** _____
	$80.01–$100.00	$9.00	**Shipping (for book orders only)** _____
	$100.01 and up	$10.00	**TOTAL** _____
	No shipping charges for newsletter		

☐ My check or money order is enclosed (make payable to Beginning Press and send your order to:

Beginning Press, 13075 Gateway Drive, #160, Seattle, WA 98168)

☐ Please charge my credit card (account number listed below)

Printed Name _____

Address _____

Phone # _____

Signature _____

Credit Card # _____   Expiration Date _____

(Visa, MasterCard, American Express, and Discover Accepted)

Call (800) 831-4088 to order now
www.cosmeticscop.com

DG4AD

Editors: Sigrid Asmus, María Brown
Art Direction, Cover Design, and Typography: Studio Pacific, Inc.
Printing: Publishers Press
Research Assistants: María Brown, Julie Dertinger, Kristin Folsom, Andrea Gleason, Carrie Goodman, Laura Kraemer, Sabine Kunkel, Kelly Muldoon, Melissa Roeder, and Jill Wasberg

Publisher: Beginning Press
             13075 Gateway Drive, Suite 160
             Seattle, Washington 98168

First Printing for this edition: November 1998

ISBN   1-877988-23-5
           3 4 5 6 7 8 9 10

This book is distributed to the United States book trade by:
             Publishers Group West
             1700 Fourth Street
             Berkeley, CA 94710
             (800) 788-3123

and to the Canadian book trade by:
             Raincoast Books
             8680 Cambie Street
             Vancouver, B.C. V6P 6M9
             (800) 663-5714

Publisher's Note

Acknowledgments

I want to personally thank María Brown, my main research assistant, for her dedication and loyalty to getting this book to print. Her organizational skills and focus were truly a godsend. Without her feedback, contributions, and love of cosmetics this book would not have been possible.

Contents

Chapter Three—Product-by-Product Reviews......... *67*

The Reviews

Contents

Contents

Contents

CHAPTER ONE

Through the Looking Glass

A Different Point of View

Is there a woman anywhere who hasn't purchased a cosmetic that didn't do what it said it would? Haven't most of us felt upset when we bought an all-day lipstick that didn't last all day, a wrinkle cream that didn't change a wrinkle, or an oil-control product that didn't control oil? How many "look younger" products have we purchased, only to buy the next "look younger" products launched the following season?

Those of you who have read my books *Blue Eyeshadow Should Be Illegal,* or *The Beauty Bible,* or previous editions of *Don't Go to the Cosmetics Counter Without Me,* or who subscribe to my newsletter, *Cosmetics Counter Update,* or read my syndicated newspaper column (I'm in about 30 newspapers across the country), or who have seen me on television know that I have strong feelings about the quality of information and products the cosmetics industry provides for women. My research has proven that, from almost every corner of the $45 billion cosmetics industry, women receive an immense amount of misleading, deceptive, or just plain false information, in one form or another. Whether it comes from cosmetics advertising, cosmetics salespeople, cosmetics companies' brochures, or so-called editorial pieces in fashion magazines, distorted, inaccurate, and specious explanations about skin care and makeup products are continually being given to women.

I draw my information and conclusions from many sources, which I encourage all of you to check out for yourselves. My primary references for the conclusions drawn and assessments used throughout this book are from *Drug and Cosmetics Industry* magazine, *Cosmetics & Toiletries* magazine, and *The Pink Sheet* report. All of these are industry publications that print ongoing cosmetic research, U.S. Government Food and Drug Administration (FDA) regulations, state-of-the-art formulations, and opinions from people making the products. I also constantly refer to medical journals such as *Cosmetic Dermatology, The Journal of the American Medical Association, The New England Journal of Medicine,* and *The Lancet* (a British medical research journal), as well as to press releases from the American Academy of Dermatology, and published studies from the biochemistry world found in *The Blue Sheet* (a health and biomedical publication). Two of my favorite sources of late have been the FDA's

Web site at *www.FDA.gov* and the medical research site at *www.Medscape.com*. I also use several dermatology journal Web sites, including *Dermatology Online Journal http://www.matrix.ucdavis.edu/DOJdesk/desk.html* and the *American Academy of Dermatology* at *www.AAD.org*. But despite the fact that written, published information is integral to my work, I spend a great deal of time interviewing cosmetic chemists, dermatologists, cosmetic ingredient manufacturers, biochemists, oncologists, and plastic surgeons.

This accumulated research provides me with abundant sources of information that you may not get a chance to hear because the fashion magazines leave out much, if not all, of what this kind of information reveals. My goal has always been to tell you everything the cosmetics companies won't tell you and everything the fashion magazines leave out or can't tell you because of the control that cosmetics and fashion companies assert via their advertising dollars. There's a lot to tell. Some of it you may find shocking, funny, enlightening, and, depending how much money you've wasted, disheartening.

People who sell cosmetics usually find my work both awful and wonderful. My book is considered insightful and helpful when I recommend the products they sell, but if I suggest that some of the products in their line are a waste of money or potentially damaging to skin, then their opinion is that I don't know what I'm talking about and I should mind my own business.

Dear Paula,

I read with interest your comments in your newsletter regarding your negative experiences with salespeople at upscale cosmetics counters. I had a similar experience with a saleswoman at Robinsons-May in Santa Barbara, California, last year. While trying on foundations at Lancome, I struck up a conversation with the young woman behind the counter. I mentioned that I had read your book and used your comments as guidelines when buying cosmetics. Rolling her eyes, she spat back, "Don't listen to her! She compares OUR products to stuff at the drugstore! Everything she says is garbage. Garbage!" "But," I said, "she generally likes Lancome products. In fact, that's one of the reasons I'm here today." "Oh ... really?" She then paused for a long time and finally gulped and said, "Sorry." She shut up after that and proceeded to ring up my sale.

Alvina, via e-mail

Dear Alvina,

Your story was great! Thanks for sharing your experience with me!

By the way, it seems quite convenient that the Lancome salespeople have a rough time remembering that Lancome is owned by L'Oreal, which now also owns Maybelline.

What I can assure you is that I will always be as straightforward and thorough as possible. I do the best I can to present both sides of the picture, so you can make more informed decisions about dealing with an industry in which the consumer is so vulnerable and easily taken advantage of. In the long run, this book will help you save money, take better care of your skin, and look more beautiful—all at the same time.

This edition of *Don't Go to the Cosmetics Counter Without Me* presents product-by-product reviews of cosmetics from more than 175 of the most popular lines, which is 75 more lines (and thousands more products) than I covered in the first edition of the book.

If you've ever felt uncertain about a product, or too short of time or energy to figure out for yourself which foundations are too pink or too orange, which eyeshadows are too shiny or too difficult to use, which powders went on too chalky, which cleansers are too greasy, which toners are too harsh, or what makes one moisturizer different from another, or how wrinkle creams differ, look no further. As you read the reviews in this book, you will start to get a better understanding of how the cosmetics industry really works. I've also included a summary chapter of best finds and best buys, but don't jump to that one first. It is important to read the individual product reviews so you understand *exactly* what you are buying. I might recommend twenty good mascaras, but each one might be good for a different reason.

In the reviews, each product is described in terms of its reliability, value, texture, application, and effect. Within every category of product—foundations, mascaras, blushes, eyeshadows, concealers, pressed powders, lipsticks, and pencils—I have established specific criteria, and I evaluate products using those standards. For example, a foundation meant for someone with oily skin, according to my criteria, should be matte, contain minimal to no oil, blend easily, leave a smooth, even finish, and have no ingredients known to cause breakouts. All foundations must match skin tones exactly: They cannot be any noticeable shade of orange, peach, rose, pink, or ash, because people are not orange, peach, rose, pink, or ash. I made the same determinations for mascaras, blushes, eyeshadows, concealers, pressed powders, lipsticks, and pencils. I relied on my ten years as a professional makeup artist to help establish guidelines for the quality of a product.

Skin-care products were evaluated almost entirely by analyzing the ingredient list and comparing it to the claims made about the product. If a toner asserts that it is designed for sensitive skin, it shouldn't contain ingredients that irritate the skin. If a moisturizer claims it can hydrate the skin, it should contain ingredients that can do just that. In addition, I have made a point of challenging the inflated claims made about such ingredients as yeast, herbal extracts, botanicals, seaweed extracts, placenta extracts, alpha hydroxy acids, vitamins, DNA, RNA, hyaluronic acid, liposomes, and other much-hyped ingredients. I also explain why some of these and other seemingly impressive-sounding ingredients might indeed benefit the skin, but more complete explanations for product claims and miracle ingredients are found in my book *The Beauty Bible*.

Never Say Never

Several times during the research for this edition of *Don't Go to the Cosmetics Counter Without Me,* I found myself saying, "I'm never going to do this again. It's insane out there, I refuse." On each occasion, one of the women I work with would sit me down and say, "You always go through this and you know you'll keep on doing the work, so calm down, we'll get through this one just like we got through the other books and every edition of your newsletter for the past eight years." I need that kind of pep talk every now and then because the work my staff and I do can be so frustrating.

For more than a year, I was out with my research staff (there are three of us now) working almost exclusively on the book (I can hardly believe this is the fourth edition). Perhaps the most disturbing aspect of our work is trying to get information from the cosmetics companies regarding their products. Almost without exception, any time we ask for ingredients listings, despite the fact that the FDA legally mandates that they are to be available to the consumer, we are thwarted at every turn. Either we are told they can't release that information to us or we are told it will be forthcoming, and then it never arrives! Even more frustrating are the responses we get when requesting verification or substantiation for a claim. If a cosmetics company does agree to send something, we often get press releases and not what we originally asked for: established data or published research.

Obviously a large part of compiling the information and products for an effort like this requires spending a lot of time shopping for cosmetics. When it comes to dealing with cosmetics salespeople, I always have a litany of war stories, just as many of you do. Outfitted in a baseball cap, T-shirt, and khaki pants, I try to be as inconspicuous as possible. But once my notepad comes out, the salespeople quickly wonder what is going on and then I am on the offensive, hoping that a few purchases will distract their attention. Thankfully, that usually takes the pressure off—but not all the time. I still can get a pretty cold shoulder or be asked to leave.

Making matters somewhat worse, or at least more intriguing, were two incidents that happened while my researchers were checking cosmetics counters in San Francisco and Dallas. At the Clinique counter in Dallas, as one member of my staff pulled out her notepad to write down an ingredient listing, she was reproached with a curt, "Why do you need to write down ingredients? You don't work for that *psycho* up in Seattle, Paula what's-her-name, do you? We've been warned about her and we're told not to help." A woman at the Prescriptives counter in a San Francisco department store, who turned out to be incredibly helpful, told another of my staff members that part of her training over the past year included how to handle comments from women who have read Paula Begoun's books.

I'm not sure whether I should be flattered or concerned that my job just got harder. Regardless of how you look at it, it's an interesting position to be in. Researching the cosmetics industry is what I do for a living, and I have every intention of continuing as long as women want to know what I have to report (and, according to the letters I receive and my book sales, they definitely do). Whether my job is easy or hard isn't really the point, but I just thought you might like to know how we're doing out there. And for those of you who stopped to say hello when you saw me out at the counters working, thank you for your words of encouragement and for keeping a low profile!

The Never-Ending Story

How is it possible that every time I finish reviewing a new line of cosmetics, I receive requests to review another ten lines I've never even heard of before! Will it never end? Remede, Darphin, Rejuvennis, Collagen Plus, Dermatique, Rozelle, Dionis, DHC, Earth Science, Elite Skin Care, Ella Bache, Exuviance, Repechage, Ilona, Doctor's Dermatologic Formula, Lancie, E International, Lisse, Mill Creek, Neoderma, Nutri-Tonic, Peter Roth, Pevonia, Pola, Rejuvaderm, Reviva, Sea Minerals, Farouk, Skin Life, and ZA are only a some of the lines from which I received requests for product reviews over a one-week period. From plant products galore to dermatologist- or pharmacist-formulated, natural, botanical, pure, completely nonchemical cosmetics (gosh, everything is labeled natural, botanical, and pure in today's cosmetics marketplace, of course no one uses chemicals any more), to aromatherapy and spa formulas, women want to know if these lines work or can live up to their claims. Each and every one of these lines—and many, many, many more— make elaborate promises, often with very scientific, extravagant, appealing language, promising everything from healing acne to feeding skin, eliminating lines, getting rid of scars, wiping out cellulite, and erasing skin discolorations, and when they include hair care products, those claim to make hair grow, fix damage, and anything else your heart desires.

And as if all the lines I haven't yet reviewed weren't already so overwhelming, more than 1,700 new anti-aging products were launched in 1997, with at least that many more slated for 1998! Of course, the question to pose is, if all those wondrous, anti-aging products launched in 1997 worked, what happened to the ones you bought the year before? And what about the new anti-aging products you'll start seeing advertised in 1999 and again in the year 2000? Do those replace the ones that didn't work in 1998 and 1997? Don't we ever get tired of the recycled products with expensive price tags—or inexpensive price tags, for that matter—making endless, empty promises? Do our lines or the puffiness under our eyes ever go away, the cellulite disappear, or the sagging skin firm up?

I can't tell you the number of letters I receive that say something like, "I've seen this new skin-care line being recommended by dermatologists, plastic surgeons, or some celebrity as an alternative to Retin-A, alpha hydroxy acids, chemical peels [I don't recommend chemical peels, by the way, and I explain this in *The Beauty Bible*], and laser resurfacing. I can't wait to hear what you think about it!" I know these women are waiting for me to tell them that finally a line of products has been created that will, at long last, live up to its claims and be well worth the investment. So what do I think about all this? Actually, what I think isn't as important as what I know to be true. There are indeed great products out there that can do wonderful things for our skin; but there are absolutely no miracles, no plants, no botanicals, no patented formulations, no cures, no lotions, no potions, no vitamins, no European formula, not one secret ingredient in the world of cosmetics that will erase wrinkles, smooth out cellulite, cure acne, get rid of scars, or terminate any other beauty ill. As soon as it happens, believe me, I will let you know; we can all invest in the company and retire!

The First Time

A number of you have asked how I happened into this unusual line of work. It's not as if you can answer an ad for this kind of job! Clearly, the cosmetics industry and fashion magazines aren't interested in hiring someone to do what I do (for the same reasons the insurance industry doesn't want to employ Ralph Nader or someone like him to do what he does), but somewhere along the line it became clear to me that someone needed to be doing this work.

It all started in 1977, when I took my first job at a department-store makeup counter to supplement my income as a freelance makeup artist. As a young makeup artist in Washington, D.C., I had built up a list of celebrity clients and was doing quite well, both financially and professionally. I found the artistry of creating beautiful makeup styles for women intriguing, and the world of fashion and glamour thoroughly exciting. At the age of 24 I was thrilled with my career. My clients wanted only me, and they were some of the most powerful and formidable women in Washington. The constant ego reinforcement was great. But, as with any business, it had its ups and downs, and shoring up my income once in a while became necessary. A store at a mall in Silver Spring, Maryland, had an opening for a cosmetics salesperson. They hired me on the spot because, I was told, I looked the part, wearing nice makeup and dressing well. It was also made crystal clear that, while my previous experience was a plus, it was completely unnecessary for employment as a cosmetics salesperson.

Even though I was enthusiastic and loved the dynamic and glamorous world of makeup and skin care, I already knew something was awry with a substantial number of cosmetics and their advertising, particularly in the skin-care area. Having struggled for years with oily skin and acne, I knew from personal experience that astringents didn't close pores, that products claiming not to cause breakouts made me break out, and that most products that promised to clear up acne only made my skin more red and irritated. I didn't yet know all the technical details of why this was so, but it was blatantly obvious that plenty of mascaras that claimed to be flakeproof weren't, toners that boasted they could close pores didn't, and creams that were supposed to eliminate scarring and lighten "age spots" didn't. The claims made about the products rarely matched their performance. However, while it seemed unquestionable that much of the cosmetics industry was grossly misrepresenting its products, at the time I had no way to confirm my suspicions.

On my first day on the job, I was assigned to work behind the Calvin Klein (in those days, Klein had a makeup line) and Elizabeth Arden counters. With no previous training or information about these lines, I was told to sell the products. I did the best I could. Unfortunately, my notion of how to help customers was completely different from that of the other salespeople and the line manager. My first mistake was telling several customers not to bother using an astringent because alcohol-based products could cause something called a "rebound effect." By irritating the skin, these products could actually stimulate oil production and make oily skin worse. I then recommended 3% hydrogen peroxide, available then for 50 cents at the drugstore. By the end of the second day, the woman working next to me was mortified. She called in the line representative, who made it clear that I should keep my personal opinions to myself and just sell the products. I said I would do my best. This was only my second day. Things had to get better, I thought.

The fourth day on the job, thinking I was doing what I was supposed to do, I assisted a customer who wanted help putting together a makeup look. I went about this seemingly ordinary task by assembling a selection of products from several different lines. I noticed that the saleswomen behind the other counters didn't appear happy as I took products from their stock, but I thought maybe it was because I was making the sale instead of them. That was only the half of it. Although the women I helped that day bought almost everything I suggested, the other saleswomen complained to the head of the department, who subsequently ordered me to stay behind the counters I was assigned to. I protested that the two lines I was assigned to didn't always have the best makeup colors or skin-care products for every woman I talked to. Without hesitation, she said, "That's just the way it is, so you'd better get used to it." That was the fourth day. It couldn't get any worse, I thought, sighing. But it did.

At the end of my second week, I finally met the woman who was responsible for training. At last, I was going to learn how to sell the products assigned to me, and what to say about each product's benefits. I truly wanted to find out everything I could, but apparently my approach was unacceptable. When the trainer explained that I was supposed to sell Elizabeth Arden Eight Hour Cream as a product designed to help heal the skin, I asked her what the product contained that made it able to do that. She said what it contained wasn't important. I disagreed, saying that it would help me sell the cream better if I knew what made it heal skin; surely the customer would want to know. She said, "All the customer wants to know is what you tell her; the customers never ask questions, because they trust the products."

"How can that be," I insisted, "when all the cosmetics lines say the same thing? Why should they trust us any more than someone else?"

"Because they do," she said. Finally, she threw the product down and said, "Just say it! There's nothing else to discuss." To my dismay—but not surprise—that turned out to be my last day on that job. It was a relief to return to the world of freelance makeup.

Shortly after that incident, I read *The Great American Skin Game* by Toni Stabille. It changed my life. This landmark book conveyed in clear, concise terms the processes and techniques the cosmetics industry used to sell hope to gullible and uninformed consumers. In fact, Ms. Stabille was largely responsible for proposing many FDA regulations involving cosmetics, including advertising guidelines, safety regulations, and mandatory ingredient lists. Her work confirmed what I had already reasoned must be true, and significantly changed the way I approached cosmetics.

Although it sounds a bit melodramatic, I couldn't continue selling something I knew to be a waste of money or bad for the skin. Consumers (including myself) deserved better. I wasn't anti-makeup—just the opposite—but I was (and am) anti-hype and against misleading information. As one newspaper reporter recently commented, "She's not Mother Teresa, but it does seem to be just Ms. Begoun against these huge cosmetics companies." Thus I took my first steps on a long career path— longer than I ever imagined—that went from owning my own cosmetics stores to working as a TV news reporter to owning my own publishing company, and back to owning my own skin-care company. With every step, my goal has been to do what it takes to find out and expose the truth behind the ads and the literally unbelievable claims thrown about by the cosmetics world. After all, one good sales pitch about an "exclusive patented secret" or a revolutionary new formula, and your pocketbook could easily be $50 to $250 lighter for a 1-ounce jar of standard cosmetics ingredients or ingredients that can't live up to their claims.

It's Getting Expensive Out There

One of the more amazing trends in the world of cosmetics is how expensive it's getting out there, and not just at department-store cosmetics counters, but for products found at all venues, including drugstore products and those sold by infomercials. Even Avon has been raising its prices.

Take Almay's Time-Off Wrinkle Defense Capsules with Micro-Fillers, which costs $12.49 for 0.29 ounce. That turns out to be an unbelievably expensive product. When you do the math, this stuff comes out to be $44.96 an ounce! And for what? Not much. In this case it's merely silicones, a slip agent, water, water-binding agents, and some vitamins. Avon's Anew Formula C Treatment Capsules cost $19 for 0.41 ounce in 30 capsules—that's almost $42 an ounce! Wow! These prices aren't that different from department store prices.

Price still has nothing to do with quality, nor does the name on the product have anything to do with whether you are getting an effective product that can live up to its claims. In the above case, the vitamin C Avon adds to its product isn't any better than Lancome's Vitabolic Deep Radiance Booster at $45 for 1 ounce. If you were thinking the Avon product was a better buy, think again. Price should be an issue when products are equal; why spend more than you have to? But when price *is* the concern, don't be misled by a low price tag on a product with a ridiculously low content. Avon's vitamin C is no bargain. (I should point out that vitamin C is one of the most overhyped cosmetic ingredients these days, which I explain in Chapter Two, Skin-Care Update, so don't consider any of this a rationale for purchasing any vitamin C product.) I'm pointing out this issue of cost versus contents as an encouragement for you to start paying attention to ounces as well as cost. Sometimes just comparing the dollar amounts alone is quite misleading in terms of whether you are getting a reasonably priced product.

The Crazy Things Cosmetics Salespeople Say

I can barely keep myself from reeling every time I hear or read some of the inane cosmetic information women are handed on a daily basis. From cosmetics counters to fashion magazines and infomercials, it is enough to make me scream, "I can't take it anymore!" Here is a sampling of some of the amazing stories that I'm sure you've run into as often as I have.

Overheard at an Estee Lauder counter: Our foundations are specially formulated to make light reflect away from the face, which hides lines.

In reality: There are a lot of great foundations out there, but none that reflect light in a way that reduces the appearance of lines. If anything, foundations and concealers of all kinds tend to make lines look more apparent. You can do your own test by placing the "light-reflecting" or line-diminishing foundation on one side of your face, and leaving the other side without any makeup. The foundation side will have a more even color tone, but the lines will also look more noticeable. I wish it were different, but that miracle hasn't been invented yet.

I overheard one woman at an Estee Lauder counter, who was trying on their Lucidity Foundation, exclaim, "It looks like it did before I put it on; I can still see my lines." The salesperson agreed and suggested she check it out in the daylight, saying, "Perhaps there's not enough light in here to reflect away from the lines." The woman proceeded to walk outside to see if there was a difference. She returned a few minutes later, saying dejectedly, "I guess there's not enough light outside either." It never occurred to the woman shopping for foundation that it had nothing to do with daylight but everything to do with a misleading sales pitch.

Explained to me by an Elizabeth Arden representative: Cleanliness is so important; for example, if you don't get all your foundation off at night, it will make your skin age.

In reality: Aging is a very complicated and intricate process, but of all the things associated with aging (and 95% of them are connected with sun damage), it absolutely has nothing whatsoever to do with dirt. You could be covered in dirt, awash in pollution every day of your life, and if you received no sun exposure (which the dirt would surely block), you would have few or no lines on your face.

Told to me at an Origins counter: Our under-mascara treatment provides essential nutrients to help make eyelashes grow.

In reality: Vitamins can't make hair grow on the eyelids any more than they can on the head. While it sounds plausible that vitamins can be absorbed into the skin and make us healthier and stronger, it just isn't possible.

Overheard at a Lancome counter: This concealer will prevent lipstick from bleeding.

In reality: Most concealers, which usually have a consistency similar to lipstick, won't stop bleeding in the least; they melt and move as readily as most lipsticks do. However, if the concealer has an ultra-matte consistency (say, like Almay Amazing Lasting Concealer or Maybelline Great Wear Concealer), it can work as a barrier.

Heard on a talk show from a makeup expert: Line your lips with a pale blue pencil to create a striking look.

In reality: Blue-lined lips do look striking, but only in the same way blue-streaked hair looks striking. There is nothing about a blue line around the mouth that looks like anything other than a blue line.

Recommended in a fashion magazine: To apply a natural blush, hang your head downward for a few seconds to see where the natural flush appears; that's where you should apply your blush.

In reality: This isn't much of a trick, because it all depends on how you naturally blush. For many of us, that would mean putting blush all over the face, or in big circles from the jaw up to the eye area.

Suggested by a makeup artist at a makeup store: One way to keep lashes curled all day is to warm an eyelash curler under your blow dryer before you use it.

In reality: If the metal gets hot enough to alter the shape of the lashes, you would be running the risk of possibly burning the very delicate skin of the eyelid. Not a good idea! Heat is definitely capable of setting a shape, but it is also capable of damaging the very delicate, fragile eyelash. You may end up with fewer eyelashes than you started with.

Recommended in a fashion magazine: Use a cotton ball to smooth out your foundation after you've applied it.

In reality: If you want little pieces of cotton on your skin or want to run the chance of getting some flecks in your eyes, go for it. A smooth sponge is by far the best tool for applying and smoothing out foundation.

Told to me by an Elizabeth Arden salesperson: You'll need our cleanser to take off our foundation, because no other one can get it off, and if you don't get all your foundation off at night, it will cause your skin to wrinkle.

In reality: Foundation doesn't age skin, sun does. The Arden cleanser is not the only one capable of removing the Arden foundation; however, if it was, I would strongly suggest that such a foundation would be the wrong one to buy. Anything that difficult to get off the face could cause problems such as skin irritation or clogged pores.

Told to me by a Borghese salesperson: Our products are all pure and natural; there isn't one chemical in any of them.

In reality: All cosmetics contain a host of "unnatural" ingredients, Borghese's included.

Overheard at a Lancome cosmetics counter: A woman mentioned to a salesperson that she had heard that many of L'Oreal's products were the same as Lancome's. The salesperson responded by saying that was a nasty rumor, that Lancome had nothing to do with anything sold at the drugstore.

In reality: Lancome has everything to do with L'Oreal—L'Oreal *owns* Lancome. It would only take a glance to notice that the ingredients lists and product types of Lancome and L'Oreal are more often than not virtually identical. And now that L'Oreal owns Maybelline, you'll start seeing those products looking more and more like L'Oreal's and Lancome's.

Conversation with a Shaklee sales representative: Our new skin-care line is the only one that can legally make claims about stopping and improving wrinkles. Our patented formulations are completely unique and we have independent studies proving this.

In reality: The ingredients in the Shaklee line are hardly unique and they cannot stop or change wrinkling. Shaklee's studies are not independent in the least; they come out of a claim-substantiation lab that comes up with any results the company consulting it is looking for, and all companies have these types of studies. Shaklee's so-called study merely demonstrates that their product performed better than some unknown moisturizer. That's easy to prove, especially if brand X is a bad moisturizer or contains irritants. Also, no long-term studies or sun-exposure studies were done. Their products aren't bad, they just aren't miracles or worth the cost.

Dear Paula,

One year after you reported on the importance of screening UVA [ultra violet A] rays with avobenzone, titanium dioxide, or zinc oxide, *Glamour* magazine is now encouraging the use of these products (a lot of damage can be done in a year). In the June issue, a sunscreen article warns against wearing AHA under your sunscreen because "these products form a coating that interferes with a sunscreen's ability to bind to your skin. It's also a bad idea to layer an AHA over sunscreen, because the AHA also needs to bind to skin to be effective. Your best bet: a daily-use product that contains both a sunscreen and an AHA (such as Neutrogena Healthy Skin Face Lotion with SPF 15)."

Help, Paula. I use a glycolic lotion in the morning, wait a few minutes, and then apply your nongreasy sunscreen. Then I apply Estee Lauder SPF 10 foundation. In the evening, I apply Renova. I live in Florida, have fair skin, and must wear sunscreen. Have I been doing it all wrong? What's your take on *Glamour*'s advice?

Mary, Jacksonville, Florida

Dear Mary,

I think *Glamour*'s article sounds like a plug for Neutrogena. Did Neutrogena have a lot of advertising in *Glamour* that month or something? Nevertheless, let's sort out the information presented. I am glad to hear the fashion magazines are finally discussing the UVA issue that I've been talking about for more than a year now. However, Neutrogena Healthy Skin SPF 15 doesn't contain any of the established UVA-protecting ingredients like avobenzone, zinc oxide, or titanium dioxide. Plus, Healthy Skin doesn't have a low enough pH to make it a reliable AHA product either (it would need a pH of 4 or less and it has one of 5 to 6). On both counts, this product comes up short.

In terms of applying AHAs and sunscreens separately, whether or not the AHA blocks the sunscreen depends on the product you use and how you apply it, but there is nothing about an AHA in and of itself that should block the absorption of a sunscreen product. If you apply too much of an AHA product or one that is too thick, or you didn't allow the AHA to be absorbed first, then the sunscreen would have problems binding to the skin. This is one of the reasons I recommend gel- or toner-type AHA or BHA products. Those kinds of products never have heavy thickening agents or emollients that would get in the way of other products you may want to apply, such as sunscreen or foundation during the day, or other moisturizers over dry areas at night (remember, not all skin types need to use a moisturizer all over). If you want to use both a sunscreen and an AHA in one, that would be the best, but there are only a handful available that meet that criterion and they are extremely pricey. Check Exuviance for some formulations of that kind.

Crazy Things on the Web

The following letter from a reader really caught my attention and summed up so much of what I hear about the misleading information from cosmetics salespeople and cosmetics companies. She was searching for information on skin-care ingredients and came across a Neways Web site. I think many of you will appreciate the more involved answer I provided.

Dear Paula,

I have been trying to "research" skin-care companies and products using the Internet. I came across a site (*www.livebetter.com/myths.html*) that contains some very thought-provoking information. Whether it's true, I do not know. I would be interested in your response to the information contained in this site. There are several different Web pages with this same information; one of them references you in the bibliography. Do you agree with all the contents?

Jean, Knoxville, Tennessee

Dear Jean,

I was able to locate the site, and it turns out that the information there is really a very long advertisement for Neways—the same line that brought you Neways thigh cream with its claims of eliminating cellulite. Neways talks quite a bit about the company's ethics, but a company that claims efficacy for a cellulite cream is hardly one to brag about noble principles and factual information.

As you might expect, there are lots of problems with quite a bit of the information listed on their Web site. They quote several people out of context, including me, and they also quote people whose information is, at best, no more reliable than what you might read in a fashion magazine or hear at a cosmetics counter (which is almost always in complete support of whatever the cosmetics industry does). Here are a few examples excerpted from the site and my comments on what I think is problematic or untrue. I should mention that Neways is not the only company to perpetuate many of these erroneous, misleading cosmetic fabrications and falsehoods.

What appears on the Neways Web site: "Propylene glycol, called a humectant in cosmetics, is really industrial anti-freeze, and the major ingredient in brake and hydraulic fluids. Tests show that it can be a strong skin irritant. Material Safety Data Sheets (MSDS) on propylene glycol warn users to avoid skin contact, as systemically it can cause liver abnormalities and kidney damage."

My comments: It is true that propylene glycol is antifreeze, but—and this is a very big *but* (no pun intended)—in cosmetics it is used in only the smallest amounts to keep products from melting in high heat or freezing when it is cold outside. It also helps active ingredients penetrate the skin. In the minuscule amounts used in cosmetics, propylene glycol is not a concern. Women are not suffering from liver problems because of propylene glycol in cosmetics.

I have seen several studies indicating that propylene glycol is not a problem as it is used in cosmetics, while I have seen no studies indicating the opposite. The Material Safety Data Sheet warning concerned 100% concentrations of propylene glycol for industrial or manufacturing purposes only, not the extremely diluted form used in cosmetics. Furthermore, many other cosmetic or pharmaceutical ingredients, from alpha hydroxy acids to tretinoin (the active ingredient in Retin-A) and standard cleansing agents, would make your skin miserable if they were used in 100% concentrations.

However, to consider the other side of the coin, there are dermatologists who worry that too much penetration into the skin is a bad thing. Getting things into the skin, especially irritating ingredients (even plants and vitamins can be irritating), may not be best for skin. Penetration into the skin gets talked up a lot in cosmetics sales pitches, and overpenetration may be a concern, but even so that doesn't make small amounts of propylene glycol bad for skin.

What appears on the Neways Web site: Mineral oil "comes from crude oil (petroleum), used in industry as metal-cutting fluid. May suffocate the skin by forming an oil film. Healthy skin needs oxygen, and to release carbon dioxide it should not be inhibited. Holding too large amounts of moisture in the skin can 'flood' the biology and may result in immature, unhealthy, sensitive skin that dries out easily." Also on the Neways Web site is a comment that petroleum has the "same properties as mineral oil. Industrially it is use[d] as a grease component."

My comments: I hate this foolish, recurring misinformation about mineral oil and petroleum. If people knew how decaffeinated coffee is made, no one would drink the stuff. Pretzels are browned with urea (which is also a popular skin-care ingredient) that is derived from urine. Is any of that bad? Hardly, although it doesn't sound great. Lots of ingredients are derived from awful-sounding sources but are nevertheless benign and totally safe. Salt is a perfect example. Common table salt is sodium chloride, composed of sodium and chlorine, but salt doesn't have either the poisonous gas–emitting properties of chlorine or the unstable explosiveness of sodium. In fact, it is a brand-new compound with properties of neither of its components.

Mineral oil and petrolatum are considered to be the safest, most nonirritating moisturizing ingredients ever found. Yes, they can keep air off the skin, but that's what a good antioxidant is supposed to do! In addition, in an article in *Cosmetics & Toiletries* magazine, Dr. Albert Kligman said, "Petrolatum is known to help in wound healing."

Yes, overmoisturizing can "flood" the skin, but that is true for a host of ingredients, including a number of waxy thickening agents that are much more occlusive than mineral oil or petrolatum. I would be much more concerned about ingredients such as triglycerides, myristates, palmitates, and fatty acids than about mineral oil or petrolatum for occluding the skin.

What appears on the Neways Web site: On sodium lauryl sulfate (SLS) and sodium laureth sulfate (SLES)—"Potentially, SLS is perhaps the most harmful ingredient in personal-care products. SLS is used in testing labs as the standard ingredient to irritate skin. Industrial uses of SLS include garage-floor cleaners, engine degreasers, and car-wash soaps, just to name a few. Studies show its danger potential to be great when used in personal-care products. A study from the Medical College of Georgia indicates that SLS is a systemic, and can penetrate and be retained in the eye, brain, heart, liver, etc., with potentially harmful long-term effects. It could retard healing and cause cataracts in adults, and can keep children's eyes from developing properly. (Summary of report to Research to Prevent Blindness, Inc. Conference.)

"Other research has shown that SLS and SLES may cause potentially carcinogenic nitrates and dioxins to form in shampoos and cleansers by reacting with commonly used ingredients found in many products. Large amounts of nitrates may enter the blood system from just one shampooing. SLES is the alcohol form (ethoxylated) of SLS. It is slightly less irritating but may cause more drying. Both SLS and SLES can enter the bloodstream. They are used in personal-care products because they are cheap. A small amount generates a large amount of foam, and when salt is added, it thicken[s], giving the illusion of the product being thick and concentrated."

My comments: Talk about exaggeration. I agree that SLS can be a problem. The research about it being sensitizing is well-known, and I have written about this in the past. However, irritation as such isn't dangerous—it is just irritation, and while it is indeed harmful to the skin, it is not lethal. The doctor who did the research mentioned is Dr. Keith Green from Georgia Medical College. I spoke with him and he told me the following: "My work is completely misquoted. There is no part of my study that indicated any development of cataract problems from SLS or SLES and the body does not retain those ingredients at all. The Neways people took my research completely out of context and probably never read the study." The statement about SLS forming nitrosamines isn't true, though it is true for TEA lauryl sulfate (TEA stands for triethanolamine). The amine exists in a free state, and if it meets up with a formaldehyde-releasing preservative like quaternium-15, carcinogenic nitrosamines can be formed. However, though this is problematic, it does not produce nitrosamines in large amounts, and the nitrosamines do not enter the bloodstream after one or even thousands of uses. It turns out the research as to the impact of nitrosamines from skin-care products in any form on humans is actually quite conflicting. Still, consumers can easily avoid products with nitrosamine-forming ingredients, and it doesn't take using Neways's products.

What appears on the Neways Web site: Bentonite "is a naturally occurring mineral used in facial masks. It differs from true clay, kaolin, in that when it is mixed with liquid it forms a gel. It can have sharp edges that scratch the skin. Most bentonites can be drying to the skin. Bentonite is used in formulations and facial masks. It forms films that are gas-impermeable, effectively trapping toxins and CO_2 in the skin that need to vent and escape, suffocating the skin by shutting out the vitally needed oxygen."

My comments: This is just bizarre and a complete distortion of fact. Bentonite, like any mineral, can have hard edges, but when it is crushed and blended into cosmetics, this isn't a problem any more than the walnut shells or ground-up seashells used in other products are.

And then there's this continuing nonsense about toxins lurking under the skin, waiting to get out. What are these toxins anyway? Has Neways taken samples of harmful substances escaping from the skin? If so, what are they? Various companies and people selling cosmetics or spa treatments love throwing around the term *toxins*, yet there is no substantiation of this notion anywhere.

Also, any earth mineral can place an occlusive layer over the skin. That is why sunscreens containing the preferred ingredients of zinc oxide and titanium dioxide work so well. Suffocating the skin is an interesting notion, but in essence that could be said of any foundation, lipstick, or powder that leaves a visible layer over the skin. While the layer might be occlusive, it is hardly solid, and the skin is not dying underneath. If anything, the extra layer can prevent the sun from damaging the skin. For example, one of the reasons dermatologists feel that women have fewer occurrences of lip cancer and skin cancer than men is because women wear lipstick and foundation.

What appears on the Neways Web site: "Collagen and Elastin of High Molecular Weight—Derived from animal skins and ground-up chicken feet. Both of these ingredients form films that may suffocate and overmoisturize the skin."

Neways also comments on bar soaps: "Made from animal fat and lye. May let bacteria feed and grow in it. May corrode the skin and dry it out.

"Many of the 'hyped' ingredients procollagen, collagen, elastin, cross-linked elastin, and hyaluronic acids found in most cosmetic brands cannot penetrate the skin because of high molecular weight and are of little benefit."

My comments: Corrode the skin! Come on, what woman has corroded skin? First of all, rarely, if ever, do companies use collagen and elastin derived from animal sources anymore; plant sources are much more typical in the cosmetics industry. Yes, these ingredients have high molecular weights, as do most skin-care ingredients, but if everything were absorbed into the skin, what would be left on top to protect it? Penetration, as I mentioned above, is not the most important criterion, nor is it required for a skin-care product to be effective.

Bar soaps are made from lard and lye, which is the legal definition of soap, but the fat isn't what is causing bacteria proliferation. Studies indicate that the high pH (alkalinity) of the soap breaks down the skin's intercellular layer, allowing bacteria to enter and flourish.

What appears on the Neways Web site: "Other virtually useless ingredients are insoluble, oil-based vitamin A (Retinyl Palmitate), Placental Extracts, and Royal Bee Jelly."

My comments: I agree about placental extracts and royal bee jelly being useless, but not vitamin A. Vitamin A is a fine antioxidant and can be helpful as a skin-care ingredient. Yes, the claims made for it are often overblown, but it is hardly useless.

What appears on the Neways Web site: Humectants are "ingredients that draw moisture to the skin and aid in moisturization. Most moisturizers contain humectants that act as water attractors; they actually pull moisture out of your skin. The problem with humectants, including propylene glycol and glycerin[,] is that although they are most effective when you are in areas with high humidity, if you are going to be in an extremely low-humidity atmosphere, such as in an airplane or even a dry room, they can actually take moisture from your skin. Here's why: Humectants are on the search for moisture that can be absorbed from the environment. If the environment is so drying that there is no moisture to be had, they will get it from the next best source—your skin. When this happens, the ingredient, which is supposed to help your skin retain moisture, instead does the opposite."

Humectants are "a substance used to preserve the moisture content of materials, especially in hand creams and lotions."

Humectants "are natural or synthetic compounds that are used to prevent water loss and drying of the skin. They also form a smooth feel to cosmetic lotions. Some are safe, some aren't."

My comments: This long technical discussion just doesn't, if you'll excuse the pun, hold water. Rarely is glycerin used in concentrations of more than 5% to 8% in cosmetics—1% to 2% at most. It mostly keeps the moisture in the product stable and keeps the product attached to the skin so it doesn't evaporate. Glycerin molecules are too large to penetrate the skin and take moisture out of it. The notion that glycerin (at least as used in cosmetics) is dehydrating in low-humidity environments just isn't true. Besides, this fear of dry skin reinforces the myth that dry skin is evil, yet it is not. Dry skin and wrinkles are not associated, while on the other hand skin that is too moist won't heal.

What appears on the Neways Web site: Albumin is the "chief ingredient in artificial face-lifts. It is being touted as a wrinkle treatment. The last time a serious case concerning consumer claims came up was in the 1960s. Both of these products were temporary wrinkle removers. The formulas contained a bovine serum albumin that, when dried, formed a film over wrinkles, thus making wrinkles less obvious."

My comments: Albumin is merely egg white and absolutely a waste for the skin. However, there is nothing bad or harmful about albumin; egg white doesn't cause skin damage. Complaints about instant face-lift products spring up repeatedly for the Food and Drug Administration, but serious complaints about cosmetics occur every year, and many, many skin-care ingredients have been withdrawn from the market over the years.

What appears on the Neways Web site: "Advertisers have found that the words 'contains Lanolin' help to sell a product and have promoted it as being able to 'penetrate the skin better than other oils,' although there is little scientific proof of this. Lanolin has been found to be a common skin sensitizer causing allergic contact skin rashes. . . . Lanolin usually contains pesticides used on sheep and wool."

My comments: How can so much bad information be floating around out there? First, lanolin isn't all that common a skin sensitizer. Many other cosmetic ingredients are far worse, including fragrance from natural, so-called essential oils, preservatives, vitamin E, and lots and lots of plant and fruit extracts. Lanolin can cause problems for about 10% of the population, and if you have a tendency to break out it can clog pores, but that leaves a lot of people risk-free. Further, cosmetic-grade lanolin is devoid of any pesticides or other impurities. Just think of the insects and pesticides that would be retained in plant extracts if they weren't purified before going into a cosmetic.

What appears on the Neways Web site: Liposomes, nanospheres, or micellization are supposedly the "ultimate anti-aging agent[s]. Liposomes are one of the newest entries in the 'fountain of youth' arena. According to one recent theory, cellular aging involves the rigidification of skin cell membranes. Liposomes, which are tiny bags of fat and thymus gland extract suspended in a gel, are supposed to merge with your aging skin cells, revive them, and add moisture to them. Current scientific understanding does not support the rigidification theory. The cell membranes of young and old persons are alike. As a result, it is likely that liposome-containing moisturizers represent nothing more than another expensive allure."

My comments: This information is so convoluted that it is meaningless. Liposomes are hardly new—they have been around for more than 15 years and were created by a division of L'Oreal—and are a delivery system, not an ingredient. They are simply a way of suspending water and oil so they disperse on the skin over time and not all at once. Other companies, in an attempt to compete with L'Oreal/Lancome's liposomes, created their own forms and gave them names like nanospheres. These are all interesting ways to keep moisturizers around longer, but they did not catch on with the consumer.

Yes, current research does not support the notion of rigidification (a fancy way of describing severe dry skin), but the cell membranes of old and young people are not alike in the least, at least not if you're looking at older people who have endured repeated, unprotected exposure to the sun over the years. Sun-damaged skin, which shows up clearly when we are older but is evident microscopically even in very young skin, is identified by abnormal skin cells. Rather than skin cells being smooth and round when produced in the lower layers of the dermis, sun-damaged skin cells are irregular, misshapen, and flat. As a result of this abnormal cell growth, sun-damaged skin cells become thickened, rough, and stiff, and are difficult to shed, while normal, non-sun-damaged skin cells remain pliant and smooth and are shed evenly.

What appears on the Neways Web site: "The term pH stands for the power of the hydrogen atom. Skin and hair do not have a pH. A scale from 0 to 14 is used to measure acidity and alkalinity of solutions. pH 7.0 is neutral. Acidity increases as the pH number decreases, and alkalinity increases as the pH number increases. Usually the pH of a cosmetic will not change the natural pH of the hair or skin because the hair and skin contain keratin, fatty acids, and other substances that adjust the pH levels with which they come into contact. As long as a pH is not unusually high or low, there is no problem—pH-wise—with a cosmetic. Naturally, the high pH of cold-wave solutions and hair straighteners can damage the hair and skin, but even this is rare, providing a proper conditioner or moisturizer is used after such pH alterations. There is no such thing as a 'pH balanced' product because a product's pH will drift during shelf life and alter when applied to the hair and skin. A product's pH is not a danger to the body, but the synthetic chemicals used in cosmetics often [are]."

My comments: I'm starting to see red. Is there no end to this craziness? The first statements about pH are completely true, but the rest are a complete and total departure from reality. While pH is indeed a rating of how alkaline or acid a substance is, hair and skin can be compromised by a product that is too alkaline or too acid. After all, sulfuric acid (with a pH of 1) will eat through metal, and lye (with a pH of 12) will eat through wood, not to mention hair and skin, and all the moisturizers and conditioners in the world will not be able to stop or repair that damage! I agree that the term pH balance is misleading, because skin and hair do seek their own natural pH level; however, if you compromise the pH of the skin or hair with a product whose pH goes too high or too low, you can encourage bacterial growth, dry out the skin, damage the skin (by destroying the pH-sensitive intercellular layer of skin, the "mortar" between skin cells that keeps skin intact), or inhibit the skin's healing process. As it turns out, most skin-care and hair-care products, except for bar cleansers and soaps, have a pH of about 3 to 6, which is fine for most skin types and allows the natural pH of skin to remain intact. (By the way, skin does have a pH, reflected by its oil and water content.)

What appears on the Neways Web site: Seaweed is "promoted to nourish and moisturize the skin. This plant has gelatinous properties. It is the major ingredient of the thin, clear masks that peel off in one piece. These masks allow the skin to build up a supply of water. Seaweed is also used in face creams and lotions, where it gives body and substance to the products, not to the skin. . . ."

My comments: This is an interesting mix of misinformation. First, most peel-off masks use hair spray–type ingredients, and they have nothing to do with seaweed. Seaweed and algae are plants that can indeed thicken cosmetics, but I would not write them off quite so quickly. Many universities around the world, including Tufts University and Maine University, are studying myriad forms of seaweed for many purposes. The research process is still young, but early reports are encouraging and fascinating. Seaweed may not be quite so mundane as Neways makes it sound. I wouldn't suggest that smearing the stuff on your face in a cosmetic has any great benefit, but I am keeping an eye on this research.

What appears on the Neways Web site: AHAs (alpha hydroxy acids—such as glycolic acid, lactic acid, and others) exfoliate "the skin to remove wrinkles and expose young skin. Removing the outer layer of the skin exposes the young skin to the harsh aging and damaging environmental agents. Use of AHAs could make you age much faster. You could look better today but may not be such a pretty sight in ten years. Your outer layer of skin is your first and most important line of defense. Everything should be done to make it healthy and keep it, NOT LOSE IT. The FDA reported their deep concern with exfoliating the stratum corneum, and the aging and health risks associated with this potentially dangerous procedure. . . ."

My comments: The FDA is concerned about AHAs and long-term irritation. However, when the outer layer of skin is furrowed and wrinkled, it is hardly healthy; it is simply a reaction to severe sun damage. Yes, you could say that the old skin protects the new skin, but if you are already protecting your skin from more sun damage by using a good sunscreen, you don't need this damaged outer layer. That would be like saying you need to keep calluses and corns on your feet as protection from overly tight shoes instead of taking off the shoes and removing the calluses and corns. Revealing new skin and improving cell turnover rates (which are slowed and distorted by sun damage) can absolutely improve the appearance of skin. That is the whole purpose behind facial peels and laser resurfacing. It is not dangerous; if anything, it removes potentially cancerous skin growths. Bottom line: Sun damage causes thickened, uneven skin, and getting that stuff off the face is good, not bad.

Crazy Things Dermatologists Say

Let me first say, I have the utmost respect for the field of dermatology. For many different skin problems from acne to rosacea, seborrhea, psoriasis, infections, and rashes of all kinds, dermatologists are an essential resource and are too often neglected in favor of cosmetic-counter advice. Yet I have encountered my own share of misinformation from dermatologists, and the letters I've received from women about their experiences make my heart sink.

Little more than five to ten years ago, most dermatologists eschewed cosmetics as being silly and a waste of time for women. How many times did I hear dermatologists say, "Oh, just use bar soap and Eucerin; everything else is a waste of time"? Somewhere along the way something changed, and dermatologists stepped into the sphere of cosmetic sales. Over the past several years, dermatologists in search of better or more profitable patient care began selling skin-care products, often in tandem with makeup products. Fifteen years ago, when I first started my cosmetic research work, there were maybe 4 skin-care lines being wholesaled to dermatologists for retail sales; today there are more than 50.

I am hardly against anyone making money selling cosmetics; I am, however, very concerned about the way many dermatologists are diving into the fray. Dermatologists often portray their products as having special or unique formulations and that is not always, if ever, the case. Rather I find the same shortcomings in products sold by dermatologists that I find in the rest of the cosmetics industry: overpriced formulations promising miracles they can't live up to. I've seen the same "trend hysteria" run amok among dermatologists. Much like any consumer, dermatologists will read a study from some researcher about an ingredient revelation and, without any further information or substantiation, begin selling products that contain the showcase ingredient. And, of course, every skin-care revelation has to sell for at least $40 an ounce.

Some dermatological lines are also known for their remarkably potent strengths of AHAs. A well-formulated AHA product is great, and most dermatological lines have them, but the value of higher and higher concentrations of AHAs (typically being sold by dermatologists via such lines as M.D. Formulations and GlyDerm) is questionable. If you refer to my section on AHAs in Chapter Two, you'll see that the FDA has serious concerns about effective AHA formulations and their potentially harmful side effects. Why aren't dermatologists equally concerned? Why aren't dermatologists warning their patients that there are no long-term studies demonstrating the effects that continued use of high concentrations might have on the skin?

Possibly dermatologists' worst offenders are their wrinkle creams, which have expensive price tags, standard cosmetic formulations, and no proof of efficacy. I find that intolerable. I have heard dermatologists recommend things that make my hair stand on end. A reporter from *Self* magazine called me concerning an article she was writing. She wanted to check out information she received from a dermatologist who told her that the best moisturizing ingredients were beeswax and chamomile. My response was, "That's sheer nonsense, that is just crazy." Beeswax is not all that emollient in comparison to a host of other ingredients, and while chamomile may work as a mild anti-irritant, it has no moisturizing properties whatsoever.

Recently I was personally interviewing a dermatologist who was selling a $26, 2-ounce jar of sunscreen (one I thought was a good formulation). I asked how long he expected that product to last a consumer. The doctor said at least three months. The SPF factor of a product is ensured by a liberal application, and, rated on a 1-ounce application per use, that means that if someone is using that 2-ounce product correctly, it wouldn't last more than a day or two for the parts of the body exposed to sun and therefore only slightly longer for just the face. When I mentioned this, he just shrugged and said he had never heard that about SPF. All he needed to do was call the cosmetic chemist who formulated the product; he or she would have the FDA requirements for SPF testing right there.

Here are a few sample letters from the "Dear Paula" section of my newsletter; I think you will find them interesting, and they speak directly to this topic:

Dear Paula,

My dermatologist is selling a product called Phase 16-C Cream (*$37.50 for 2 ounces*) with the following ingredients: deionized water; organic citrus blend; cornflower, cress, ivy, rosemary, and sage extracts; stearic acid; cetearyl alcohol; ceteareth-20; carboxymethyl cellulose; glyceryl stearate; dimethicone; alpha bisabolol; cetyl alcohol; allantoin; ascorbyl palmitate, magnesium ascorbyl phosphate; lactic acid; sodium PCA; royal bee jelly; triethanolamine; phenoxyethanol; methylparaben; and propylparaben. What is this supposed to be about? Is there anything really special in here?

Curious, via e-mail

Dear Curious,

I think your dermatologist didn't look at the ingredients listing. There are several plant extracts in here that can cause allergic reactions or skin sensitivities. Why would any dermatologist want his or her patients to be putting orange juice on their face, or ivy? What purpose could that possibly serve except irritation? And no dermatologist should be selling any product that contains royal bee jelly; that nonsensical, gimmicky ingredient is just embarrassing coming from a physician.

Dear Paula,

I am a plastic surgeon practicing in Honolulu. The *Honolulu Advertiser* published an article of yours regarding skin-care products sold by physicians. You stated that products sold by dermatologists are not necessarily any better than what one can find in the cosmetics section of a drugstore or department store.

I would like to correct what I feel is misinformation. First of all, the Obagi regimen is available only to physicians who have trained with Dr. Obagi. These formulations, it is true, have some characteristics in common with other cosmetic products. However, this is one of the only skin programs manufactured to be integrated and have what is necessary to correct many skin problems; [some of the ingredients are] not available in over-the-counter products. This includes the incorporation of Retin-A into the program and a hydroquinone product for pigmentation problems. I have found Dr. Obagi's program to be exceptional.

Dr. Jon, Honolulu, Hawaii

Dear Dr. Jon,

Physicians who sell cosmetics are still just selling cosmetics. It is misleading to suggest that when physicians are merchandising cosmetics of any kind that they are somehow selling specially regulated products or products that contain ingredients you can't get anywhere else. They are not. Cosmetics are all regulated the same, no matter where they are sold. While you may have found that many of his products are good, and some of them indeed are, there are lots of good (and generally much less expensive) cosmetics on the market that can perform equally as well as Obagi's. The ingredients included in the Obagi products are not unique, and to suggest that this line is somehow more "integrated" than other product lines—meaning, I take it, that the products work magically together or in tandem with Retin-A or other prescription products—is just not true. No matter how good Dr. Obagi might be, he's not the only game in town, as your letter implies—just the one you happen to be selling.

Dear Paula,

I am a faithful reader of your newsletters and books, and user of your products. You have always been helpful. I have had rosacea now for about eight years. I've seen several different dermatologists until I found one who didn't try to sell me their products or give me the impression that there was not much they could do for me other than MetroGel. I had been using MetroGel and seeing very little in the way of controlling my rosacea (my skin was red, flaky, broken out, and dry). The dermatologist that I see currently said that MetroGel doesn't work for everyone. He had me try a couple of different products and we settled on Emgel. It is a topical gel that is 2% erythromycin. I used it morning and night for about four weeks. The results were amazing! He said I could continue to use it with no side effects, either as needed or on a regular basis. I use it mostly at night and have found that I can use either my MetroGel or MetroCream in the mornings; my skin looks ten times better. (I use your moisturizers/sunscreen, either dry or oily, depending on the season, over the Emgel.)

Kim, Chicago, Illinois

Dear Kim,

Thank you for the great feedback; I will share your comments with my readers. I am impressed by your doctor's diligence in helping you find something that works. I can't tell you the number of readers I hear from who are handed a prescription by a dermatologist, given little or no information about what it is, what it does, or how to use it, and then, when it fails, are given no other options. A dermatologist who is willing to work with you and test alternatives is a blessing! I wish I got more letters like yours in this regard!

One More Wrinkle Cream

Is collagen the answer? What about gold, algae, lotus seed, AHAs, proteins, amino acids, DNA, a newly created unknown molecule of some kind, mink oil, emu oil, kalaya oil, myriad plants ranging from ginseng to *Ginkgo biloba*, vitamin C, vitamin A, or perhaps vitamin E? What about aloe, chamomile, beta glucan, superoxide dismutase, or selenium? How many secret formulas can there be for wrinkles? All of them? None of them? Do we ever get tired of the onslaught?

Every few years, there is another cosmetic miracle promising women perfect skin. And every few years, women purchase another cache of products believing they've bought the answer to erase their wrinkles or stop their breakouts. Some doctor or renowned scientist will introduce a line, or some new natural, all-botanical line will be launched, and I'll get a horde of letters asking, "What do you think of this? It sounds so good, surely this must be it." Usually there is some interesting research behind many popular skin-care ingredients, but I haven't seen any research indicating that "the answer" or the fountain of youth is finally out there. I wish it were, because then this book would be one page long, about one product, and we would all look 20 again without a blemish in sight.

The entire issue reminds me of the vitamin E craze from the early '80s, the collagen and elastin frenzy from the late '80s, and the AHA mania from the early '90s. Women thought those were the answers to their skin-care woes; hundreds of these products were created and millions of units were sold—and women still had their wrinkles. It's not that vitamin E, collagen, elastin, and AHAs weren't good ingredients, and aren't still good skin-care ingredients, but they weren't the fountain of youth. For some unknown reason, it seems women need to believe there is a magic potion out there that will restore their youthful appearance or get rid of any and all skin flaws. To that end they will accept whatever sales pitch they're handed as long as the promise is for miraculous results. Actually, the more unbelievable the claim, the more expensive the product, or the more well-known the celebrity endorsing it, the more likely it is to be bought by women. Vitamin E, collagen, elastin, and AHAs are now merely memories, and vitamin C, vitamin A, and a host of plant extracts from weeds to flowers are now the big deal everyone is buying. But the next fad is on the horizon, and it will have its swarms of devotees, and vitamin C and vitamin A, along with all the other by then has-been skin-care miracles, will be hardly a memory.

The Signs of Aging

One of the best ways to curb our appetite for wrinkle creams is to understand that the skin's aging process is more complicated than we can ever imagine. Researchers generally agree that the visible signs of aging on the surface of the skin—deep wrinkles, lines, and discolorations—are only one aspect of a multilevel composite of events. Surprisingly, furrowed, leathery skin and brown "liver" spots are directly caused by sun exposure and are not genetically predetermined. What does seem to be genetically predetermined is a vast range of occurrences in the skin that can cause it to look older.

Looking at the issue objectively can help us to better understand what is happening to our skin, and therefore gain some insight into why wrinkle products can almost never really live up to their claims. For example, while we know that collagen and elastin are the support structures of the skin and that they break down and flatten as a result of exposure to the sun, we should realize that they also become less pliant and more hardened with age, so the skin becomes less elastic. Even if a product could build more collagen or elastin in our skin, if our skin isn't pliant and flexible, what good is the product? Some products claim to build only collagen or only elastin. That is much like building a house with only cross-beams and no support beams. One without the other is useless, because the house won't stay erect. Additionally, the process that builds collagen isn't the same as the one that builds elastin. But, for the sake of argument, let's say there are products that *can* selectively build more collagen or elastin. Regardless, just rebuilding elastin or collagen or any other single part of the skin isn't enough to halt or reverse the intricate, convoluted aging process and its effect on our face, because collagen and elastin represent only a part of the skin's aging.

One notable difference between older skin and younger skin is that younger skin has more fat cells in the dermis than older skin. That is one reason why older skin looks more transparent and thinner than younger skin. But of course no one is going to sell an anti-wrinkle product by saying it increases fat content in the skin, despite the fact that if a product could do that, it would absolutely make the skin look younger.

Furthermore, for some unknown reason, the skin keeps growing and expanding as we age, despite the fact that the fat tissue in the lower layers of skin is decreasing. That is why the skin begins to sag. Too much skin is being produced, but there isn't enough bone (remember, bone also deteriorates with age), fat, or muscle to shore it up. Simultaneously, facial muscles lose their shape and firmness, giving the face a drooping appearance. All the exercise in the world can't stop that from happening; it isn't that the muscles of the face aren't toned or strong—facial muscles are the most used muscles of the body. Instead, with time, use, and sun damage, the facial muscles begin to sag away from their original position on the face. One way that plastic surgeons deal with the issue of sagging muscles is to anchor them back to the position they had before they began to be pulled down by gravity.

Furrowing the brow is also a major reason that part of the face gets horizontal or vertical lines. All the cosmetic lotions and potions can't change facial expressions. That is why an injection of Bo-Tox, a medical procedure which paralyzes the facial muscles of the forehead, smooths out the wrinkles in that area.

Certain components of the skin also become depleted with age. The water-retaining and texture-enhancing elements, such as ceramides, hyaluronic acids, polysaccharides, vitamins, enzymes, coenzymes, and proteins, are exhausted. Older skin is also more subject to allergic reactions and skin sensitivities than younger skin, which suggests that older skin is less capable of defending itself against irritants because of a weakening autoimmune system.

On a deeper molecular level, the DNA codes within the skin cells can get lost or rearranged, either from sun damage or from aging itself. This change in the DNA (the fundamental cornerstone that controls aging throughout the entire body) prevents our skin cells from reproducing as they did when we were younger. Cells become abnormally shaped, which further changes the skin's texture and also prevents the cells from holding onto water. This inability to retain water is why older skin tends to be drier than younger skin. Companies that stick DNA and RNA in their products want you to believe they can help rectify this deterioration. They can't, and even if they could do something, do you really want to mess around with your genetic coding? If those ingredients really could change cell growth, it could put your skin at serious risk of cancer.

Cosmetics companies target many of these factors of aging by adding cosmetic ingredients that claim to counteract the effect of these specific depletions. Ceramide, hyaluronic acid, vitamins, proteins, and other components of skin are popular in wrinkle creams. The problem is, you can't put ceramide or hyaluronic acid back into the skin from the outside in (or even from the inside out); their molecular structure is too large to penetrate the skin. Moreover, even when these ingredients are chemically altered so they can penetrate skin, how much of the ingredient does skin need? A gram? A milligram? No one knows. Plus, the quantity of skin substances being depleted numbers in the thousands. Simply put, no product anywhere can handle all the multitudinous nuances of skin aging.

Like collagen and elastin, ceramide and hyaluronic acid are good water-binding agents and therefore are useful in moisturizers. Unfortunately, the cosmetics industry loves to use phrases such as "Replaces what skin has lost," leading you to believe that these ingredients can affect skin structure when all they are doing is working as a good moisturizer—which is great for skin; it's just not worth $25 to $325 an ounce.

Growing old cannot be reversed by the right skin-care routine, by jerking your face into funny shapes, or by stimulating muscles with machines. As far as anti-aging products are concerned, you are never going to get what you think you've paid for, unless you're buying a sunscreen, because sunscreens can truly prevent a great deal of sun damage, and that's what is primarily causing our skin to wrinkle.

Cosmetics Seduction

You see an ad for a new wrinkle cream or skin-care line. The promises and the enthusiastic endorsements about the results you can expect to see make you start to think, "Well, just maybe this one will be the right one." Despite the fact that the ad you are looking at is about a product that is only one of thousands like it, your mind has to do some fast work to validate your reason to spend your hard-earned money and risk your skin.

Whenever you shop for makeup or skin-care products, the choices are dazzling, provocative, and extensive, and the sales methods fetching and slick. You notice the display for a new foundation or eye cream at the department store, or you hear enthusiastic exclamations from a celebrity endorsing an infomercial line of skin-care products, or a friend selling a new line of cosmetics rattles off a litany of scientific-sounding information that sounds too good to be true. Enticing names and colors suggest the very essence of beauty. Tantalizing claims sound too good to pass up. The thoughts flicker up: "If I buy that, I will look really great; if I use that, my skin may really look younger." Elegance, glamour, and sensuality, all in one small bottle. How can you not at least try it? What difference does price make when all that matters is looking and feeling beautiful? Your're reaching for your wallet before you know it.

That is when the déjà vu should begin. You should be saying to yourself, "Didn't this happen a few months or a year ago? Did the last wrinkle cream I bought really make a difference? Why should this one work? Didn't the last lipstick I bought, which said it wouldn't bleed but did, convince me to be more skeptical?" Even if you like the products you are using, the next eye-catching ad can make you doubt them. Perhaps there is something better out there that you're missing. Another $50, $75, $100, or $200 later, you have a collection of new products at home, and the cycle continues.

I understand the pull generated by creative cosmetics advertising. But chasing after every new anti-wrinkle product or anti-acne product that comes on the market would cost thousands upon thousands of dollars a year. At the Lancome counter, the salespeople tout the miraculous results of their new Primordial Lotion, giving it the same kind of hype they gave their Bienfait Total a few months before. In fact, you can hear similar claims no matter where you stop to get advice, whether from Chanel, Prescriptives, Arden, Orlane, Christian Dior, L'Oreal, Nivea, Almay, Amway, Murad, or Cellex-C. All cosmetics companies promote their skin-care products as "miracles." How many miracles can there be in the world, and why are all of them generated by the cosmetics industry?

The industry also uses vague language that can neither be proven nor refuted, so they don't have to worry about claim substantiation. How does skin "act young"? That can be defined in a hundred different ways. Additionally, even if the company can substantiate the claim, what they substantiate may not be what you were hoping for. This cycle gets you nowhere, and that's why you need me.

There are several major obstacles to overcome when tackling the cosmetics-buying process: (1) the vast number of choices; (2) the vast number of products that are a waste of time and money; (3) the vast number of products that really work and help you look wonderful; (4) salespeople who are trained to sell products, and not how to honestly evaluate your skin-care needs or apply makeup colors; and (5) the difficulty of knowing what really works and what doesn't, as well as what looks good on you and what doesn't.

The purpose of this book is to help you narrow down the choices. Yes, it's hard to know what looks the best and what skin-care products really do work, but the more information you have, the easier it gets and the less money you will waste. In all honesty, shopping the cosmetics counters may never be truly easy, but it can be a fun, challenging adventure that you can approach with confidence and more knowledge than most any salesperson you will ever meet.

Please keep in mind the following facts:

1. According to the FDA, cosmetics companies do not have to prove their claims. That means that they get to say just about any little thing they want about their products and these claims absolutely do not have to be true or have any proof.

2. The FDA also does not require safety documentation for cosmetics until after the product has been brought to market and the FDA starts receiving consumer complaints.

The only part of the cosmetics industry that is strictly regulated for the consumer is the ingredients label. Unfortunately, the vast majority of consumers don't know how to read a cosmetics label, or they just don't care about it and would rather rely on the unregulated claims and assertions the marketing copy boasts about.

The Artists Down the Block

It was no secret to professional makeup artists that pink, orange, peach, and rose colored foundations were about as loathsome a beauty mistake as blue or shiny eyeshadow. But most cosmetics lines were clueless about these beauty concepts and assumed that women wanted a "rosy" glow to their skin, regardless of how artificial it looked. They also sold shiny eyeshadows because iridescence catches a woman's attention and looks more appealing in the package than a drab matte shade. Forget that it wears poorly and enhances the appearance of wrinkles; as far as Estee Lauder, Lancome, Clinique, and the others were concerned, what was eye-catching was more important than fashion and common sense. That is, until, in a relatively short period of time, M.A.C. took off, because it gave women the kind of makeup information they were longing for. Fashion-conscious consumers lined up to get what the other lines didn't have, or had in short supply.

In less time than it takes to say "profit margin," executives in cosmetics sales began to realize that launching color lines with M.A.C.'s kind of voguish style was the way to go. Makeup artists who could attractively represent their own line became hot properties in New York, resulting in a veritable explosion of new cosmetics companies. Bobbi Brown, Trish McEvoy, Carol Shaw, Laura Mercier, Nars, and Stila are no longer unknown makeup artists with tiny credits alongside photographs in ads or fashion spreads in magazines—they are cosmetic lines sold across the country. Lines bearing their official seals are now heralded with bold captions in the *Recommended Product* sections of fashion magazines. It is hard to miss them if you've shopped lately at department stores such as Barneys, Neiman Marcus, or Nordstrom.

What they all have in common is a glaring similarity to M.A.C., only with a higher price tag. Surprisingly, it's hard to tell the difference between any of these lines. Of course, the salespeople carry on at length about exclusive formulations and one-of-a-kind textures, but they aren't apparent to me or even to many of the salespeople I talked to. I was impressed by the soft, neutral blush colors, great foundation colors, impressive (though pricey) brush selections, wonderful eyeshadow colors and textures (for the most part—they do have their shiny assortment), and the fairly long-lasting lipsticks with stains. However, these lines have some serious drawbacks and, unquestionably, less-expensive alternatives can be found (like M Professional—a drugstore line of color products). I encourage you to take the time to check out a few of these lines to get a clearer sense of what a truly neutral, non-iridescent color palette looks like, but beware the trends and allure of expertise fronting good old-fashioned overmarketing of cosmetics.

"Shine Is Hip"

Many of you know that I get plenty of criticism for the work I do in the cosmetics industry. Some of the criticism is merely a nuisance: "Why come down so hard on the cosmetics industry? Women just want to have fun." "Women can make up their own minds; they don't need you." "You're not a cosmetic chemist." "How can you recommend drugstore products? They use ingredients inferior to the department stores'." Those remarks are hardly worth commenting on because they are so uninformed and reflect someone who has been completely seduced by advertising and cosmetic marketing distortions. My question back is, "Why not come down so hard on the cosmetics industry when they create products that can hurt your skin or waste your money and legally lie to you about it at the same time?" It doesn't take a cosmetic chemist, only a diligent researcher (I list all my sources at the end of this book in the appendix) to discover that ingredient quality has very little to do with where you shop for cosmetics. Plus, if you don't want to take my advice, don't read my books.

Then there are those comments I take very seriously. I worry about my accuracy and being up to date on the latest relevant (meaning valid) research. In addition, I pay close attention to maintaining my objectivity, to be sure I'm basing my comments on fact and not emotion. I also care a great deal about how fashion and looking one's best affect a woman's image in the world. I try constantly to blend my technical knowledge with the part of me that is a professional makeup artist.

This last concern is sometimes the trickiest thing for me to come to terms with, because it is based more on opinion and intuition than factual information. For me, the one critique I am most puzzled about addressing is the one that says I don't take the needs of younger women into consideration when I review products. I am sometimes told that my work focuses on older women, while leaving the twenty- and early-thirtysomething crowd in the dust. One young woman wrote a great letter to me saying, "I know you don't like shiny eyeshadows, blushes, or powders because they make wrinkles look more obvious, but I don't have any wrinkles and I think shine looks great on those of us under thirty. Why don't you add comments for us?"

And I recently received this letter via e-mail:

Dear Paula,

I love the idea of what you are doing. As someone who doesn't have enough money to make more than a few select, higher-end purchases a year, it's nice to have such great descriptions of products to help me decide what to buy. The only thing is, I like some of the things that you don't. The Estee Lauder Two-In-One Eyeshadow is one of my favorites. I LOVE a shiny eye! I'm twenty-seven, and most of my friends use Vaseline over their eyeshadow to give them a more iridescent, shiny look. You also said that a "problem" with Avon eyeshadows was that they were slightly iridescent (I'm talking about the cream-to-powder). That look is sooo beautiful. I think you should be more open to new looks in makeup. The fact that it is somewhat iridescent is not a mistake on Avon's or Lauder's part; it is the look they were trying to achieve—it is what is "in" right now. Shiny is hip. Shiny lips, shiny eyes, shiny cheeks. I agree that if you're shiny all over, it is overkill and can look really bad, but pick up an issue of *Vogue* or *Marie Claire* or *Bazaar*. I think it's time you opened up to new products and looks. What you dislike could be another person's like. State the facts: ingredients are ... slightly iridescent ... ; leaves skin looking shiny ... ; etc. And don't judge so harshly.

Was I actually ignoring the needs of a younger audience? And if that's true, what should I do to correct this oversight? Philosophically, how do I come to terms with the fashion trends that maybe do look great on younger girls and women? I've thought about this a lot lately, and especially in regard to the product line called Urban Decay. Pondering this dilemma has been an interesting one and a source of much discussion in my very twentysomething office and among the readers I polled.

I have come to this conclusion: while I do think I have calmed down in my chastising of shine in cosmetics, I am still not going to set aside what I believe to be the best way for a woman of any age to dress her face. After all, I'm the woman who wrote the book *Blue Eyeshadow Should Be Illegal* back when blue eyeshadow was the number one selling color at the cosmetics counters!

In response to the young woman's letter above, I do read practically every fashion magazine that's published, every month. More than I care to count. I am completely aware of the trends put forth by the fashion world. I am very aware of the four-inch high heels, plunging necklines, skin-tight pants, cellulite creams, and a host of other "in" products and looks espoused monthly. It is every woman's right to choose what she likes best on herself. I am the last person to suggest otherwise. But I would be betraying my strong beliefs to suggest that shine on women of any age, or multicolored prismatic eyeshadows, or overglossed lips, or thick foundation, or peach-colored foundation, or greasy magenta eye pencils, or overly defined brown lips, or smeary, thick black eyeliner, or blue eyeshadow—on and on—are things women should consider. Trends aplenty can be found that turn women into "dolls" or mannequins, not women. I can only offer what I know and then let women choose from there. Let fashion magazines hand women trends by the bandwagonful; I choose to offer women some pointers toward empowerment—with an eye toward sophistication and elegance—but the final decision is up to you. I have often said, even if you don't agree with me you can still figure out what your options are out there, in all price ranges, but to leave my opinion out would be to leave out why I do what I do.

Having said all that, how do I comment on shiny cranberry mascara and lime green lipstick? What am I supposed to say about black metallic nail polish, glittery peacock blue eyeliner, or gold lamé body paint? I would encourage women of all ages to think about why they get dressed in the morning and what they want from their life, and then figure out how metallic black, sparkling nail polish fits into that plan. In the meantime, I'll review those types of products with an eye toward quality and application, as I always do, but I will continue to comment about what I think and let the consumers make the final decision for themselves.

For Women of Color

Many cosmetics lines are trying to make up for their past inequities by adding makeup products appropriate for women of color. Previously, the foundations offered in this area were too orange and greasy, the eyeshadows were strictly shiny, and the skin-care products were fairly drying. It seems unbelievable that it has taken so long for the major cosmetics companies to finally acknowledge and try to meet the needs of such a large group of women. Revlon, Prescriptives, M.A.C., Clinique, and Lancome are the leaders in this area, and they are to be commended. Not only are their color products appropriate, but they offer a large number of choices. Although some lines designed specifically for women of color, such as Flori Roberts and Fashion Fair, offer limited options and problematic colors, other lines, including Black

Opal, Posner, and Iman, have incredible color selections and high-quality products.

One area in which these specialty lines often fail is when it comes to skin care. Although Black Opal or Flori Roberts would like to lead the consumer to believe that their products are specially formulated for African-American skin, there is nothing in their formulations supporting that claim. In fact, products for African-American women are often formulated to be either greasy, with heavy moisturizers and wipe-off cleansers, or drying, with alcohol-based toners. Both of these product types pose problems for darker skin tones. Alcohol can dry out the skin and increase ashiness, and greasy products can cause breakouts and make skin look dull.

A handful of cosmetics lines coming on the scene claim they are designed for Asian women. Their brochures say Asian skin is supposedly so different from Caucasian, Latin, and African-American skin that it requires a separate product line. Nothing could be further from the truth, and the products in these lines are just like those in all the other lines on the market, and the formulations just as problematic. Creating a special marketing niche where none exists might be good business, but it isn't necessarily good for the consumer. As it turns out, according to marketing surveys, most Asian and African-American women do not want a line directed specifically at them; they would rather just buy mainstream cosmetics that include them too.

When it comes to skin-care routines, the differences having to do with your skin color are minimal to nonexistent. Product choices need to be based on skin type, not skin color. As surprising as this may sound, skin color does not affect skin type. If you have a blemish or dry skin, the treatment is the same regardless of your skin color. Darker skin tones may have more problems with keloidal scarring or ashy skin tones, but these problems are not addressed differently from those of scarring or freckling for Caucasian women. Many cosmetics lines aim their makeup and color products at Caucasian skin, but their skin-care routines can be suitable for any skin color. If anything, I find that skin-care routines from lines specifically aimed at darker skin tones tend to leave out sunscreen, or include products with alcohol and irritants, or, more often than not, offer extremely greasy moisturizers. All those things can create ashy skin tones (alcohol creates flaky, gray skin tones), damage skin (irritants can exacerbate scarring), and impede the healing process (heavy moisturizers can hurt the skin's ability to produce new skin cells). As long as a product line has gentle, effective cleansers, reliable sunscreens (SPF 15 with UVA protection), nonirritating toners, effective blemish products, and lightweight moisturizers, there is little risk to any skin type or skin color.

International Readers

For those of you who shop for cosmetics outside of the United States, let me give you a heads-up—that's American slang for advanced warning—about how this book applies to where you live. For the most part, most cosmetic products sold here in the United States are identical to those sold in Europe, Canada, and Australia. Occasionally there are minor differences in formulations, but they rarely affect a product's actual performance. Sunscreens are the one product in which there are major differences between formulations found in the United States versus the rest of the world. Sunscreen formulations outside of the United States, for the exact same product, are more often than not vastly different. European, Canadian, and Australian formulators have been using the UVA-protecting ingredients avobenzone (Parsol 1789), titanium dioxide, zinc oxide, and Mexoryl SX™ (a UVA-protecting ingredient not available in the United States) for years. Also, the international sunscreen formulations allow for very different combinations of active ingredients. Whether the products are from L'Oreal, Lancome, or Lubriderm SPF 15, they will all have radically different sunscreen formulations than their U.S. counterparts and, when there are differences, the international versions are preferable.

International regulations for sunscreen agents allow for larger concentrations of zinc oxide and titanium dioxide. For some reason, U.S. regulations do not allow for avobenzone to be formulated with zinc oxide or titanium dioxide, while international formulations do. Because of this discrepancy in sunscreen formulations, you cannot judge my SPF reviews as being universal. You must always check the active ingredient list to be sure the UVA protecting ingredients are included, and then be sure you are also buying an SPF 15, a universally important sunscreen number.

In terms of ingredients, a reminder to my Canadian readers: You still don't have a mandatory ingredient listing. The rest of the western world does. All of Europe, Australia, and the United States (since 1978) have compulsory cosmetic ingredient labeling laws. Come on, Canadian women, call Health Canada and tell them you aren't going to take this anymore. Health Canada's excuses are unsatisfactory. They say the dual-language requirement makes it impossible to get the listing on the products. That doesn't wash. European products have more than seven languages to get on a label or insert, and they all do it. Canadian women can also bring pressure to bear on the cosmetics companies themselves. Simply do not buy products or shop cosmetics lines that do not disclose complete ingredient listings. If a $3 can of soup can have a complete ingredient listing and dietary breakdown, then a $75 moisturizer can do the same. After all, these companies are merely changing their packaging when they get to your part of the world, and just replacing the ingredients label.

When to Throw Out Makeup?

Skin-care and makeup products are generally formulated and tested for a shelf life of one to three years under normal storage conditions, depending on a product's composition, packaging, preservation, and other factors. However, there are no regulations under current law that require cosmetics manufacturers to print expiration dates on the labels of cosmetic products. Consumers should be aware that expiration dates are simply rules of thumb, and that a product's safety may expire long before its expiration date if the product has not been properly stored. Cosmetics that have been improperly stored—for example, exposed to high temperatures or sunlight, or opened and examined by consumers prior to final sale—may deteriorate substantially before the expiration date. On the other hand, products stored under ideal conditions may be acceptable long after the expiration date has been reached.

In general, it is best to toss out cosmetics placed near the eye (mascara is a good example) after four to six months, and to dispose of face products after one to two years. But those are merely suggestions, and not based on any established research or guidelines.

CHAPTER TWO

Skin-Care Update

The Beauty Bible

I tried to address every makeup and skin-care problem, doubt, curiosity, argument, issue, style, and fad I could possibly think of in my book *The Beauty Bible*. It is as comprehensive a compilation of what I've learned about the world of skin care and makeup as I could possibly assemble. I spent two years being sure every question I had ever been asked was addressed in some way in that book. If you bought this edition of *Don't Go to the Cosmetics Counter Without Me* hoping to find out answers to such questions as how to tell what your skin type is, what vitamins can really do for the skin, what tea tree oil is, how AHAs work and whether you should use them, whether Retin-A or Renova is worth it, or how much oxygen your skin needs—you bought the wrong book. This book is strictly a product guide that answers vital questions about whether a specific product can live up to its claims. Answers to questions about current beauty issues, how to select the right foundation, whether you need a moisturizer, and what the latest treatments are for acne are all found in *The Beauty Bible*.

I would like to share the following letter—which represents the type of letters I've received from women who have read *The Beauty Bible*. Most of the mail I receive has been wonderfully supportive. Some of the following comments might help you decide if the information in *The Beauty Bible* is for you.

Dear Paula,

I just want to thank you for your sane, good advice about skin care. I have suffered from acne for years and have tried so many different products that I don't want to know how much money I've spent! Then I got your book, *The Beauty Bible*, and was amazed at how simple your "battle plan for blemishes" really is. By using only over-the-counter products, I have gained clearer skin than I have ever had (even than when I was on oral antibiotics)! Best of all, I am not spending a fortune for products that hurt my skin. But what I was most impressed with was your suggestion to use Milk of Magnesia to combat oiliness. I thought it sounded really strange, but I tried it anyway—it really works! And it's a whole lot cheaper than those oil-controlling moisturizers (does that make sense or what?) that are on the market right now. I hope others will try your suggestion, too, even if it sounds strange at first. Thanks again for all your hard work, which benefits us all.

Sincerely, Jennifer, via e-mail

The following are excerpts from *The Beauty Bible* that reflect some of the more salient points, and highlight how I go about evaluating a variety of products.

It Really Is Irritating

I started my career as a cosmetics consumer advocate by warning women about the damage being done to their skin by irritating skin-care ingredients. Over the years, my fears about irritation have been confirmed and reinforced by many dermatologists and cosmetic chemists. Indeed, irritation is a bigger problem for the skin than even I had suspected. As many already know, irritation can stimulate an already overflowing oil production by activating nerve endings attached to the oil gland; it can dry up skin cells that need to retain water; it can cause increased dryness, which adds to cell debris that can clog pores; it can cause breakouts like a diaper rash over the skin; it can cause redness; and it can bring out surface capillaries on the face. In short, irritation is hell on the skin.

It also appears that irritation can destroy the skin's integrity by breaking down the skin's protective barrier, which, over time, damages the skin's structure and impairs the skin's natural immune/healing ability. Additionally, breaking down the skin's protective barrier can allow the introduction of bacteria, therefore raising the risk of breakouts. What's more startling is the histological evidence that even if your skin doesn't feel irritated when you apply a cosmetic or skin-care product containing irritants, it is still being irritated and the breakdown of the skin's protective barrier is nonetheless taking place. That means if a product contains potentially irritating or sensitizing ingredients, the irritating ingredients can still harm the skin, even if it doesn't sting or burn. Not paying attention to the irritation potential of ingredients can be damaging to the health of your skin.

Stop the Moisturizing Mania

Not everyone needs or should be using a moisturizer, especially women with oily, combination, or acne-prone skin! And women with dry skin only need one moisturizer (not including sunscreen). That sums it up. As we approach the next millennium (and it's getting closer all the time), I can't think of one skin-care product that is more misunderstood, misused, and abused than moisturizer. How did things get so out of hand? The only answer is that things tend to get out of hand in the world of cosmetics.

I like more moisturizers than I dislike (putting aside the nasty debate over cost versus performance), but because moisturizers are overused by most women, they can cause some pretty surprising skin problems. A lot of women (maybe most) still cling to the erroneous belief that moisturizers somehow prevent wrinkles. Not just moisturizers with a high sun-protection factor (SPF), which do stop further skin damage if they contain titanium dioxide, zinc oxide, or avobenzone, but all moisturizers. The mistaken notion that dry skin is more prone to wrinkles than oily skin remains firmly implanted in the mind of the consumer, and that's on top of all those claims about firming, toning, repairing, and lifting the skin with all sorts of creams, gels, and lotions.

The only reason to use a moisturizer is if you have dry skin or wrinkled skin you want to look smoother (moisturizers can smooth over, not change, wrinkles). If you don't have dry skin, there is no reason to use a moisturizer. If you have oily skin or skin that breaks out, the worst thing you can do is use a moisturizer of any kind. It's that simple. What happens when you overuse a moisturizer? Pores get clogged and blackheads can develop; dead skin cells get trapped and have a harder time naturally sloughing off, which can leave the skin looking dull; and you run a higher risk of getting patches of dermatitis, increasing the number of breakouts, and creating your own combination-skin predicament. Additionally, oversaturating the skin can turn off the skin's own immune/healing response. Overdoing moisturizers can actually prevent the skin from repairing itself.

What Works and What Doesn't?

By now your skepticism about cosmetics and the cosmetics industry should be firmly in place. However, you must be wondering, if the cosmetics industry's promises and claims aren't real—then what is real? What is and isn't possible when it comes to your skin? If you can accept the following premises, you are much less likely to waste money on overpriced or ineffective skin-care products or be swayed the next time you hear a sales pitch for a miraculous (or even semi-miraculous) sounding skin-care product or routine. I base a great deal of my evaluation of skin-care products on the following facts:

1.   **You can clean your skin, but you can't "deep-clean" it.** You can't get inside a pore and clean it out like a dentist with a drill. And even if you could get inside, the damage to the skin would negate any benefit of deep cleaning. (I know a blackhead looks like it's dirty, but dirt isn't what's making it look black!) Expensive water-soluble cleansers will not make your face any cleaner, nor are they necessarily any gentler than the less-expensive water-soluble cleansers. In fact, the handful of standard cleansing agents used in cleansers are the same across the cosmetics spectrum. What is essential is to find a gentle, water-soluble cleanser that doesn't dry out the skin or

leave it feeling greasy and that can remove eye makeup without irritating the eyes. Many cleansers that claim to be water-soluble are really too greasy to rinse off completely and can cause clogged pores.

2.   **Spending more money does not affect the status of your skin.** The amount of money you spend on skin care has nothing to do with how your skin looks. However, what product you use does. An expensive soap by Erno Laszlo is no better for your skin than an inexpensive bar soap such as Dove (though I would suggest that both are terrible for the face); on the other hand, an irritant-free toner by Neutrogena can be just as good as, or maybe even better than, an irritant-free toner by Orlane or La Prairie, and any irritant-free toner is infinitely better than any toner that contains alcohol or other irritants, no matter how natural-sounding the ingredients and regardless of the price. Spending less doesn't hurt your skin, and spending more doesn't necessarily help it.

3.   **Even minimal sun exposure is damaging to the skin.** Women clamor for the latest skin-care products that contain antioxidants, vitamins, plants, and a host of other exotics, yet all of that is meaningless if you are not using an effective sunscreen every day of your life. If you are exposed to the sun, even for as little as a few minutes every day, which includes walking to your car, walking to the bus, or sitting next to a window (sun's damaging UVA rays come through windows), that cumulative exposure over the years will wrinkle your skin. No skin-care product except a sunscreen with a high SPF and appropriate UVA protecting ingredients (see the section on Sun Reflections, later in this chapter) can change that. If exposure that minimal can wrinkle the skin, imagine how much worse the impact of sunbathing is. In short, there is no such thing as careful, safe, or wrinkleproof tanning or sun exposure of any kind.

4.   **Sun damage is such an important issue, I will say it one more time:** Due to the fact that any amount of sun exposure at any time of year is so damaging to skin, any daytime moisturizer that doesn't contain an effective SPF 15 is jeopardizing the health of your skin and is a complete waste of money.

5.   **A great number of skin-care problems are caused by the skin-care products used to prevent them.** Overly emollient moisturizers can clog pores, temporary face-lift products can cause wrinkles because of the irritation they generate on the skin, and products designed to control oily skin often contain ingredients that can make skin oilier (oil-free products often contain pore-clogging ingredients that don't sound like oils). Allergic reactions are often caused by products that contain plants because plants are inherently potent sources of allergens. Lots of skin-care products from the most expensive lines contain irritating ingredients such as fragrance, alcohol, witch hazel, and on and on. All of those things can contribute to the very skin problems you want to eliminate from your life and face.

6. **Dry skin doesn't wrinkle any more or less than oily skin.** Oily skin may look less wrinkled, which means it can have a smoother, more fluid appearance, but wrinkles are caused by sun exposure, genetic inheritance, muscles sagging (not from lack of exercise but from gravity—they slip down on the face), or other facial trauma— but not because of dry skin. All the moisturizers in the world won't change a wrinkle on your face, or prevent one, regardless of the amount of vitamins or plants they contain. That's not to say moisturizers can't temporarily, day to day, make dry skin look smoother, because they absolutely can. But stop using the miracle lifting moisturizer and in a day or two, very unmiraculously, your skin will be back the way it was.

7. **Your skin may become inflamed, dry, and blemished if you use too many scrubs, products that contain potentially irritating ingredients, or several AHA or BHA products, either at the same time or in combination with one another.** For example, the following combinations can hurt the skin: a granular cleanser used with a loofah, a washcloth used with an abrasive scrub, an AHA product used with a granular scrub, or an astringent that contains alcohol used with an AHA product. If you use too many irritating products at the same time, you are likely to develop skin irritations, breakouts, dryness, and, possibly, wrinkles.

8. **Exfoliating the skin does not regenerate skin or build collagen.** It is good to exfoliate the skin, and it is very important for many skin types, but exfoliation doesn't create new skin or get rid of wrinkles. Exfoliation can smooth the skin and help moisturizers be better absorbed, but the effects are temporary, and it doesn't alter the actual structure of the skin.

9. **For the most part, the fewer products you use on your skin, the better.** The more you use, the greater your chances of allergic reactions, cosmetic acne (from product buildup in the pores), and/or irritation.

10. **Worry about skin-care products that "smell" nice or have pretty colors.** Coloring agents and fragrance may seem attractive, but they are problematic and unnecessary in skin-care products. Ingredients that add fragrance to a product, even natural fragrances, are notorious for causing allergic reactions or skin sensitivities. Coloring agents may be great in a lipstick or foundation, but a blue or pink moisturizer is not great for taking care of skin and protecting it.

11. **Do not automatically buy skin-care products based on your age.** Many products on the market are supposedly designed for women who are 30, 40, or more than 50. Before you buy into these arbitrary divisions, ask yourself why the over-50 group always gets lumped together. Isn't it odd that women between the ages of 20 and 49 have skin that requires three or four categories, but women over the age of 50 need only one? There are a lot of years between 50 and 90. According to this logic, someone who is 40 shouldn't be using the same products as someone who is 50, but

someone who is 80 should be using the same products as someone who is 50. Categorizing products by decades is nothing more than a marketing device that sells products; it does not correlate with benefits to the skin. Skin has different needs based on how dry, sun-damaged, oily, sensitive, thin, blemished, or normal it is, all of which have little to do with age. Plenty of young women have severely dry skin, and plenty of older women have oily skin and breakouts (particularly those women experiencing peri-menopausal systems). Turning 40 or 50 does not mean a woman should assume that her skin is drying up and that she should begin using overly emollient moisturizers or skin creams.

12. Do not automatically buy skin-care products based on your skin type. I know that sounds strange, but there are several reasons for this. It's not that skin type isn't important, but more often than not, your skin type is not what you think it is. Possibly your skin type has been created by the products you are already using. Soap can severely dry the skin; a wrinkle cream can clog pores and cause blemishes; an alcohol-based toner can irritate the skin and cause combination skin. The only way to know what your skin type really is, is to start from square one with the basics that won't alter or adversely affect your skin, such as: a water-soluble cleanser, an irritant-free toner (or a disinfectant if you break out), an exfoliator (such as an AHA product if you have sun-damaged skin and a BHA product for breakouts), a sunscreen for the daytime (which can be included in your moisturizer or foundation), and a moisturizer at night (but only if you have dry skin). Please understand that the intense cosmetic hype that insists that everyone needs a moisturizer is absolutely not true. (I discuss this at length in *The Beauty Bible*.) If your skin is truly dry or you really are prone to breakouts, you can do the extra things, such as using a more-emollient moisturizer at night, or a more-emollient foundation or a moisturizer with sunscreen during the day. For breakouts, you can try varying topical disinfectants and oil-absorbing masks.

13. Treat the skin you have today, not the skin you had last month, last week, or yesterday. Skin type can fluctuate. Skin-care routines based on a specific skin type don't take into consideration the fact that your skin changes according to the season, your emotions, the climate (humidity, dryness, cold, and heat all affect your skin), and your menstrual cycle. Pay attention to what your skin tells you it needs at any given time. This month you might need an extra-moisturizing sunscreen during the day, and an emollient nighttime moisturizer. Next month you may only need a lightweight sunscreen or a foundation with sunscreen during the day and no moisturizer at night. The same is true for oily skin and breakouts. Don't hold fast to the idea that your skin fits into only one group—it changes, and so should your skin-care routine. That doesn't mean you need new products every month, it just means you may need to use less of one item or more of another.

14. **Teenagers are not the only ones who have acne.** One of the biggest fallacies around is that women over the age of 20 should not have blemishes. What a mistaken belief that is! Women in their 30s, 40s, and 50s can have acne just like teenagers. Not everyone who has acne as a teenager will grow out of it, and even if you had clear skin as a teenager, that's no guarantee that you won't get acne later in life.

15. **Oily skin types rarely, if ever, require a moisturizer.** Specialty products such as oil-free moisturizers are rarely if ever good for someone with oily skin, because even though they may truly not contain oil, they include plenty of ingredients that don't sound like oil but that can make the skin feel oily and clog pores. Furthermore, if you don't have dry skin you don't need a moisturizer. The notion that the skin needs moisture even if it's oily may sound nice, but moisturizers contain a lot more than water, and those ingredients can clog pores and make skin look and feel like an oil slick. You only need moisturizer where you have dry skin. Oil-free moisturizers can be good for someone with normal to slightly dry skin, but they are often a waste for someone with truly oily skin or someone who tends to break out. If the dryness is caused by other skin-care products, stop using those first before you decide to use a moisturizer.

16. **There are great skin-lightening products to be found that can have an impact on sun-damage spots.** You can expect about a 20% to 40% improvement if you use these products in association with an effective sunscreen. However, plants are not a source of skin lightening properties; the ingredients to look for on the label are hydroquinone, kojic acid, or kojic palmitate. Moreover, there are plenty of effective, inexpensive skin-lightening products to be found.

17. **AHAs can smooth skin but they can't stop wrinkling.** A well-formulated AHA product (meaning one having a 4% to 10% concentration of AHA with a pH of 3 to 4.5) can help encourage cell turnover, that is, help remove built-up surface skin cells. But it can't affect actual cell production.

18. **Tretinoin, the active ingredient in Retin-A and Renova, can change abnormal cell growth back to some level of normalcy.** In discussing anti-wrinkling products or skin products designed to improve the appearance of sun-damaged skin, it is important to consider the use of a retinoid such as tretinoin. What retinoids deliver to the skin is significant because of the way they can positively affect cell production. But all retinoids need to be prescribed by a physician; the over-the-counter vitamin A products cannot perform like Retin-A or Renova.

Vitamin A

As this book goes to print the hoopla around skin-care products containing vitamin A has replaced the AHA craze and the vitamin C mania. It is quite certain no other vitamin has generated as much public, medical, and media attention over the past ten years as vitamin A and all its counterparts have. Vitamin A and its derivatives, called retinoids, exploded into consumer awareness in 1988 when headlines and talk shows heralded a study conducted by Dr. John Voorhees, professor of dermatology at the University of Michigan, which demonstrated tretinoin, a form of vitamin A (the active ingredient in the prescription-only cream Retin-A), could effect a marked improvement in wrinkles.

Back in 1987, before all the publicity, Retin-A was a popular but low-profile acne drug, with sales totaling about $16 million a year. Today, sales of Retin-A and its spin-offs (primarily Renova, the only prescription medication approved by the FDA for wrinkles) are well over $175 million. It turns out that extensive subsequent and independent research from a diverse range of medical fields reveals that many forms of retinoids are potent mediators of healthy cell production.

According to the inventor of Retin-A, Dr. Albert Kligman, professor of dermatology at the University of Pennsylvania School of Medicine, "Some retinoids can change abnormal cell growth back to a level of normalcy." When asked how retinoids actually work, Kligman explained, "There is no single mechanism that explains how any of them work; in fact, we aren't exactly sure how they do what they do."

While tretinoin and other acid forms of vitamin A exist in the realm of medicine, retinol and retinyl palmitate exist in the world of cosmetics. Cosmetic companies from Estee Lauder to Neutrogena and Avon all have their assortment of products containing retinol or retinyl palmitate, and their claims mirror those made for Retin-A. But can cosmetics containing retinol or retinyl palmitate perform like tretinoin? Dr. Gary White, Chief, Department of Dermatology at Kaiser Permanente, San Diego, doesn't think so. He said, "There are no formal studies verifying any information on the topical use of retinol. The only studies I've seen used no control groups, they weren't done double blind, only small groups of patients were observed [fewer than ten], and the results were rated primarily by someone's visual assessment. That might sound good, but you can probably get the same results with just about any moisturizer. Visual improvement without a placebo-base [meaning without comparison of the product being tested with the use of a placebo in a control group] is useless information." But more studies are coming.

Dr. Anne R. Haake, assistant professor of dermatology at the University of Rochester School of Medicine and Dentistry, indicated that the yet-unpublished studies she's heard discussed had her "convinced that retinol may be less potent than tretinoin, but [retinol] can be taken up and metabolized in the cell, so it does become the effective form, but probably higher concentrations are then needed to get it to work. Plus, the advantage of retinol is that it is less irritating than tretinoin."

Should you give up your tube of Renova or Retin-A for a cosmetic containing retinol? Probably not, because the research just isn't there to support that change.

However, if retinol does prove to be as effective, the same concerns about sun damage and possible birth defects would apply. Retin-A and Renova can both make the skin more vulnerable to sun damage and come with a clear warning about sun protection. Oral forms of tretinoin—such as isotretinoin, better known as Accutane—can cause birth defects if a woman becomes pregnant while taking them. All prescription forms of vitamin A require extensive research to prove their safety and function, but cosmetic products require none of that very expensive investigation or documentation. Active forms of vitamin A are about changing cell production, something that goes well beyond superficial cosmetic changes to affect the very essence of the skin's structure.

Vitamin C

I don't know about you, but I'm really getting tired of this whole vitamin C skin-care craze. I thought for sure the vitamin A craze would take its place, but it hasn't seemed to dampen the fire; vitamin C products and claims keep on coming. You wouldn't think that one nebulous little ingredient would cause so much commotion but, then, we're talking about the cosmetics industry. It only takes one ingredient to start a furor. Especially one ingredient that promises instant youth, and vitamin C is such an ingredient. This time the new angle with vitamin C appears to be more politically motivated than anything else, which in some ways does make it more intriguing, just not skin worthy.

I've discussed at length the research surrounding vitamin C. It started with Dr. Sheldon Pinnell from Duke University, who looked at the effect of sun exposure in relation to applying L-ascorbic acid (a specific form of vitamin C) on hairless pigs. It seems the pigs with L-ascorbic acid applied to their skin did not get sunburned. From this study, and following theoretical models of vitamin C and its role in healthy skin, it was assumed by Pinnell that L-ascorbic acid was an exceptional antioxidant that could suppress sun damage. Yet, Pinnell also knew at the time that L-ascorbic acid was an exceptionally unstable ingredient. However, Pinnell didn't tell anyone that the $70-an-ounce bottle of Cellex-C containing L-ascorbic acid decomposed when exposed to air, sun, or heat. Despite this known drawback, dermatologists and the cosmetic world became enthralled with Cellex-C, and the bottles were flying off the shelf. Not to be left out of the running, other cosmetics lines, from Lancome with its Vitabolic to Avon's Anew Formula C Treatment Capsules and La Prairie Cellular Defense Shield with SPF 15 to companies selling vitamin C patches, all launched products containing forms of this now famous vitamin.

The story has become more complicated since I originally researched these issues surrounding vitamin C. I tried to get information from Dr. Pinnell back in 1996 when I first wrote about Cellex-C, but he neither returned my calls nor did I receive any of the documentation I requested from his company. All the data I have used over the past two years were obtained from other sources, including Pinnell's own published research and articles. I am pleased to say that this time, a representative from Pinnell's new company, SkinCeuticals, contacted me and was willing to provide me with some information.

It turns out that in 1997 Pinnell stopped endorsing Cellex-C (he never endorsed the entire Cellex-C product line, by the way, which included more than 20 additional products). Yes, Pinnell has always recognized that the original L-ascorbic acid he researched was unstable. He now claims to have a stabilized version of L-ascorbic acid available only through his company, SkinCeuticals. Not surprisingly, this stabilized form of L-ascorbic acid is not available to Cellex-C. Of course, why we are supposed to believe Pinnell now is anyone's guess.

Vitamin C in the form of L-ascorbic acid may have its place in skin care, and Pinnell stands to do quite well if his research stands up under peer review. Actually, he may do well regardless, because his version of stabilized L-ascorbic acid is selling well through his skin care line. With or without the proof, Pinnell's brochure states "Each product contains a unique blend of botanical extracts that help restore a youthful, radiant experience." So much for his vitamin C being the be all and end all for wrinkles. Any time researchers start bandying about cosmeticbabble like *botanicals* and *looking younger,* I suggest that medical and ethical lines have been crossed. And where is the research that substantiates any long-term effects of any of Pinnell's rather expensive products? The original question I posed some time ago in regard to Cellex-C applies to SkinCeuticals: If L-ascorbic acid, stabilized or otherwise, is supposed to be so amazing for building collagen and repairing skin, why do there have to be all these other products making more miraculous claims? Why would you need AHAs, toners, and other wrinkle creams if one product was doing all the work? There are some good products in this line, but the prices are stupefying, the claims are exaggerated beyond belief, and the misleading notion that a combination of several products will make a difference on the skin is farcical.

What is true for any issue involving skin aging is that aging is more complicated than just the loss of vitamin C or any other vitamin, enzyme, protein, or fatty acid in the skin. It is the whole picture we should be concerned about, not one small aspect. Besides, there are many other antioxidants that are as good as or even more impressive than vitamin C, including beta glucan, vitamin E, and vitamin A, to name a few; and, according to many researchers dedicated to the study of antioxidants, there are probably thousands of undiscovered antioxidants out there that may be even more significant.

The entire arena of antioxidants is new and there is nothing definitive to warrant the current cost or tumult. They won't get rid of wrinkles or replace sunscreen, so calm down! They can offer increased sun protection, which is important, but that's it. Of course, that doesn't stop the companies selling products that contain vitamin C from making claims about reversing aging, building collagen, feeding the skin, and healing sun damage, despite the fact that, as Pinnell states in his own paper published in *Les Nouvelles Esthetiques,* February 1996, "conclusive studies of the effect of [topical vitamin C to reduce sun damage] have not yet been conducted."

More Oxygen?

If you're a fan of celebrity magazines or if you caught the Jay Leno show some time ago, you may have heard stories about actress Kirstie Alley toting around a canister of oxygen as a way to take care of her skin. With all due respect to Kirstie, the only benefit she is getting from the oxygen is from schlepping it around. Hauling that extra weight would burn off a few extra calories, and that would be a healthy benefit.

Oxygen is perhaps the most confusing element among health concerns for the body. While we need oxygen to live, oxygen (oxidation) also causes free-radical damage. You may be aware that free-radical damage is an activity on the molecular level that causes aging. But there is no way to reconcile the issue of free-radical damage caused by the presence of oxygen in the environment with our basic need to breathe oxygen!

Strong evidence exists that skin damaged by smoking (smoking chokes off the blood supply to the skin) as well as seriously wounded skin can be helped by oxygen delivered in a hyperbaric chamber (like the ones divers use), but only if ongoing damage is stopped. You can't have it both ways. You can't smoke and then get a shot of oxygen (especially from a canister; you need the booth) to fix the skin. Besides, you can spend only so much time in a hyperbaric booth before it starts hurting you. Too much pure oxygen over time can actually cause damage to the body. But don't worry about Kirstie: She can't get enough oxygen from a canister to cause problems—or to help reverse the damage from her daily smoking habit, for that matter.

Asking whether products that contain vitamin C or oxygen can offer the skin some special miracle begs the question. It assumes that any of these ingredients can shore up skin from the outside in, and do it better or more so than other vitamins, enzymes, proteins, or a variety of components found in skin, from hyaluronic acid to mucopolysaccharides to yet-undefined enzymes, coenzymes, and proteins. While there is a lot of vitamin C in skin, and it does deteriorate upon exposure to sunlight, so do lots of other elements in skin deteriorate with sun exposure and age. You simply can't put everything the skin loses because of sun damage or age back into the skin! Not only would you need an unbelievably long ingredient list to accommodate all those components, but how much of any of these ingredients would be needed is still a complete unknown!

Let's say you *could* get all those necessary but depleted skin elements back into the skin; there is no research explaining how much is needed for the surface of skin, particularly not in cosmetics. Is 0.5% enough? What about 1%? And when is that amount used up? Do you need to reapply it every few minutes? Once an hour? Even drugs like Retin-A or Renova (or other acid forms of retinoids) that have clear, substantiated evidence of improving cell production can't change wrinkles the way we want them to. There is nothing wrong with wanting to put back what the skin has lost, but trying to undo damage with a healthful-sounding ingredient list isn't going to do the trick.

Sun Reflections

Media headlines sometimes have a way of creating news sensations where none exist, or making something sound new and eye-popping when the information is really well-established and even dated. You may have seen a brouhaha in the media in the spring of 1998 regarding a new study claiming that sunscreens do not help in protecting a person from skin cancer. According to an epidemiological review of ten previously published studies, recently presented at the American Association for the Advancement of Science meeting in Philadelphia by Dr. Marianne Berwick, an epidemiologist at Memorial Sloan-Kettering Cancer Center in New York, "based on the evidence, we conclude that sunburn itself probably does not cause melanoma, but that it is an important sign of excessive sun exposure, particularly among those who are genetically susceptible because of their skin type." Well, duh!

Dermatologists have long been aware that sunscreen protection is probably not related to skin melanomas, which are most likely directly linked to basal cell carcinoma. Further, the issue of sunburn *not* being implicated in some skin cancers has long been settled in Europe and Australia, and recently here in the United States. But that's about UVA protection versus UVB protection. The importance of protecting skin from UVA rays (which cause skin cancer and wrinkling) as well as UVB rays (sunburning rays) has been demonstrated. I'm not sure how Berwick missed this one, but she did. Her study looked at sunscreen use over the past ten years. She should have checked into the formulations that were used over that period. It is only recently that cosmetic chemists have started formulating sunscreens with ingredients that can protect equally from both UVB and UVA damage. People who used traditional sunscreens over the past ten years were putting their skin at risk because they would have been getting sunburn protection only, while still being exposed to harmful UVA rays.

Others have raised questions about how Berwick's study was done and the conclusions her team reached. Dr. Roger Ceilley, past president of the American Academy of Dermatology, refuted the suggestion that long-term sunscreen users derived no benefit from sunscreen. "That would be like saying more people are using condoms and more people are getting AIDS, therefore condoms cause AIDS," said Dr. Ceilley. "The study asked only about sunscreen use in the prior ten years, whereas skin cancer typically occurs many decades after the damaging sun exposures. To be most effective, sun protection should begin in childhood and continue throughout life. An overwhelming number of studies in recent years demonstrate that UV light causes DNA mutations leading to skin cancer and that sunscreens protect against the development of skin cancer in animals and humans."

Studies also abound regarding the appearance of thickened, yellowed, mottled, sun-damaged skin versus the smooth, even, wrinkle-free appearance of the skin of someone who has stayed out of the sun; the contrast is a classic in dermatological annals. Staying completely out of the sun isn't possible (nor would it be healthy), but good sun protection is now very possible, and available.

Sun Damage: What's Happening

The most insidious result of sun exposure is that it does serious damage to the entire system, beyond the problems that eventually take place on the surface. The skin contains components that are integral to the body's immune system. The Langerhans cells in the epidermis prevent bacteria from attacking the system and also prevent cell mutation. These Langerhans cells are indispensable to good health. Yet a few minutes of unprotected sun exposure can damage the Langerhans cells in ways that can last for weeks.

In addition to damaging the immune system, sunlight also attacks the collagen structure of the skin, changing it from a cohesive network of support into a disorderly, weakened mass. And while the sun is busy destroying collagen underneath the surface of the skin and the Langerhans cells throughout, it also thickens the exterior of the skin, chokes off the skin's blood supply, and reduces the skin's elasticity. (And you thought suntanning was attractive.)

For similar reasons, wearing sunglasses on a regular basis is a significant protective measure. The lens of the eye turns out to be a pretty good absorber of UVA rays, but, unlike the skin, the lens cannot slough off damaged cells. That means there is no way for the lens to ever repair itself. Protecting the eyes isn't just cosmetic, it is about keeping your sight undiminished for as long as possible.

To Tan or Not to Tan: NOT

Tanning is a problem. Turning brown or darkening is the skin's defensive response to sun damage. It may look nice, but it isn't nice for the skin. Melanocytes are skin cells that contain the brown-colored protein called melanin. These brown skin cells determine a person's natural skin tone. Surprisingly, the difference between the lightest skin color and the darkest is only a very small amount of melanin. With exposure to sun, the melanocytes produce more melanin, and tanned skin is the result. But here's another shock: despite the fact that tanning is a protective response, it isn't all that helpful. By some estimates, a tan provides an SPF of only about 2 or 4! Sorry, there just isn't any way a tan of any kind can be considered healthy. As one dermatologist described it, a tan is the same as a callus on your foot. Yes, it protects the foot, but who wants that kind of protection and why continue doing what caused the callus in the first place?

Because melanin isn't a very reliable sunscreen, dark-skinned people still suffer negative effects from sun exposure. Ashen skin color, mottled skin, wrinkles, and even skin cancer can happen to those with dark skin. Skin cancer is less likely, but the risk of skin aging is certain.

If you're determined to tan, the only safe way to do it is with the self-tanning products sold by cosmetics lines of all kinds. Whether you choose a self-tanner made by Revlon or Estee Lauder or Decleor Paris, **all of them are created equal. The active ingredient in every one of these products is dihydroxyacetone.** That's what turns the surface layer of skin brown. You may not like the smell of one product versus another, but that is merely a function of the fragrance added to the product to mask the smell of the dihydroxyacetone. A masking fragrance might be pleasant, but it doesn't change how the product functions, and the natural odor of the product is transient.

UV Overview

The sun feels great, especially when it's out shining. But even on a cloudy day, when you can't see the sun, the sun's rays are ever-present and attacking the skin. Infrared rays (IR) from the sun keep us warm, and the visible rays provide daylight. But while the sun's ultraviolet radiation (UVR) is also important, its effects are serious for skin and eyes.

UVR is divided into three different bands: UVA, UVB, and UVC. Virtually all UVC radiation is filtered out by the atmosphere, so that none actually reaches the Earth's surface (although ozone depletion has some researchers worried about this one too). In direct contrast to UVC, UVB and UVA rays both reach the earth in significant amounts.

UVB radiation, the burning rays of the sun, is much stronger in some ways than UVA radiation, and has a considerable capacity to cause instant skin damage in the form of blistering sunburns. However, the Earth is bombarded with about a hundred times as much UVA as UVB, so, while it may be weaker, UVA radiation still has a potent impact on the skin.

All UVR is strongest between 10 A.M. and 2 P.M. Clouds filter some, but not most, of the UVR, which is why you are still likely to get burned on an overcast day. Different surfaces, such as water, cement, sand, snow, and even grass, can reflect UVR, causing a double whammy for the skin. Altitude is also a sun enhancer; for every 1,000-foot increase in altitude, the UVR potency increases by 4%.

Pollution's effect on the ozone layer, located many miles above the Earth's surface, is serious business for many reasons, but this discussion is about what that means for skin. When intact, the ozone layer filters out much of the sun's UVB radiation (although it has relatively little effect on UVA). It is the quantity of sunburning UVB rays that increases when the ozone layer is eroded, which means more serious burns for those who dare to go outside without protection.

By the way, UVB rays can't get through glass, so there's no risk of sunburn when you sit in a car or next to a window, but that's the good news. The bad news is that UVA rays can get through windows. Glass doesn't protect skin from UVA damage, so sitting in a car or next to a window that lets daylight through offers no protection whatsoever.

We all know about sunburn. Spending too much time in the sun, which for some of us is only 15 to 30 minutes, can cause a serious, painful burn. More bad news: A sunburn continues to develop for 12 to 24 hours after the initial burn takes place.

Treat a sunburn the same as you would treat any other burn. Do not cover it with thick salves (butter is the worst). That will trap the heat and cause more damage. Get the skin in contact with cool water immediately (do not put ice directly on the skin—that's too much cold and can cause a different kind of burn on the skin). Then keep applying the cool water on and off for several hours. Do not soak the skin with water; too much water in the skin can inhibit the skin's healing response.

PLEASE NOTE: Many products make claims about UVA protection that are truly misleading. While titanium dioxide, zinc oxide, or avobenzone offer protection from about 80% to 90% of UVA radiation, other formulations that don't contain these ingredients only protect from about 20% of UVA radiation.

Factoring in Protection: SPF Explained

Ever since I learned about the extensive research concerning UVA protection I have been carrying on about the importance of using avobenzone, titanium dioxide, and zinc oxide for UVA protection. A product's sun-protection factor (SPF) relates only to how long it takes you to get a sunburn. The SPF gives you important information as to how long you can be in the sun before you start to burn. If it normally takes you 20 minutes in the sun before you start turning pink, an SPF 15 product will let you stay in the sun for five hours without burning. The formula is 20 (minutes) x (SPF) 15 = 300 (minutes), or five hours. But that five hours applies only if you aren't swimming or perspiring. If you are active or if you get wet, you need to reapply the sunscreen after 60 to 90 minutes. Waterproof sunscreens are generally assumed to last for 90 minutes to two hours, or as specified on the label.

It is important to realize that an SPF 2 product blocks about 50% of the UVB rays and an equal amount of UVA rays when the appropriate UVA ingredients are included. An SPF 10 filters out about 85% of the UVB rays and an equal amount of UVA when the appropriate UVA ingredients are included. An SPF 15 stops about 95%, and an SPF 30 stops about 97%. Evidently, the increase in protection between SPF 15 and SPF 30 is not the great improvement many think it is, which is why most dermatologists and oncologists feel that SPF 15 is more than enough for the skin. I also strongly recommend SPF 15, with the caveat that a product must contain UVA protection. However, occasionally I do recommend foundations with SPF 10 to SPF 12. For casual use or minimal exposure to the sun, SPF 10 to SPF 14 is not a problem and can definitely protect the skin. (What is a problem is the limited number of options for reliable sunscreen protection, especially for women who tend to break out.) Despite my recommendations, you can always choose to stay to the higher side of the SPF number range. I hope that the cosmetics industry will take more notice of the Skin Cancer Foundation's and the American Academy of Dermatology's recommendations regarding SPF 15 and create more products that meet those standards.

SPF is assuredly important, but it is only a measurement about sunburn. There are no numbers to tell you about protection from UVA radiation, which causes wrinkles and some forms of skin cancer. For that you have to check the active ingredient list. Basically, there are two types of sunscreen agents: chemical (inorganic) and mineral (meaning physical blocks or popularly referred to as nonchemical). Chemical sunscreens are absorbed into the skin and refract or absorb the UVR. Mineral sunscreens—zinc oxide and titanium dioxide—provide a cover over the skin to block out the sun's rays. You can expect sunblocks with titanium dioxide and zinc oxide to be far less irritating than chemical sunblocks, though they do tend to leave a whitish cast on the skin. But the occlusive nature of physical sunscreens means they can clog pores, although for those people who tend to break out, all sunscreens can pose problems. Chemical sunscreens can irritate the pores and physical sunscreens can clog them. I wish it were different (I'm in the same breakout-prone boat), but sunscreen is just one of those skin-care musts that leave little room for options.

Just for the record: Always apply sunscreen at least 15 to 20 minutes before going outside. This gives the sunscreen time to be absorbed and to spread over the skin. And when it comes to application, here's something else that's startling. A cosmetic chemist told me that when SPF testing is done in the lab, the standard method is to use an ounce of sunscreen per adult from head to toe! Think about that. A 4-ounce tube of sunscreen (standard at the drugstore and cosmetics counters) would allow for only four applications. And if you are outside for long periods and have to apply the stuff twice, that would be only two days' worth of protection per tube. Is anyone out there applying the right amount? Please, stay away from the expensive sunscreen; you are much less likely to liberally apply the pricey stuff than the less expensive brands (which are equal in efficacy if they have the same SPF and the appropriate UVA-protection ingredients).

L'Oreal's Mexoryl SX™

L'Oreal has a patented sunscreen ingredient called Mexoryl SX™. It is a sunscreen agent that has been approved for use in countries outside of the United States for some time now. Mexoryl SX™ is not approved by the FDA for use as a sunscreen ingredient in the United States. According to L'Oreal spokespeople, "There is only one sure and stable UVA sun filter" and to them it is their Mexoryl SX™. L'Oreal claims that Mexoryl SX™ "provides long-lasting, effective protection because the molecule is virtually impervious to the action of solar energy."

L'Oreal is correct when it says that "it isn't enough to protect against UVBs; skin must also be protected against UVAs. These two components of sunlight differ by virtue of their electromagnetic spectrum, their intensity, and their wavelength (290/320 nanometers for UVBs, 320/400 nanometers for UVAs), which indicates their ability to penetrate deeply into the skin. True, UVAs are intrinsically less powerful than UVBs, but they are more numerous and more penetrating. Mexoryl SX™ was the molecule finally selected. It brings together all of the essential required features [with] maximum absorption of 345 nanometers."

While I completely accept L'Oreal's research in regard to UVA protection and the effectiveness of Mexoryl SX™, the research I've seen from Hoffman-LaRoche, the manufacturers and patent holder of avobenzone, indicates that avobenzone absorbs up to 400 nanometers. The manufacturers of zinc oxide have shown their micronized zinc oxide to be effective at 380 nanometers. And the manufacturers of titanium dioxide have shown it to be effective at up to 360 nanometers. This may seem like hairsplitting, but when it comes to protecting the skin from UVA damage, every nanometer counts.

It is clear that L'Oreal is aware of the UVA issue, and its Mexoryl SX™ seems to be a player against that kind of sun damage. It is also nice to know that there may be another option besides avobenzone, zinc oxide, and titanium dioxide in sunscreen formulations to address true broad-spectrum protection, but from the data I've seen, it doesn't look like Mexoryl SX™ is a must-have ingredient to fight against sun damage.

I do have one question for L'Oreal, given the fact that Mexoryl SX™ is not allowed in the United States: You seem to have extensive information about UVA sun damage, but why don't any of your U.S.-formulated sunscreens contain avobenzone, zinc oxide, or titanium dioxide? It would seem to me that that would have been a nice way to protect the consumer until Mexoryl SX™ was approved here.

Sun Care for the Little Ones

If you have babies or small children, the issue of sunscreen protection should absolutely be of primary concern. Their delicate skin is even more sensitive to the sun's damaging energy. Whether or not you are diligent about using sunscreen for yourself, you must be diligent when it comes to the health of your children. It's easy to be attracted to the child-oriented products with pictures of cute babies on the label, but I have yet to see a formulation variance between products aimed at children and those for adults. Of greater concern to me is that I haven't seen a child's formula that contains any amount of avobenzone, titanium dioxide, or zinc oxide. Sea & Ski for Kids SPF 30, Coppertone Water Babies SPF 45, and Coppertone Kids Colorblock SPF 40 all sound great for children, but not one offered appropriate protection from UVA damage when I reviewed them.

All sunscreen formulations that have an SPF are closely regulated by the FDA; the formulations don't differ in any way because of the age of the intended user. The only difference I've ever noted in baby products is the use of fragrance. Certain fragrances may make you think of little ones, but fragrance can be irritating for all skin types, and baby formulas tend to add more than most. If you are looking for a less-irritating sunscreen for your kids, choose one that contains only pure titanium dioxide or zinc oxide as the active ingredient, which will definitely be less irritating than a product with other inorganic sunscreen agents.

Sun Risk with AHAs or Retinoids

As I mention above, one of the major signs of sun-damaged skin is that the outer layer of skin becomes browned and thickened. To some extent that does serve as protection, but it isn't very good protection (it barely rates an SPF 2), nor is it very attractive protection. AHAs (because they exfoliate the surface of the skin) and retinoids (because they change abnormal cell production back to some level of normalcy) can help remove some of that thickened, damaged exterior. That change in the exterior of the skin does leave the skin more vulnerable to the effects of sun exposure. It isn't the AHAs or the retinoids that cause the skin to be more sensitive to sunlight, but the effect they have on the skin. Sunscreen is always important, *always*, but it becomes even more essential if you are using AHAs or retinoids on a regular basis.

Speaking of AHAs

I thought you might find this information from the FDA's Web site (*www.fda.gov*) on AHAs quite intriguing. According to the FDA, "Cosmetics that contain alpha hydroxy acids (AHAs) have become widely used in recent years despite many unanswered questions about their safety. The [FDA] has received about 100 reports of adverse effects with AHA products, ranging from mild irritation and stinging to blistering and burns. If you use cosmetics with AHAs and experience skin irritation or prolonged stinging, FDA advises you to stop using the product and consult your physician.

"The extent of exfoliation depends on the type and concentration of the AHA, its pH (acidity), and other ingredients in the product. Most cosmetics sold to consumers contain AHAs at levels of up to 12%." It is the FDA's understanding that products with AHA concentrations of 20% or higher are used by trained cosmetologists for salon "mini-peels."

The Cosmetic Ingredient Review (CIR) panel concluded at its December meeting that AHAs are "safe for use in cosmetic products at concentrations of less than or equal to 10%, at final formulation of pHs greater than or equal to 3.5, when formulated to avoid increasing the skin's sensitivity to the sun, or when directions for use include the daily use of sun protection." For salon-use products, the panel said that the products are "safe for use at concentrations of less than or equal to 30%, at final formulation pHs greater than or equal to 3.0, in products designed for brief, discontinuous use followed by thorough rinsing from the skin, when applied by trained professionals, and when application is accompanied by directions for the daily use of sun protection."

These conclusions were made final at a June 1997 meeting of the CIR panel in spite of serious safety questions submitted by a consumer group and a major manufacturer. The FDA is reviewing these CIR conclusions, as well as the other available data about these products. Consumers should be aware that AHA concentration and pH are generally not noted on all products. (The FDA does not require it.) However, the information should be available from the manufacturer.

Cosmetics manufacturers are not required to submit safety data to the FDA before marketing products, although they bear the responsibility for manufacturing safe products.

Consumers should report any adverse reactions, such as irritation or sun sensitivity, associated with the use of AHAs to their local FDA office, listed in the Blue Pages of the phone book, or to the FDA's Office of Consumer Affairs at (800) 532-4440.

Plants, a Growing Problem

The cosmetics industry wants women to believe that a plant extract of any kind, short of rubbing broccoli or asparagus on our faces, must be good for skin and synthetic ingredients must be bad. It doesn't matter if it is a completely unknown plant; if it grows, there must be an excellent reason to use it. It also doesn't matter that the plant ingredients are less than 0.5% to 3% of the total product and the other unnatural ingredients account for more than 47% (the rest being water) of the contents. Regardless of the facts, the image of plants in cosmetics is overpowering for the consumer. Aveda has made a religion out of plants, and The Body Shop has turned it into a political issue.

But why use *Prunus persica* (peach extract) over *Hordeum distichon* (barley extract); *Betula alba* (birch extract) versus *Brassica oleracea capitata* (cabbage extract); or *Cananga odorata* (ylang ylang oil) instead of *Anthemis nobilis* (chamomile extract) or *Pseudopterogorgia elisabethae* (sea whip extract—actually this one is a marine invertebrate, but you get my drift)? There are literally thousands and thousands of potential extracts that can be used in cosmetics. Do they all perform equally well or at all? And what about overdoing it? Can you overdose on plant extracts?

The issue of natural versus synthetic is one I've written about extensively over the years. To sum it up succinctly, natural does not mean good and synthetic does not mean bad. Each group has its shortcomings and strengths, but I would no sooner accept any plant as being good for my skin than I would walk naked through a patch of poison ivy assuming that because it's a plant, it must be OK.

"Natural" simply defines the source of the ingredient; it tells you nothing about the ingredient's effectiveness or risks. Menthol and peppermint may have a natural source, but both are serious skin irritants and absolutely terrible for the skin. Ingredients like silicone and stearyl alcohol are synthetic but they are remarkably silky-soft ingredients vital to a vast array of cosmetic formulations. And the opposite is true too. Licorice extract (in the form of glycyrrhetinic acid) is an excellent anti-irritant and sesame oil is a great emollient. Yet C16-14 olefin sodium sulfate is a very irritating synthetic cleansing agent, as is sodium lauryl sulfate.

"Synthetic" merely tells you that the ingredient was derived in a laboratory, and though that kind of origin may sound artificial and unhealthy, it often means that the resulting ingredient is going to be purer than a natural ingredient. Natural ingredients can be made up of hundreds of known and unknown ingredients. Plus, the ingredients it took to create the plant extract—the chemical process used to extract the oil or other natural substance from the plant—are almost always a completely synthetic, unnatural process.

As seductive as it may be to get trapped by the plant craze in cosmetics, please think again. "Natural" doesn't give you any information about the quality of the formulation.

Choosing a Really Great Skin-Care Routine

Most skin-care regimes are at best unrealistic. They are either too complicated (too many steps, such as two or three cleansing steps), too contrived (such as layering products or applying too many moisturizers, which can clog pores and make skin look dull), too irritating (toners that contain alcohol, lotions that contain peppermint or menthol, which can obstruct the skin's healing process) or absurdly and unnecessarily expensive. Choosing a really great skin-care routine isn't about the parochial notion of getting back to basics, because what is the definition of basic? A lot of women think of soap as basic, but the pH of most soaps increases bacteria in the skin, and the same ingredients that keep the bar in its bar form can clog pores. Is sun protection part of getting back to basics? And what about exfoliation? Skin care doesn't have to be complicated, but it does have to address what is best for your skin, and depending on your skin type that can be complicated. Choosing a really great skin-care routine also doesn't mean looking for plants and natural ingredients. There are lots and lots of natural ingredients that can be damaging to skin, and for the most part adding plants or foods to a cosmetic just increases the need for a stronger preservative base and more fragrance to mask the smell of rancid, molding ingredients. After all, how long do plants of any kind last in your refrigerator? Choosing a really great skin-care routine means doing what it takes to be good to your skin without wasting money, and buying only products that live up to their claims.

The following is a realistic, viable skin-care routine that's free from gimmicks and selling techniques.

Step 1

Even at night, when you're removing makeup, always wash your face with a gentle water-soluble cleanser that rinses off completely and doesn't irritate the eyes. Your eye makeup should come off with the same water-soluble cleanser that cleans your face. Do not use an extra product to wipe across the eye, pulling the skin and eyelashes unnecessarily. (Wiping off makeup is never good for the skin; it pulls at the skin, and rubbing with a tissue or washcloth, no matter how gentle you try to be, can irritate skin.)

Use only tepid to slightly warm water. Hot water burns the skin, and cold water shocks it. Repeated use of hot water, saunas, or Jacuzzis can cause broken capillaries to surface on the nose and cheeks and cause unwanted irritation that damages skin.

If you are wearing one of the new ultra-matte foundations, you may need to use a washcloth to help remove makeup. This is an exception to the rule but may be necessary for the new breed of stubborn foundations that are very effective for oily skin types.

Step 2

Exfoliating the skin helps unclog pores and removes dead skin cells, benefiting both dry and oily skin. There are two ways to exfoliate: with a physical exfoliant such as a scrub, and with a chemical exfoliant such as AHAs or BHA. For many skin types only one of these two types of exfoliant is necessary. Overdoing the exfoliation bit with scrubs and several AHA or BHA products is at best overkill, and I do mean kill. You only have so much skin, and too much exfoliation can start causing damage and negate any of the positive effects you were hoping for.

Scrubs: If your skin is oily and tends to break out, after you've rinsed off your water-soluble cleanser but while your face is still wet, pour a scant handful of baking soda into the palm of your hand. Add a small amount of water to create a paste, gently massage your entire face with this paste, then rinse generously with tepid water. (You can also mix 1 or 2 teaspoons of baking soda with 1 or 2 tablespoons of a good water-soluble cleanser such as Cetaphil Gentle Skin Cleanser. This alternative is good for any skin type.) Be extra careful not to get carried away: overscrubbing can cause more problems than it solves. The operative word for all skin care is "gentle."

If you have combination skin, massage only those areas that tend to break out, and avoid the areas that are dry. If you have normal skin, use the baking soda scrub only two to three times a week. If you have dry skin, use the baking soda mixed with Cetaphil Gentle Skin Cleanser only about once or twice a week, and rinse very well. If you have extremely dry skin, follow the advice for dry skin, but use more Cetaphil Gentle Skin Cleanser and just a pinch of baking soda in your mixture, and be very, very gentle when massaging your face.

Chemical exfoliates: An effective alternative to scrubs (or in conjunction with scrubs, depending on your skin type), are products that contain at least a 5% or greater concentration of AHAs or 0.5% to 2% BHA. (AHA and BHA products with an emollient base can double as moisturizers or can be the only product your skin needs besides a cleanser and sunscreen.) The AHA or BHA product is applied after the face is washed and dried (see Step 6).

Step 3

Once your face is clean, gently squeeze any blackheads or blemishes you want to remove. One way to get rid of blackheads is to squeeze them (see my review for the Biore Strips if you were wondering whether or not to consider that kind of product). Blackheads usually don't leave on their own. They can be stubborn even if you are using a good AHA or BHA product or Retin-A. Blemishes, on the other hand, can heal on their own, but relieving the pressure and removing the contents can help them heal faster. If you are shocked by this suggestion, that's OK; you don't have to do this, but it does help. This is what most facialists do best for your skin; however, it is cheaper to do it yourself. Many people worry about making matters worse. The only way to prevent that from happening is to NEVER, absolutely NEVER, oversqueeze. If the blemish or blackhead does not respond easily, stop and leave it alone. Squeezing does not cause problems on the face; in fact, it is one of the best ways to clean out the skin and remove pressure from a swollen lesion. The problems occur when you massacre the skin by squeezing until you create scabs and sores.

Step 4

Toners are an optional step after the cleanser and mechanical scrub. Depending on your skin type and the toner you choose a toner can help soothe the skin and add some good water-binding agents to the skin. For someone with normal to oily skin it can be the only moisturizer needed. For someone with normal to dry skin it can be a good addition to the regular moisturizer. If you have acne or blemish-prone skin, this toner needs to be an effective disinfectant to kill blemish-causing bacteria.

When your face is completely rinsed and dried, take a cotton ball and apply the appropriate toner for your skin type. Please keep in mind that toners (as well as any skin-care product that comes near your face or body for that matter) need to be as irritant-free as possible. There are many irritant-free toners to choose from, but the more-expensive ones are absolutely not worth their exorbitant price tags, especially when you consider that their basic ingredients are almost always the same as those in the less-expensive versions.

Step 5

If you have extremely oily skin or skin that breaks out frequently, try a facial mask of plain Phillips' Milk of Magnesia (the stuff in the blue bottle that you normally take for indigestion; just ask your pharmacist). Milk of magnesia is a mixture of magnesium and water. Magnesium is a good disinfectant, and it can absorb oil.

The clay masks for oily skin have no disinfecting properties, and their ingredients cannot absorb oil as well as magnesium can. Your skin type and reaction to the mask will determine how often you can use it. Those with severely oily skin can use it every day; those with slightly oily skin may need to use it only once a week.

Step 6

After your face is clean (cleanser and scrub) and you've applied the toner, this is the time to apply an AHA or BHA product or Retin-A and Renova. If you have chosen to use both an AHA and Retin-A or Renova, the AHA is applied first and then the Retin-A or Renova. This can be done once or twice a day or every other day, depending on your skin type.

Step 7

During the day it is essential to wear a sunscreen with an SPF of 15 that contains UVA protection. You must be certain that the product you choose contains one of the following in the list of active ingredients: avobenzone (Parsol 1789), zinc oxide, or titanium dioxide. If you have normal to dry skin, wear a sunscreen that comes in a moisturizing base (actually, most sunscreens come in a moisturizing base). If you have normal to oily skin, you do not need a moisturizer, but you still must wear a sunscreen with an SPF of 15 that includes UVA protection. In this instance you can choose a matte foundation with an effective sunscreen. **Remember: The only way to prevent wrinkles is sun protection.**

Step 8

Moisturizing is a step in skin care most women obsess over, and the cosmetics industry is certainly glad they do. Loading up on moisturizers and anti-wrinkle potions is big business. Yet, in truth, you only need to wear a moisturizer if you have dry skin. In short, not everyone needs a moisturizer! The biggest myth you've been sold by the cosmetics industry is that there are wrinkle creams and moisturizers out there that will undo or prevent wrinkles. It just isn't true. Every month a host of new anti-wrinkle creams are launched with more promises and supposedly newfangled formulations. And every few months our hope is renewed until the next round of lies and misleading claims are thrown at us. You can choose not to believe me on this one, but unless you have dry skin or want to improve the appearance of your wrinkles (not change them), it is not necessary to wear a moisturizer! Even more to the point, dry skin and wrinkles are not associated. Yes moisturizers help to make skin look smoother, but they don't alter wrinkles, their effect is gone the next day, and no moisturizer supplants the need for sunscreen (sunscreens come in moisturizing bases so you only need one product, not two). During the day, if you have dry skin, wear a moisturizer with a reliable SPF. At night, if you choose to wear a moisturizer, it is only necessary over dry areas. Do not use moisturizer of any kind over areas that tend to break out. Oil-free moisturizers still contain waxy thickening agents that can clog pores. Heavy, rich, creamy moisturizers are best only for extremely dry skin. Try the less-expensive moisturizers before you venture into the higher-priced brands. The formulations do not differ because of price!

At night, if you want to use an AHA or BHA product that comes in a moisturizing base, apply it after the toner. If you use a liquid- or gel-type AHA product, apply it after the toner but before the moisturizer.

Step 9

If you have melasma or chloasma, which are brown or ashen discolorations caused by sun damage or hormonal changes (usually the result of birth control pills), then you may want to consider adding a skin-lightening product to your routine. These products need to contain at least 1% hydroquinone, and as an option they may also contain kojic acid and a small amount of BHA and AHA. This step would come after the toner and AHA or BHA product steps, but before the Retin-A and Renova or sunscreen. This layering process can be tricky for some skin types, but it can prove to be quite effective in the lightening process. Please keep in mind that no lightening process works if you do not use an effective sunscreen day in and day out.

Cosmetics Cop On-Line

Surfing the Internet is much like floating around in the middle of the ocean. The water is refreshing but there is so much of it that you're not sure you will ever reach shore and fear you might drown first. Floating around in cyberspace, surfing from location to location, is amazing. Cyberspace is truly a universe unto itself, with a language, protocol, and navigating systems that are complex and frustrating, yet utterly simple and convenient once you find what you are looking for. What is truly exasperating is trying to sort through the amazing amount of appalling, erroneous information you encounter. And if you think cosmetics counters, drugstores, specialty boutiques, television, and fashion magazines are filled with makeup and skin-care choices, wait until you see the Internet. A recent search for the words "skin care" brought up more than 1.6 million possible Web pages! There are more home pages selling anti-wrinkle products, acne systems, cellulite cures, and weight-loss promises than you can fathom.

As someone who owns a publishing company, writes books, and does extensive research, I find the information superhighway completely fascinating (and "fascinating" is a lot better than "intimidating," which is how I regarded it when I first got started). Despite my shock at the abundant amount of disturbing cosmetic information, I am also impressed at the plethora of medical research, published studies, and professional expertise available. As I mention above, my favorite Web sites are *www.Medscape.com, www.FDA.gov,* and *www.ncbi.nlm.nih.gov/PubMed* (this is the National Library of Medicine Web page, with a search engine that looks through more than 9 million published medical studies).

I have also developed my own Web page. I would never consider myself equal to the brilliance of these medical and government regulatory Web sites, but I do try to provide answers to readers' questions; I also post interesting articles from previous newsletters that include the research I've gleaned from the published studies I've surveyed and my years of experience in the field of cosmetics. For those of you who surf the Net, my URL (address) is *www.cosmeticscop.com.*

Animal Testing

I am proud to say that my skin-care company, Paula's Choice Distinctive Skin Care, does not test any aspect of its products on animals, and I donate a portion of its earnings to The Humane Society of the United States (HSUS) every year. Please check out HSUS's Web site at *www.hsus.org.* Their mailing address is The Humane Society of the United States, 2100 L Street N.W., Washington, D.C. 20037 (they can use your financial help as well).

HSUS's approach to the issue of animal rights and animal testing is one I agree with most strongly. The Spring 1998 issue of *HSUS News* stated, "The HSUS shares with these scientists [the many who are opposed to or are uncomfortable with animal testing] the desire to eliminate the harmful use of animals in laboratories. In the meantime The HSUS is planning a campaign to urge the scientific community to adopt, as a priority goal, the elimination of all animal pain and distress in the laboratory. The HSUS believes that an emphasis on humane issues will lead to good science and will benefit, rather than harm, the advance of human knowledge."

For those of you unfamiliar with my full position on animal testing in cosmetics and in the medical research field, the following offers a discussion of the topic from my book *The Beauty Bible.*

Politically, I'm a moderate. I haven't always been. I grew up in the 1960s, and my politics have ranged from idealistic liberal to confused bipartisan. Now, as I stand loosely planted in the '90s, leaning into the millennium, I can earnestly say I am convinced that few, if any, issues in life are black and white, or all or nothing. More and more often, I find that there is truth on both sides of the issues and the middle ground is often the only reasonable position. At least the middle ground is the only position that acknowledges the whole picture and not just one side. I vote both Republican and Democrat, depending on the individual and his or her voting record.

This middle position also reflects my perspective on animal testing as it pertains to cosmetics products and the health-care industry. While I unquestionably advocate the humane and ethical treatment of all life, especially unprotected and dependent life, I am not in favor of eliminating all forms of animal testing when it comes to health-care issues or human safety issues.

I feel terrible pain and anguish when I think of animals suffering in any way so I can put on mascara or clean my face. Many animal tests that are used to ascertain whether a cosmetic will hurt people are cruel and gratuitous. No one is ever going to eat 50 pounds of mascara. Forcing animals to do so in order to demonstrate how much mascara people can eat before they die makes me want to resign from the human race. How can anyone put an animal through such torture?

On the other hand, my older sister, who had breast cancer, my father, who had prostate cancer, my dearest friend's mother, who has Alzheimer's, and my husband, who has high blood pressure, all take medication and have undergone medical procedures that have prolonged and improved their quality of life—and all of these medications and procedures have been proven effective and safe as a result of animal testing. I absolutely do not want to see even one animal die by being force-fed foundation or eyeshadow to prove a favorable cosmetic formulation. And it would be my absolute preference in life that no animal suffer for any reason; yet if sacrificing an animal's life can help find the cure for Alzheimer's, prevent more cancers, or reduce the risks of high blood pressure and a host of other illnesses, I would and do support that research. Simultaneously, I actively donate money to animal rights groups that are helping to encourage the creation of alternative testing methods so that eventually no animals will be needed for any kind of medical research.

Most of us are aware of the dramatic pictures distributed by animal-rights groups showing the terrible torment of animals in research laboratories. This is indeed a grotesque and painful exposé that all of us should be sickened by and do our best to change. But this narrow, shocking display does not address the results of animal research (the creation of safe products and medical treatments), nor does it represent the labs that treat animals humanely by caring for them and anesthetizing them.

Children who survive leukemia owe their lives to animal testing. Arthritis patients who can walk again owe their agility to animal testing. Successful excisions of brain tumors are due to animal testing, and on and on. Human health-care advancement and the use of animals to test various protocols and risks are inextricably linked and cannot be separated. This is the dilemma of animal testing.

There are many arguments from both points of view surrounding this issue. On one side are the animal rights activists who claim there is no need or reason to ever use animal testing (or eat meat, use leather goods, or employ animals for any purpose other than as pets). When it comes to animal testing, they point to alternative methods of research assessment that can be used. Spokespeople for People for the Ethical Treatment of Animals (PETA) and the National Anti-Vivisection Society (NAVS) claim that a preponderance of research proves that all animal testing is inconclusive and has no relation to what takes place in humans. Animal activists insist that all animal testing is motivated by financial profit and stubborn old-fashioned doctors or "good old boys" who refuse to change. Their reasoning is that animal testing is big business, and no one wants to alter what they are doing and potentially lose money.

On the other side are a vast majority of physicians, medical research groups from most major universities, national medical organizations representing everything from cancer to heart disease, and pharmaceutical companies, all of which believe the use of animal models for research is essential to the evaluation of new and old medical treatments and procedures. These physicians and organizations often agree that in vitro (test tube–oriented) tests and computer model studies can replace some animal testing.

However, no one among these countless medical professionals would concede that all or even most animal testing is futile and immaterial. They can point to thousands of chemical substances and operations that were first determined to be safe and effective or dangerous and deleterious because of animal testing. Suggesting that these be stopped would halt most medical research, from AIDS to Alzheimer's, and the development of any new drug. Even physicians deeply involved in finding alternative research methods to replace animal testing would not agree that we close the door to that ultimate and desirable goal.

The truth probably exists somewhere in the middle. Medical, pharmaceutical, and cosmetics industry experts freely admit that they were doing far more animal experiments than were needed to prove safety. Animal rights activist campaigns inspired a vocal consumer base to force a major change in the number and type of animal tests being done. Many companies responded by reducing animal testing, changing to alternative methods whenever possible, and instituting humane treatment of their animals. Yet all or nothing is the goal of animal rights activists, and it may not be the goal of all consumers buying makeup, taking medicines, or considering medical procedures. Consumers should look at the whole issue and not just shocking pictures.

For example, according to an article in the January 1997 issue of *Drug and Cosmetic Industry* magazine, Gillette has been a boycott target of PETA since 1986. What PETA does not acknowledge is that, since its boycott, Gillette has reduced tests on animals by more than 90%, has contributed millions of dollars to alternative research, and has donated more than $100,000 to the Humane Society. You would think PETA would ease up on Gillette, but that isn't the case. It still lists Gillette among its companies to boycott. As long as a company does any animal testing, humane or otherwise, it is a target for PETA's condemnation. That is regrettable, because as a consumer you get only a limited perspective.

As a result of PETA's and NAVS's black-or-white position, you may be led to believe that The Body Shop is the greatest ally of animal rights since the inception of the concept. Yet, when faced with the publication of an article exposing The Body Shop's ambiguous animal-testing policy, owner Anita Roddick had her cabal of attorneys suppress the story from running in *Vanity Fair.* That only fueled the ire of reporter Jon Entine, who was then able to get his story published in *Business Ethics* and *Drug and Cosmetic Industry* magazines. It seems The Body Shop didn't want people to know its product development included use of ingredients that had been tested on animals; in fact, The Body Shop was banned from using the phrase "not tested on animals" on its products by West German courts in 1989. (The company subsequently began using the phrase "against animal testing.") According to a January 1997 article in *Drug and Cosmetic Industry* magazine, a research executive at The Body Shop in 1993 was quoted as saying that "the technology of alternative testing for raw materials has not yet sufficiently advanced to guarantee product safety." This story about The Body Shop was overlooked or completely ignored by both PETA and NAVS.

Most of us are against animal testing, but we also have the right to safe products and straight information about how that can best be accomplished. It would be wonderful if alternative, computer-based, and test-tube models were sufficient for establishing a cosmetic, drug, or medical procedure's safety, but that doesn't seem to be true, at least not now or in the near future. If alternatives become common practice, it will probably happen in the world of cosmetics first, mainly because cosmetics are not ingested, and alternative research methods for irritation studies are showing promise.

Frank Fairweather, head of clinical and pathological programs at the British Industrial Biological Research Association, is a frequent spokesperson in Europe on alternatives to animal testing of cosmetics. In a presentation Fairweather made at the Second World Congress on Alternatives to Animal Use in the Life Sciences, 1996, he said that "none of the alternative techniques could yet be reliably substantiated." He is hoping that research protocols can be quantified and then mimicked via in vitro methodology, but at this point, they don't exist, though he feels optimistic that in the next several years tests will be developed that finally do away with the need for testing cosmetics on animals. I hope so too.

I will continue to earnestly support the humane and ethical treatment of animals, but I do not at this time support a complete ban on animal testing. I personally do not use animal testing for any of my Paula's Choice skin-care products, either directly or indirectly (meaning I don't hire third-party testing facilities to do my testing for me). I use only proven, long-established formulations and ingredients, as do many other companies that make claims about no animal testing. But because all of the cosmetics ingredients currently in use have at some point been tested on animals, no one can claim that the ingredients in their products involved no animal testing.

By creating products that are not tested on animals and by my support through financial contributions to such organizations as animal welfare groups and legal groups that fight for animal causes, I feel I am doing my part to help create a world in which fewer and fewer animals will be used for testing, and those that are will be treated humanely and ethically every step of the way.

I want my readers to know that I believe that their decisions and consumer activism in this area have been and continue to be vital. Cosmetics companies only started changing and looking for alternative methods because you, the consumer, brought pressure to bear and forced them to change. It is important to keep up this pressure. However, I feel it would be foolish to follow organizations like PETA and NAVS blindly unless you truly agree completely with their goal of abolishing all animal testing and creating a completely vegetarian society. **Instead, I encourage you to support organizations fighting for the welfare and safety of all animals, limited and humane animal testing, and continued research to find alternatives to animal testing in hopes that eventually someday no animal will have to be used in any research experiments.** This is completely in your power, because you, the consumer, have everything to say about what you buy and whom you buy it from, and that speaks loudly and clearly to all kinds of corporations and enterprises the world over.

CHAPTER THREE

Product-by-Product Reviews

The Process

You may well be wondering how I go about deciding what distinguishes a terrible product from a great one, or a good product from a fantastic product. Above all, you need to know that I do not make this up as I go, nor do I base the decisions on my own personal experience, or let my personal feelings about a particular company blur my judgment. In other words, just because I like the way a cleanser feels on my skin doesn't translate to how thousands of other skin types will feel about it. Rather, I base my decision on the individual product's formulation via published research about the ingredient(s) being used and their possible resulting interactions with the skin. From that I can assess the potential for irritation, dryness, breakouts, sensitivities, greasiness, and other issues of texture and performance. If I think a company is absurdly overcharging for its products or is exceedingly dishonest in their claims and literature, no matter how unethical I find it, that won't prevent me from saying its product is good for a particular skin type (though I do often say, "This is a good product but what a shame the price has to be so absurd and the claims so offensive!").

Almost without exception, my evaluation process for this edition was the same as for previous editions of this book. I reviewed each cosmetic line for several different elements. The first consideration was overall presentation and how user-friendly the displays or company literature were. For those lines available at retail locations, I always considered it an asset if their display units were set up with convenient color groupings, such as colors divided into yellow and blue tones, or were easily accessible. Skin-care and makeup products that were convenient to sample without the help of a salesperson were also rated high. For drugstore lines, colors had to be easy to see, and samples or tester units were also considered a bonus.

For infomercial and in-home shopping channel companies, my major criterion was the organization of their skin-care routines. Generally, ordering from sources like these means you are buying a set of products, not picking and selecting from what is being offered. If these prefab kits do not include an adequate sunscreen, or the kit for someone with breakouts is only minimally different from the kit for dry skin, then the overall rating would go down dramatically (dry-skin–care products are never suited for someone with oily, acne-prone skin).

The fundamental determination for each individual product's rating was based on a specific criterion I've established for each product category. Every category, from blushes to eyeshadows, concealers, foundations, cleansers, toners, scrubs, moisturizers, facial masks, AHA products, brushes, and wrinkle creams, has its own standards for garnering a happy, unhappy, or neutral (meaning unimpressive but not bad) face.

Makeup products were assessed mostly on texture (was it silky smooth or grainy and hard?), color (was a wide range of colors available, and was there an adequate selection for women of color?), application (could it be applied easily or was it difficult to spread or blend?), ease of use (was the container poorly designed; were colors placed too close together in an eyeshadow set; was foundation put in a pump container that squirted too much product or didn't reach to the bottom of the jar?); and, finally, price.

Skin-care products were evaluated almost exclusively on the basis of content versus claim. If a product said it was good for sensitive skin, it therefore couldn't contain irritants, skin sensitizers, or drying ingredients.

I also asked the following questions to see if a product could hold up to its claims, based on established research: (1) Given the ingredient list, could the product do what it promised? (2) How did the product differ from other products? (3) If a special ingredient or ingredients were showcased, how much of them were actually in the product, and was there independent research verifying the claim? (4) Did the product contain problematic preservatives, fragrances, coloring agents, plants, or other questionable ingredients? (5) How far-fetched were the product's claims? (6) Do I feel this product is safe? Are there risks such as allergic reactions or increased sun sensitivity?

I wish I had the space to challenge and explain every single exaggerated claim and lofty explanation that accompanies the products listed in this chapter, but there is just not enough room (or time) to tackle that prodigious task. I tried to cover many of the distortions and some of the hyperbole about products in my book *The Beauty Bible*, but even that book can't keep up with the hundreds and hundreds of miraculous-results skin-care ingredients and the vast number of miraculous-results products available. For this book, I chose to include all the information I could to overcome the sales and advertising pitches so you can focus on a product's quality, realistic performance, and feel.

You Can't Judge a Product by Its Label?

At this point, aside from makeup products—and I do test each one personally and survey my readers for their feedback—you may wonder if I can really judge a skin-care product from the ingredient listing. You may be thinking, "Perhaps it would be like judging food by only its ingredient list? What about taste?" As it turns out, I absolutely judge food by an ingredient list. It is no longer wise for any of us to consume any food without a clear understanding of how much fat, sodium, preservatives, coloring agents, or calories it contains, along with many other details pertinent to our health. Without that information, regardless of taste (everyone has their own bias), you would never know what you were putting in your body. You could be causing yourself harm by eating more fat, calories, or salt than you should, leading to weight gain, cancer, high blood pressure, and so on. If you don't eat enough fiber, you could end up with gastrointestinal distress or other serious problems. If you aren't getting appropriate nourishment you could get very sick, and what about food allergies or sensitivities? How would you ever know what you were doing to yourself? The food label is every consumer's best friend, whether you're shopping at a discount grocery or the fanciest gourmet shop.

Food labels are incredibly important, as are skin-care labels. If a skin-care product says it is good for sensitive skin or won't cause breakouts but contains ingredients known to cause irritation or breakouts, that is essential information. If a skin-care product sells for $100 but contains the same ingredients as a product that costs $10, that is, to say the least, very important information. Perhaps even more significant, if a $100 product contains fewer or less-effective ingredients than a $10 version, I think that is crucial consumer information.

The ingredient list helps you sort through the jungle of choices. Besides, it is a far better starting point than basing decisions strictly on advertising mumbo jumbo or promises that are never delivered.

Evaluation of Makeup Products

FOUNDATION: My fundamental expectation for any foundation, regardless of type (liquid, pressed powder, loose powder, stick, or cream-to-powder), is that it not be any shade or tone of orange, peach, pink, rose, green, or ash. Consistency, coverage, and feel are also important. All foundations, regardless of texture, need to go on smoothly and evenly, not separate or turn color, and be easy to blend. Foundations that claim to be matte must be truly matte, meaning no shine or glossy finish, and they have to have the potential to last most of the day. Foundations that claim to moisturize have to contain ingredients that could do that. Many foundations that claim to be oil-free contain silicone, which is an ingredient that has a definitely slippery, somewhat oily feel. It is most unlikely that silicone will cause breakouts, but in some formulations it can leave a slippery or slightly greasy feel on the skin. I also expect foundations with SPFs to have the same UVA protection ingredients as any other sunscreen. That means I consider that foundations without avobenzone, zinc oxide, or titanium dioxide cannot be relied upon for complete sun protection.

There is a new generation of shiny, iridescent foundations on the market today from many cosmetics lines. They come either in a sheer, moisturizing-type formula or with a slight amount of tint. What they provide is some amount of iridescence or sparkle on the face. While I generally do not care for sparkly makeup, especially for daytime, these products were rated on ease of use, how well they lasted, how much they flaked (controlling where the shine is placed is important—you don't want sparkles falling on your clothes), and how sheer and easy they were to blend.

Beauty Note: Color suggestions for all makeup products were often based on tester units available at the cosmetics counter, samples (including gifts with a purchase or discounted promotions), but mainly from products that were purchased. The color, shade, or tone of a particular product can fluctuate for a number of reasons. If I refer to a particular foundation as being "too peach" and you find that it's just right, it may be that we simply disagree, or it may be that the product I tested or bought is different from the one you ended up buying.

<u>CONCEALER:</u> Concealers should never be any shade of orange, peach, pink, rose, green, or ash, and they should not slip into the lines around the eye. I look for creamy-smooth textures that go on easily without pulling the skin, don't look dry and pasty, and, perhaps most important, do not crease into lines. I generally do not recommend using concealers over blemishes, but there is rarely a problem with using most concealers on other parts of the face if they match the skin.

Despite claims a product may make that recommend it for oily skin versus dry skin, please keep in mind that companies can make these claims regardless of ingredient content. In general, the thicker and greasier the product, the more likely it is to be problematic for oily, acne-prone skin. However, anything you apply over skin can cause problems. Just because a product does or doesn't contain oil is no guarantee one way or the other that it won't cause problems for the skin. There are lots of ingredients that don't sound like oil that can cause problems for skin. Generally, a matte-finish product is best for oily skin, but that still won't assure a lack of breakouts.

<u>COLOR CORRECTOR:</u> I am not a fan of color correctors in any form. Color correctors are usually a group of concealers you apply before you apply your foundation color. They generally come in shades of yellow, mauve, pink, or green. Color correctors are marketed as a way to change skin color, so that if your skin has pink undertones, a yellow color corrector is supposed to even that out. All these products do is give the skin a strange hue; does anyone think the colored layer isn't noticeable? That yellow or mauve layer then mixes with your foundation, giving it a strange color. Another problem with this kind of product is that it adds another layer on the skin, and the buildup of cosmetic ingredients on the face can be suffocating and pore-clogging. A well-chosen foundation color and blush can easily provide the color

balance you are looking for without adding another layer of strange makeup colors on the skin.

POWDER: Finishing or setting powders come in two basic forms: pressed and loose. I evaluated them on the basis of whether they went on sheer, chalky, or heavy, and whether they are too pink, peach, ash, or rose. I consistently gave higher marks to powders that went on sheer and had a silky soft texture with a natural beige, tan, or rich brown finish. Talc is the most frequently used ingredient in powders in all price ranges, and it is probably one of the best for absorbing oil and giving a smooth finish to the face. Other minerals are used for the same purpose, and though they may sound more exotic, they are not any better for the skin. Cornstarch or rice starch in powders can be a skin concern, as there is some evidence that it can clog pores and cause breakouts. I tried to screen for these as much as possible.

I should mention that the mineral talc often gets showcased as being an awful cosmetic ingredient that should be avoided and I do not agree in the least with that assessment. While it is true that prolonged inhalation of talc can cause lung problems because it is similar in chemical composition to asbestos (asbestos is a known lung irritant and cancer causing agent), that is only true for those working in the manufacture of talc or talc-related products. But that kind of exposure is radically different than the tiny amounts of talc found in makeup application.

When it comes to bronzing powders, I generally suggest using them as a contour color and not an all-over face color. Darkening the face almost always looks overdone. After all, if a foundation is supposed to match the skin, how can the use of a powder that darkens the skin be rationalized? The face will be a color decidedly different from the neck, and there will be a line of demarcation where the color starts and stops. Also, most bronzing powders are iridescent. Dusting a color over the face that is darker than your skin tone is bad enough, but why make it more obvious with particles of shine all over, particularly in daylight?

As I mention above for foundations, there is also a new generation of shine products on the market in powder form. Much like their foundation counterparts, the idea is to shine up the face. These products were rated on ease of use, how well they last, how much they flake, and how sheer and easy they are to blend. Shiny powder as an oil absorbent was never judged a good idea. If the idea is to powder down shine, applying more shine doesn't make sense.

Powders are often designated as being for dry or oily skin. Those designations by the cosmetics companies are often bogus; I rated a product as being good for oily skin if it contained minimal waxy or oily ingredients. Cornstarch or rice starch in powders is considered problematic for causing breakouts, despite its dry feel on the skin. I indicate which powders contained these ingredients as they could be a potential problem for acne-prone skin.

BLUSH: I considered it essential for blushes to have a smooth texture and to blend on easily, and the silkier the feel, the better the rating. I don't recommend shiny blushes. Although they don't make cheeks look as crepey or wrinkly as shiny eyeshadows do the eyes, sparkling cheeks look out of place during the day. Blushes that go on with a sheen or shine but did not sparkle are described with a warning, but are not rated as highly as matte blushes. This is more a matter of personal preference than a problem; you simply should know exactly what you are buying and what you can and cannot expect.

Cream blushes were rated on their blendability, whether they streak, how greasy they feel, and how well they last. I also describe which cream blushes tend to work better over foundation and which ones work better directly on the skin.

EYESHADOW: It won't surprise most of you who have read any of my previous books or newsletters to find out that I don't recommend shiny eyeshadows of any shade, or vivid shades of blue, violet, green, or red, whether they shine or not. Intense hues may be a personal preference, but I don't encourage anyone to use them. Makeup that speaks louder than you maybe kicky and fun, but it doesn't help empower a woman or help her to be taken seriously. If that's not your goal in life, ignore my color or shine recommendations. Regardless of color or shine, all eyeshadows were evaluated on texture, and ease of application played the largest part in determining my eyeshadow preferences. I point out which colors have heavy, grainy textures, because they can be hard to blend and can easily crease. Eyeshadows that are too sheer or powdery are also a problem because the color tends to fade as the day wears on, while they can also be difficult to apply, flaking all over the place. I am also leery of eyeshadow sets that include difficult-to-use color combinations. Many lines have duo, trio, and quad sets of eyeshadows, with the most bizarre colors imaginable. Sets of colors must be usable as a set, coordinated in complementary colors; they should never paint a rainbow or kaleidoscope of color across the eye. However, if you are looking for a kaleidoscope, I've pointed them out; they just have an unhappy face next to them. Generally, it is best to buy eyeshadow colors singly, not in sets. That way you can be assured of liking all the colors you buy, not just two out of three or four.

Specialty eyeshadow products such as liquids, creams, powdery or creamy pencils, and loose-powder eyeshadows were evaluated on ease of use, blendability, staying power, and how well they work over and with other products. My reviews indicate a clear bias toward matte eyeshadow powders as opposed to any other types of eyeshadow. I find liquids and creams hard to control and even more difficult to blend with other colors. However, some women are quite adept at using this kind of product and should balance my preference against theirs.

EYE AND BROW SHAPER: Basically, all pencils, regardless of brand, have more similarities than differences. Most eye pencils, lip pencils, and eyebrow pencils are manufactured by the same company (meaning the same manufacturing plant) and are then sold to hundreds of different cosmetics lines. Whether they cost $30 from Chanel or $4 from Almay, they are likely to be exactly the same product. Some pencils are greasier or drier than others, but for the most part there are few marked differences among them. Eye pencils that smudge and smear and eyebrow pencils that go on like a crayon—meaning thick and greasy—are always rated as ineffective, because they can get very messy as the day goes by. (Keep in mind that whether an eye pencil smears along the lower eyelashes depends to a large extent on the number of lines around your eye, how much moisturizer you use around the eye area, the type of under-eye concealer you use, and how greasy the pencil is. The greasier the moisturizer or the under-eye concealer, the more likely any pencil will smear, and you can't blame that on the pencil. But pencils do tend to smear more than powders, which I explain in my book *The Beauty Bible*.)

As a general rule, I do not recommend pencils for filling in the brow. Eyebrow pencil almost always looks matte and artificial next to an eyebrow. I use only powder, and I encourage you to do the same (this too is explained in *The Beauty Bible*). Any eyeshadow color that matches your eyebrow color *exactly* can do the trick, applied with a tiny eyeliner or angle brush. Brow gel and eyeshadow or brow shadow work superbly together to fill in the brow. A handful of companies make a clear brow gel meant to keep eyebrows in place without adding color or thickness. This works well, but no better than hairspray on a toothbrush brushed through the brow.

LIPSTICK AND LIP PENCIL: Every woman has her own needs and preferences when it comes to lipstick. Some women like sheer applications; others prefer glossy or matte finishes. Colors are also difficult to recommend because of the wide variation in taste. Given those limitations, I primarily reviewed the range of colors and textures available, commenting on texture rather than critiquing it, because personal preference is vital to a final decision. The general groupings are gloss, creamy, creamy with shine or iridescence, matte, and ultra-matte. As a matter of preference, because of staying power and coverage, I gave highest marks to creamy or semi-matte lipsticks that went on evenly and weren't glossy, sticky, thick, or drying. The ultra-matte lipsticks (introduced first by Ultima II with its LipSexxxy and then made overwhelmingly popular by Revlon's ColorStay, which is virtually identical to the former) are unique because of their dry, flat finish, and because they don't easily come off on coffee cups or teeth. I evaluated them for how dry their finish is, how much they chip and peel, and how well they last during the day. Please note that ultra-matte lipsticks can dry out the lips and peel off during the day. I usually don't recommend lip glosses, because they don't stay on longer than an hour or two, while most women want long-lasting lip makeup. I evaluated lip pencils according to whether they went on smoothly without being greasy or dry.

MASCARA: Mascaras should go on easily and quickly while building length and thickness. Brush shape has improved phenomenally over the years. A brush can be awkward to use if it is too big or too small. Mascara should never smear or flake, regardless of its price. A $4 mascara is no bargain if it doesn't go on well. However, no mascara can hold up to a heavy layer of moisturizer around the eyes. If you pile on any kind of moisturizer, whether it be oil-free, a gel, or a product designed especially for the eyes, your mascara will be affected.

Except for swimming and special occasions that may produce tears, I don't recommend waterproof mascaras. Trying to remove waterproof mascara is awful for the eyes and worse for the lashes. All that pulling and wiping isn't good for the skin and tends to pull lashes out. There are dozens of waterproof mascaras out there, but only a handful are truly reliable. Plus, waterproof mascaras do not stay on any better than water-soluble ones, given that both break down in contact with emollients from moisturizers, sunscreens, under-eye creams, foundations, creamy under-eye concealers, and other specialty products applied around the eye.

Beauty Note: I should mention that I have a personal preference for mascaras that produce long, thick lashes. I admit that my own preference in this regard can get in the way of my evaluations. For example, I rate Maybelline Volum' mascara as excellent because it can build incredibly long, thick lashes; unfortunately, it can also go on clumpy and thick, not something every woman wants to deal with when applying mascara.

BRUSHES: Brushes are essential to applying makeup correctly and beautifully. Blush and eyeshadow brushes are offered by some of the major cosmetics lines, and most department stores sell brush sets of some kind. Brushes were rated on overall shape and function as well as on the softness and density of the bristles. An eyeshadow or blush brush with scratchy, stiff, or loose bristles was not recommended. Also, let me warn you against buying brush sets. They almost always include brushes you don't need or can't use. It is best to buy brushes individually so you can select the best ones for your needs and for the shape of your face and eyes.

Evaluation of Skin-Care Products

The following are the criteria I used to evaluate the quality of varying groups of skin-care products. For those of you who are familiar with my reviews, you may notice that I am much more cautious about products that contain any amount of irritating ingredients, particularly those containing lemon, grapefruit, mint, peppermint, menthol, camphor, eucalyptus, ivy, fragrant oils, and overly drying detergent cleansing agents. My more exacting criteria on this subject relate to the growing research indicating that irritation damages skin and hurts the skin's healing process. In the midst of our daily battle against sun damage, wrinkles, and the causes of breakouts, there is never a reason to unnecessarily irritate the skin with ingredients that provide no benefit whatsoever for the face or body.

My reviews of skin-care products in each line are, with a few exceptions, organized in the following categories: cleanser, eye-makeup remover, exfoliant (scrubs or AHA products), facial mask, toner, moisturizer (of all kinds regardless of the claim), eye cream, specialty products (serums), sunscreen, and acne products.

<u>CLEANSER:</u> In reviewing facial cleansers, I was primarily interested in how genuinely water-soluble they were. Facial cleansers should rinse off easily, without the aid of a washcloth, and be able to remove all traces of makeup, including eye makeup. Once a water-soluble cleanser is rinsed off, it should not leave skin feeling either dry, greasy, or filmy. And it should never burn the eyes, irritate the skin, or taste bad. Removing makeup with a greasy cleanser is an option for some women with extremely dry skin; however, it is not a preferred method of makeup removal. Wiping at the skin pulls at it and causes the skin to sag. Plus, wiping at the skin with a washcloth or tissue can be irritating. Wiping off makeup with cotton balls is less irritating but the pulling is still problematic.

<u>EYE-MAKEUP REMOVER:</u> Using a separate eye-makeup remover more often than not is completely unnecessary. An effective but gentle water-soluble cleanser should take off all your makeup, including eye makeup, without irritating the eyes. The problem with wiping off makeup is simply that you have to wipe and pull at your skin to get the stuff off. That pulling and wiping causes the skin to sag faster than it would otherwise. Another problem is the tendency for makeup to get wiped into the eye itself as opposed to splashed away, and that can cause irritation. Unless you are wearing waterproof mascara or can't get the knack of removing your eye makeup with a water-soluble cleanser, there are many reasons to avoid this step.

Some women who find using a water-soluble cleanser ineffective for removing eye makeup can saturate a large cotton pad with eye-makeup remover, close their eyes, and very gently place it against eyebrows and eyelids, holding it there for a few seconds. This way, you won't be tugging or pulling but, rather, loosening and dissolving the eye makeup. Then you follow with a water-soluble cleanser and more easily remove your eye makeup. Most every eye-makeup remover I've seen is either water with a lightweight surfactant (detergent cleansing agent) or some form of oil. More so than with any other skin-care category, there is no reason to waste money on this group of products. My tendency is to rate these products with a "neutral" face regardless of the product's effectiveness. Almost all of these products are formulated similarly, with no surprises or real cautions needed other than telling you that they are not the best way to remove makeup on a daily basis.

EXFOLIANT—SCRUB: With the advent of alpha hydroxy acids (AHAs) and the increased use of beta hydroxy acid (technical name, salicylic acid), there is little reason to use a mechanical exfoliant on the skin. Mechanical exfoliants are scrubs that remove skin cells by rubbing them over the skin. Even when the scrub particles are small and uniform in size, this can still abrade the skin and be harsher than necessary. Some women prefer the feeling of a scrub on the skin, but I've yet to see one that can supersede using plain baking soda mixed with Cetaphil Gentle Skin Cleanser. My strong suggestion, if you do want to try a scrub, is to start with Cetaphil Gentle Skin Cleanser and baking soda mixed together before shopping a cosmetics line for a scrub.

ALPHA HYDROXY ACID—BETA HYDROXY ACID PRODUCTS: I expect products containing AHAs or BHA to be exfoliants because that is how they work to smooth skin and help cell turnover. I wish you could tell whether an AHA or BHA product will be effective by its label, but that just isn't possible. All the claims and promises on the sticker, and even the ingredient label, won't tell you whether you are purchasing an effective AHA or BHA product. Unfortunately, effectiveness is based not only on ingredient content (which I explain in the next section, on ingredients) but also on the percentage (how much of the AHA or BHA is in the product) and the pH level (how acid or alkaline it is). I have two major considerations for alpha hydroxy acid (AHA) and beta hydroxy acid (BHA) products. First, the percentage of AHAs or BHA used in the product is assessed, with 5% to 10% being preferred for AHAs—more in this regard does not mean better because of the resulting irritation it can cause—and 1% to 2% being preferred for BHA—more does not mean better here, either. Then I measured the pH of the product (pH is significant because these ingredients can work only when they are in an acid base). If the base is too neutral or too alkaline (a higher pH), the acid becomes ineffective for exfoliating the skin. AHAs and BHA both work best in a pH of 3 to 4. By the way, an AHA or BHA product with a high pH is not a harmful product, just an ineffective one for exfoliation.

From my perspective, as I explain at length in my book *The Beauty Bible,* I do not recommend products that use AHAs and BHAs together. Each has its preferred action and that does not translate to all skin types. AHAs work on the surface of the skin and are best for sun damage or a thickened outer layer of skin (as often happens with dry skin). BHAs, on the other hand, can cut through the lipid layer of skin and work better in the pore, helping skin to shed cells and loosen plugs in there, improving the size of the pore. If you don't have breakouts, you don't need that kind of penetration; if you have breakouts, AHAs may help to some extent, but the penetration from the BHA can be more effective.

One word of caution: Any time you use a well-formulated AHA product that contains more than 5% AHAs, some stinging can occur; also, you should not let the product come in contact with the eyes or any mucous membranes. You may have an irritation or sensitivity to AHAs. Slight stinging is expected, but continued stinging is not. Discontinue use if this should happen.

FACIAL MASK: Most facial masks contain claylike ingredients, which absorb oil and, to some degree, exfoliate the skin. The problem with many masks is that they contain additional ingredients that are irritating or that can clog pores. Although your face may feel smooth when the mask is first rinsed off, after a short period of time problems may be created by the mask's drying effect. As a rule I don't recommend most facial masks. The few clay masks that contain emollients and moisturizing ingredients can still be too drying for dry skin and can cause oily skin to break out. Despite this, for those who are interested, I've pointed out the ones that do not contain any additional irritating ingredients except for the clay.

TONER: Toners, astringents, fresheners, tonics, and other liquids meant to refresh the skin or remove the last traces of makeup after a cleanser is rinsed off should not contain any irritants whatsoever. I evaluated these products primarily on that basis. Claims that toners can close pores or refine the skin are not realistic, so I ignored such language and looked primarily for toners that leave the face feeling smooth and soft, are able to remove any last traces of makeup, and do not irritate the skin. Some toners may also contain water-binding and anti-irritant ingredients, and these were listed as being preferred for normal to dry skin. Toners with lightweight detergent cleaning agents, minimal water-binding agents, and anti-irritants were rated high for normal to oily skin. However, toners are always considered an optional step for most skin types. For someone with normal to oily skin, they can be the only moisturizer the skin needs; for someone with dry skin, they can be a great lightweight start to add extra water-binding agents to the skin.

MOISTURIZER: In spite of all the fuss surrounding wrinkle creams and moisturizers as a way to make skin look and stay young, this category was actually quite easy to review. Wrinkle creams and moisturizers all do the same thing—they keep the skin from looking and feeling dry—so I expected the same thing from all of them: they must contain ingredients that could smooth and soothe dry skin and keep water in the skin cell. Most other claims are exaggerated and misleading. Remember that dry skin and wrinkles are not associated, so you can't stop wrinkles or get rid of wrinkles by applying a moisturizer, despite the claims.

Lots of moisturizers boast that they can penetrate layers of skin cells better than others do, which is a meaningless claim. Skin cells are quite permeable, so claims of penetrating layers of skin would be true for most products if they contained even one drop of water. Nonetheless, it is essential that some moisturizing ingredients be left on the surface of the skin to prevent the air from drinking up the water in your skin cells. My reviews show a preference for formulas that utilize unique or interesting water-binding agents and antioxidants.

I also list the ingredients I think are more hype than help, such as brewer's yeast; bee pollen; gold; animal extracts from thymus, spleen, placenta, and fish collagen; many plant extracts ranging from algae to flowers, and countless weeds. Additionally, I was interested in what order the "good" or "hyped" ingredients were listed on the container. Often the percentage of the most interesting or the most extolled ingredients is so negligible that those ingredients are practically nonexistent. Just because an ingredient is in there doesn't mean there's enough to make a difference.

There are moisturizers that claim they are great for combination skin because they are able to release moisturizing ingredients over dry areas and oil-absorbing ingredients over oily areas. This is categorically impossible. A product cannot hold certain ingredients back from the skin—where would they go? Imagine a lotion touching your skin, and the ingredients for the oily parts get up and run over here and the ones for the dry area get up and head over there. It just isn't feasible in any way, shape, or form.

MOISTURIZER FOR OILY SKIN: The only time to use a moisturizer is when you have dry skin; if you don't have dry skin, you don't need to use a moisturizer. When a product, particularly a moisturizer, claims to be "oil-free," more often than not it misleads consumers into thinking they are buying a product that won't clog pores. There are plenty of ingredients that don't sound like oils but can absolutely aggravate breakouts. Almost all cosmetics contain waxlike thickening agents that are notorious for clogging pores. Simple, standard moisturizing ingredients that are great for dry skin can wreak havoc on someone with oily skin or breakouts. Triglycerides, palmitates, stearates, myristates, stearic acid, plant oils, plant waxes, shea butter, vitamin E, acrylates (film-forming agents), and many other ingredients can all clog pores. These ingredients are used in moisturizers because they duplicate the natural lipids (sebum or oil) in our skin or prevent dehydration, and that's great. But if you have problems with the oil already being created in your pores, adding more of the same kind of substance will only make things worse. Despite the problems these ingredients can cause, they show up in lots and lots of so-called "oil-free" products. To that end, I've judged all moisturizers on their effectiveness for some level of dry skin. Never use a moisturizer over areas of the face that are oily, that break out, or that have blackheads—it will only make matters worse. Moisturizers are only needed where you have dry skin.

DAY CREAM VERSUS NIGHT CREAM: The only difference between a daytime moisturizer and a nighttime moisturizer is that the daytime one often has sunscreen; other than that, there are no formulation variances that make one preferable over the other. There are many moisturizing formulations that have great sun protection, and that is the only way you should differentiate a daytime product from a nighttime version. All other claims on the label are rhetoric you should ignore.

EYE, THROAT, CHEST, NECK, AND OTHER SPECIALTY CREAM AND SERUM: Buying a product for a special area of the body or face, whether it is in the form of a cream, gel, lotion, or serum is altogether unnecessary. Almost without exception, their ingredient lists and formulations are identical to other face creams, gels, serums, and lotions. That doesn't mean there aren't some great products out there for different skin types in the form of some specialty products, especially eye products, but why buy a second moisturizer for the eye area when the one you are already using on the rest of your face is virtually identical? Even more bothersome is the fact that most cosmetics companies give you a tiny amount of the so-called specialty product but charge you much more for it than for an equal amount of nonspecialty face creams, despite the similarities.

What do sometimes show up in eye-care products are irritating ingredients such as witch hazel. These types of ingredients temporarily swell the skin around the eye, creating an appearance of diminished wrinkles. Swollen skin can temporarily look smooth, but the resulting irritation is, in the long run harmful, not helpful, for the skin.

SUNSCREEN: Please refer to Chapter Two, Skin-Care Update, for more information about sun care. My main criterion for evaluating sun-care products is the SPF rating, with SPF 15 being preferred, though an SPF 8 is minimally acceptable and SPF 10 to 14 is OK for limited daily sun exposure. If you are only going from your car to the office and then to the store, and then driving home, you will probably be just fine in terms of sun protection with a lower rating. Nevertheless, I still strongly recommend using SPF 15 on a daily basis, because you never know how much sun you're really going to get on any given day.

Because of the difference between UVA damage and UVB damage, to be assured you are getting adequate UVA protection, your sunscreen must contain one of three ingredients. Those ingredients are avobenzone, titanium dioxide, and zinc oxide. No sunscreens received a happy face unless one of those is listed on the active ingredient part of the ingredient listing.

Sunscreen ingredients can be irritating no matter what a product's label says, because the way these ingredients work can cause a reaction on the skin. You just have to experiment to find the one that works best for you. Although purely nonchemical sunscreens that use only titanium dioxide or only zinc oxide as the active ingredient are considered almost completely nonirritating, they can still pose problems for someone with oily or acne-prone skin because their occlusive composition can clog pores and aggravate breakouts.

Although I've said this before it still bears repeating: Many products make claims about UVA protection that are truly misleading. While titanium dioxide, zinc oxide, or avobenzone protect from about 80% to 90% to UVA radiation, other formulations that don't contain these ingredients only protect from about 20% of UVA radiation.

SELF-TANNER: For the most part I did not review self-tanning products individually. All of these products, whether you choose one made by Revlon, Estee Lauder, Clarins, Decleor Paris, or Estee Lauder, are created equal. The active ingredient in every one of these products is dihydroxyacetone. That's what turns the surface layer of skin brown. The ingredient acts on the skin cells and their amino acid content, and the chemical reaction is what turns the skin a darker color. Self-tanners do not add a tint of color to the skin. You may not like the smell of one product versus another, but that is merely a function of the fragrance added to the product to mask the smell of the dihydroxyacetone. A masking fragrance might be pleasant, but it doesn't change how the product functions, and the natural odor of the product is transient. Where sunscreens do differ is in the amount of dihydroxyactone used. There is no way to judge that from the ingredient list. However, you can assume that those self-tanners rated as light, medium and dark have the correct corresponding amount of dihydroxyacetone. Self-tanners without any stated level you can assume have a light to medium concentration of dihydroxyacetone.

ACNE PRODUCTS: From all the research I've seen, particularly in dermatological journals and literature from the American Academy of Dermatology, acne products need to deliver three categories of performance to deal with breakouts: effective exfoliation, disinfection, and absorbing excess oil. I delved into this subject at length in my book *The Beauty Bible*. I base my reviews on how well over-the-counter products (as opposed to those available by prescription only) respond to those skin-care needs.

Exfoliating: For exfoliating the skin with an over-the-counter treatment, it is best to start with either a 5% to 8% alpha hydroxy acid (AHA) product or a 1% to 2% beta hydroxy acid (BHA) product. For blemishes or oily skin, these products were rated especially high if they were available in gel or very lightweight lotion form.

When it comes to cosmetic scrubs, I almost never prefer them for exfoliating the skin, because they are almost all formulated with waxy thickening agents that can clog pores and cause breakouts. That's not to say they can't be effective for exfoliation, because they can be, but I find most of these formulations faulty for blemish- or blackhead-prone skin. For all skin types, if you are looking for a mechanical scrub, I still have yet to find a product that can beat mixing baking soda with Cetaphil Gentle Skin Cleanser.

Cleanser: Using a gentle, water-soluble cleanser is standard for any skin-care routine, but even more so for oily skin because it reduces irritation and redness. After all, what color is acne? Red. So why use any product that makes skin redder? I also never recommend bar soap for acne or breakouts. Bar soaps of any kind are kept in their bar form by ingredients that can absolutely clog pores. Research also shows that high pH cleansers (soaps are usually over a pH of 8) can increase the presence of bacteria in the skin. To that end, gentle cleansers were rated high if they did not contain irritating or excessively drying ingredients.

Disinfecting: In order to kill the bacteria in the skin that cause blemishes, you need a reliable disinfectant. There aren't many options when it comes to disinfecting the skin. Alcohol, when used in very high concentrations (more than 60%—thankfully, never found in skin-care products) and sulfur can be good disinfectants, but they are way too drying and irritating for most skin types, and can just make matters worse. Other ingredients that repeatedly show up in products for problem skin, such as lemon, grapefruit, acetone, witch hazel, peppermint, menthol, eucalyptus, and camphor, have no effect at all on bacteria and can cause unnecessary irritation. Currently popular plant-derived disinfectants such as tea tree oil (from *Melaleuca alterniflora*) are not present in high enough concentrations to reliably kill bacteria. The best over-the-counter disinfectants are: 3% hydrogen peroxide, 2.5% benzoyl peroxide, 5% benzoyl peroxide, and 10% benzoyl peroxide. Only the types of products containing these ingredients, with no additives, were given high ratings.

Absorbing excess oil: While most people think clay masks are the only way to absorb excess oil on the skin, these are my last choice for that purpose. Using milk of magnesia (yes, like the Phillips' Milk of Magnesia that you take for indigestion) as a facial mask is by far the best way to absorb oil I have ever found or personally used. Milk of magnesia is nothing more than liquid magnesium hydroxide, which is known to soothe skin and reduce irritation, and it has incredible oil-absorbing properties. Magnesium absorbs more oil than clay, and clay has no disinfecting or soothing properties. How often you use the milk of magnesia has to do with how oily your skin is. Some use it every day; others, once a week. Only you and your skin can determine what frequency works best for you.

The Ingredients for Skin Care

While I want to emphasize the extent of the misleading portrayals of skin-care products made by the cosmetics industry, I also want to underscore what great products *do* exist for all skin types. However, it is difficult for me to describe my elation or enthusiasm about any product without always being careful to let you know what can really be expected and how out of line the price often is for what you are getting.

Just because I think a formula can be amazing for dry skin, that doesn't mean I concur with its claims about firming, lifting, anti-wrinkling, reducing lines, fighting stress, erasing cellulite, building collagen, and on and on and on…

Every skin-care product was evaluated on the basis of what it contains. The ingredients are the basis for whether a claim can be verified. Unlike earlier editions of *Don't Go to the Cosmetics Counter Without Me*, **I do not summarize the ingredient listing for every skin-care product** in this edition. I wanted to include as many new lines as possible in this book and the repetitive "this product contains" listing was not everyone's cup of tea—and it took up an astounding amount of room. Unless I felt this kind of information was needed to help understand a product's performance, I provided just a general summary of the product's contents and then described what it could and couldn't do. When I did describe a product's ingredients, it was always **in the order they appear on the ingredient list.** I also let you know how it compares to similar products that cost much less. Of course, you will have to test for yourself how any specific product feels on your skin and how you react to its fragrance or lack thereof.

In the product reviews, when I do describe a product's contents, I frequently use the phrase "contains mostly," often followed by one or all of the following terms: **thickener** or **thickening agent, slip agent, water-binding agent, film former, detergent cleansing agent** or **standard detergent cleanser, preservative, fragrance, plant extract** or **plant oil, vitamin, antioxidant,** and **anti-irritant.** It was easiest to summarize groups of ingredients by using these general terms, but they need more explanation before you read the reviews.

Beauty Note: When reading ingredient lists, remember that the closer a specific ingredient is to a preservative (such as methylparaben, propylparaben, ethylparaben, imidazolidinyl urea, or quaternium-15) or a fragrance (listed as fragrance or often as an individual essential oil like lavender or bergamot oil), or the closer it is to the end of the ingredient list, the less likely it is that any significant amount is present in the product.

When I use the term "**thickeners**" to describe an ingredient, the term refers to those components that add texture, thickness, viscosity, spreadability, and stability to a product. Thickeners are also vital for helping to keep other ingredients mixed together. **Thickening agents** often have a waxlike texture or a creamy, emollient feel, and can be great lubricants. There are literally thousands of ingredients in this category, and they are the staples of every skin-care product out there, regardless of the product's price or claims about "natural" ingredients.

Slip agents help other ingredients spread over or penetrate the skin. These include propylene glycol, butylene glycol, polysorbates, and glycerin. They are as basic to the world of skin care as water.

Water-binding agents are known for their ability to help the skin retain water. These ingredients range from the mundane glycerin to the more exotic hyaluronic acid, sodium hyaluronate, mucopolysaccharides, sodium PCA, collagen, elastin, proteins, amino acids (of which there are dozens), cholesterol, glucose, sucrose, fructose, glycogen, antioxidants, phospholipids, glycosphinglipids, and on and on. For the most part, they all work equally well. Looking for a specific one is a waste of your time and energy. They are what they are: good water-binding ingredients.

Film formers are ingredients such as PVP, methylacrylate, and polyglycerylacrylates presently being used in a vast number of moisturizers, wrinkle creams, and eye gels to help the skin look smoother. Film formers are usually found in hair sprays and hairstyling products like gels and mousses because they place a thin, transparent, plasticlike layer over the skin (and hair) and leave the face appearing smoother. These film-forming ingredients do a good job, but they can be irritants for some skin types, though they are generally used in such tiny amounts that it is unlikely to be a problem for most skin types. When these film-forming ingredients are found higher up on a product's ingredient list, it can leave a slightly sticky feeling on the skin.

For products in which an ingredient is included primarily for its sudsing or degreasing ability, such as in skin cleansers, I use the phrase "**detergent cleansing agent**" or "**standard detergent cleanser.**" Ingredients in this category include sodium lauryl sulfate, sodium laureth sulfate, TEA-lauryl sulfate, cocamide DEA, ammonium laureth sulfate, and ammonium lauryl sulfate, to name a few (though these tend to be the most typical). Because sodium lauryl sulfate, TEA-lauryl sulfate, and sodium C14-16 olefin sulfate are very strong detergent cleansing agents and are known for their serious irritation potential, I warn against using a product that contains these ingredients when they appear in the first part of its ingredient list.

When **fragrances** are listed in the ingredients, I indicate this simply by stating it as such. Fragrance is used in cosmetics either to mask the smell of a product's ingredients or to add a specific fragrance. My strong recommendation is that skin-care products not contain fragrance. Fragrances of all kinds, including essential oils, are irritants and serve no function for skin. Because of that I would prefer that all skin-care products be fragrance-free. Nevertheless, women like their products to smell nice. It is up to every woman to make her own decision on that matter. Even if I thought fragrance was OK in a skin-care product, fragrance is still a very tricky thing to comment on because smell is such a personal experience. Avoiding fragrance is easy to do by checking the ingredient label. If fragrance (listed as "fragrance") or essential oils like lavender, cardamom, lemon, ylang ylang, bergamot, or other fragrant oils are listed on a product you know it has fragrance and you can choose what to do, make your nose happy or make your skin happy.

There are **preservatives** that some people feel are more problematic than others. I have not included specific warnings for preservatives such as quaternium-15, 2-bromo-2-nitropane-1,3-diol, phenoxyethanol, or dmdm hydantoin. There is research indicating that these ingredients pose a higher potential for irritation than other preservatives. Recent data, however, strongly dispute that conclusion. After discussing this matter with several cosmetic chemists, I have concluded that all preservatives can be a problem for many different types of skin, so it would be unfair and misleading to pinpoint one specific preservative as a problem. If you are concerned, you can easily avoid any of these ingredients; however, as several cosmetic chemists warned me, a reliable preservative system is better for the skin because microbial contamination of a product can cause more problems for the eyes, lips, and skin than the risk of a reaction to a preservative.

On a related matter, some of you may be familiar with research that warns against using cosmetics that contain DEA, triethanolamine, or TEA-lauryl sulfate mixed in the same product along with formaldehyde-releasing preservatives such as imidazolidinyl urea, quaternium-15, 2-bromo-2-nitropane-3,1-diol, or dmdm hydantoin. There is evidence that suggests these combinations can form nitrosamines in a cosmetic, creating a potential carcinogen (nitrosamines, as you may recall, are carcinogenic substances). There is substantial disagreement among the cosmetic chemists I spoke to as to how significant a problem this is for the skin (or even whether it is a problem). They suggested that going out of the house without a sunscreen or sitting in a bar exposed to secondhand cigarette smoke poses more risk to the skin than any combination of skin-care ingredients ever could. However, you should be aware that there are those who consider this nonchalant attitude to be mere apologetics for and sidestepping around a very serious question. As someone who has looked at this issue for some time, I actually understand both viewpoints and have no definitive position to share. To that end, I leave the final decision up to you. All you need to do is check the ingredient list of any product you are considering to determine whether it excludes amines as well as the questionable preservatives mentioned above.

It is impossible to list all the individual **plant extracts** used in cosmetics. As far as the world of cosmetics is concerned, if it grows it can change skin. Yet there is no consensus on which plant is the most amazing. According to the various cosmetics companies, the plants they use have the most astonishing merits. When plants are an issue in a skin-care product, I point out those plants' known benefits; otherwise, I mention all plants only under the generic category of plant extracts.

Plant oils (other than those called essential oils) are almost always beneficial as emollients and lubricants. The debate whether or not emu oil, mink oil, sunflower, canola, or a myriad of other oils or blends of oils are superior is a marketing game to showcase a product, it has nothing to do with skin sense.

Some plant oils, often referred to as essential oils, are highly fragrant, volatile oils and are almost always irritants or photosensitizers, and I indicate when this is the case. However, I attribute no superiority to one over another, because none exists. **Essential oils** are nothing more than a way to get fragrance into a skin-care product. The cosmetics industry knows that many women are aware that fragrance can be a strong source of skin irritation and sensitivities, so they use the term "essential oils" as a way to put fragrance in a product without saying "fragrance." Women may know that fragrance ingredients are bad, but they still want their products to smell nice. Caught between a rock and a hard place, the cosmetics industry came up with essential oils as the way around the dilemma. But the notion that plants can save the skin from wrinkles, stress, sun damage, scars, and a host of other skin ills is sheer fantasy and has no legitimate substantiation. That doesn't mean that natural ingredients can't be helpful, but they can't perform the miracles attributed to them by sales pitches, and fragrant oils such as clove, peppermint, citrus, ylang ylang, cinnamon, coriander, and lavender, among many others, can cause irritation.

I often list the exact name of any **vitamin** included in a product. Regardless of the individual vitamins—whether it is vitamin A, C, or E—vitamins in skin-care products can't feed the skin, but they can work as antioxidants when the product contains enough, and theoretically that can benefit the skin.

When specific antioxidant ingredients such as superoxide dismutase, selenium, glutathione, vitamin E, vitamin A, and vitamin C are included, I sometimes refer to these specifically as **antioxidants**. I describe antioxidants and their function at length in *The Beauty Bible.* To sum up, while research indicates that antioxidants may have much benefit for the skin, a vast amount is still not known. For example, even if antioxidants do have definitive benefits, there are no amounts established for effectiveness. Is 0.25% enough or 3% too much? Is there such a thing as too much? Should we be putting vitamins only on the skin? What about oral supplements? For many of the more popular antioxidants, like vitamin A or vitamin C and other plant extracts that can work as antioxidants, stability is a problem. Vitamin C deteriorates in the presence of air or sunlight and doesn't mix well with other ingredients. Ascorbic acid is considered a poor antioxidant because of its irritating effect on the skin. Until there is more information, we can only assume that antioxidants are good guys because they keep the drying effect of the air off the skin and help protect skin cells; other than that, it is all guessing and hoping.

If you are still sold on the hype around antioxidants, don't worry; most cosmetics in all price ranges contain them. These aren't secret ingredients to which only some cosmetics companies have access. Everyone knows about them and they are widely used in the industry.

Anti-irritants are **soothing** ingredients known for their ability to reduce inflammation on the skin. A small group of ingredients can perform this function and they do so quite nicely. When these types of ingredients—such as bisabolol, allantoin, burdock root, aloe, licorice root, or green tea—are present in a product, I refer to them by the term "anti-irritant(s)."

Many products use an assortment of exclusive-sounding adjectives—**deionized, purified, triple-purified, demineralized**—to describe what is actually just plain water. These terms indicate that the water has gone through some kind of purification process, which is standard for cosmetics. You will also find phrases such as "infusions of" or "aqueous extracts of," followed by the name of one or more plants. That means you're getting plant tea, or plant juice and water. Though this description indicates that you are getting mostly water and a hint of plant, they sound so pure and natural that it creates the impression that it must be better for the skin. Water is water. The kind of water used does not affect the skin or the final product. After the water is combined with other ingredients, its original status is unimportant.

Silicone is a skin-friendly ingredient that shows up repeatedly in skin-care, makeup, and hair-care products. I would venture a guess that the ubiquitous silicone appears in about 80% of all cosmetic products being sold. In the past, I have referred to silicone as silicone oil, which I have recently learned is incorrect terminology. While silicone may look, act, and feel like oil, and though every cosmetic chemist I've spoken to refers to it as silicone oil, this ingredient is still not an oil. Chemically speaking, silicone as a chemical compound is related to fluid technology. Either way, regardless of the precise name, silicone is an elegant skin-care ingredient that has an exquisite, silky, somewhat slippery feel. Its popularity in formulations reflects its versatility and the finish it gives products. It is also a cheap ingredient, and standard to all kinds of cosmetics in all kinds of price ranges. **For someone with oily or acne-prone skin, silicone is not necessarily a problem, at least when it comes to breakouts, though it can leave a residue behind on the skin that someone with oily skin might not like.**

Antibacterial ingredients: While cleanliness has merit, there are limitations to how clean a person can be. In the battle against germs and other loathsome microorganisms floating about our environment, the desire to wash with zest is valid (do not take that as a plug for Zest bar soap; I just couldn't resist the pun). We are also greatly influenced by news programs that ballyhoo the horror of bacteria being spread through less than scrupulous ablutions. It isn't surprising, then, to hear that antibacterial soaps have recently had an upsurge in sales. Unfortunately, this attention to antiseptic skin care is misplaced. It's not that I'm against cleanliness—far from it—and it goes without saying that disinfecting the skin is absolutely necessary in the battle against acne. The problem is that antibacterial cleansers of any kind, even the kind used in a doctor's office, regardless of the active ingredient, can't really kill germs and bacteria. At least, not any better than regular soaps and cleansers.

Here's the issue. In order for any disinfectant to work, it must be in contact with the skin for at least several minutes, and ten minutes or more is best. How many of us are scrubbing our hands and face for that long with an antibacterial cleanser? Hopefully, none of us, because that much contact with such potent disinfecting cleansers would destroy the skin in short order. But that's what it takes for antibacterial cleansers to do their job. When physicians scrub up for a surgical procedure, they wash their hands vigorously for several minutes, depending on the type of wash they use. They know that contact and scrubbing are the key to effectively disinfecting the skin. They also know that it makes their skin raw and dry, but there is no way around this one. Washing your hands and face with an antibacterial cleanser for a few seconds is fine, but don't expect your skin to be totally disinfected.

I'm not encouraging everyone to start scrubbing, because it is certainly detrimental to anyone's skin in the long haul, and for many skin types in the short haul. It hurts the intercellular layer of skin (the mortar that holds skin together), and that, ironically, is what keeps bacteria and germs out. Generally speaking, I do not encourage the use of antibacterial products for the face if you don't have a problem with breakouts. If you do have a problem with breakouts, I still think bar cleansers are a poor option because, though you may be getting some minimal benefit from the disinfecting ingredient, you're stuck with the ingredients that keep the bar soap in its bar form, and which can clog pores. Liquid or lotion water-soluble antibacterial cleansers are an option, but again, the contact with the antibacterial agent is so brief that I find it a poor option, given the other types of topical disinfectants available.

Alpha hydroxy acids and beta hydroxy acid: I absolutely do not recommend products that claim an association with AHAs or BHA but contain ingredients such as fruit extracts or sugarcane extracts, which sound like they can work like AHAs or BHA, but cannot. There are a host of legitimate AHA ingredients, the two most popular and most well-researched being glycolic acid and lactic acid. The only acceptable BHA ingredient is salicylic acid. While glycolic acid can be derived from sugarcane and BHA from wintergreen leaves, that doesn't mean that the original source has the effect of what is separated out from it. The analogy I use repeatedly is that just because penicillin is derived from moldy bread doesn't mean you would want to eat moldy bread when you are sick.

Aside from glycolic acid and lactic acid, the following are acceptable forms of AHA on an ingredient label: malic acid, ammonium glycolate, alpha-hydroxyethanoic acid, ammonium alpha-hydroxyethanoate, alpha-hydroxyoctanoic acid, alpha-hydroxycaprylic acid, and hydroxycaprylic acid.

Just a reminder: Any time you use a well-formulated AHA product that contains more than 5% AHAs, some stinging can occur; also, you should not let the product come in contact with the eyes or any mucous membranes. You may have an irritation or sensitivity to AHAs. Slight stinging is expected, but continued stinging is not. Discontinue use if this should happen.

The Ratings

The following are the rating symbols for the products reviewed in this book. These simple but succinct (and albeit cute) symbols depict my approval or disapproval of a specific product:

☺ This indicates a great product that I recommend highly and that is also low in price. This face means the product is definitely worth checking into and potentially worth buying.

☺ This indicates an OK but unimpressive product, or an OK product that can cause problems for certain skin types. I often use this neutral face to portray a dated or old-fashioned product formulation. That doesn't mean it's a bad or poorly formulated product, but it just isn't very interesting or is lacking some of the newer water-binding ingredients, antioxidants, anti-irritants, emollients, or nonirritating ingredients for dry skin. I also use the neutral face to reflect a makeup product that isn't really bad, but that is completely unnecessary, or unnecessarily overpriced for such an ordinary product that could easily be replaced with a far less-expensive version from the drugstore. Depending on your personal preferences, products rated with this face may be worth checking out, but are nothing to get excited about.

☹ For many reasons, this symbol reflects a product that is truly bad from almost every standpoint, including price, performance, application, texture, potential for irritation, skin reactions, and breakouts.

☺ $$$ This symbol designates a great product that I would recommend without a doubt were it not so absurdly overpriced, either in comparison to similar products or in relation to what you are getting for the money.

☺ $$$ this symbol indicates an ordinary, boring product whose excessive price makes it ludicrous to consider.

Prices: Because the cost of drugstore cosmetics often fluctuates from store to store, and because cosmetics companies often change prices every six months, the prices listed in this book may not be up to date or match what you find when you are shopping. Use the prices as a basis for comparison, but realize that they may not precisely reflect what you will find when you go shopping.

Up-to-date information: My staff and I struggle to make sure all the information we have is accurate and current. **However, cosmetics companies frequently and without notice change or reformulate their products, sometimes in a minor way and sometimes extensively.** To keep abreast of these changes that cannot be kept current in a book, I report all revisions and new product launches that occurred after this book went to press in my newsletter, *Cosmetics Counter Update.*

Foreign names: For the most part, I give only the English names of foreign-produced products. The French and Italian names are pretty, but they don't tell you anything about the product if you don't speak the language.

No endorsements: Neither the information nor the evaluations included in any of my work are to be misconstrued as endorsements, nor do they represent a particular company's sponsorship. None of the cosmetics companies paid me for my remarks or critiques. This includes the listing of my own products. While I clearly like my products, they are only options—just like any of the other products I've reviewed for this book—and I do not recommend them above any others. All "Best Choices" are just that, choices, with the final decision up to you.

Order of presentation: The cosmetics are listed alphabetically by brand names, so the order in which they appear does not represent my preference. There is no implied winner among any of the cosmetics companies included; no one line has all the answers or the majority of great products (even my own). Almost every line has its strong and weak points.

Don't go shopping without me: I encourage you to take this book with you on shopping trips to the cosmetics counters or the drugstore. Then you will have all the information you'll need readily at hand. There is no way you can remember the details of each product, color, and brand. Do try to be discreet at the department-store cosmetics counters—don't be surprised if you find that using the book in clear view of the salespeople makes them defensive or irritated. There are always risks when a consumer comes prepared with information that disagrees with the salesperson. I urge you to persevere. Nothing will change at the cosmetics counters if you don't change first.

You Don't Have to Agree

If you're just now reading this section, it is probably after you have picked up this book and quickly looked up the products you are presently using, have used in the past, or are thinking of using in the future. You went to those sections first because my credibility with many women hinges on whether you agree with my assessments of the products you are using. However, be aware that you need not agree with all my reviews to obtain benefit from this book. As you read my comments, you may indeed find yourself disagreeing with me. That is perfectly understandable and as it should be, because the criteria you use to evaluate cosmetics may differ from mine. Or, for any one of a dozen reasons (personal preference, different expectations, actual usage—once a week versus twice a day), a product I dislike may work well for you, or just the opposite can be true: a product I love, you may hate. What I cannot account for is how millions of women will feel about a particular product.

What I present in the following pages are merely guidelines, based on my extensive research and experience about what works and what doesn't. If you decide to follow any of my suggestions, be aware that my recommendations are not a guarantee, but a suggestion as to how to narrow down the endless options the cosmetics industry sells. It is my earnest desire to help you chose from this very crowded field so you can make the best choices possible, but the final choice is up to you.

Your Feedback

I want to tell you how much I appreciate the feedback I've received from many of you regarding my research and product reviews. As I've mentioned before, your input keeps me on my toes and helps me obtain information and opinions on a wide variety of makeup, skin-care, and hair-care issues. Your criticisms and compliments have also helped me improve in numerous areas, including boosting my spirits when the cosmetics industry gets the better of me, or helping me to grasp a differing point of view. In regard to improvement, I want to thank those of you who have written to me with corrections on some details of my research. I am wowed beyond words at the thoroughness of your analysis and the value of your input.

Women who have read previous editions of this book may notice that my reviews for some products have changed. There are four basic reasons why this happens: I was wrong the first time I checked out the product; I have acquired new research that supports a different evaluation; the company changed the product since I last tested it or looked at the ingredient listing; or, based on new information, I've changed my criteria to include a different perspective than I did when I last updated this book.

For example, in the last edition of this book, one woman noticed that I included Borghese's liquid-to-powder blush when it had already been discontinued. Another longtime reader pointed out that Estee Lauder's Fresh Air makeup was long gone, but there it was in my product review, even though my notes indicated it had been discontinued. Whenever I receive information I can confirm, I quickly include it in the next edition of my newsletter and in subsequent reprints of my book, but sometimes, trying to compile thousands of product reviews, oversights do happen.

With the fourth edition, you may notice that many reviews of still-existing products have changed. For example, one reader pointed out that some of my recommendations, particularly regarding L'Oreal mascaras, had changed wildly from one edition to another. She asked, "Could formulations change that much?" My response: Absolutely. Other possibilities are that my impressions changed, or the competition got better (meaning the standard of excellence changed). This is a major reason I continue to update my books and write my newsletter.

One woman wrote that although she was looking forward to my new book and loved my skin-care products (she replaced her Chanel routine with my products), she felt the book had not been completely updated. She mentioned that I had missed the change in colors for Lancome Anticernes Waterproof Undereye Concealer that were introduced almost a year ago. She also pointed out that I said Lancome's only matte eyeshadow was Les Mats Naturel and Soft Taupe, but she discovered that Lancome had several others, and she was right.

I'm sure there are other problems of this nature that you may find in this edition, as there were in the previous three; though I work diligently to make sure everything is correct, things do get by me. My staff (and several freelance researchers) have worked on the new edition for more than a year, practically day and night, living at computers surrounded by cosmetics, visiting cosmetics counters and drugstores, talking with in-home sales reps, checking out shopping infomercials and in-home shopping channels (and you all know how much I love doing that!) as well as poring over technical journals research papers and abstracts, and interviewing cosmetic chemists and dermatologists.

One of the dilemmas of doing a consumer product guide about the cosmetics industry (aside from the sheer plethora of products) is that products and product lines change. Every month new items are added to and deleted from almost every line out there. That means if I finished researching a line in, say, January, by July, when I finish this manuscript, newly launched products or product changes occurring after those dates won't be in this edition. That is why I do my newsletter—the cosmetics industry is ever-changing and for those of you who want to keep abreast of all those changes, my newsletter is an option you may want to consider.

Please, keep your letters coming, both the good and the bad. One personal request, for those of you who are angry with my views or information: please address the information and leave out the personal attacks. I unconditionally consider all the feedback I receive and delve further when given the data and resources to do so. I am not out to get anyone; I just want to share what I know from my research. Here is an example of a less than enthused reader:

Dear Paula,

I just spent the last ten minutes reading your third edition of *Don't Go to the Cosmetics Counter Without Me*. Although you do have a tiny bit of good information, your book is riddled with mistakes, incorrect statements, and useless information. For example, if you felt that it was so important to include prestigious lines, then why did you leave out Givenchy and Nina Ricci, yet take the time to mention Monteil, which sold maybe one product last year?

Let me point out a few mistakes that I found, and keep in mind that it only took minutes to sight these. First of all, you should not use the word *moisturizer* in reference to serums such as Dior's Capture for the face and Chanel's Lift Serum Extreme; they are not intended to moisturize. In both cases you have to use a moisturizer over the top for the serums to be effective; therefore it is incorrect to suggest that these would be effective moisturizers for someone with dry skin. They would not supply enough moisture to the face of a greasy preteen.

In reference to Trish McEvoy, there are too many mistakes to mention. You said you liked the cream-to-powder foundation, but it would not be good for an oily skin. That is why she also makes an oil-free cream-to-powder foundation.

You praised Radiant Touch from Yves St. Laurent, yet only liked one color. There is only one color; the other product is called Sunny Touch and it is used like a bronzer.

Perhaps the most heinous mistake was to say that McEvoy's brush No. 23 was for contouring the nose (ridiculous). It is an awesome brush that can do the entire eye, under the brow, the crease, and the lid.

I don't know if you got your information from a brochure or from a stock person, but one thing is for certain: if you are so concerned with average women not getting taken at the cosmetic counter, then you should also not want them to get taken at the bookstore. After viewing your book I am left with one thought: is the return policy at Waldenbooks as liberal as the return policy in the cosmetics department at Nordstrom?

Anonymous, via e-mail

Dear Anonymous,

I bet you work for a cosmetic company's line at a department store, don't you? The tone of those letters I receive often tends to be the same. Nevertheless, you are right, I am concerned about women feeling ripped off, which is why if the bookstore where you bought my book won't take it back, I would be glad to refund your money via my publishing company. Simply send the book back to me at Beginning Press, 13075 Gateway Corporate Center, Suite 300, Tukwila, WA 98168.

Now I'd like to set the record straight. I chose the companies reviewed in my book according to a survey of a number of my readers (more than 2,000) on the lines they wanted me to include, and Monteil was on that list. That was more than three years ago. Monteil isn't in the fourth edition, but neither is Nina Ricci. Even though you may think it is an important line, I have never received a question about it, and I receive hundreds of letters and e-mails a week.

Your comment about serums versus moisturizers is classic cosmetics doublespeak. No matter what you've been told about what these serums are intended to do, as far as the formulations are concerned (and you only need to look at the ingredient list on the label to check this out), they are nothing more than moisturizers. They have no capability to do anything else, despite the hype about toning, nourishing, reducing stress, healing, and a litany of other meaningless, unsubstantiated claims. Besides, layering products, moisturizer over moisturizer (what you call a serum), is a problem for skin. According to research published in *Cosmetic Dermatology* magazine, *Drug and Cosmetic Industry* magazine, and *Cosmetics & Toiletries* magazine, overmoisturizing the skin can inhibit the skin's healing process.

You're right, I grouped the two YSL Touch products together because of their similarity in consistency and performance, but, yes, technically they are different products. Why and how that matters I'm not sure, but I will correct it in future editions of my book.

In regard to my "most heinous" crime of describing the McEvoy brush incorrectly (at least according to you; I was relying on the saleswomen who helped me at the counter), if that's my most horrendous mistake, I am relieved that I must be doing much that is right. However, I do understand and share your concern about trusting what I am told at cosmetics counters.

But speaking of heinous mistakes, the cosmetics industry makes more heinous mistakes than I can count, not the least of which are: continuing to sell sunscreens that can cause skin cancer because they don't contain ingredients that protect skin from UVA radiation; moisturizers that supposedly won't clog pores but contain pore-clogging ingredients; products labeled as good for sensitive skin that contain seriously irritating ingredients; so-called anti-aging products (more than 1,700 launched last year, with another couple of thousand planned for this year) that can't prevent aging in any manner; and, well, the list is too long to recite in a letter, but you get my drift.

On the other hand, many of you find my work helpful, and I receive thousands of these comments a month; while this may sound a bit selfish, don't hold back, the good thoughts are greatly appreciated!

Dear Paula,

I just finished reading your book *Don't Go to the Cosmetics Counter Without Me*, and I have to admit that I'm a little depressed. You wouldn't believe what I calculated I have spent on ineffective, outrageously priced cosmetics purchased over the last two decades. (I guess you would believe it, given your experience, but it shocked the heck out of me!) The number of wasted dollars totals in the thousands (several of them), making my mild malaise more than understandable. I've regrouped only because I'm the kind of person who tends to look forward, not behind me. I am—as we speak—bouncing back and saving money, and taking better care of my skin than ever before.

My quick recovery is due to the fact that I feel educated and armed to deal with the cosmetics companies in a manner that I did not think was possible. As a sales and marketing executive myself, in another industry, I always knew that I was being sold to with claims of questionable validity. However, the advertising is so damn slick and convincing that even I, seasoned professional that I am, just wasn't able to stop myself!

If you really begin to peel back the layers of the onion, what nearly all of these ad campaigns are promising is not only glorious skin, but a change in the quality of your life! The infomercials and TV shopping networks have perfected this to a science, not only on cosmetics, but on every single product that they sell! Listen carefully, and before you know it, you too will begin to believe that, although you were unattractive before, your new purchase of the Super Duper Wrinkle Cream will change all that. Heck, it's even going to change how other people react to you! My comments might sound a bit ridiculous, but they're only a slight exaggeration of what actually goes on in the world of cosmetics.

All I can say is a heartfelt thank you, and a request to please keep up the great work. You are providing an invaluable consumer service. I only wish I had found you years ago!

Depressed but Smarter

Dear Smarter,

Thank you for your wonderful, supportive comments. I'm glad my work has been helpful for you. The best news is that you are now an informed woman who won't be hurting her skin or wasting her money.

The Reviews

I decided early on in organizing this book that the best way to organize the list of companies was alphabetically. There were many reasons for this but primarily it was because women instinctively turn first to the products they are using to see if I agree with their impressions and alphabetical is the easiest way to make your way through a list. The second major reason was that alphabetical would imply no hierarchy, which is how I truly feel. Unfortunately these first two lines are not the ones I would have selected to start with. They are two disappointing acne lines that can't help skin and may actually cause more problems. Still it's a start—and there are a lot more happy, unhappy, and so-so faces to come.

Aapri (Skin Care Only)

Aapri is owned by the Gillette Company; for more information about Aapri products call (617) 463-3000.

☹ **Aapri Apricot Facial Scrub Gentle Formula** *($4.29 for 2 ounces)*. Sodium lauryl sulfate (SLS) is the third ingredient in this scrub, which hardly makes this gentle; if anything it is considered one of the more sensitizing detergent cleansing agents around. This product also contains lanolin oil and waxes known for causing breakouts.

☹ **Aapri Apricot Facial Scrub Original Formula** *($4.61 for 4 ounces)* is similar to the one above and the same review applies.

Acne-Statin (Skin Care Only)

This line is still being sold and it has been around for years. Does that indicate a modicum of success? Yes, but does it mean it's good for you? I doubt it. **Acne-Statin** *($39.95 for the 4-ounce Skin Cleanser and Moisturizer and the 4-ounce Cream)*. How does Acne-Statin claim to deal with acne? Well, not very directly that's for sure, because Acne-Statin doesn't list ingredients on its label. Due to a grandfather clause in the FDA's mandatory ingredient listing rules, Acne-Statin doesn't have to list any of its nonactive ingredients. Nevertheless, they do have to list the active ingredients, so what isn't a mystery is that Acne-Statin's Cleanser & Moisturizer contains 0.5% triclosan, a standard disinfectant found in many antibacterial products. The Cream contains 0.5% salicylic acid. The other 99.5% of these products is composed of standard cosmetics ingredients that hold no hope for acne sufferers, and the consistency of both is suspect for containing ingredients that are probably not the best for someone with breakouts or oily skin.

It turns out the Federal Trade Commission (FTC) seems to agree with my conclusions. According to a press release from the FTC "Acne-Statin ... has agreed to pay a $200,000 civil penalty to settle Federal Trade Commission charges that ads touting the product as an effective treatment for severe or cystic acne were deceptive. The claims also violate a 1979 order prohibiting Dr. Atida H. Karr from making unsubstantiated claims about the effectiveness or superiority of any acne preparation she markets, the agency alleges. Karr and her Beverly Hills, California, based companies sold Acne-Statin and currently sell the Acne-Statin Kit.

"The 1979 order prohibits Karr and her firms from advertising the effectiveness or superiority of any acne preparation unless the claims are supported by competent and reliable scientific or medical evidence. Karr paid $175,000 into a consumer refund account as part of the 1979 settlement of the initial case."

Acne-Statin's claims sound sweeping and impressive. But as consumers, we are given only advertising and hype to help us make a decision. The ingredient list, the only verifiable truth on any cosmetics label, is kept a secret. If the Acne-Statin products could cure acne, as the ads and infomercial claim, who would have acne? Bottom line: The active ingredients listed can't do what the product claims it can do, and moreover, despite the age of these formulations (they've been around for more than a decade) they haven't updated their formulation either.

Adrien Arpel/Signature Club A (Skin Care Only)

Adrien Arpel sold her department-store line and the right to use her own name in any publicity or marketing ventures. So, when Arpel started selling a new line of cosmetics on the Home Shopping Network, she legally could not use her own name for endorsement purposes, hence her infomerical line is called "Signature Club A." It is interesting to note that whenever Arpel is on HSN, she is never introduced as "Adrien Arpel." She is always introduced as just "Adrien." Due to this legal technicality "Adrien Arpel" has nothing to do with the department-store cosmetics line bearing her name. There are only a handful of these left in the U.S. and Canada, and they have not changed in years, though they have been and still are in desperate need of a face-lift.

Adrien Arpel has been very busy on the Home Shopping Network (HSN) selling her Signature Club A skin-care products, especially her instant-lift products and Skin Vacuuming Home Facial Kit. There are also a host of scrubs and AHA products in that line, which all combined (and you are supposed to use all of this stuff) would take off every inch of skin you have.

Like most infomercial lines, the promise being sold is either about curing acne or erasing wrinkles. Arpel excels in the latter, but there is also the guarantee of blemish-free skin as well. Arpel sells her products as miracles that deliver newly smooth, flawless skin with instant success. But there are no miracles to be found in this line, and I have yet to hear Arpel discuss sunscreens. To find so many instant-lift products with no sunscreens is about as funny as finding cars without brakes. Maybe even funnier is the vacuum machine with a rotation device and pumice head for massage, and a suction device for who knows what. Either way, the trauma this machine delivers to the skin is problematic for surfaced capillaries and general irritation. Overmanipulating and scrubbing the face isn't anything I would ever recommend, and that's what this vacuum machine does. The pumice stone might as well be sandpaper; the skin just doesn't need that kind of abrasion.

Arpel also promotes the effectiveness of her Big "7" Wondercover Compact as being the only skin perfecting makeup you need. This group of seven concealers in a range of colors from blue to mauve, peach, shiny, beige, medium beige, and dark tan is a greasy mess that may be OK for very dry skin, but which will easily crease if you place it around the eyes or other lined areas of the face. Mauve, peach, and blue only give the skin a strange cast; to cover face problems, all it takes is one concealer and one good foundation that doesn't crease. For more information about Adrien Arpel please call (800) 627-9126 or (212) 333-7700.

Signature Club A by Adrien Arpel

☹ **Signature A French Vanilla Meltdown, Cleansing Creme for Face & Eyes** *($18 for 4 ounces)* contains mostly water, thickeners, silicone, vanilla extract, more thickeners, fragrance, vitamin A, thickener, and preservatives. This is just a wipe-off, cold cream–type cleanser with a tiny amount of vitamin A thrown in for effect. Even if the vitamin could help, you would be wiping it away before it had a chance to work. And I never recommend wiping off makeup.

☺ **$$$ Signature A Vitamin C Complex, Illumination Source** *($24.50 for 6 ounces)* contains mostly water, slip agent, vitamins, plant extracts, preservatives, coloring agents, and fragrance. This toner is OK, but don't expect much from the vitamins in this one either. The vitamin C used here is ascorbic acid, which is not one of the forms recommended in the research I've seen. Other than that, it shouldn't be a problem, but it also won't be of much use.

☺ **Signature A AHA Daily Face Wash** *($15.50 for 6 ounces)* is a standard detergent-based cleanser that can be somewhat drying depending on your skin type. It has an assortment of AHAs and some vitamins thrown in, but the pH is wrong for it to be an effective AHA, and even if any of the ingredients were effective they would be rinsed off before they had a chance to have any effect.

☹ **AHA Toner** *($15.50 for 6 ounces)* contains mostly witch hazel, salt, vitamin A, and AHAs. It also contains some peppermint and spearmint. Between the salt and the mints, the irritation for the face would be significant. Salt should never be left on the skin.

☺ $$$ **The 5 Essentials Creme Face and The 5 Essentials Creme Eye** *($24.95 for 4 ounces of face creme and 0.5 ounce of eye creme).* The Creme Face and Creme Eye are virtually identical and have the same assortment of AHAs as the toner and the cleanser above. If these products had the right pH, you would be well into AHA overkill by now. No need to worry, this is not an effective AHA product, though it would be a good moisturizer for someone with dry skin.

☹ **Soft Resurfacing Peel** *($14.50 for 2 ounces)* contains mostly very thick, heavy waxes. Rubbing wax over the skin can take off skin cells, but it can also clog pores and cause breakouts. There are much better ways to exfoliate the skin than with this product.

☺ $$$ **Alpha Hydroxy and Retinol Soft Scrub with Vanilla Bean** *($14.50 for 2 ounces).* Not another AHA product? But don't worry, the pH isn't right for the AHAs to be effective. This is a standard, water-soluble cleanser, and the scrub particles in it come from ground-up vanilla beans. This isn't terrible, but why bother? Cetaphil Gentle Skin Cleanser mixed with baking soda would be far more effective.

☹ **Instant Lift and Hold for Face and Neck** *($21.95 for 8 vials)* contains plenty of alcohol so the resulting slight swelling should make your skin look smoother. Other than that, this is just plant extracts and water-binding agents; it won't lift or hold any part of your skin anywhere.

☹ **Instant Lift and Hold for Eyes** *($24.95 for 8 vials)* is similar to the lift for the face and the same review applies.

☹ **The Big "7" Wondercover Wheel** *($20)* is a group of seven concealers in a range of colors from blue to mauve, peach, shiny, beige, medium beige, and dark tan. This is a greasy mess that may be OK for very dry skin, but if you place it around the eyes or other lined areas of the face it will easily crease. Mauve, peach, and blue only give the skin a strange cast; to cover face problems, all it takes is one concealer and one good foundation that doesn't crease.

Adrien Arpel

☺ $$$ **Adult Oily Skin Sea Foam Gel Cleanser** *($19 for 4 ounces)* is a standard, detergent-based, water-soluble cleanser that can be for anyone, not just adults, with normal to oily skin.

☺ $$$ **Aromafleur Petal Daily Cleanser** *($21 for 4.5 ounces)* is a detergent-based, water-soluble cleanser that would work well for someone with normal to oily skin. It has its share of plant extracts, which are at the end of the ingredient list, but even if they could benefit the skin (they can't) it wouldn't matter, since they all get washed down the drain.

☹ **Foam Cleanser** *($20 for 8 ounces)* is a plant oil–based cleanser that doesn't quite take off all the makeup and can leave a greasy film on the face. It has its share of interesting plant extracts and water-binding agents, but in a cleanser any benefit from these is washed away. It also contains peppermint which can cause significant skin irritation.

☹ **Freeze-Dried Collagen Protein Cleanser, Super Dry Skin Formula** *($20 for 4 ounces)* has changed its name; it was "Embryonic Collagen," though the ingredient listing has remained the same. I imagine the notion of associating an embryo with younger skin is no longer something a consumer can swallow. Regardless, this is merely a detergent-based, water-soluble cleanser using sodium lauryl sulfate, which is known for causing irritation. There are also several thickening agents that are difficult to rinse off without a washcloth. The showcase ingredient is calf skin, and although it may be a good water-binding agent, in a cleanser any benefit is washed down the drain.

☹ **Sea Kelp Cleanser** *($20 for 4 ounces)* contains mostly water, mineral oil, thickeners, petrolatum, more thickeners, and pumice (scrub agent). This cleanser is a fairly greasy scrub that uses a rather formidable abrasive. Despite the name, there's only a small amount of sea kelp, and the mineral oil and petrolatum can leave a greasy residue on the skin.

☹ **Coconut Cleanser** *($20 for 4 ounces)* is a cold cream that contains mostly water, plant oils, and some lanolin. This is a wipe-off cleanser that can leave a greasy film on the skin.

☹ **Honey and Almond Scrub** *($32 for 5 ounces)* has almonds that will help slough skin, although Cetaphil Gentle Skin Cleanser and baking soda mixed with a little water will do the same thing for a lot less. The lemon in this product can be a significant skin irritant.

☹ **Lemon & Lime Freshener** *($18.50 for 8 ounces)* is an alcohol-free freshener that instead delivers several other potential skin irritants, including balm mint, lemon peel, and lime extract. Ouch!

☹ **Flower Extract Freshener** *($18.50 for 8 ounces)* is nothing more than witch hazel and plant extracts, several of which, such as lemon flower, lemon grass, and geranium flower, can be skin irritants.

☺ **$$$ Bio Cellular Night Cream with AHA** *($35 for 1.25 ounces)* contains about 4% AHAs and an entire arsenal of water-binding agents. It is a far better moisturizer for dry skin than it is an AHA product. The scientific name won't impress your skin cells and the price is unwarranted for what you get.

☺ **$$$ Bio-Cellular Anti Serum with Alpha Hydroxy Complex** *($52.50 for ten 0.23-ounce vials)* is essentially some thickener agents, AHAs, and water-binding agents. Much like the night cream above, this serum doesn't have the right pH to make it an effective exfoliant, though it can be a good lightweight moisturizer for someone with dry skin.

☺ **$$$ Bio-Cellular Night Eye Gelee with AHA Complex** *($26 for 0.4 ounce).* How many AHA products does one face need? Thankfully, none of these are effective exfoliants, so don't worry. Basically this product is the "greasy kid stuff," containing mostly mineral oil, lanolin, plant oil, petrolatum, and thickeners. If you have extremely dry skin, this product would be just fine.

☹ **Eyelastic Lift** *($40 for 30 capsules and 0.5 ounce of the creme)* is a two-part product: you're supposed to mix the **Extra Strength Puff Deflator Capsules** with the **Eyelastic Lift and Firm Creme.** It won't lift the eye anywhere. The Puff Deflator (do you believe that name?) contains mostly silicone, water-binding agents, placental extract (doesn't say whose, but whatever kind of placenta it is, give me a break), and preservatives. The rather common ingredients make for a good moisturizer, but that's about it. Placenta extract can't make your skin one hour younger, no matter where it comes from. The Lift and Firm Creme contains mostly water, water-binding agent, silicone, mineral oil, oat flour, plant extract, and more thickeners. It works as a paste and contains some moisturizing ingredients. All this is a complete waste of time and money.

☺ **$$$ Skinlastic Lift Daily Transparent Tightening & Firming Lift** *($40 for 1.7 ounces—18 vials)* is a good lightweight moisturizer for normal to slightly dry skin, but that's about it. If you believe it will lift your skin, though, I have a bridge I'd like to sell you.

☺ **$$$ Moisturizing Blotting Lotion** *($23.50 for 2 ounces)* is a greasy mix of mineral oil, lanolin, lard, and water-binding agents. This is a very rich, thick moisturizer, best for someone with extremely dry skin.

☹ **Morning After Super Moisturizer, SPF 20** *($32.50 for 1 ounce)* does not contain any UVA protecting ingredients, and is not recommended.

☹ **Oil Control Moisturizer, SPF 15** *($32.50 for 3 ounces)* does not contain any UVA protecting ingredients, and is not recommended.

☹ **Skin Correction Complex Four Cremes in One with Alpha Hydroxy Complex** *($34.50 for 2 ounces)* calls itself "the only creme you will ever need." What about a sunscreen? It also contains *minimal* AHAs. This is an overpriced but good moisturizer for someone with dry skin.

☺ **$$$ Swiss Formula Day Cream #12 with Collagen** *($50 for 1 ounce)* is a very emollient, rich moisturizer for someone with very dry skin. It claims to be nongreasy, but that doesn't jibe with the inclusion of mineral oil and lanolin, both fairly greasy ingredients. It also contains brewer's yeast, but that has no effect on wrinkles.

☺ **$$$ Swiss Formula Day Eye Creme, with Vitamin A Palmitate and Col-**

lagen *($27.50 for 0.5 ounce)* is similar to the cream above, only with a tiny amount of vitamin A added. The same review applies.

☺ $$$ **Vital Velvet Moisturizer** *($23.50 for 2 ounces)* contains mostly water, standard water-binding agent, lanolin, thickeners, mineral oil, more thickeners, oils, collagen, and preservatives. This is a fairly emollient moisturizer and would work well for extremely dry skin only.

☺ $$$ **Adult Oily Skin Detoxifying Spray** *($18.50 for 8 ounces)* is a toner with some plant extracts, water-binding agents, and detergent cleansing agents. It won't detox anything, but it is a decent toner for normal to dry skin. It isn't appropriate for oily skin or acne.

☹ $$$ **Aromafleur Flower Petal and Botanical Extract Masque** *($24 for 4 ounces)* does contain plenty of plants, so if you have allergies this mask could be a problem. Other than that, it is an OK lightweight mask, with no real benefit for the skin.

☹ **Aromafleur Flower Petal Mini-Facial in a Jar** *($29.50 for 4.5 ounces)* is basically a good moisturizer with several plant extracts that can be a problem for the skin.

☹ **Bio-Cellular Lip Line Cream with Alpha Hydroxy Complex** *($22.50 for 0.5 ounce)*. No one needs a specialty AHA product just for around the lips, but then this one doesn't contain enough AHA or have the right pH to qualify, so it doesn't matter anyway. This is just a very emollient moisturizer for any part of the face.

☺ $$$ **Freeze-Dried Protein Lip Peel and Salve** *($39.50 for 1 ounce of peel and 0.25 ounce of salve)* is a two-part system quite similar to BeautiControl's Lip Apeel that I have recommended quite often (which is also half the price of this one), and I have a similar one for slightly less. All of these work the same; the peel is a wax you rub over the lip and the salve is just a good lip gloss. It's great for preventing dry lips but none of these will do anything for wrinkles.

☹ **Sea Mud Mask** *($24.50 for 4 ounces)* is just clay, alcohol, and film former. To sum it up, this is a lot of money for little to no skin benefit.

☹ **Underglow Line Minimizing Moisturizer** *($35 for 1.25 ounces)* places a hairspray-like layer of film over the face. That can make skin look smoother, but also has a somewhat tacky feel. Other than that, this is a lightweight moisturizer for someone with normal to slightly dry skin.

☹ **Vegetable Peel Off** *($20 for 2 ounces)* does peel off, but that serves no function, and it contains peppermint, which is a potent skin irritant.

☹ **Wrinkle Peeling Gel** *($32.50 for 3.25 ounces)* contains mostly alcohol and film former. The film former leaves a plastic-like layer over the face that, when peeled off, does exfoliate a layer of skin, but the irritation from the alcohol and film former is not worth it.

Alexandra de Markoff

Alexandra de Markoff has had its problems of ownership. It was owned by Revlon, then sold to a small company called Parlex, and was recently sold again. The change in ownership and the lack of direction has hurt this line and the number of stores carrying it has declined. Despite the change in owners, for some women Alexandra de Markoff has retained its image as a prestige line of cosmetics offering the same illusion of affluence as do Chanel or Borghese. However, don't expect anything new; there are no lightweight moisturizers, no AHAs or BHA here, and most of the sunscreens are at best described as poor.

Markoff remains attractive for a longtime older clientele who like the elegant mental picture this line exudes. What this line does have lots of are products aimed at women with parched, dry skin. This is most apparent in the foundations, which are either very greasy or very emollient. Even the matte-finish foundation is not all that matte, but feels very moisturizing, and the ingredient list supports that contention. In general, the line is limited and, for the money, relatively unimpressive. For more information about Alexandra de Markoff, call (800) 366-7470.

Alexandra de Markoff Skin Care

☺ **Balancing Cleanser** *($28.50 for 6 ounces)* is a mineral oil–based cleanser that also contains a detergent cleansing agent, thickeners, and a group of fragrant oils. This can be a good cleanser for someone with very dry skin, but it may leave skin feeling greasy. The fragrant oils can be a problem for sensitive skin.

☹ **Comfort Cleanser** *($40 for 4 ounces)* is a standard mineral oil–based wipe-off cleanser. This is a lot of money for oil and standard waxy thickeners. The cleanser also contains protein and elastin, but they are only emollients and are useless in a cleanser because they are wiped away.

☺ **$$$ Complete Foaming Cleanser with Ivy and Birch** *($28.50 for 6 ounces)* is a standard detergent-based wash-off cleanser. Several of the cleansing agents are more drying, which makes this cleanser more of a problem than most. There are a host of fragrant oils in here which can be skin sensitizers.

☹ **Luxury Cream Cleanser, with Aloe and Rosewater** *($40 for 6 ounces)* is a cold cream–type cleanser with a host of thickening agents, plant extracts, and vitamins. Even if the plant extracts could have an effect they would be wiped away, but these plants are useless, and several of them are potential skin irritants.

☹ **Luxury Facial Cleansing Bar** *($20 for 4 ounces)* is a very overpriced, standard bar cleanser. The ingredients that keep bar cleansers in their bar form can clog pores and the cleansing agents can be drying for most skin types.

☺ **Eye Makeup Remover Pads** *($18 for 60 pads)* contain a standard detergent-based eye-makeup remover with plant extract. They also contain witch hazel, which can be a skin irritant.

☹ **Fresh Solution with Sage and Witch Hazel** *($26 for 7.5 ounces)* contains mostly water, water-binding agent, calamine, clay, witch hazel, plant extracts, more water-binding agents, vitamin B, mineral salts, thickeners, plant oils, and pre-servatives. This is a lot of money for what is essentially calamine lotion. Several ingredients here—calamine, clove oil, witch hazel, and sandalwood oil—are serious potential irritants.

☺ **$$$ Luxury Skin Toner, with Aloe Vera and Comfrey** *($28.50 for 6 ounces)* is a very good irritant-free toner with a handful of plant extracts and water-binding agents.

☺ **$$$ Soothing Lotion, Alcohol Free, for Dry or Sensitive Skins** *($48 for 4 ounces)* is a very good irritant-free toner with a handful of plant extracts and water-binding agents.

☺ **$$$ Compensation Skin Serum** *($65 for 2 ounces)* contains mostly water, silicone, plant extracts (tea water), mineral oil, thickener, plant oils, vitamins, water-binding agents, and preservatives. This is a very good emollient oil for someone with very dry skin, and it contains a small amount of antioxidant, but the $65 price tag doesn't make sense.

☹ **Countess Isserlyn Moisture 364 +, with SPF 15** *($45 for 1.8 ounces)* doesn't contain titanium dioxide, zinc oxide, or avobenzone, and is not recommended.

☺ **Daytime Moisturizer** *($32 for 2 ounces)* contains isopropyl myristate, noto-rious for causing breakouts; in fact, it's the first ingredient on the list. Otherwise, it is just a standard ordinary moisturizer for dry skin. However, because this product does not contain sunscreen it is best to wear it only at night.

☺ **$$$ Fresh Moisture Lotion** *($45 for 4 ounces)* contains mostly water, plant extracts, glycerin, several thickeners, vitamins, plant oils, water-binding agents, silicone, and preservatives. This is an OK lightweight moisturizer for someone with normal to slightly dry skin, and it contains a small quantity of antioxidants. There are several fragrant oils in this product that can be problem for sensitive skin types.

☹ **Moisture Reserve Cream SPF 8** *($55 for 2.25 ounces)* does not contain titanium dioxide, zinc oxide, or avobenzone, and is not recommended.

☹ **Oil-Free Matte Moisture** *($38 for 4 ounces)* is a confused product. It con-tains water, talc, witch hazel, thickeners, vitamins, and water-binding agents. The talc can absorb oil but that's what pressed powder is for. All this product does is lay down some waxy ingredients that aren't needed for oily skin, while the talc probably just ends up absorbing the emollients in the product.

☺ **$$$ Skin Renewal Therapy Restorative Eye Cream** *($42 for 0.5 ounce)* won't renew anything, but it can be a good, though absurdly expensive, moisturizer.

It contains mostly water, thickeners, plant oil, more thickeners, water-binding agents, silicone, anti-irritants, and preservatives.

☺ **$$$ Skin Tight Firming Eye Cream** *($50 for 0.4 ounce)* won't firm skin, but it is very emollient—good for someone with dry skin. It contains mostly water, thickeners, slip agents, shea butter, a long list of additional thickeners, film former, antioxidants, several water-binding agents, plant oil, silicone, and preservatives.

☺ **$$$ Sleep Tight Firming Night Cream with Comfrey** *($60 for 1.7 ounces)* doesn't contain enough comfrey to warrant a mention. It is a standard moisturizer with thickeners and water-binding agents. It also has a long list of fragrant oils, of which several are strong potential skin sensitizers.

☹ **Vital 10 New Age Skin Complex with Marigold, SPF 6** *($65 for 2 ounces)* isn't vital, it's pointless. SPF 6 isn't adequate to protect the skin from sun, and it doesn't contain titanium dioxide, zinc oxide, or avobenzone for UVA protection.

☺ **$$$ Weekly Revitalizing Clay Mask, with Green Tea and Sage** *($30 for 2 ounces)* is a fairly standard clay mask with thickeners, witch hazel, water-binding agents, vitamins, and plant extracts. For a clay mask it's just fine.

☹ **Weekly Revitalizing Exfoliating Mask, with Pineapple and Papaya** *($30 for 2 ounces)* contains mostly water, thickener, plant extracts, and preservatives. The plant extracts here are supposed to sound like they are connected to AHAs and enzymes. They aren't. This is just a mask with little benefit.

☹ **Weekly Revitalizing Moisture Mask, with Jasmine and Avocado** *($30 for 2 ounces)* is a moisturizer with some talc and some very irritating plant oils, including menthol, clove, and rose oil. This mask is not recommended.

☹ **Extra Help Gel for Lips** *($20 for 1 ounce)* offers minimal help for dry lips. It has almost no emollients or skin-softening ingredients. It can put a film over the lips to make them look temporarily smooth but it won't feel very good, particularly in the winter.

Alexandra de Markoff Makeup

☹ <u>FOUNDATION:</u> **Countess Isserlyn Liquid Makeup** *($45)* is a mineral oil–based foundation in which the mineral oil floats to the top and the color lies at the bottom. You have to shake this product really hard to get it to mix together, and even then it tends to separate on the skin. All of the colors for this line are just too peach or pink, and the colors also tend to darken once applied.

☹ **Countess Isserlyn Moisturizing Matte Makeup** *($45)* is identical to the makeup above except that it uses silicone instead of mineral oil. Although it feels less greasy, it is hardly matte. The oil in this foundation still rises to the top, and the color sits at the bottom of the bottle. Chances are pretty good the color will streak or separate on the skin when blending.

☺ **$$$ Countess Isserlyn Creme Makeup** *($45)* is more than creamy—it is very rich and emollient. The third ingredient is lanolin oil, which makes it appropriate only for someone with extremely dry skin. It has a rich texture and provides medium coverage. **Colors to consider: 82+, 88+, 91+, 92+. Colors to avoid because they are absurdly peach or pink: 71+, 72+, 76+, 86+, 89+, 96+, and 98+.**

☺ **$$$ Countess Isserlyn Soft Velvet Makeup Oil-Free** *($42.50)* is a fairly emollient liquid foundation providing medium coverage that feels quite soft and relatively velvety. Like all of the foundations in this line, the color selection is awful. Of all the shades only three have any relation to skin tone. The only ones to consider are: 81+, 82+, and 92+.

☹ **Countess Isserlyn Powder Creme Finish Makeup** *($32.50)* is a very soft cream-to-powder makeup that has a wonderful feel on the skin. However, the foundation colors are exceedingly poor, being either too peach or pink for most all skin tones.

☺ **CONCEALER:** The **Concealer** *($18.50)* is a tube concealer that comes in three very good colors and has a good consistency, though with a slight tendency to crease. **Disguise for Eyes** *($25)* is supposed to help eyeshadow stay on better. It doesn't.

☺ **$$$ POWDER: Countess Isserlyn Pressed Powder** *($30)* is a standard powder that comes in six very good colors (though Dusty Rose can be too peach for most skin tones). It has a wonderful soft, silky texture. **Moisturizing Loose Powder** *($35)* has a soft texture but is on the dry side, not moist, though the colors are OK.

☺ **$$$ BLUSH: Outlasting Moisturizing Powder Blush** *($30)* has a very soft silky finish and some amount of shine, too, though it's not all that intense. The price doesn't make sense for this very standard formulation but the colors are nice. **Face Shapers** *($30)* is a group of pressed-powder blushes, each one with two shades, one a tone of brown for contouring, the other a highlighter shade. It's a good idea, but there are far less expensive ways to create the same effect.

☹ **Moisturizing Powder Blush** *($30)* isn't even slightly moisturizing; all the colors are shiny, and I do not recommend any of them.

☹ **EYESHADOW:** The line offers a selection of duo eyeshadow sets called **Eye Shaper Duets** *($27)*. While the consistency is nice, all of the colors are shiny, and the color combinations are strange.

☺ **$$$ EYE AND BROW SHAPER: Smooth Stroke Eyeliner** *($18.50)* is a standard, twist-up eye pencil similar to dozens of other pencils on the market. You guessed it: overpriced and nothing to write home about. **Easy on the Eyes Eyeliner** *($18.50)* has a slightly smoother finish than the Smooth Stroke, but that's splitting hairs. The only difference is that this one has a smudge tip at one end. **Professional Secret Liquid Eyeliner** *($18)* is just a standard liquid eyeliner with a too-stiff applicator. This product is identical to Almay's I-Liner, which sells for, you guessed it, one-fourth the price. **Brow Finisher** *($18.50)* is essentially identical to the Smooth Stroke Eyeliner, except that one end has a brush to smooth out the line.

☺ **$$$ <u>LIPSTICK:</u>** It was easy to predict that Alexandra de Markoff would have a lipstick similar to Revlon's ColorStay because at one point Revlon owned this line. It's called **Lips Like Hers** *($17.50)*. It is nothing more than a knockoff with a higher price tag and less impressive colors. **Lasting Luxury Lipsticks** *($17)* are fairly glossy, cream lipsticks with a slight tint, so they have some staying power. **Under Color for Lips** *($25)* comes in two colors: Clear and Neutral. It is designed to keep lipstick from bleeding but it doesn't do a very good job. **Outlasting Smooth Stroke Lip Liner** *($18.50)* is a standard, very overpriced twist-up pencil. **Lip Definer** *($18.50)* is a standard pencil with a lip brush at one end. Max Factor has the exact same thing for one-fourth the price.

☺ **$$$ <u>MASCARA:</u>** **Professional Secrets Mascara** *($20)* builds surprisingly long lashes with a good deal of thickness.

☹ **Lash Amplifier** *($18.50)* is a clear mascara that is supposed to enhance the lashes, but it's no better than an extra coat of mascara. Besides, if the regular mascara is any good, why would it need an amplifier in the first place?

Almay

Almay has a long-standing reputation for being one of the few lines that is 100% hypoallergenic. Given that the FDA has never issued specific guidelines about which ingredients are less likely to cause allergic reactions, this is an admirable marketing feat. For the most part, Almay does a good job of eliminating well-known irritants such as fragrance, formaldehyde compounds, lanolin, and lauryl sulfate compounds. But those may not be the ingredients that cause your particular skin problems.

Almay excels in several areas. It makes some good mascaras, great blushes and lipsticks, two excellent under-eye concealers, and two very good foundations. Almay's Amazing Lasting line has some of the best ultra-matte products on the market, which is not so surprising when you know that Almay is owned by Revlon, the company that originated ultra-matte technology. On the other hand, it is possible to take the matte craze too far.

The line also has some excellent skin-care products and one of the largest selections of them in the business. Unfortunately, many of the products listed are not found reliably at every drugstore, which makes finding the product you're interested in a 50/50 proposition.

Almay Skin Care

☺ **Anti-Bacterial Foaming Cleanser** *($2.91 for 7.75 ounces)* is a standard detergent-based water-soluble cleanser that contains a small amount of triclosan, an antibacterial agent (the same one found in Acne-Statin products), but the effects of this or any disinfectant are lost in a cleanser because it is so quickly washed away.

☹ **Clear Complexion Clarifying Cleanser** (*$8 for 5 ounces*) is a standard, detergent-based water-soluble cleanser that is more drying than most. This one also contains BHA (salicylic acid), which is unnecessary in a cleanser because it is washed away before it can get inside a pore and have an effect. It isn't good to get this in your eyes.

☹ **Clear Complexion Clarifying Facial Bar for All Skin Types** (*$5.89 for 4 ounces*) is a standard bar cleanser that can be fairly drying for most skin types, while the ingredients that keep the bar in its bar form can clog pores. This one also contains BHA (salicylic acid), which is unnecessary in a cleanser because it is washed away before it can get inside a pore and have an effect. It isn't good to get this in your eyes.

☺ **Deep Cleansing Cold Cream** (*$2.60 for 4 ounces*) is a traditional mineral oil–based cold cream that needs to be wiped off and that will leave the skin feeling greasy. I don't recommend wipe-off cleansers, although if you're looking for cold cream, this is as good as any.

☺ **Deep Cleansing Cold Cream Pump (Water Rinseable Formula)** (*$2.72 for 8 ounces*) isn't all that rinseable. It contains mineral oil, and that's hard to rinse off with water. It may be good for someone with very dry skin, but only maybe.

☹ **Cold Cream Cleansing Bar** (*$2.25 for two 4-ounce bars*) is a standard bar soap that contains mineral oil to help cut the irritation from the soap. However, the soap is still irritating due to the cleansing agent, and the ingredients that keep the bar in its bar form can clog pores.

☺ **Moisture Balance Cleansing Lotion for Normal/Combination Skin** (*$7.69 for 7.25 ounces*) is a mineral oil–based cleanser that does not rinse off well without the aid of a washcloth, and it leaves some makeup behind. If you have normal skin you will find this cleanser somewhat greasy; if you have combination skin, it will feel terrible. If you have extremely dry skin and use a washcloth (which I don't recommend because of irritation), it is passable.

☺ **Moisture Renew Cleansing Cream for Dry Skin** (*$4.50 for 4.75 ounces*) is similar to the cleansing lotion above, and the same review applies.

☺ **Sensitive Care Cleansing Cream for Super Sensitive Skin** (*$4.48 for 3.75 ounces*) is almost identical to the cream above, and the same review applies.

☺ **Sensitive Skin Foaming Cleanser** (*$2.79 for 7.75 ounces*) is a detergent-based water-soluble cleanser that isn't all that special for sensitive skin, except that it does contain a small quantity of anti-irritants. This would be good for someone with oily skin, but it could also be drying and irritating, particularly for someone with sensitive skin.

☺ **Oil Control Cleansing Gel for Oily Skin** (*$7.59 for 7.25 ounces*) is a standard detergent-based water-soluble cleanser that can be good for someone with oily skin. However, it is only a cleanser, and nothing in it will control or stop oil. It does contain a small amount of menthol, which serves no purpose whatsoever for skin care, but can irritate the skin and eyes.

☺ **Time-Off Age Smoothing Cleansing Lotion** *($8.39 for 7.25 ounces)* is a standard mineral oil–based cleanser that contains methoxypropylgluconamide, which is a good water-binding agent that doesn't have much to do in a cleansing lotion. This cleanser doesn't rinse off all that well, and it tends to leave a greasy film on the skin.

☺ **Moisturizing Eye Makeup Remover Lotion** *($4.39 for 2 ounces)* and **Moisturizing Eye Makeup Remover Pads** *($3.29 for 35 pads)* are just mineral oil and some slip agents. They will wipe off eye makeup, but they also make a greasy mess.

☺ **Moisturizing Gentle Gel Eye Makeup Remover** *($4.03 for 1.5 ounces)* is similar to the lotion above, only in gel form. It's still mineral oil, and it's still fairly greasy. It does contain vitamins but you would just be wiping them away.

☺ **Non-Oily Eye Makeup Remover Lotion** *($4.49 for 2 ounces)* and **Non-Oily Eye Makeup Remover Pads** *($2.80 for 35 pads)* are indeed non-oily; they are just lightweight detergent cleansing agents that cut through makeup. They are good, but the numerous other cleansers in this line should be fine for removing eye makeup. If you are stuck on eye-makeup remover, this one is just fine.

☺ **Non-Oily Eye Makeup Remover Gel** *($4.03 for 1.5 ounces)* is similar to the lotion above, and the same review applies.

☺ **Oil Control Complexion Scrub** *($6.89 for 4 ounces)* is a detergent-based water-soluble cleanser with abrasive scrub particles. It can be irritating to some skin types, and it won't stop or control oil. I wouldn't choose this over Cetaphil Gentle Skin Cleanser mixed together with some baking soda.

☺ **Clear Complexion Clarifying Tonic for All Skin Types** *($8 for 7.25 ounces)* isn't totally alcohol-free as the label claims because the second ingredient is witch hazel, which has some alcohol content. Nevertheless, this is could be considered an OK BHA product.

☹ **Moisture Renew Balance Toner for Dry Skin** *($7.69 for 7.25 ounces)* contains mostly water and alcohol, and the only thing it can do for the skin is cause irritation.

☹ **Moisture Balance Toner for Normal Skin** *($7.69 for 7.25 ounces)* contains ingredients almost identical to those in the toner above, and it too can irritate the skin. A completely useless product.

☹ **Oil Control Astringent for Oily Skin** *($7.69 for 7.25 ounces)* contains mostly alcohol and salicylic acid. The salicylic acid may be effective, but the alcohol just hurts skin.

☹ **Time-Off Age Smoothing Toner** *($8.39 for 7.25 ounces)* would be a rather soothing toner with its methoxypropylgluconamide (among several other good water-binding agents), but the second ingredient is witch hazel, and that can be a skin irritant.

☹ **Sensitive Care Toner for Super Sensitive Skin** *($6.57 for 7.25 ounces)* is similar to the toner above, and the same review applies.

☹ **Clear Complexion Eye Gel-Cream SPF 4** *($10.49 for 0.25 ounce)* does contain titanium dioxide as the active sunscreen agent but an SPF 4 is only 30 minutes of sun protection, so why bother? Anything less than an SPF 15 is a waste of your money and potentially damaging to your skin.

☹ **Clear Complexion Moisture Lotion SPF 8 for Normal to Oilier Skin** *($11.49 for 2 ounces)* doesn't contain zinc oxide, titanium dioxide, or avobenzone for UVA protection, and is not recommended.

☹ **Clear Complexion Moisture Cream SPF 8 for Normal to Drier Skin** *($11.49 for 1.7 ounces)* doesn't contain zinc oxide, titanium dioxide, or avobenzone, and is not recommended.

☹ **Double Action Daily Moisture Lotion SPF 8** *($7.29 for 4 ounces)* doesn't contain zinc oxide, titanium dioxide, or avobenzone, and is not recommended.

☺ **Moisture Balance Eye Cream for Normal Skin** *($6.79 for 0.5 ounce)* is a standard petrolatum-based moisturizer that would be good for someone with dry skin. It contains all the requisite vitamins and water-binding agents.

☺ **Moisture Balance Moisture Lotion for Normal/Combination Skin** *($9.99 for 4 ounces)* lists mineral oil as the second ingredient, and also contains several thickeners, film former, plant oil, vitamins, and even a small amount of petrolatum. Now, who in the world with combination skin would be happy with this formula? It could be good for someone with dry skin, though.

☺ **Moisture Balance Night Cream for Normal/Combination Skin** *($10.39 for 2 ounces)* is similar to the lotion above and the same review applies.

☹ **Moisture Balance Moisture Lotion SPF 15 for Normal/Combination Skin** *($7.39 for 4 ounces)* doesn't contain zinc oxide, titanium dioxide, or avobenzone, and is not recommended.

☺ **Moisture Renew Cream for Dry Skin** *($7.99 for 2 ounces)* is a standard mineral oil–based moisturizer with small amounts of vitamin A and water-binding agents. This would be a good moisturizer for someone with dry skin. The label suggests that it is greaseless, but calling mineral oil greaseless is just not accurate.

☺ **Moisture Renew Eye Cream for Dry Skin** *($6.79 for 0.5 ounce)* is a good moisturizer for dry skin, with mineral oil, plant oils, water-binding agents, and a tiny amount of vitamin A.

☺ **Moisture Renew Moisture Lotion for Dry Skin** *($9.99 for 4 ounces)* is almost identical to the Renew Creams above, and the same reviews apply, which means it is just fine for someone with dry skin.

☺ **Moisture Renew Night Cream for Dry Skin** *($7 for 2 ounces)* is almost identical to the Renew Creams above, and the same reviews apply, which means it is just fine for someone with dry skin.

☹ **Moisture Renew Moisture Lotion for Dry Skin SPF 15** *($10.59 for 4 ounces)* doesn't contain zinc oxide, titanium dioxide, or avobenzone, and is not recommended.

☺ **Perfect Moisture** *($5.68 for 4 ounces)* causes me to ask, if this one is perfect, what are all the other Almay moisturizers for? This is a good, simple moisturizer for someone with dry skin, with all the vitamins your skin could want, but it isn't perfect or all that different from many other moisturizers in the Almay lineup.

☺ **Sensitive Care Cream for Super Sensitive Skin** *($6.78 for 2 ounces)* is similar to many of the above moisturizers, which makes this one a good ordinary moisturizer for someone with dry skin.

☺ **Sensitive Care Moisture Lotion** *($8.48 for 4 ounces)* is a good but rather ordinary moisturizer for someone with dry skin.

☹ **Sensitive Care Eye Gel for Super Sensitive Skin** *($5.77 for 0.5 ounce)* contains witch hazel, which makes it suspect for sensitive skin, much less for someone with super-sensitive skin.

☺ **Stress Eye Gel** *($8.29 for 0.5 ounce)* contains mostly water, film former, slip agent, water-binding agents, and preservatives. Like many products that contain film-forming agents, this gel can temporarily make skin look smooth. It is a good lightweight moisturizer.

☺ **Time-Off Age Smoothing Moisture Lotion** *($11.49 for 2 ounces)* is a rather good, lightweight moisturizer for someone with normal to dry skin, and it has antioxidants. It contains mostly water, water-binding agents, several thickeners, vegetable oil, vitamins E and A, anti-irritant, more thickeners, and preservatives.

☺ **Time-Off Age Smoothing Eye Cream** *($8.49 for 0.5 ounce)* is almost identical to the moisturizers above, only somewhat more emollient. An eye cream isn't necessary, but this is still a good moisturizer.

☺ **Time-Off Age Smoothing Night Cream** *($9.69 for 2 ounces)* is similar to the lotion above, with the addition of a few fancy water-binding agents. This would be a very good moisturizer for someone with dry skin.

☹ **Time-Off Age Smoothing Moisture Lotion SPF 15** *($11.69 for 4 ounces)* doesn't contain zinc oxide, titanium dioxide, or avobenzone, and is not recommended.

☺ **Time-Off Lasting Moisture SPF 25** *($14.99 for 3.8 ounces)* is a good sunscreen with titanium dioxide for someone with dry skin. It has a similar base as the Time Off Age Smoothing Moisture Lotion. It contains salicylic acid, but the pH isn't low enough for it to be effective as an exfoliant.

☺ **Time Off Revitalizer Daily Solution** *($18 for 0.72 ounce)* and **Time Off Daily Solution Pads** *($18 for 112 pads)* contains a good concentration of salicylic acid (BHA) at the correct pH, making it a good exfoliant. However, it comes in a mineral-oil base, which isn't great for someone with skin prone to breakouts or skin that is oily. Because of the way BHA penetrates pores I only recommend these products for breakouts and blackheads.

☺ **$$$ Time-Off Wrinkle Defense Capsules with Micro-Fillers** *($12.49 for 0.29 ounce)* is an unbelievably expensive product. This stuff comes in at $44.96 an ounce! And for what? Not much. The contents are merely silicones, slip agent, water, water-binding agents, and some vitamins. It is a good moisturizer for someone with normal to somewhat dry skin.

☹ **Time-Off Wrinkle Defense Cream with Micro-Fillers** *($12.49 for 2 ounces)* is similar to the capsules above, but with sunscreen. The sunscreen ingredients do not include UVA protection, and the cream is not recommended.

☺ **Vitalizing Moisture Night Cream** *($7.29 for 2 ounces)* is a standard mineral oil–based moisturizer that also contains vitamin A and water-binding agents. It would be good for someone with dry skin.

☹ **SPF 15 Waterproof Moisturizing Lotion** *($5.40 for 4 ounces)* doesn't contain titanium dioxide, zinc oxide, or avobenzone and isn't recommended.

☺ **SPF 30 Waterproof Sunblock Sensitive Skin Formula** *($5.40 for 4 ounces)* is a part titanium dioxide sunscreen and can provide good, extended-wear sun protection. It also has some antioxidants which can be helpful for sun protection.

☹ **Oil Control Lotion for Oily Skin SPF 15** *($10.39 for 4 ounces)* doesn't contain titanium dioxide, zinc oxide, or avobenzone and isn't recommended.

☺ **Oil Control Anti-Blemish Gel for Oily Skin** *($4.75 for 2.3 ounces)* contains salicylic acid in a base of silicone that also contains talc and clay as oil absorbers. It is definitely absorbent and the pH is low enough for this to be effective.

☹ **Oil Control Lotion for Oily Skin** *($9.99 for 4 ounces)* is a confused product. It contains silicone, water-binding agents, and talc. The talc can absorb oil, but that's what pressed powder is for. All this product does is lay down some slick ingredients that aren't needed for oily skin, while the talc probably just ends up absorbing the emollients in the product.

☹ **Oil Control Overnight Treatment for Oily Skin** *($5.32 for 4 ounces)* can be a problem for oily skin for many reasons, but primarily the alcohol in here can be a skin irritant, while there is really nothing present to absorb oil.

☹ **Oil Control Clay Mask for Oily Skin** *($5.50 for 2.5 ounces)* contains water, clay, preservative, detergent cleanser, slip agents, more clay, and more preservatives. It won't control oil, and it is potentially irritating.

Almay Makeup

☺ **FOUNDATION:** Almay's foundations include **Time-Off Age Smoothing Makeup** *($5.52)*, **Sensitive Care Formula SPF 15 Cream to Powder Foundation** *($4.89)*, **Sensitive Care Formula SPF 8 Liquid Makeup** *($4.70)*, **Powder Wear Pressed Powder Foundation** *($5.71)*, **Clear Complexion Light & Perfect Makeup** *($6.79)*, **Clear Complexion Light & Perfect Compact Makeup SPF 8** *($7.29)*, and **Liquid** to Powder Makeup *($5.64)*. Unfortunately, testers are not available for any of them. That's regrettable, because most have excellent textures and very good color selections. But no matter how good the foundation, if you get the color wrong, it looks bad. By the way, Almay, if you are listening, consider reducing this overwhelming list of foundations and concentrate on just a few types while expanding the color selection. Maybe then you could invest in some testers, make things less confusing for the consumer, and help a more diverse group of women!

☺ **Amazing Lasting Makeup SPF 6** *($7.35)* comes awfully close to being amazing, at least in terms of staying power and color choices, but SPF 6 is a very unamazing number. Other than that, the colors, though limited to light to medium skin tones, are wonderfully neutral. It provides a smooth, dry, unmovable, ultra-matte finish. If the SPF could be at least a 10 with titanium dioxide, I would give this one a much better rating, but as it is, for someone with oily skin, which is the skin type this makeup is best for, it would require an additional sunscreen underneath and that would negate the ultra-matte finish. There are often testers for this line so it is one you can try on for size.

☺ **Amazing Lasting Sheer Makeup SPF 12** *($8.37)* is definitely sheer—actually it's beyond sheer to almost nonexistent. The nonchemical (titanium dioxide) SPF is great and the application smooth and even. Because the appearance is so sheer, it would be hard to make a mistake with this stuff, but you also don't get any coverage. One concern: the texture is slightly sticky. It has the "lasting finish" texture of the other Amazing Lasting products (similar to Revlon's ColorStay foundations, which isn't surprising given Revlon owns Almay). If you want transparent coverage with a good SPF and no moisturizing feel, this one is a definite option. Most of the ten colors are superior; the ones to avoid are Pale, Naked, and Warm.

☹ **Moisture Renew Foundation for Dry Skin** *($6.79)*, **Moisture Balance Foundation for Normal to Combination Skin** *($6.79)*, and **Moisture Oil-Control Foundation for Oily Skin** *($6.79)* have a poor color selection and wouldn't be recommended even if you could them try on.

☺ <u>CONCEALER:</u> **Cover-Up Stick** *($3.43)* is a good concealer that comes in three workable shades: Light, Medium, and Dark. The lipstick-like applicator helps it go on creamy, but not greasy, and it tends not to crease in the lines around the eyes. This one is definitely worth looking into, although the consistency may be too moist for someone with oily skin. **Extra Moisturizing Undereye Cover Cream** *($6.50)* comes in three excellent shades: Light, Medium, and Dark. It goes on somewhat greasy, though it is anything but extra-moisturizing. It dries to a matte, almost powdery finish. It isn't best if you have lines around the eyes or dry skin, but it doesn't crease in the lines around the eyes, and that's great. **Time-Off Age Smoothing Concealer** *($6.18)* doesn't erase wrinkles, but it goes on smoothly and doesn't crease. The color selection, though small, is terrific. **Amazing Lasting Concealer** *($6.19)* is amazing. It doesn't crease and it goes on smoothly and evenly! **Sensitive Care Concealer** *($5.95)* is actually a decent concealer with good color choices, but nothing about it makes it any better for sensitive eyes than any other concealer.

☹ **Clear Complexion Acne Blemish Concealer** *($4.57)* contains sulfur, which is drying and irritating and can cause problems for someone with acne-prone skin.

☺ <u>POWDER:</u> **Moisture Renew Pressed Powder for Dry Skin** *($6.60)*, **Moisture Renew Pressed Powder for Normal to Combination Skin** *($6.60)*, **Moisture Renew Oil-Control Pressed Powder for Oily Skin** *($6.29)*, **Time-Off Age Smoothing Pressed Powder** *($7.99)*, and **Clear Complexion Light and Perfect Pressed Powder** *($7.29)* are all good possibilities except that each is packaged in a box that prevents you from getting a peek at the real color. Without being able to at least see whether or not a color comes close to your skin tone, you can end up with the absolute wrong product and that is neither attractive nor a bargain. **Amazing Lasting Powder** *($9.95)* does have staying power, at least more so than your average powder, but the cream-to-powder application does not work well over dry skin because any flakes will look exaggerated; it is also tricky to blend on evenly. Initially it has a lot of slip, leaving some areas streaked if you're not careful, but once this stuff dries into place it doesn't move and can make the skin feel very tight. That can be good and bad. If you have normal to oily skin and want a real matte finish from a powder (as opposed to the more creamy finish you get from most cream-to-powder foundations), this is a definite option, but one to check very carefully in the daylight before you decide to wear it in public. It does not work well over foundation.

☺ **Luxury Finish Loose Powder** *($7.79)* has a very satiny shiny finish. If you are using loose powder to reduce shine, this is not the way to go about it. But if you want a shiny look for evening then this is a very good option.

☺ <u>BLUSH:</u> **Cheek Color** *($4.99)* and **Brush-On Blush** *($6.50)* are very similar and both are excellent; the Brush-On comes with an attractive mirrored compact. Most of the colors are matte.

☺ **Amazing Lasting Blush** *($7.59)* is a cream-to-powder blush that has very impressive staying power and goes on relatively smoothly and evenly, but only if you can get the knack of blending it on. Note that the compact can dry out quickly, too, making it impossible to use. This is not for everyone.

☺ <u>EYESHADOW:</u> **Long Lasting Eyecolor Singles** *($3.45)*, **Duos** *($3.82)*, and **Quads** *($5.95)* come in a small but good color selection; they go on soft and blend nicely. The shades labeled matte actually have a slight amount of shine, but not enough to show up. The shades labeled shiny are indeed shiny, though, and should be avoided. **Amazing Lasting Eyecolor** *($4.50)* comes in a lipstick-like applicator, goes on very smooth and creamy, and dries to a powdery finish. It comes in a small but exceptionally neutral group of colors. It is supposed to last up to 12 hours, but most eyeshadows last that long and then some. I don't prefer this type of eyeshadow because blending or layering can be tricky, but it is an option for a one-shadow look. **One Coat Gel Eye Color** *($6.29)* is, as weird as it sounds, a chubby eyeshadow pencil that goes on somewhat wet, spreading on easily. Then it dries to a matte, powdery finish that doesn't smear. Don't ask me how they do it, but for a pencil/eyeshadow this is a very interesting formula. I only wish the colors were more varied and that you could actually see the pencil color. As it is, you have to judge this one by a color swatch on the end of the pencil. One caution: you have to keep the tip clear of the powder it picks up while coloring to retain a smooth application.

☹ **Amazing Lasting Eye Color** *($6.50)* does have amazing staying power, at least more so than your average powder shadows; these colors actually seem to stick to the skin. Application is another story. The eyeshadows have a cream-to-powder finish with a hard-to-control slippery texture and they also tend to streak when applied. These are not recommended.

☺ <u>EYE AND BROW SHAPER:</u> **Eye Defining Liquid Liner** *($4.79)* is a standard, tube liquid liner that can create a very dramatic line. It doesn't budge once it dries, and it does dry matte. **I-Liner** *($6.50)* is a good liquid liner that goes on smoothly and easily, creating a thick, dramatic line without flaking or looking crinkled, and I think you will find it identical to many of the more expensive versions at the department store. **Amazing Lasting Eye Pencil** *($6.50)* is a standard pencil in a twist-up, no-sharpen pen applicator. It's nice but not amazing. **One Coat Gel Eye Pencil** *($6.29)* is quite similar to the Gel Eye Color above. This version goes on slightly less smoothly, but it still goes on somewhat wet, then dries to a matte, powdery finish that lasts all day without smearing. Again, don't ask me how they do it, but for a pencil this is an interesting formula, although with the same color drawbacks as the one above. One caution: you have to keep the tip clear of the powder it picks up while coloring to retain a smooth application.

☹ **Kohl-Formula Eye Pencil** *($5.75)* is an incredibly greasy pencil that smudges and smears easily. **Wetproof Shadow Liner** *($3.57)* is another greasy pencil. It isn't all that waterproof, and it wipes off easily and tends to smear and smudge. **Soft Brow Color** *($3.51)* is a standard pencil that tends to be greasy rather than soft; it has a brow brush on the cap.

☺ <u>LIPSTICK AND LIP PENCIL:</u> **One Coat Lip Color** *($7.69)* is just a very greasy lipstick. It works well enough, but it doesn't go on any more reliably in one application than any other lipstick with the same glossy finish. **One Coat Lip Shine** *($6.29)* is a standard but very emollient and shiny lip gloss, but the name is misleading. If one-coat coverage is what you like, you can put on one coat of most any lip product; if you like more, then you have to apply more. **Amazing Lasting Lip Color**

($7.95) is Almay's version of an ultra-matte lipstick, and this is one of the better ones. The automatic **Lipcolor Pencils** *($4.95)* are excellent, with a dry but smooth texture, and the **Amazing Lasting Lip Liner** *($6.85)* is just a good lip liner.

☹ **Stay Smooth Lip Color SPF 25** *($8.79)* doesn't contain UVA protection and is not recommended for sun protection but it does contain menthol which can cause irritation and chapped lips!

☺ <u>MASCARA:</u> **One Coat Mascara** *($4.95)* and **Mascara Plus** *($4.95)* create beautiful lashes without clumping or smearing, and the price is right! However, the term One-Coat isn't exactly accurate; it does takes several applications to get the length and thickness you want. **Triple Thick Mascara** *($4.99)* builds long, thick lashes and has good staying power.

☺ **Amazing Lash** *($6.29)* is unreliable. Of the four tubes purchased to review, each one performed differently. They all built some amount of length, but with this kind of inconsistency I don't quite know what to say. **Longest Lashes Mascara** *($5.79)* is a good mascara, but doesn't stand out in comparison to those reviewed above. **Perfect Definition Mascara** *($5.50)* is slow going; it takes forever to get even a little thickness, but if length and thickness aren't your goal this isn't bad. **Super Rich Mascara** *($5.50)* is just OK, but why bother with OK when there are so many great mascaras out there?

☹ **One Coat Waterproof Mascara** *($4.95)* is not in the least a one-coat mascara. It can take many coats and then you still won't look like you have any lashes. The lashes also tend to clump together when wet, which isn't the best result from a waterproof mascara. **Amazing Lash Waterproof Mascara** *($4.95)* isn't amazing or waterproof. It takes forever to build length and it then it comes off with water!

Aloette (Skin Care Only)

Evidently the heart of these formulas is aloe as a cosmetic ingredient, which may have some benefit for the skin as an anti-irritant, though nothing more. Every other aspect of these formulations, however, is so ordinary and commonplace that it is almost bewildering. I imagine Aloette thought there was enough fascination with aloe that nothing else would matter. I think many consumers may be waylaid by the aloe content in these products, but they should know that every line, from Avon, Mary Kay, Pond's, and Neutrogena to Clinique, Lancome, and even Oil of Olay (a line I find wanting in many respects) has better formulations than those in these Aloette products. Aloette's ordering number is (800) 256-3883.

☹ **Cleansing Lotion** *($10 for 8 ounces)* is a very standard mineral oil–based cleanser, more like cold cream than anything else. I never recommend wiping off makeup, because pulling at the skin causes it to sag. But if you tried to rinse this stuff off, it would leave a greasy film on the skin.

☹ **Cleansing Creme** (*$10 for 4 ounces*) is similar to the cleanser above, only this one has more ingredients that can cause breakouts.

☹ **Cleansing Oil** (*$13 for 2 ounces*), as the name implies, is mostly plant oil that must be wiped off the face, and that's a problem. Using this product is in no way different from taking some pure safflower or sesame oil from your kitchen cabinet and using it on your face, though I wouldn't recommend that either.

☹ **Scrub 'n Sluff** (*$11 for 4 ounces*) contains mostly ground almonds, honey, and clay, making this a rather passé scrub. No one is formulating this kind of facial scrub anymore because it is so problematic for skin. You can't get a smooth edge on the ground almonds, so they are too hard on the skin; clay is drying and doesn't rinse well; honey doesn't do anything for skin; and the other ingredients are just waxy thickeners, preservatives, and fragrance.

☺ **Moisture Creme** (*$12.50 for 2 ounces*) is almost identical to the cleansers above. It is a standard water and mineral oil moisturizer with no other water-binding agents or emollients. Oil of Olay and Pond's have far better formulations than this do-nothing product does.

☺ **Performance Plus** (*$16.50 for 2 ounces*) is merely a list of waxy thickening agents, emulsifiers, and that's it! It doesn't get much more ordinary and insubstantial than this! It can't perform much of anything, and I can't imagine what skin type would find any benefit from it.

☺ **Moisturizing Lotion** (*$12.50 for 4 ounces*) is almost identical to Performance Plus above, only in a lotion form. The same review applies.

☺ **Alcohol-Free Toner** (*$11 for 8 ounces*) is a rather decent irritant-free toner for someone with normal to dry skin.

☹ **Skin Refining Toner** (*$11 for 8 ounces*) is nothing more than alcohol with some slip agents. It can only irritate and dry out the skin, nothing more.

☹ **Oil Control Toner** (*$11 for 8 ounces*) contains a serious amount of alcohol, which can only irritate the skin. It also contains camphor and zinc phenosulfonate, which will cause further irritation and redness and potentially stimulate oil production.

☺ **Skin Conditioner** (*$14 for 8 ounces*) won't do much conditioning. This product is almost entirely slip agents, emulsifiers, thickeners, and some animal protein. Not only isn't this an "animal-friendly" product, but animal protein won't do much for the face—not in this tiny amount anyway. It isn't a bad product; it just won't do much for the skin.

☺ **Night Creme** (*$14 for 2 ounces*) is similar to all the other moisturizers in this line, only this one is more emollient, which would be good for someone with dry skin. It is still extremely ordinary, and if it were priced any higher it would be a real rip-off.

☺ **Eye Beauty Creme** (*$10 for 0.5 ounce*) is similar to the cream above, and the same review applies. Be careful with this one around the eyes; there are lots of pore-clogging ingredients.

☺ **Nu-Trish** *($14.50 for 8 ounces)* contains 89.6% aloe vera gel, which means a small percentage of aloe and a lot of water. "Aloe gel" indicates that you will not be getting a pure ingredient, but if you want aloe, this is your best option. You can put this on first and then use some really good skin-care products from another line over it.

☹ **Tender Touch** *($18 for 2 ounces)* isn't the least bit tender. It is just a bunch of wax and preservatives with a tiny bit of animal protein, which can be an emollient. This product will just clog pores, although—and this is a big "although"—it could be a mediocre moisturizer for someone with dry skin.

☺ **Advanced Hydrating Formula** *($18.50 for 1 ounce)* isn't in the least an advanced formula, at least not by my standards. All you get are thickeners, slip agents, and preservatives. There are minuscule amounts of vitamins and other conditioning agents, but they are hardly present enough to warrant the term "advanced."

☺ **Visible Aid** *($11 for 2 ounces)* will indeed aid breakouts and clogged pores— that is, it will make matters worse. It could be a good moisturizer for someone with very dry skin, though.

☹ **Oil-Free Face Makeup** *($10 for 1 ounce)* isn't even vaguely oil-free; it contains lots of silicones (cyclomethicone and dimethicone), and the second ingredient, isopropyl myristate, is known to cause breakouts.

☹ **Translucent Finishing Powder** *($17.50 for 0.8 ounce)* is a standard talc powder that uses formaldehyde resin as the preservative base. That's rather shocking; you never see this anymore. It is considered quite irritating for the skin.

Alpha Hydrox by Neoteric (Skin Care Only)

Alpha Hydrox Lotion and Alpha Hydrox Face Creme were two of the more reasonably priced and effective alpha hydroxy acid products that first appeared on the market when the AHA craze was launched back in 1992. While other companies often hedge when telling you how much AHA their products contain, Alpha Hydrox is more than forthcoming. The AHA in its products is glycolic acid, which is considered one of the best, and the pH of the products is at an effective level. If you are interested in trying an AHA in a moisturizing or gel base, this is a great place to start. The prices and the product quality are excellent. One word of caution: To capitalize on the success of its two showcase products, Alpha Hydrox has introduced an additional 15-plus products to its line, including several that have no AHA content. The non-AHA products are nowhere near as impressive, but there are some interesting and reasonably priced products to check out. For more information about Alpha Hydrox, call (800) 447-1919.

☺ **Foaming Face Wash, for All Skin types** *($5.57 for 6 ounces)* is a standard detergent-based water-soluble cleanser that does not contain AHAs. It can be good for someone with normal to oily skin, but may be too drying for other skin types.

☹ **Toner-Astringent for Normal to Oily Skin** *($5.50 for 8 ounces)* contains mostly water, alcohol, witch hazel, slip agent, glycolic acid, chamomile extract, menthol, pH balancer, and preservatives. The chamomile can't counterbalance the irritation caused by the alcohol and menthol.

☺ **AHA Creme, 8% AHA Facial Treatment for Normal Skin** *($7.64 for 2 ounces)* contains mostly water, glycolic acid, slip agent, thickeners, pH balancer, more thickeners, silicone, and preservatives. This is a very good AHA moisturizer for normal to dry-skin types.

☺ **AHA Enhanced Creme, 10% AHA Facial Treatment, for Dry to Normal Skin** *($9.50 for 2 ounces)* contains mostly water, glycolic acid, pH balancer, slip agent, thickeners, silicone, more thickeners, and preservatives. This is a good high-percentage AHA product, but it is not appropriate for all skin types. The thickening agents could be a problem for someone with normal to combination skin.

☺ **AHA Lotion, 8% AHA Facial Treatment, for Dry Skin** *($8.64 for 6 ounces)* contains mostly water, glycolic acid, pH balancer, water-binding agent, thickeners, petrolatum, more thickeners, and preservatives. This is a very good 8% AHA moisturizer, but it is best for someone with normal to slightly dry skin.

☺ **AHA Sensitive Skin Creme, 5% AHA Facial Treatment** *($7.89 for 2 ounces)* contains mostly water, slip agent, thickener, glycolic acid, more thickeners, pH balancer, silicone, and preservatives. It's a simple but emollient base for someone with dry, sensitive skin who wants a less intense concentration of AHAs.

☺ **Extra Strength AHA Oil-Free Formula, 10% AHA Facial Treatment** *($10.95 for 1.7 ounces)* is virtually free of any ingredients that could clog pores and is little more than water, glycolic acid, pH balancer, thickener, anti-irritant, slip agent, and preservatives. I would be happier if it were still an 8% concentration of AHA, but for those looking for more exfoliation this is a definite option.

☺ **Hydrating Eye Gel** *($9.50 for 0.5 ounce)* is an average lightweight gel that contains mostly water, slip agent, water-binding agent, aloe, thickener, and preservatives.

☹ **SPF 15 Moisturizing Daily Lotion** *($7.58 for 4 ounces)* doesn't contain avobenzone, titanium dioxide, or zinc oxide, and is not recommended.

☺ **Night Replenishing Creme for Normal to Dry Skin** *($7.95 for 2 ounces)* contains mostly water, mineral oil, thickener, glycerin, plant oil, more thickeners, silicone, vitamin E, water-binding agents, and preservatives. This would be a very good, though standard, moisturizer for someone with dry skin (but not normal skin, as the name implies).

☺ **Purifying Clay Masque 4% AHA Facial Masque, for Normal to Oily Skin** *($8.35 for 4 ounces)* is a standard clay mask with a small amount of AHA. You don't need more than one effective AHA product. There is no reason to use an AHA cleanser, an AHA toner, an AHA eye cream, and an AHA face lotion or cream. It's best to use only one effective AHA product on a regular basis, rather than in a face mask you use once or twice a week. This is an OK clay mask for occasional use if you have oily to combination skin, but be careful not to overdo the number of AHA products you're using.

☺ **Lasting Lip Treatment, SPF 8 Sunscreen, All-In-One Care** (*$3.85 for 0.35 ounce*) doesn't contain avobenzone, titanium dioxide, or zinc oxide, and is not recommended.

☺ **Blemish Solution** (*$7.99 for 0.5 ounce*) would be an excellent 2% salicylic acid (BHA) product if the second ingredient weren't alcohol (ethanol to be exact). I have much respect for Alpha Hydrox and their formulations, but the alcohol in here is just not necessary for skin.

☺ **$$$ Retinol Night ResQ Anti-Wrinkle Firming Complex** (*$11.99 for 1.05 ounces*) contains mostly water, thickeners, glycerin, retinol, vitamin E, vitamin C, more thickeners, silicone, and preservatives. If you are interested in finding out if all the talk about retinol is true (I'm referring to the notion that vitamin A can work just as well as the active ingredient in Retin-A or Renova), for content and price this is one of the better options you will find!

AlphaMax (Skin Care Only)

Where do I begin? This line of products that touts their AHA content is AHA overkill at best. At least three of the five products contain the correct pH and a decent amount of glycolic and lactic acid, but the face needs only one competent AHA product. There are a lot of excellent AHA products available from many venues for under $10 for several ounces; paying $139.95 for a kit of them that doesn't even add up to eight ounces is just one more layer of absurdity. To add insult to injury, the AlphaMax brochure presents consumer questions about their products that are answered by two dermatologists endorsing the line. Here is an example. "**Q.** Can AlphaMax be used with Retin-A? **A.** Personally, we think AlphaMax is comparable to Retin-A and Renova in effectiveness." Retin-A and Renova are prescription items that can alter cellular growth, have detailed safety studies, and can increase collagen (to what extent is still under dispute) after two years of use. AHAs have no such studies or effectiveness. Moreover, the doctors literally don't answer the question asked: "Can this product be used WITH Retin-A . . ."

Here is another gem. "**Q.** Will the use of AlphaMax result in increased sun sensitivity of my skin? **A.** There is no ingredient in the AlphaMax program that would make your skin sensitive to the sun." That statement is incredibly misleading. Yes, there are no ingredients that would create a phototoxic reaction, but continued use of effective AHAs absolutely makes the skin more susceptible to sun damage because it removes older skin that can be a protective layer. This issue is a serious concern of the FDA. AlphaMax's doctors' suggestions to the contrary are unconscionable. Please note that some of the following products are sold in a kit for a total of *$139.97*. You can order by calling (800) 716-2266.

☺ **$$$ Collagen and Elastin Facial Cleanser** (*2 ounces as part of the $139.97 kit*) is a standard detergent-based, water-soluble cleanser that can feel drying to some skin types. It contains a tiny amount of collagen and elastin, but even if there were more, these two ingredients can't change a wrinkle on anyone's face. You are supposed to use this cleanser with a sponge like Buf-Puf. Clearly, this company thinks skin can handle a large amount of abuse. It can't. Between this cleanser and the sponge, watch out for some serious dryness and irritation.

☹ **$$$ Intensive Exfoliator Pads** (*$49.97 for six pads*) is a series of six pads soaked with varying concentrations of AHAs, but the company is not forthcoming about what those concentrations are. I was not able to test the pH because the liquid took the color off my pH paper. I assume it is a decent enough pH to make the pads effective, but since I don't know the concentrations, I worry that this product may deliver more irritation than a face needs. If it is a high concentration, as they suggest—high enough to eliminate the need for a peel—you should not be using these pads at home. Of course, I doubt that this company would take the risk of selling a product with that high a concentration, but who knows; they've said many things that have led me to believe they are not interested in truthful information.

☹ **$$$ Weekly Intensive Exfoliator** (*60 pads, as part of the kit*) is similar to the above product and the same review applies.

☺ **$$$ Daily Renewal Lotion with AHA and SPF 15** (*$29.97 for 2 ounces*) is a decent mix of AHAs and sunscreen. It even has a pH low enough to make the AHAs effective. For someone with normal to dry skin, this is one of the first products I've seen that contains a good sunscreen formula (titanium dioxide is one of the active ingredients) and glycolic acid with a pH of 3 to 4. This lotion is worth considering if you want to try to kill two birds with one stone. Keep in mind, though, that when you can't separate your AHA product from your sunscreen, nighttime use becomes an issue, and you may not want to use AHAs twice a day. I should mention that this cream has a noticeable medicinal smell that lingers for some time.

☹ **$$$ Moisturizing Cream** (*$19.97 for 1.7 ounces*) contains mostly water, glycerin, several thickeners, aloe, silicone oil, anti-irritant, more thickener, plant oil, still more thickeners, vitamins, plant extracts, and preservatives. This is an OK but rather ordinary moisturizer for someone with normal to slightly dry skin. The amount of vitamins and plants in it is too minuscule to have any real effect on the skin.

☹ **$$$ Renewal Eye Cream with AHA** (*$19.97 for 0.5 ounce*) doesn't have a low enough pH to make it effective. That's a relief; at least it won't cause more irritation to the face than is necessary.

☹ **$$$ Intensive Hand and Body Lotion with AHA and SPF 15** (*$14.97 for 6 ounces*) is a good sunscreen with titanium dioxide for someone with normal to dry skin. It contains a tiny amount of glycolic acid and a handful of plant extracts; the label makes them sound like AHAs when they aren't. Glycolic acid is the only one that counts, but in this tiny amount it won't help exfoliate the skin.

☺ **$$$ Fade Out with Kojic Acid** *($22.97 for 1 ounce)* is an interesting product. Research has found that kojic acid can help lighten skin by inhibiting melanin production; but hydroquinone, which is not included in this product, is still considered the best ingredient for performing this function, especially when combined with kojic acid.

Amway

There are a lot of people selling Amway products throughout the world, and unless you have been living in a shell or on a mountaintop, someone by now has likely approached you with the opportunity to either share in the theoretical wealth or at least become a customer. Talk about company loyalty! As one Amway sales representative said to me, "Why would the company make anything that wasn't wonderful?" Obviously, no cosmetics line is perfect, or they wouldn't discontinue "old" products and introduce "new" ones. If you want to shop in the privacy of your own home and enjoy being able to test the products, there are things I encourage you to consider taking a look at in Amway's skin-care and makeup lines. I hope this doesn't mean I've unleashed a monster on any of you who have an Amway representative in your area. Make it clear from the beginning that you are interested only in buying products and not in becoming an Amway representative.

What I found most startling since I last reviewed this line was the steep price increase. This line is not a bargain in the least—it is up there in price with the high-end department stores—yet the formulations, especially for skin care, just don't warrant it. There also hasn't been much improvement; the formulations are almost all the same. Still, there are some good products here, but watch out for the shiny eyeshadows and blushes, overpriced moisturizers, and the concealer pencil. For the money, you can do better elsewhere, but if you know someone selling Amway you don't want to insult them there are options to check out. For more information about Amway call (800) 926-9293.

Artistry by Amway Skin Care

☹ **Moisture Rich Cleansing Creme for Normal to Dry Skin** *($15.60 for 4.2 ounces)* is a standard mineral oil–based cleanser that needs to be wiped off, and that can leave a greasy residue on the skin. It also contains isopropyl palmitate, which can cause breakouts in some skin types.

☺ **$$$ Delicate Care Cleanser for Sensitive Skin Types** *($15.60 for 4.2 ounces)* is an OK cleanser that won't do a great job of removing makeup (it doesn't have enough cleansing agents), and it can leave a greasy film on the skin. It can be OK for someone with dry skin.

☺ $$$ **Clarifying Cleansing Gel for Normal to Oily Skin** *($15.60 for 4.2 ounces)* is a very good facial cleanser that cleans well without drying out the skin or irritating the eyes, and can remove all of your makeup.

☺ **Moisture Rich Toner for Normal to Dry Skin** *($16.60 for 8.1 ounces)* is a very good, irritant-free toner that contains mostly water, glycerin, aloe, plant extracts, water-binding agents, and preservatives. Ignore the avocado and rose extracts; they are window dressing and have little impact on the skin. The same is true of the essential oils at the end of the ingredient list, which add fragrance to this product and a risk of irritation for sensitive skin types.

☹ **Clarifying Astringent Toner for Normal to Oily Skin** *($16.60 for 8.1 ounces)* is a standard alcohol-based toner with some plant extracts thrown in for good measure. The alcohol is too irritating for most skin types.

☹ **Delicate Care Toner for Sensitive Skin Types** *($16.60 for 8.1 ounces)* would be an OK toner except that the third ingredient is benzoyl alcohol, which is a skin irritant and not something I would recommend for someone with sensitive skin.

☺ $$$ **Eye Makeup Remover Gel** *($9.20 for 0.9 ounce)* is mostly mineral oil, thickeners, and a small amount of plant oils. It will take off eye makeup, but I never recommend wiping off eye makeup. Essentially, this is a fairly pricey, standard mineral oil–based cleanser that could easily be replaced for pennies with a bottle of pure mineral oil.

☹ **Exfoliating Scrub** *($21.05 for 3.4 ounces)* is a mineral oil–based cleanser that contains some scrub particles. It will exfoliate the skin gently, but it can leave a greasy film on the skin.

☹ **Moisture Rich Moisturizer for Normal to Dry Skin SPF 8** *($21.15 for 2.5 ounces)* doesn't contain avobenzone, zinc oxide, or titanium dioxide, and is not recommended.

☹ **Clarifying Moisturizer for Normal to Oily Skin SPF 8** *($21.15 for 2.5 ounces)* doesn't contain avobenzone, zinc oxide, or titanium dioxide, and is not recommended.

☺ $$$ **Delicate Care Hydrating Fluid for Sensitive Skin Types** *($21.15 for 2.3 ounces)* contains mostly water, plant oil, thickener, several water-binding agents, plant extracts, more thickeners, and preservatives. It would be a very good moisturizer for someone with dry skin.

☺ $$$ **Eye Balm** *($14.20 for 0.5 ounce)* is a good moisturizer for slightly dry skin. It contains water, film former, thickeners, water-binding agents, and preservatives.

☺ $$$ **Advanced Daily Eye Creme** *($20.30 for 0.5 ounce)* is a very good moisturizer for dry skin, containing mostly water, thickeners, film former, plant oil, water-binding agents, vitamins, and preservatives.

☺ **Deep Cleansing Masque** *($16.15 for 3.3 ounces)* is a standard clay mask that also contains a small amount of alcohol, but probably not enough to be a problem for the skin.

☺ **Hydrating Masque** *($17.10 for 2.6 ounces)* is an emollient face mask for someone with dry skin that is more a moisturizer than a traditional mask. It contains mostly water, glycerin, petrolatum, several thickeners, plant oil, and preservatives.

☺ $$$ **Revitalizing Night Treatment** *($33 for 2.5 ounces)* contains mostly water, petrolatum, glycerin, several thickeners, aloe, several water-binding agents, plant oil, vitamins A and E (antioxidants), more thickeners, and preservatives. This would be a very good moisturizer for someone with dry skin.

☺ $$$ **Progressive Emollient** *($33 for 2.5 ounces)* is almost identical to the moisturizer above, and the same review applies.

☺ $$$ **Alpha Hydroxy Serum Plus** *($40.20 for 1 ounce)* is an AHA lotion at about a 6% concentration with a pH of 4. That makes it a good AHA solution but the price is nonsense; there are formulations equally as good, if not better, available for far less.

Artistry by Amway Makeup

☺ <u>FOUNDATION:</u> **Liquid Foundation** *($17.05)* is a very emollient foundation for dry skin that contains mineral oil and lanolin oil. It still has a sheer, light texture and some good colors. **Avoid these colors because they are too peach, pink, or rose:** True Beige, Shell Beige, Sand Beige, and Cappuccino.

☹ **Creme Foundation** *($22.15)* may be good for someone with dry skin, but it tends to be greasy and very thick. Because there are only five shades, finding the right color isn't going to be easy. **The colors to avoid are:** Shell Bisque and True Beige.

☺ **Oil-Free Foundation** *($18.90)* is a very good, creamy foundation for someone with normal to oily skin. It has a soft matte finish with sheer to medium coverage without being too heavy or drying. **Avoid these colors because they are too peach, pink, or rose:** Honey Beige, Shell Bisque, Warm Amber, and Cappuccino.

☺ **Versatile Matte Pressed Powder Foundation** *($18.20)* is really a standard talc-based pressed powder that has a silky-smooth feel, though it can go a bit too powdery if you have dry skin. All of the shades are excellent; only Shell Bisque may be too peach. For Amway, these are both pressed powder as well as an option for foundation, but they are best as pressed powders.

☹ **Base Controllers** *($17.50)* are standard lavender and green under-makeup color correctors that are supposed to camouflage yellow or red skin tones. It shouldn't take an extra product to do that, because if the foundation is a good neutral color, it should be able to even out skin tones. If you apply too many products—moisturizers, concealers, skin-tone correctors, and then a foundation—your skin can't handle it for very long without either breaking out or feeling heavy and uncomfortable.

☺ **Eye Foundation** *($13.75)* is OK, but basically contains just talc and waxes. It comes in only one color, which is not the best for all skin tones. A matte foundation with powder over it can do the same thing this product does.

☹ <u>CONCEALER:</u> **Concealer Pencil** *($12.95)* comes in four fairly peach shades, which is a problem, but an even bigger problem is having to sharpen them to apply concealer. These offer no additional convenience, and they go on rather heavily and tend to crease.

☺ <u>POWDER:</u> The **Loose Powder** *($17.50)* is a standard talc-based powder with good colors and a dry finish.

☹ <u>EYESHADOW AND BLUSH:</u> Amway's eyeshadows and blushes come in individual tins that are placed into a compact you purchase separately, either a **Two Pan Compact** *($11.25)* or a **Four Pan Compact** *($12.85)*. That means you can create your own makeup-collection compact that includes blushes and eyeshadows. It's a nice idea. The prices given below for the Powder Blush and Eye Colour are for the tins only, without a compact. Unfortunately, the blush and eye colors all have some amount of shine. The handful of **Powder Blush** *($10.50 refills)* colors have a silky texture that goes on soft and even, but all the colors have some amount of shine, as do the **Eye Colour** *($7 refills)* eyeshadows, which have a lovely soft texture and go on smoothly and evenly; here even the so-called matte ones have shine.

☺ <u>EYE AND BROW SHAPER:</u> **Softstick for Eyes** *($11.90)* are standard pencils in seven good shades, though these aren't all that soft. One end of the stick has a sponge applicator to soften hard lines. A brow pencil called **Softstick for Brows** *($8.95)* is available in five colors identical to the pencils for eyes. **Fine Liner** *($13.45)* is just a standard tube liquid liner that goes on smooth and doesn't chip or flake; it comes in only two shades.

☺ <u>LIPSTICK AND LIP PENCIL:</u> **Sheer Colour SPF 15** *($12)* is a very glossy, sheer lipstick. The SPF is there, but there's no UVA protection. **Lip Colour** *($12)* is opaque and has a very good creamy consistency. Standard lip pencils called **Softstick for Lips** *($10.60)* come in a nice range of colors and all are good possibilities.

☺ **Jumbo Lip Pencil** *($12)* is a very soft lipstick in pencil form. This one may be too soft and can smush down to nothing fairly fast.

☺ <u>MASCARA:</u> **Smudgeproof Mascara** *($14.20)* is indeed fairly smudgeproof, and it builds decent length and thickness quite quickly.

☹ **Waterproof Mascara** *($14.20)* builds great length and some amount of thickness but it isn't all that waterproof. It can start coming off after a few splashes with water, and it easily smears even when you aren't wet.

☹ <u>BRUSHES:</u> The **Cosmetic Brush Set** *($32.95)* is disappointing and shockingly overpriced for what you get. It comes with six brushes, of which three are OK; the other three are not worth the money. The powder brush is fine, but the bristles are a little too loose, so the powder can be hard to control on the face. The eyeshadow and angle brushes are also OK and usable. The eyebrow/eyelash comb is like those found everywhere; an old toothbrush would work equally well. The lipstick brush is a good six inches long and wouldn't fit easily in most makeup bags; the smaller, retractable lipstick brushes are much better. The blush brush is too small to be suited to anyone's cheeks.

Aqua Glycolic (Skin Care Only)

Herald Pharmacal has a small line of drugstore AHA products called Aqua Glycolic. Aqua Glycolic products are, for the most part, a disappointment. The only option is the Advanced Smoothing Cream for someone with normal to dry skin. Of the other two products, one has skin-irritating ingredients and the other is a risk for the eyes. For information, call Aqua Glycolic at (800) 253-9499.

☹ **Facial Cleanser Advanced Cleansing Care 12% Glycolic Compound** *($9.99 for 8 ounces)* resembles Cetaphil Gentle Skin Cleanser, but with a strong concentration of AHAs. I do not recommend washing the face with an AHA product because of the risk it poses for the eyes. Additionally, if you do want the exfoliation effect from an AHA, in a cleanser most of the potential effectiveness is washed away.

☹ **Astringent Advanced Oily Skin Therapy 11% Glycolic Compound** *($7.09 for 8 ounces)* is an alcohol-based AHA product; the alcohol compounds the irritation of the glycolic acid. It also contains eucalyptus oil, another seriously irritating skin-care ingredient.

☺ **Face Cream Advanced Smoothing Therapy 10% Glycolic Compound** *($11.29 for 2 ounces)* is a good basic AHA in a lightweight moisturizing base. It would be suitable for someone with normal to somewhat dry skin.

Arbonne

This is one exceedingly expensive line, ranking up there with those found at many department stores, yet the offerings are not all that impressive and are definitely not worth the cost. Like many in-home sales lines from Nu Skin to Shaklee, Arbonne boasts more about what their products do not contain than about what they do. That isn't necessarily good or bad, but I happen to like some of the ingredients Arbonne warns against. Much of its literature states that things such as mineral oil, lanolin, collagen, artificial fragrances, and artificial colors are *not* used in any Arbonne products. I disagree strongly with Arbonne's argument that mineral oil, petrolatum, and collagen are inherently bad for the skin because their molecular structure is too large to be absorbed into the skin, and therefore they can clog pores, cause blemishes, and interfere with skin respiration. The molecular structure of many other cosmetic ingredients, including elastin, mucopolysaccharides, waxes, and other thickeners, is also too large to permit absorption into the skin. Yet one of the best ways to prevent dehydration is to keep air off the face, and one of the best ways to do that is with a cosmetic ingredient that works as a barrier between your skin and the air. If everything were absorbed into the skin, what would be left on top to keep air off the face? Mineral oil, petrolatum, and collagen are not so totally occlusive that the skin suffocates; they simply protect it from the air. Besides, just because a cosmetic ingredient is absorbed into the skin doesn't mean it won't clog pores. Quite the contrary: once inside the pore, the ingredient is trapped and can't easily be washed or wiped away.

Arbonne also doesn't like beeswax. The company's theory is that because beeswax is sticky, bacteria and dirt will stick to the skin. However, like many waxes in cosmetics, beeswax is just another thickener, and there is rarely very much of it in a product. Moreover, beeswax isn't all that different from the synthetic waxes used in cosmetics to keep the product blended. Arbonne's products contain ingredients such as myristyl myristate and cetyl alcohol, which are quite similar to beeswax.

I do agree totally with Arbonne's recommendation against alcohol because of its drying and irritating effect on the skin. If only the company excluded all other irritants, such as witch hazel and certain plant extracts, the line would be even better.

I could go on, but to sum up, none of my reservations mean I don't like some of these products, and I am glad that Arbonne does not use animal products or perform animal testing. But the rather misleading marketing language is not convincing, and the prices are just not in touch with reality. All of the natural-sounding ingredients in the world can't keep you from reacting to an irritating preservative or fragrance or from breaking out due to cosmetic waxes such as stearic acid or myristyl myristate. For more information about Arbonne International, call (800) ARBONNE.

Arbonne Skin Care

☹ **Cleansing Lotion** (*$14.50 for 3.25 ounces*) is supposed to be a water-soluble cleanser, but oils are listed among the first ingredients, and it will leave a greasy film on your face.

☺ **Cleansing Cream** (*$15.50 for 2 ounces*) contains mostly water, plant oils, thickeners, plant extracts, and preservatives. It is a fairly greasy cleanser that leaves an oily film on the skin and doesn't take off all the makeup without the aid of a washcloth.

☺ **Freshener for Normal to Dry Skin** (*$18.50 for 8 ounces*) contains mostly water, witch hazel, water-binding agents, aloe vera, preservatives, and plant extracts. Witch hazel is an irritant.

☹ **Toner** (*$18.50 for 8 ounces*) contains water; witch hazel; glycerin; peppermint, lemon, and papaya extracts; and preservatives. Witch hazel, peppermint, and lemon are very irritating and drying, and they won't change the amount of oil your skin produces.

☺ **Facial Scrub** *($17 for 2 ounces)* contains mostly water, thickeners, ground nuts, plant oil, slip agents, and preservatives. The plants and vitamin E come well after the preservatives and are barely present. This is an OK scrub, but ground nuts are not the best way to exfoliate and can scratch the skin.

☺ **$$$ Bio Hydria Gentle Exfoliant** *($23 for 4 ounces)* is a good, relatively gentle scrub, at least compared to the one above, but I would only recommend it for someone with dry skin; it is really too emollient for any other skin type.

☺ **Moisture Cream for Normal to Dry Skin** *($18.50 for 2 ounces)* contains mostly water, plant oils, thickeners, water-binding agent, vitamins, plant extracts, and preservatives. This is an excellent emollient moisturizer for dry skin; however, I would not recommend a product this rich for someone with normal skin.

☹ **Moisture Cream for Normal to Oily Skin** *($18.50 for 2 ounces)* contains mostly water, standard water-binding agents, thickeners, plant oils, and preservatives. There are more ingredients following the preservatives, but their position so far down on the ingredient list makes their presence insignificant. Arbonne recommends this cream for someone with normal to oily skin. Why they think that someone with oily skin would be interested in putting more oil on her skin is beyond me! And this product also contains peppermint oil, a completely unnecessary skin irritant.

☺ **Night Cream for Normal to Dry Skin** *($20.50 for 2 ounces)* contains mostly water, sunflower oil, water-binding agent, thickeners, almond oil, more thickeners, jojoba oil, vitamins A and E (antioxidants), plant oils, plant extracts, yeast, anti-irritants, and preservatives. The plants do nothing for the skin, but all the other ingredients make this an excellent moisturizer for dry skin. I would not recommend a product this rich for someone with normal skin.

☹ **Night Cream for Normal to Oily Skin** *($20.50 for 2 ounces)* has almost the same ingredients as the Moisture Cream for Normal to Oily Skin, and the same review applies.

☺ **Rejuvenating Cream for All Skin Types** *($30 for 2 ounces)* won't rejuvenate anything. It is a good moisturizer for someone with normal to dry skin (but definitely not for all skin types). It contains mostly water, plant oils, standard water-binding agents, thickeners, more plant oils, vitamins A and E (antioxidants), aloe vera, plant extracts, amino acids, more thickeners, and preservatives.

☺ **Skin Conditioning Oil** *($16 for 1 ounce)* is a blend of several plant oils, aloe vera, vitamin E (an antioxidant), and some plant extracts. For someone with very dry skin, this would be a nice extra for problem areas, but any plant oil from your kitchen cabinet would work as well for far less money.

☺ **$$$ Bio Hydria Night Energizing Cream** *($58 for 2 ounces)* contains mostly water, several plant extracts, thickeners, sesame oil, more thickeners, several plant oils, aloe vera, anti-irritants, more thickeners, more plant oils, vitamins A and E, and preservatives. This is a good emollient moisturizer for someone with dry skin, but it won't energize the skin or "retard the formation of wrinkles," as the label claims. And the price tag is completely ludicrous for what you get.

☺ **$$$ Bio Hydria Eye Cream** *($24.50 for 0.75 ounce)* is very similar to the cream above, and the same review applies.

☹ **Bio Hydra Alpha Complex SPF 8** *($34.50 for 2 ounces)* has a dismal SPF, doesn't contain avobenzone, zinc oxide, or titanium dioxide, and is not recommended.

☺ **Mild Masque** *($17 for 5 ounces)* contains mostly water, clay, glycerin, anti-irritant, plant oil, vitamin E, and preservatives. For a clay mask, this is indeed fairly mild, but it is still just a clay mask. It can leave the skin feeling soft, but it could also make extremely dry skin feel even drier.

☺ **Extra Strength Masque** *($17 for 5 ounces)* is a fairly standard clay mask that contains mostly water, clays, glycerin, scrub agent, witch hazel, jojoba oil, cornmeal, ginseng, vitamin E, anti-irritants, and preservatives. Someone with oily skin won't be pleased with the oil in this product, and the grains can be rough on the skin. The ginseng and anti-irritants sound good, but they won't protect your skin from the irritation caused by the other ingredients.

Arbonne Makeup

☹ **Match Perfect Oil-Free Foundation SPF 8** *($20)* is a cream-to-powder foundation with a more creamy than powder finish. It is a titanium dioxide–based sunscreen which is great, but the SPF number is too low to be taken seriously for sun protection. The compact for this foundation comes packaged with two colors that are supposed to be blended together to create your perfect skin color. That's a tricky thing to have to do every morning, and for most of the duo sets one of the shades is either too peach or too ash.

☺ **$$$ True Colour Soft Finish Makeup SPF 8** *($17)* is a liquid foundation with a titanium dioxide–based SPF 8. While the titanium dioxide is great, the SPF number is too low to be considered reliable sun protection. Of the 12 shades available most have a peach tone. **The best colors are:** Beige, Taupe, Toasty, and Mahogany.

☹ **Cream Concealer** *($11.50)* comes in only one shade and it is exceedingly pink.

☺ **$$$ Translucent Pressed Powder** *($16)* has a soft, smooth, slightly powdery finish; the choices for color (two) are limited, though they are good.

☹ **Translucent Finishing Powder** *($18.50)* comes in two shades; both are fairly peach.

☹ **Bio Matte Oil-Free Powder Personalizer** *($21)* is a strange shade of green that contains mostly clay, oat flour, and wheat starch. While it does have a dry finish, the green builds a strange color on the skin, and the oat flour and wheat starch are not the best idea for preventing breakouts—it's sort of like feeding the bacteria that cause the problem.

☺ **$$$ Global Color Blushes** *($12.50)* have an impressive array of blush colors that go on smoothly though slightly powdery.

☺ **$$$ Global Color Eyeshadows** *($12.50)* come in an impressive range of matte shades in very workable, soft, more natural toned colors. Be careful, some of the shiny shades are hard to detect. **These colors are excellent** (but don't ask me to explain the bizarre names): Techno Tokyo, China Silk, California Raisin, Thunder Down Under, London Fog, Valencia Grape, German Chocolate, Seville Suede, Klondike, Havana Road, and Irish Cream.

☺ **$$$ Global Color Eye Pencils** *($8.50)* are standard, somewhat dry texture pencils that need sharpening.

☺ **$$$ Global Color Lipsticks** *($12)* have a great creamy texture, with only a slight glossy finish. The colors have a slight stain that helps keep the shades around somewhat longer than normal. **Sheer Shine** *($12)* is just a very standard, overpriced lip gloss. **Global Color Lip Pencils** *($8.50)* have a great range of colors and an application that is soft and easy.

☺ **$$$ Lash Colour Mascara** *($11.50)* is a decent mascara that creates somewhat long lashes but very little thickness.

Aubrey Organics (Skin Care Only)

If you haven't heard of Gale Hayman, Zia, Rachel Perry, or Aubrey Organics, you haven't been paying attention to the world of natural cosmetics, which of course is fine by me. The products manufactured under the names of this group of "natural" notability contain enough plants and herbs to make me wonder how anything can still be growing on this earth. These gurus of the "natural" skin-care and makeup craze sell a plethora of foliage-based concoctions that are supposed to deliver every woman's deepest desire for her face: namely, flawless skin. Of course, none of their formulas are the same. Each company has its own "natural" recipes that guarantee wrinkle-free, acne-free, smooth, even-toned, glowing skin. (This may sound a bit tacky, but Zia claims to come by her beauty naturally. Well, I've met her, and though she is stunningly beautiful, I suspect her 50-year-old visage and part of her well-endowed figure are attributable to a very skilled plastic surgeon. Not that there's anything wrong with that—but her skin-care routine has probably had some unnatural assistance.) But I digress. The subject of this review is Aubrey Organics.

If there is any such thing as a "natural" true believer, Aubrey Hampton is indeed one. His books *Natural Organic Hair and Skin Care* (Organica Press) and *What's in Your Cosmetics* (Odonian Press) articulately express his convictions. Foremost is his philosophic position regarding his products: "For almost 30 years I have collected herbs from around the world and combined them in 100% natural hair- and skin-care products. I make my natural shampoos, conditioners, soaps, lotions, masks, and so forth the way my mother taught me almost 50 years ago—without chemicals, using herbs known to be beneficial to the hair and skin."

While I'm sure Hampton's mother was a wonderful woman, what she didn't know about sun protection (we've only learned about it over the past few years), cell turnover (the life and death process of every skin cell is a recent discovery), the physiology of skin (the formation of the intercellular layer and its functions are still being investigated), and the nature of skin disease can, and does, fill volumes, and these volumes are being rewritten almost monthly as new research reveals astonishing information that has altered everything we once thought to be true about the skin. It's nice to think mom knew it all, but I wouldn't make a skin-care decision based on such obsolete and fanciful thinking.

Hampton also lauds his position on animal testing: "I don't believe in animal testing and never use it. None of my products are formulated with data obtained from animal testing, and yet I know they're safe to use because they contain ingredients that have been used for hundreds, sometimes thousands, of years by people all over the world. That's the best track record, don't you think?"

Well, I don't think so in the least. As nice as all that sounds, much of such thinking doesn't hold water, and in some ways it's actually dangerous. By his own admission, Hampton has only anecdotal past history to go by, and that is just too risky for my taste. "Natural" powders laced with "natural" lead were used by fashionably correct women centuries ago, causing necrotic skin and sometimes death. And what about sun exposure, which causes skin cancer and pervasive wrinkling? No one knew about that until very recently. So much for history being an arbiter of good health. Furthermore, while I abhor animal testing, scientists have ascertained the benefits of most new skin-care ingredients over the past 20 years, from water-binding agents and the new anti-irritants to AHAs, BHA, Retin-A, and sunscreens that provide UVA protection, mostly based on animal research. If Hampton is truly telling us that he ignores all that information, his products would be risky to use.

Another Hampton phobia, shared by many other "natural" eccentrics in the world, is petrochemicals. (I assume Hampton doesn't drive a car, take a taxi, or fly anywhere.) He states, "Petrochemicals, [which] are infinitely cheaper and much more convenient for mass manufacturers to use . . . [make] our hair and skin suffer as a result. What's worse, the long-term effects of these harsh chemicals on both the body and the environment are still unknown . . . "

Suggesting that all petrochemicals are harsh and all plants are good is as uninformed as thinking that eating any plant you encounter in the wild won't kill you because it is natural. And when will the zealots out there stop ignoring the fact that petrochemicals have a decidedly natural source: they come from decomposed plant and animal life and have an organic base! But I've belabored these subjects before. More to the point is Aubrey Organics' arsenal of skin-care recommendations.

One of the steps in Hampton's skin-care routine is steaming the face. "Applying steam is an excellent way to detoxify and deep-cleanse your skin. Pour boiling water into a heat-proof glass bowl and add four tablespoons of Face Flowers [an Aubrey Organics product]. Allow to steep several minutes, then, holding a towel over your head, put your face close to the steam. Keep your eyes closed. If your skin tends to be dry, apply [to the skin] Herbessence Complexion Oil [another Aubrey Organics product] prior to steaming; then remove oil with a warm washcloth." Nowhere does Hampton mention what kind of toxins are sweated out of the skin, nor does he discuss the potential for damage from overheating the face. One of the best and easiest ways to create surface capillaries is to repeatedly overheat the skin.

I am also very skeptical of the way Hampton handles his skin-care ingredient lists. They make no mention of standard cosmetic preservatives, and the ones that are listed—vitamins C, A, and E—have their own stability problems, with vitamin C being the most unreliable. Cosmetic chemists I have interviewed, including some who formulate "natural" skin-care products, suggest Hampton isn't revealing everything. If he is, product stability is a serious concern and the type of base he is using is questionable.

Setting aside my continuing concern about the far-fetched hype and unsubstantiated claims surrounding natural products (though Hampton is one of the few who seems to glory in the lack of real evidence), I must point out that Aubrey Organics is one of the most reasonably priced "natural" skin-care lines around, almost to the point of being cheap! If you are one of the myriad "natural" skin-care seekers out there, this line won't hurt your pocketbook. Of course, I question what it can really do for skin, but that's what my review will reveal. For more information about Aubrey Organics, call (800) 237-4270.

☺ **Rosa Mosqueta Moisturizing Cleansing Bar Normal to Dry Skin** *($5.35 for 3.6 ounces)* is supposed to be a soothing, mild bar soap without harsh synthetic detergents that can dry out your skin. It is supposed to gently cleanse the skin, keeping it soft and lightly moisturized. This is a pretty standard soap with coconut fatty acids (though the ingredient list doesn't specify which ones), which are found in most detergent bar cleansers. It also contains some plant oils, which are supposed to help in cell turnover. They can't, but they can help make the soap less drying, and that can be nice. However, coconut fatty acids can be drying and may clog pores.

☺ **Meals & Herbs Exfoliation Skin Care Bar Normal to Dry Skin** *($4.40 for 3.6 ounces)* is similar to the bar soap above, but with almond and walnut meal. While exfoliating the skin with crushed nuts is an option, it can cause problems. Nuts can scratch the skin, and a mechanical scrub affects only the very surface of the skin. While AHAs can produce a somewhat deeper, more even exfoliation and BHA can affect exfoliation in the pore, nuts can do neither.

☺ **Seaware Facial Cleanser Normal to Dry Skin** *($7 for 4 ounces)* is a standard detergent-based, water-soluble cleanser that contains kelp and other sea plant extracts. They sound nice, but this cleanser can be drying, and the sea plants have no substantiated effect on the skin.

☹ **Natural & Organic Facial Cleanser Normal to Oily Skin** *($11.10 for 8 ounces)* is a standard detergent-based water-soluble cleanser that is described as olive oil–based. Well, soap is soap, and whether it is derived from olive oil or coconut oil, it can be drying. This one also contains eucalyptus, menthol, and camphor, which can be irritating and sensitizing for all skin types.

☺ **Green Tea Facial Cleansing Lotion** *($7.25 for 4 ounces)* is a standard soap-based cleanser with undescribed fatty acids and soap ingredients. It can be drying for the skin. Green tea is a good anti-irritant, but then why would anyone add irritating ingredients like lemon peel that could irritate the eyes?

☹ **Herbal Facial Astringent Normal to Oily Skin** *($8.25 for 8 ounces)* is mostly witch hazel with some plant extracts. The nettle, rosemary, and balm-mint extracts, like the witch hazel (which is part alcohol), can be irritating or sensitizing for many skin types.

☹ **Rosa Mosqueta & English Lavender Toner Normal to Dry Skin** *($8.75 for 8 ounces)* contains mostly lavender water, glycerin, witch hazel, and a host of plant extracts. Lavender extract, witch hazel, and lemon peel can all be potentially irritating and sensitizing for most skin types.

☺ **Rosa Mosqueta Rose Hip Moisturizing Cream Normal to Dry Skin** *($14.35 for 4 ounces)* is indeed an emollient moisturizer for someone with dry skin. It contains fatty acids (which are not specified in the ingredient list, but are used in standard bases in all moisturizers), plant extracts, plant oils, and vitamins. Fatty acids are waxlike, creamy, thickening agents used throughout the entire realm of skin care. They are fine for dry skin but can clog pores when overdone. This cream has no sunscreen, which makes it appropriate for use as a nighttime moisturizer only.

☺ **Collagen & Almond Oil Hand & Body Cream All Skin Types** *($11.40 for 8 ounces)* contains the standard fatty acid base (again not specified in the ingredient list), plant oils, collagen, and elastin. Collagen and elastin can't be absorbed into the skin, but they are good water-binding agents. This cream has no sunscreen, which makes it appropriate for use as a nighttime moisturizer only.

☹ **Vegacol TMC (Vegetal Collagen Therapeutic) Moisturizer Cream Normal to Oily Skin** *($12.60 for 2 ounces)* contains a fatty acid base similar to that used in the other moisturizers in this line, and, despite the claims of what the plants in this product can do, fatty acids are notorious for clogging pores and causing breakouts.

☹ **Ultra 15 Herbal Sunblock** *($7.25 for 4 ounces)* is supposed to be a 100% vegetarian water-resistant formula with a PABA plant extract. How did this one get by the FDA? No plant form of PABA is on the list of FDA-approved sunscreen ingredients, and it is definitely not enough when used by itself. Even if it were, PABA of any kind cannot protect skin from both UVA and UVB rays. According to current research, when it comes to protecting from both UVA and UVB rays the preferred "natural" sunscreens are either zinc oxide or titanium dioxide. This product is absolutely not recommended.

☹ **Sunshade 15 Sunblock SPF 15** *($6.75 for 4 ounces)* does not contain avobenzone, zinc oxide, or titanium dioxide, and is not recommended.

☹ **Green Tea & Ginkgo Daily Moisturizer SPF 15** *($14.90 for 4 ounces)* does not contain avobenzone, zinc oxide, or titanium dioxide, and is not recommended.

☺ **100% Pure & Certified Organic Aloe Vera Gel** *($7 for 4 ounces)* is indeed aloe vera gel (which means a mixture of aloe and water) and aloe oil, which is something you don't see every day. This is fine if you want aloe, and an interesting form of it at that. I'm just not sure what you would want it for. Of course, aloe devotees believe it speeds healing and promotes regeneration of new skin cells. It is really just lightweight enough to allow skin to do its own thing.

☺ **Green Tea & Green Clay Rejuvenating Facial Mask** *($8.50 for 4 ounces)* contains mostly clay, green tea, glycerin, aloe vera, plant extracts, and plant oils. This is a standard clay mask and because of the oils, it can be OK for someone with normal to dry skin. I wonder why anyone would want this, but some women love clay masks. It does contain lemon oil, which can be a skin irritant or sensitizer.

Aveda

Headlines in fashion magazines are often different than headlines in newspapers. What you might have missed is that Aveda was purchased by Estee Lauder. It will be interesting to see how that is reflected in product changes over the next couple of years, but clearly Lauder wanted its hands in the boutique cosmetic business where Aveda has incredible style and élan. When it comes to "natural" skin-care and makeup products, the Aveda line has enough herbs, vegetables, fruits, and flowers to satisfy any plant lover's dreams and enough enlightened philosophies to satisfy anyone on a spiritual journey. The company even has an entire line of products, the Chakra line, meant to help get your body's spiritual chemistry into alignment. I wonder how the company could possibly substantiate such claims, but I suspect that if you have to ask, you shouldn't be buying those products.

Aveda's brochure poses the question, "Would you moisturize with petroleum? Enjoy the sweet smell of methyl-octine-carbonate? [Or] accentuate your eyes with a coat of tar? That's just what you do with many mainstream health and beauty products. Aveda's products are grown from a simple premise: what you put on your body should be as healthy and natural as what you'd put into it." I imagine Aveda never took a look at their own ingredient listings. Who would want to eat isostearyl benzoate, polyglyceryl-6 deoleate, diazolidinyl urea (a formaldehyde-releasing preservative), or octyl methoxycinnamate? I could go on, but you get my drift. Petroleum starts to sound pretty good in comparison to this lineup, and ends up being far better for the skin than many of the irritating and skin sensitizing-plants in Aveda's products.

Aveda's approach to beauty is an enigmatic blend of contemporary fashion and natural mania. This company portrays itself in no uncertain terms as being incapable of ever deigning to use even a hint of anything unnatural. Unfortunately, the company and I have different definitions of "natural" and "unnatural." Aveda describes many of their chemical-sounding ingredients as being derived from a natural substance, but believe me, you wouldn't want to eat those ingredients.

Most consumers are completely distracted by the aura surrounding botanicals, even though they haven't the slightest idea what infusions of cardamom, vetiver grass, albizia, turmeric, soapwort, or barberry will do for their skin. The products sound good enough to eat, and the ecology-oriented marketing is quite appealing. Naturally, when a company is charging $18 for a 4 ounce lotion, they often forget to mention that the lotion mainly consists of standard cosmetic ingredients. Furthermore, when mixed into cosmetics, plants retain little if any of their original form or purpose, and that's assuming they had a purpose in the first place.

More often than not, when you see a long list of herbs and plants on the ingredient list, what you are really purchasing is a rather expensive tea. Helpful for the skin? After these herbs have been cooked and preserved in a cosmetic, they don't contain much of whatever constituted their original promised benefit. And there is absolutely no independent evidence that proves any of the exaggerated claims on the labels. But "natural" products are very seductive, and it is hard not to conclude that you will have "natural," perfect skin if you use them. To make its products even more seductive, Aveda publishes an impressive little booklet (on recycled paper) that describes at length some of the benefits allegedly bestowed by the plants used in its products. The descriptions are exquisite, bordering on hypnotic. After reading the claims, you too will want to cover yourself in these "ancient" potions and elixirs. Aveda's boast is "2,500 years of research," although there are no Romans or ancient Egyptians around to show us their test results.

Aveda has created a line of skin-care and hair-care products called All Sensitive. Whenever I see products described as being good for sensitive skin, I am curious about how that was determined, given that there are no established guidelines for this. Some think that no fragrance, milder preservatives, and fewer ingredients (no more than eight to ten) are a basic standard for products aimed at those with sensitive skin. When I started researching Aveda's All Sensitive products, I was struck by four things: the ingredient lists are huge (small ingredient lists are considered best by dermatologists); they contain several potentially irritating ingredients; they use a mixture of plant extracts (which increases the amount of preservative needed and risks irritation for anyone with plant allergies); and they contain fragrance (ingredients like geranium oil and sandalwood are highly fragrant and have a high potential for causing skin reactions). Regardless of the product line or the claims, if you have sensitive skin you already know that it takes lots of experimenting to find products that don't make your skin react. If you are still in the process of experimenting, this line is not one I would encourage you to check out. For more information about Aveda, call (888) 288-0006 or (800) 328-0849.

Aveda Skin Care

☺ $$$ **All Sensitive Cleanser** *($19 for 5.5 ounces)* is a standard detergent-based, water-soluble cleanser. It contains lots of plant extracts (tea water), vitamins (which are washed down the drain), fragrance, and preservatives. It can be drying for some skin types, but it is water-soluble.

☹ $$$ **Purifying Cream Cleanser** *($18 for 5.5 ounces)* is supposed to be a water-soluble cleanser, but it leaves a film on the face, requiring a washcloth to get it all off. It may be OK for someone with dry skin.

☺ $$$ **Purifying Gel Cleanser** *($18 for 5.5 ounces)* is a fairly typical detergent-based, water-soluble cleanser that contains plant water and, way down on the ingredient list, some plant oils. It may be good for someone with oily skin, but the plant oils can be a problem for sensitive skin.

☹ $$$ **Pure Gel Eye Makeup Remover** *($15 for 3.7 ounces)* contains mostly plant water, detergent cleansing agents, and preservatives. It will take off eye makeup, but some of the plant extracts may irritate the eyes.

☺ $$$ **All Sensitive Toner** *($18 for 5.5 ounces)* contains a long list of plant extracts (tea water), glycerin, water-binding agents, anti-irritant, silicone, detergent cleansing agents, fragrance, and preservatives. This would be a good toner for those with normal to dry skin if they aren't allergic to the plants it contains.

☺ $$$ **Skin Firming/Toning Agent** *($18 for 5.5 ounces)* contains rose water, an herb called echinacea, anti-irritant, slip agent, and preservative. This is a good irritant-free toner, but it won't firm anything. Echinacea has a good reputation as an oral alternative medication to boost the immune system and help prevent colds. In order to get that benefit you need to take it orally not topically. Plus there is no evidence that in the tiny amount used here it can have benefit through the skin.

☹ **Toning Mist** *($16 for 5.5 ounces)* is a fairly irritating product that contains primarily a tea of white oak bark, witch hazel, aloe, and peppermint, as well as rose water, alcohol, grapefruit extract, and glycerin.

☹ **Exfoliant** *($14 for 5.5 ounces)* is a liquid toner that contains lavender water, chamomile, lemon balm, witch hazel, alcohol, and salicylic acid. Several of these ingredients can be incredibly drying and irritating for all skin types. Plus, the pH of this product isn't low enough to permit the salicylic acid to work as an exfoliant anyway.

☺ **$$$ All Sensitive Moisturizer** *($28 for 5.5 ounces)* contains a long list of plant extracts (tea water), several thickeners, glycerin, vitamins, silicone, fragrance, and preservatives. This is a fairly ordinary moisturizer with a minuscule amount of vitamins. It can be OK for someone with dry skin.

☺ **$$$ Firming Fluid** *($32 for 1 ounce)* contains tea water, water-binding agent, plant extracts, thickeners, vitamins, and preservatives. This is a good lightweight moisturizer for someone with normal to slightly dry skin, but it won't firm anything.

☺ **$$$ Hydrating Lotion** *($26 for 5.5 ounces)* contains a tea of chamomile, lavender, rosemary, and comfrey, as well as glycerin, thickeners, rice oil, and jojoba oil. Several of the thickeners are possible irritants. This lotion can be good for normal to slightly dry skin that isn't sensitive.

☺ **$$$ Miraculous Beauty Replenisher** *($17 for 1 ounce)* contains mostly thickener, plant oil, fragrance, and vitamins. I guess $17 isn't much for a miracle, but expecting one from this moisturizer can be a waste of time.

☺ **$$$ Night Nutrients** *($38 for 1 ounce)* contains mostly silicone, plant oils, and vitamins. This is a good emollient moisturizer for dry skin, but it won't feed the skin.

☹ **Oil-Free Hydraderm** *($26 for 5.5 ounces)* contains castor oil, which is hardly oil-free. It also contains lemon, which can be a skin irritant.

☺ **$$$ Pure Vital Moisture Eye Creme** *($26 for 0.5 ounce)* contains mostly plant water, thickeners, glycerin, more thickeners, several water-binding agents, vitamin E, silicone, and preservatives. This is a good moisturizer for someone with dry skin, but most of the really interesting ingredients are at the end of the ingredient list and don't add up to much.

☺ **$$$ Daily Light Guard SPF 15** *($16.50 for 5 ounces)* is a titanium dioxide–based sunscreen that would be very good for someone with dry skin.

☹ **Light Protection SPF 12** *($28 for 5.5 ounces)* doesn't contain avobenzone, titanium dioxide, or zinc oxide, and is not recommended.

☺ **$$$ Sun Source** *($16.58 for 5 ounces)*, like all self-tanning products, uses the very unnatural ingredient dihydroxyacetone. It will turn skin brown the same as any $6 self-tanner will.

☺ **$$$ Balancing Infusion for Dry Skin** *($18 for 0.33 ounce)* contains mostly plant oil, fragrance, water-binding agents, and vitamins. This is a good, but very overpriced, plant oil for dry skin.

☹ **Balancing Infusion for Oily Skin** *($18 for 0.33 ounce)* contains 0.5% salicylic acid as well as jojoba oil, plant oil, and silicone (which has an oily texture). Even if this form of BHA had the right pH to work as an exfoliant (it doesn't), the other ingredients can clog pores and make the skin feel quite oily!

☺ $$$ **Balancing Infusion for Sensitive Skin** *($18 for 0.33 ounce)* contains mostly thickener, plant oil, anti-irritant, and vitamins. While nothing about this product makes it preferred for sensitive skin, and the plants and flowers it contains are a problem for anyone with sensitive skin, it can be good for someone with dry skin.

☹ **Bio-Molecular Recovery Treatment** *($28 for 1 ounce)* contains mostly plant water, lactic acid, glycerin, salicylic acid, vitamins E and A, thickeners, fragrance, and preservatives. This is about a 5% AHA and BHA product combined; however, the pH of this product isn't low enough for it to be an effective exfoliant.

☺ $$$ **Deep Cleansing Herbal Clay Masque** *($20 for 4.5 ounces)* is, for the most part, just a standard clay mask that contains kaolin as its primary ingredient. As a clay mask it may be more gentle than most. Several ingredients in this mask can cause breakouts, and others make it appropriate only for someone with dry skin, but even then the clay may be too drying.

☹ **Intensive Hydrating Masque** *($29 for 5.5 ounces)* contains mostly a tea of aloe, kelp, lavender, and rose water, as well as glycerin, thickener, water-binding agent, anti-irritant, protein, and preservatives. It also contains a "tissue respiratory factor," described on the label as biofermentation of corn. Fermentation in this instance means the action of bacteria on corn. The bacteria break down the corn, resulting in the release of gases such as hydrogen sulfide and carbon dioxide. It sounds better when you don't know what it really is, doesn't it?

☹ **Lip Saver SPF 15** *($8 for 0.15 ounce)* doesn't contain avobenzone, titanium dioxide, or zinc oxide, and is not recommended.

Aveda Makeup

☺ $$$ <u>FOUNDATION:</u> **Base Plus Balance** *($20.50)* is an excellent foundation with a smooth, slightly matte finish. The coverage isn't what I would call natural but it does provide very good light to medium coverage. **Most of the colors are wonderful, with no overtones of peach or pink. The only colors you may want to avoid are** Amber and Mocha.

☺ $$$ **Dual Base Minus Oil** *($19.50)* is a fairly standard powder foundation with a very good color selection and a soft finish; it works better as a pressed powder than a foundation. The recommendation to wear it wet doesn't really work, as it can look streaked and choppy.

☺ <u>CONCEALER:</u> **Conceal Plus Protect** *($13.50)* goes on rather creamy, but dries to a light, matte finish. For the most part it works quite well and doesn't crease. What a shame it only comes in three shades.

☺ $$$ <u>POWDER:</u> **Pressed Powder Plus Antioxidants** *($17.50)* and **Pure Finish Loose Powder** *($18.50)* are standard talc-based powders with a silky, dry, translucent finish. The color selection is beautiful and the application sheer and soft. In the Loose Powder, Bronze can be too peach, and in the Pressed Powder, Cream can be slightly peach.

☺   **BLUSH:** **Blush Minus Mineral Oil** *($11)* comes in a beautiful selection of subtle matte shades, blends on easily, and has a smooth, dry finish. Of all the colors, only Vapor may be too shiny pink to use daily.

☺   **EYESHADOW:** **Shadow Plus Vitamins** *($10)* comes in a good assortment of neutral matte shades that go on even and soft, though perhaps too soft. Don't expect much intensity or coverage from these colors. The shiny shades are clearly iridescent and easily avoided.

☺   **EYE AND BROW SHAPER:** **Eye Pencil Minus Preservatives** *($11)* is a standard pencil that comes in an attractive range of colors.

☺   **LIPSTICK AND LIP PENCIL:** **Lip Matte Plus Fresh Essence** *($14)* is a creamy opaque lipstick with a smooth semi-matte finish and remains one of my personal favorites. It doesn't bleed, but still has a slightly creamy finish. **Lip Satin Plus Fresh Essence** *($14)* is a good creamy lipstick. **Lip Satin Plus Uruku** *($14)* makes a big fuss about using annatto, a natural coloring agent, in these slightly glossy lipsticks. Of course, they also contain good old iron oxides and manganese violet to help create a variety of colors. While those are natural metal oxides, they are standard colorings throughout the cosmetics industry, and have their own issues in terms of problems for the skin or inhalation. Not that I think they are a problem, but there are risks associated with them, which Aveda ignores, preferring to point out warnings only about those things that sound unnatural. **Lip Gloss** *($12.50)* is a small pot of very emollient, very standard gloss. **Lip Liner Minus Preservatives** *($11)* is just a standard pencil in a good range of colors.

☺   **$$$ MASCARA:** **Mascara Plus Rose** *($14.50)* is a very good mascara. It goes on easily and holds up during the day. It doesn't build much length or thickness, but if you're looking for a less noticeable application of mascara this one is just fine.

☺   **BRUSHES:** Aveda has a wonderful collection of brushes *($6.50 to $23.50)*; only a few should be avoided. The **Powder Brush** *($23.50)* is too loosely packed and the bristles are rather long for good control. The **Eye Liner Brush** *($7.50)* is too thick to create a controlled line along the lashes. The handle of the **Lip Brush** *($19.50)* is too long to be convenient; the **Retractable Lip Brush** *($6.95)* is cheaper and works better. All the other brushes are worth checking out, particularly the eyeshadow brushes.

Aveeno (Skin Care Only)

For more information about Aveeno products, call (800) 558-5252.

☹   **Aveeno Natural Colloidal Oatmeal Cleansing Bar for Dry Skin** *($2.99 for 3 ounces)* contains about 50% oatmeal, which can be a soothing agent. It also contains a detergent cleanser, vegetable oil, vegetable shortening, glycerin, lactic acid (about 4%), mineral oil, and preservatives. Although it could be a good bar soap if you have dry skin, the AHA ingredient could be too irritating if you use another AHA product afterwards.

☹ **Aveeno Natural Colloidal Oatmeal Cleansing Bar for Combination Skin** (*$2.99 for 3 ounces*) contains about 50% oatmeal, which can be a soothing agent. It also contains glycerin, lactic acid (about 5%), petrolatum (like Vaseline), and thickeners. The petrolatum makes it questionable for combination skin, and the AHA ingredient could be too irritating if you use another AHA product afterwards.

☹ **Aveeno Natural Colloidal Oatmeal Cleansing Bar for Acne Prone Skin** (*$2.99 for 3 ounces*) contains salicylic acid (BHA). While BHA can help prevent breakouts, in a soap its effectiveness is just rinsed down the drain rather than left on the skin, while all the problems of a bar cleanser remain.

☹ **Aveeno Medicated Acne Cleanser** (*$5.60 for 6 ounces*). BHA in a bar cleanser doesn't make much sense because the ingredient would just be rinsed off the face. In addition, this product contains several ingredients, including tallow, that could clog pores.

Avon

One of the major complaints I have about Avon is their sales force, and one of the biggest complements I have for the company is about their wonderful Web page (*www.avon.com*) that provides a complete ingredient listing for all their products (something most every other cosmetics line leaves out). Awesome Avon. When it comes to Avon's salespeople, though these women try hard, most of them are little more than order-takers. In fact, most of the representatives I talked to were quite honest about how much they didn't know about makeup or skin care, or specifics about the products they were selling. None of the Avon women I spoke to even had samples or testers. And there is often a great deal of confusion about what products are available during a given "campaign." If you have the wrong book or the products aren't up on the Web site, you're out of luck. That's not just confusing, it's frustrating.

Avon has an astonishing number of products. I doubt that any salesperson could keep track of them all anyway, or afford to. In addition, most of the women who work for Avon do it part-time, to earn extra money, not as a major source of income. (The average sales representative earns about $5,000 a year, top sellers earn about $10,000, and only the rare exceptions earn more than $20,000 a year.) That constitutes a sales force whose main interest is not necessarily Avon. (Avon does guarantee 100% satisfaction, and they are true to that policy.) However, if you know what you want, there are some incredible bargains, particularly in the lip and eye pencils, mascara, lipsticks, and some very good skin-care products, particularly the water-soluble cleansers and the moisturizers for dry skin.

By the way, Avon's line of AHA products, called Anew, went through quite an overhaul. While it now offers more products than ever before, for the most part the AHA content is missing, and the sunscreen additions contain no UVA protection. That isn't an improvement in the least.

I must praise Avon's commitment to consumer information. The operators at their ordering number—(800) 233-2866—and their consumer information center number—(800) 445-2866—were quite helpful. No matter how many products I requested ingredient lists for, they provided them without hesitation or question. Thank you, Avon, for great customer service.

Avon Skin Care

☺ **Anew Perfect Cleanser** *($11 for 5.1 ounces)* is a standard detergent-based water-soluble cleanser that can be good for most skin types. It does contains a small amount of orange oil, which can be a skin irritant.

☺ **Anew O$_2$ Energizer Clarifying Essence** *($14.50 for 4.2 ounces)* has no extra oxygen, unless you count water (H$_2$O). This is just a toner of water and glycerin, very ordinary and very overpriced.

☹ **Anew All-In-One Intensive Complex SPF 15** *($18 for 1.7 ounces)* doesn't contain zinc oxide, titanium dioxide, or avobenzone, and is not recommended.

☹ **Anew All-In-One Perfecting Complex SPF 15** *($16 for 1.7 ounces)* doesn't contain zinc oxide, titanium dioxide, or avobenzone, and is not recommended.

☹ **Anew All-In-One Perfecting Lotion SPF 8** *($16 for 1.7 ounces)* doesn't contain zinc oxide, titanium dioxide, or avobenzone, and is not recommended; besides, SPF 8 wasn't a convincing number for sun protection even before the new sunscreen information came out.

☺ **$$$ Anew Formula C Treatment Capsules** *($19 for thirty 0.41 ounce capsules)* is pretty pricey for an Avon skin-care product, but when you consider that Avon is attempting to compete with Cellex-C, which sells for $70 an ounce and lots of other overpriced vitamin C products, this one is truly a bargain. The form of vitamin C in this product is ascorbic acid, considered to be among the more irritating and less effective of the vitamin Cs used in cosmetics in terms of its effect as an antioxidant.

☺ **Anew Perfect Eye Care Cream SPF 15** *($12.50 for 0.53 ounce)* is a product containing about 2% AHAs with a pH of 6, which makes it a poor exfoliant. Though the AHA part is misleading, part of the SPF 15 is titanium dioxide, and that's good.

☺ **Anew Instant Eye Smoother** *($16 for 0.5 ounce)* is a good silicone-based moisturizer for normal to dry skin and would work well to smooth and soothe. It is in many ways quite similar to Clinique's All About Eyes. This moisturizer contains silicones, thickener, film former, water-binding agents, and preservatives.

☺ **Anew Moisture Supply Day Cream** *($16 for 1.7 ounces)* is a good moisturizer for dry skin, but for daytime you would need to add a sunscreen. This cream contains mostly water, thickeners, silicone, plant oils, water-binding agents, and preservatives.

☺ **Anew Moisture Supply Night Cream** *($16 for 1.7 ounces)* is just a simple moisturizer of water, mineral oil, thickeners, and Vaseline. It would be good for someone with dry skin.

☺ **$$$ Anew Day Force Vertical Lifting Force SPF 15** *($20 for 1 ounce)* won't do anything to get rid of wrinkles, but it is a very good, though very overpriced, moisturizing sunscreen with avobenzone. It basically contains water, silicone, glycerin, vitamins, thickeners, water-binding agents, plant oils, and preservatives. Both Ombrelle and Lancome (as well as my line) have avobenzone-based sunscreens for far less money.

☺ **$$$ Intensive Line Minimizer** *($12.50 for 0.13 ounce)* is a very overpriced glycolic acid–based 8% AHA product in a lightweight gel/lotion base. It does have a good concentration and a low pH, but the price! I don't know what Avon is thinking these days. At this price, it ends up being almost $100 for one ounce of this stuff. That makes this one of the most expensive AHA products on the market.

☺ **Anew Night Force Vertical Lifting Complex** *($20 for 1.7 ounces)* isn't pricey by some standards, but it is far from what I would call reasonably priced, especially for what you get. It contains mostly water, silicone, thickener, petrolatum, glycerin, more thickeners, slip agent, more thickeners, more silicone, vitamins, fragrance, and preservatives. It does have two new ingredients that I haven't seen anywhere else: ammonium trioxaundecanedioate and trioxaundecanedioic acid. At this writing, I can't find independent information about what they do, but I suspect they are some kind of thickening agent and possibly a peeling agent.

☺ **Anew Perfecting Lotion for Problem Skin** *($15.50 for 1.7 ounces)* is a standard lotion and salicylic acid–based product that also contains about 3% AHA. While the BHA part of this product would work fine, the amount of AHA isn't enough to work as an exfoliant. I'm also not one to recommend combining both AHA and BHA, although using each one alone, depending on the problem, is just fine.

☺ **Anew Retinol Recovery Complex P.M. Treatment** *($17.50 for 1 ounce)* is just a good standard moisturizer for someone with normal to dry skin, but that's it. Research does show that Retinol, a vitamin A derivative, can benefit the skin; however, it takes a lot more Retinol than this product contains—20 times as much, according to one study.

☹ **Anew Alpha Peel Off Facial Mask** *($12.50 for 2.53 ounces)* contains a film former in an alcohol base that hardens and then is peeled off. It also contains about 4% AHA, but in a pH of 5, which is too high to work as an exfoliant. This is a mask that risks too many problems for the skin.

☹ **Basics Deep Clean Cold Cream** *($4.99 for 6.7 ounces)* is, as the name implies, a standard wipe-off makeup remover. It can leave a greasy film on the skin, and pulling at the skin can cause sagging.

☹ **Basics Really Clean Gel Cleanser** *($4.99 for 5.1 ounces)* is a standard detergent-based, water-soluble cleanser. It does contain a small amount of menthol, which makes it unnecessarily irritating for all skin types.

☹ **Basics Right Balance Cream Cleanser** *($4.99 for 5.1 ounces)* is just a wipe-off cleanser that can leave a film behind on the skin; it contains mostly thickening agents and plant oil.

☺ **Basics Perfect Day Moisture Cream** *($4.99 for 3.4 ounces)* is a fairly thick but good moisturizer for very dry skin. It primarily contains thickeners, silicone, petrolatum, plant oil, vitamins, water-binding agents, and preservatives.

☺ **Basics Vita Moist Face Cream** *($4.99 for 3.4 ounces)* is similar to the cream above but contains more mineral oil. The same basic review applies.

☹ **Calming Effects Sensitive Skin Cleanser** *($9.50 for 6.7 ounces)* is a wipe-off cleanser that can leave a greasy film on the skin. There is nothing more calming about this cold cream–type product than any other you might find.

☹ **Calming Effects Sensitive Skin Toner** *($9.50 for 6.7 ounces)* is a toner that contains alcohol, which makes it absolutely not good for any skin type, much less for someone with sensitive skin.

☺ **Calming Effects Sensitive Skin Creme** *($10.50 for 1.7 ounces)* is quite similar to the Basics Perfect Day Moisture Cream above, and the same basic review applies. Why this one is far more expensive is sheer marketing, and has nothing to do with either ingredients or formulation.

☺ **Calming Effects Sensitive Skin Lotion** *($10.50 for 1.7 ounces)* is similar to the creme above, but includes more silicone and comes in lotion form. This is fine for normal to dry skin.

☹ **Clearskin Antibacterial Cleansing Cake** *($1.99 for 3 ounces)* contains sodium tallowate, which can clog pores and cause irritation.

☹ **Clearskin Cleansing Pads for Sensitive Skin** *($3.99 for 42 pads)* contains alcohol and menthol, which makes the product too irritating and drying for all skin types, especially for sensitive skin.

☹ **Clearskin Maximum Strength Cleansing Pads** *($3.49 for 42 pads)* contains salicylic acid (skin irritant and peeling agent), water, alcohol, witch hazel (skin irritant), an antiseptic, preservative, fragrance, menthol (skin irritant), aloe, and vitamin E. It is too strong and drying for most skin types, particularly when used in association with any of the other Clearskin products.

☺ **Clearskin Foaming Facial Cleanser** *($3.29 for 4 ounces)* contains water, detergent cleansers, coloring agent, preservatives, and menthol (skin irritant). It can be irritating for most skin types, but may be an OK water-soluble cleanser for younger skin.

☹ **Clearskin Medicated Gel Wash** *($4.99 for 5.1 ounces)* uses sodium C14-16 olefin sulfate as the main cleansing agent (it is the second ingredient), a substance that is very drying and irritating for the skin.

☹ **Clearskin Antibacterial Cleansing Scrub** *($2.99 for 2.5 ounces)* contains mostly water, slip agent, vegetable oil, mineral oil, thickener, glycerin, more thickener, alcohol, detergent cleanser, menthol, and a blue salt coloring agent. As a scrub it is OK, but the oils are not great for anyone with oily skin, and the menthol and alcohol are irritating.

☹ **Clearskin Clearbreeze Astringent** *($3.49 for 8 ounces)* contains mostly water, alcohol, peppermint oil, eucalyptus oil, and camphor. The number of irritating ingredients in this product is astounding and none of them are beneficial for the skin.

☹ **Clearskin Maximum Strength Astringent Cleansing Lotion** *($3.99 for 8 ounces)* contains more alcohol than anyone should even consider allowing near their face.

☺ **Clearskin 10% Benzoyl Peroxide Vanishing Cream** *($3.39 for 0.75 ounce)* contains water, slip agent, thickener, preservative, sodium hydroxide, and benzoyl peroxide. It can be an OK, but strong, benzoyl peroxide disinfectant, although the sodium hydroxide can be irritating for most skin types.

☹ **Clearskin Overnight Acne Treatment** *($3.49 for 2 ounces)* contains salicylic acid (skin irritant and peeling agent), water, alcohol, and thickeners. It will peel the skin and dry it out terribly—not a great thing to wake up to in the morning.

☹ **Clearskin Clay Mask** *($3.99 for 3 ounces)* is a standard clay mask with alcohol and cornstarch, two very problematic ingredients for acne-prone skin.

☺ **Moisturizing Gentle Creme Cleanser** *($7.50 for 6.7 ounces)* requires wiping to get makeup off. It is always problematic to wipe off makeup because that can cause the skin to sag. But this could be a good cleanser for someone with dry skin who doesn't wear much makeup.

☺ **Purifying Facial Cleansing Gel** *($7.50 for 6.7 ounces)* is a standard detergent-based, water-soluble cleanser that can be good for someone with normal to oily skin.

☹ **Eye Makeup Remover Pads** *($5.50 for 80 pads)* is a standard detergent cleanser–type eye-makeup remover. It will get makeup off, but wiping and pulling at the skin is always a problem.

☹ **Moisture Effective Eye Makeup Remover Lotion** *($3.50 for 2 ounces)* is a standard mineral oil–based makeup remover that can leave a greasy film on the skin.

☹ **Perfect Wear Makeup Remover** *($4.50 for 2 ounces)* is similar to the remover above, only this one contains mostly silicone. Silicone leaves a nicer finish on the skin but it still means makeup has to be wiped off, and that isn't good for the skin.

☹ **Skin Refiner Exfoliating Scrub** *($8 for 2 ounces)* includes a tiny bit of papaya, but so little that it couldn't refine anything. It does contain tiny bits of synthetic scrub particles that make it a decent scrub, but several of the cleansing agents in here can make it fairly drying for most skin types.

☺ **Moisturizing Alcohol-Free Toner** *($7.50 for 6.7 ounces)* contains mostly water, slip agent, plant extracts, vitamins, detergent, and preservatives. This is a good but basic toner for someone with normal to slightly dry skin.

☻ **Purifying Matte-Finish Toner for Normal to Oily Skin** *($8 for 6.7 ounces)* contains mostly alcohol, which makes it too irritating for most skin types.

☻ **Smooth Finish Alpha Hydroxy Cream** *($8.50 for 1.7 ounces)* contains less than 3% AHA, which makes it a poor exfoliant. However, everything else about this cream makes it a mediocre but OK moisturizer for normal to dry skin.

☹ **BioAdvance 2000 Skin Lotion and Fortifier** *($20 for 0.85 ounce of the skin lotion and 0.12 ounce of the fortifier)* are two separate components of one product that you mix together. The lotion contains water, film former, silicone, petrolatum, preservative, thickeners, and preservatives. The fortifier contains mostly silicone, alcohol, thickener, vitamin A, plant oil, and preservatives. The vitamin A is nice, but it can't change a wrinkle, and the alcohol can irritate the skin.

☺ **Dramatic Firming Cream for Face and Throat** *($12 for 1.5 ounces)* won't firm anything, but it is a good moisturizer for dry skin. It contains mostly water, thickeners, plant oils (one is arnica, which can be an irritant), vitamins, and preservatives.

☹ **Eye Perfector Soothing Eye Gel with Liposomes** *($8.50 for 0.6 ounce)* contains mostly water, witch hazel, slip agent, plant extracts, water-binding agents, thickeners, vitamins, and preservatives. Except for the witch hazel, which can be a skin irritant, this would be a good lightweight moisturizer for dry skin.

☻ **Hydra Gel Oil-Control Lotion** *($10 for 1.7 ounces)* is a silicone-based moisturizer that also contains too much alcohol for it to be an option for any skin type.

☺ **Hydrofirming Cream Night Treatment** *($11 for 1.7 ounces)* contains mostly water, glycerin, petrolatum, thickeners, slip agents, plant oils, plant extracts, vitamins, water-binding agents, silicone, and preservatives. This is a good emollient moisturizer for someone with dry skin. The cream won't firm anything, but it is an excellent emollient moisturizer for someone with seriously dry skin.

☺ **Hydrofirming Eye Treatment** *($9.50 for 0.5 ounce)* contains mostly water, glycerin, thickeners, plant extracts, plant oil, vitamins, water-binding agents, and preservatives. This would be a good moisturizer for normal to dry skin.

☺ **Maximum Moisture Super Hydrating Gel** *($10.50 for 2.5 ounces)* contains mostly water, glycerin, slip agents, emollient, thickeners, vitamins, plant oils, and preservatives. This would be a good moisturizer for someone with dry skin.

☻ **Moisture Generator Cream** *($8 for 2.5 ounces)* contains mostly petrolatum and alcohol, with the alcohol making it unacceptable for most skin types.

☻ **Nurtura Replenishing Cream** *($7 for 2 ounces)* does contain BHA, but the pH isn't low enough for it to be an effective exfoliant.

☺ **Age Block Daytime Defense Cream SPF 15 UVA/UVB Protection** *($12.50 for 1.7 ounces)* is a great sunscreen with avobenzone for UVA protection for someone with normal to slightly dry skin. It does contain alcohol, but most likely as an emulsifier so that shouldn't cause problems for most skin types. This is still pricey for a sunscreen though.

☺ **Avon Sun Age-Fighting Protective Sun Cream SPF 15 Waterproof** *($10 for 4.2 ounces)* is a very good avobenzone-based sunscreen for normal to slightly dry skin. It contains mostly water, slip agent, film former, thickeners, vitamins, plant extracts, and preservatives.

☺ **Avon Sun Age-Fighting Protective Sun Cream SPF 30 Waterproof** *($10 for 4.2 ounces)* is similar to the cream above only with a higher SPF; the same review applies.

☹ **Avon Sun Age-Fighting Protective Sun Gel SPF 6** *($9.50 for 4.2 ounces)* has a terribly low SPF and doesn't contain avobenzone, zinc oxide, or titanium dioxide; it is not recommended.

☹ **Avon Sun Sunless Tanning Cream SPF 8** *($9.50 for 4.2 ounces)* is a standard dihydroxyacetone-based self-tanner but with its SPF 8 without any UVA protection it's useless for outdoor use.

☹ **Skin-So-Soft Bug Guard Mosquito Repellent SPF 15 Moisturizing Sunblock Spray** *($9.95 for 4 ounces)* I can't verify that this product does or doesn't keep the bugs away, but as a sunscreen it doesn't contain avobenzone, zinc oxide, or titanium dioxide, and is not recommended.

☹ **Skin-So-Soft Moisturizing Suncare Plus SPF 15 and 30, Original Woodland & Herbal Fresh Scents** *($9.95 and $11.95 for 4 ounces)* has similar ingredients to the spray above, and the same review applies.

☹ **Skin-So-Soft for Kids SPF 30** *($11.95 for 4 ounces)* is similar to the products above and the same review applies.

☹ **Moisture Lift Protective Cream SPF 15** *($10 for 1.7 ounces)* doesn't contain zinc oxide, titanium dioxide, or avobenzone, and is not recommended.

☹ **Moisture Lift Protective Lotion SPF 15** *($10 for 1.7 ounces)* doesn't contain zinc oxide, titanium dioxide, or avobenzone, and is not recommended.

☺ **Banishing Cream Skin Lightening Treatment** *($8.50 for 2.5 ounces)* can have an effect on darkened patches of skin. It uses 2% hydroquinone in a fairly standard moisturizing base of water, thickeners, petrolatum, and preservatives. Like all hydroquinone-based skin-lightening products, it can improve pigment problems if you are using a reliable sunscreen every day; just don't expect the dark areas to go away completely.

☺ **Lighten Up** *($14.50 for 0.5 ounce)* is supposed to reduce dark circles and diminish lines, just what most women want from an eye product. This one contains mostly glycerin, water, thickeners, silicone, plant oils, vitamins, water-binding agents, and preservatives. That makes it a very good emollient moisturizer for any area of the face, but it contains nothing that makes it better than hundreds of other moisturizers.

☺ **Intensive Hydrating Facial Mask** *($8.50 for 3.4 ounces)* doesn't include anything intense; it's just a good basic dry-skin moisturizer that contains thickeners, petrolatum, plant oils, water-binding agents, vitamins, fragrance, and preservatives. That's good for dry skin, but it's no different from a lot of moisturizers in Avon's lineup.

☺ **Soothing Hydrating Mask Rose & Apple Blossom** *($4.99 for 3 ounces)* is similar to the Intensive Hydrating Facial Mask above and the same review applies.

☹ **Pore Reducer Beauty Treatment Mask** *($8.50 for 3 ounces)* is basically a clay mask (bentonite) that contains alcohol and rice starch with some glycerin. It won't reduce pores (there isn't a clay mask on earth that can), but it can dry out and irritate the skin.

☹ **Refreshing Hydrating Mask, Bay & Eucalyptus** *($4.99 for 3 ounces)* includes both bay and eucalyptus oil, which are irritating, not refreshing, and can cause problems for all skin types.

☹ **Stimulating Hydrating Mask, Peppermint & Ivy** *($4.99 for 3 ounces)* contains both ivy and peppermint, which are irritating not stimulating, which is a problem for all skin types.

☺ **Stress Shield Serum** *($12.50 for 1 ounce)* won't reduce stress on the face, but it is a good, lightweight, gel-type moisturizer with a 5% to 6% concentration of AHAs. If you're looking for a gentle AHA product, this is a good one. It contains mostly water, slip agent, glycerin, AHAs, water-binding agents, vitamins, anti-irritant, and preservatives.

☹ **On Everyone's Lips Daily Lip Refiner** *($8.50 for 0.5 ounces)* is supposed to prevent lipstick from bleeding; regrettably, it doesn't work.

☹ **Moisture Therapy Moisturizing Lip Treatment SPF 15** *($1.49 for 0.15 ounce)* doesn't contain avobenzone, zinc oxide, or titanium dioxide, and is not recommended.

☹ **New Figure Cellulite Body Cream** *($10 for 2 ounces)* is supposed to "improve the appearance of skin in cellulite-prone areas and smooth skin in areas subject to stretch marks. And it's been clinically proven to show results in as few as four weeks." All that for $10. My oh my! Of course, the copy doesn't say it will get rid of cellulite or stretch marks, just improve their appearance, which any moisturizer could. It contains mostly water, thickeners, plant oils, glycerin, more thickeners, silicone, plant extracts, salicylic acid, water-binding agents, more plant extracts, and preservatives. Salicylic acid can help exfoliate skin, but that won't change a bump on your body.

Avon Makeup

FOUNDATION: Much like shopping at a drugstore, shopping for foundations from a catalog can be incredibly frustrating. Not being able to test the color is one issue, but catalog shopping compounds the problem because you can't even see the actual color. Judging compatibility from a color swatch that is a picture of the color is at best problematic. Unless you have an Avon Lady with samples for a range of colors for the foundation you are interested in, and that you preferably can try on, think twice about going this route for foundation.

☹ **Perfect Wear Foundation SPF 6** *($8.95)* is a titanium dioxide–based sunscreen, but its low SPF 6 really makes it useless. This is Avon's version of a stay-put foundation, and it does work OK although the texture leaves much to be desired and it is not reliable for a full day of sun protection. Another warning: All of these colors have some amount of sparkle. What is shine doing in a product meant to be a matte, transfer-resistant finish? **These colors are excellent:** Creamy Beige, Rich Honey, Almond Beige, Porcelain Beige, Toasted Tan, and Warmest Beige. **These colors are too peach, pink, or orange:** Honey Beige, Soft Bisque, Ivory Beige, Cocoa, Warm Bronze, Toasted Brown, Blush Tint, Rose Beige.

☺ **Face Lifting Moisture Firm Foundation Liquid** *($8.95)* has a smooth consistency and glides over the face, providing light to medium coverage and a semi-matte finish. (Of course, this foundation won't lift the face anywhere; it does have a smattering of good water-binding agents, but those don't lift the skin.) This is a terrific product for normal to dry skin. **These colors are exceptional:** Ivory Beige, Porcelain Beige, Soft Bisque, Creamy Beige, True Beige, Warmest Beige, Honey Beige, Almond Beige, Warm Bronze, Toasted Tan, Toasted Brown, Rich Honey, Cool Copper, Cocoa, Deepest Brown, and Mahogany. **These colors are too peach or pink:** Blush Beige, Rose Tint Beige, and Rich Copper.

☺ **Face Lifting Moisture Firm Foundation Cream** *($8.95)* is a creamy foundation that would work well for someone with dry skin. It doesn't lift the skin anywhere, but some of the foundation colors are quite good. **These colors are great:** Ivory Beige, Porcelain Beige, Soft Bisque, Creamy Beige, True Beige, Warmest Beige, Honey Beige, Almond Beige, Warm Bronze, Toasted Tan, Toasted Brown, Rich Honey, Cool Copper, Cocoa, Deepest Brown, and Mahogany. **These colors are too peach or pink:** Blush Beige, Rose Tint Beige, and Rich Copper.

☺ **Clear Finish Oil-Free Foundation Anti-Acne Treatment** *($5.25)* gets its anti-acne effects with salicylic acid (BHA). BHA isn't a treatment, it's an exfoliant, and it works better in skin-care products where the pH is around 3 and you have better control over where and how often your skin type needs it. This product has a pH of 5, which means the BHA won't even exfoliate well. Still, this can be a good foundation with a soft matte finish. **These colors are very good:** Porcelain Beige, Almond Beige, Warm Bronze, Rich Honey, Toasted Brown, Deepest Brown, and Mahogany. **These colors are too peach, pink, orange, or rose:** Creamy Beige, Ivory Beige, True Beige, Soft Bisque, Blush Beige, Rose Tint Beige, Honey Beige, Warmest Beige, Cool Copper, Toasted Tan, Rich Copper, and Cocoa.

☺ **Calming Effects Illuminating Foundation** *($8.95)* isn't all that calming, but it is a very good, lightweight foundation that blends on fairly sheer and dries to a smooth matte finish. Liquidy-thin foundations like this seem to be very popular this season, with similar products being offered by Chanel, Prescriptives, and Revlon. Perhaps the only drawback for Avon's is the poor range of colors. There are more pink, peach, and rose tones than there are neutral skin tones. What a shame. Despite this limitation, there are a few excellent colors to choose from, especially for medium to darker skin tones. If you have normal to oily skin this is a real option. **These colors are beautifully neutral and are all great shades to consider:** Almond Beige, Warmest Beige, Creamy Beige, Rich Honey, Cool Copper, Toasted Brown, Warm Bronze, Deepest Brown, and Mahogany. **These colors are either too peach, too pink, or too red, and should be avoided:** True Beige, Blush Beige, Honey Beige, Rose Tint Beige, Cocoa, Rich Copper, Soft Bisque, Toasted Tan, Porcelain Beige, and Ivory Beige.

☺ **Perfect Match Wet/Dry Powder** *($5.25)* is a standard, very powdery talc-based powder that has sparkle (which isn't the best for every day). After all, isn't a powder supposed to leave a matte finish and reduce shine? Regardless, the coverage for this one is choppy and uneven, wet or dry.

☺ **Perfect Match Self Adjusting Foundation** *($5.50)* doesn't self-adjust, but it is a very creamy, smooth foundation that blends on sheer and soft with a dry matte finish. **These colors are beautiful:** Porcelain Beige, Soft Bisque, Warmest Beige, Creamy Beige, Almond Beige, Toasted Tan, Cocoa, Toasted Brown, Cool Copper, Warm Bronze, Deepest Brown, Rich Honey, and Mahogany. **These colors are too peach, pink, or orange:** True Beige, Rose Tint Beige, Rich Copper, and Ivory Beige.

☺ <u>CONCEALER:</u> **Face Lifting Moisture Firm Concealer with SPF 8** *($4.75)* won't lift or firm, has a poor texture, and creases terribly. The color selection is either peach or pink. **Concealing Stick** *($4.25)* goes on quite smooth but thick with a matte finish, but creases and looks caked under the eye. **Face Lifting Corrector Pencil** *($4.25)* is a thin version of the Big Cover Up Concealer Pen, except with a dry finish, and it doesn't hide lines in the least; if anything, it creases and makes them look more obvious.

☺ **Big Cover Up Concealer Pen** *($4.75)* is actually a decent concealer that goes on somewhat thick but blends out smooth and even with minimal to no creasing. Unfortunately, this chubby pencil-style of application is made difficult because sharpening is so time-consuming and tricky.

☺ <u>POWDER:</u> **Translucent Pressed Powder** *($7.25)* and **Translucent Loose Powder** *($7.25)* are both standard talc-based powder with a soft, sheer finish and good color selection, but every color has shine. That makes them useless for reducing shine during the day, although they are an option for an evening look.

☺ **Anew Pressed Powder** *($9.95)* is supposed to protect against free-radical damage and control oil, but it is nothing more than a standard powder with shine.

Because of the shine, it will make oily skin look oilier, while the amount of protective antioxidant vitamins is at best insignificant.

☺ **BLUSH:** **True Color Powder Blush** *($6.75)* has a moist, smooth texture, though it tends to go on somewhat powdery. Many of the colors have some amount of shine, so be careful. It blends on easily and holds up well during the day.

☺ **Natural Radiance Blush Stick** *($4.75)* is a cream blush in a twist-up stick. You can wipe this fairly greasy, iridescent blush over the cheek and blend it out fairly sheer.

☹ **EYESHADOW:** Avon's **True Color Powder Eyeshadow Quads** *($5.25)* are conveniently broken up into cool and warm tones, and there are some attractive, soft neutrals. Another apparent convenience is that the label states whether a color is shiny or matte. Yet almost all of the colors designated matte turned out to be shiny—very disappointing, since shiny eyeshadow makes skin look wrinkly. **Perfect Wear Eye Color** *($6.50)* goes on like a cream and dries to a powder. Eye colors like these are hard to control when you blend them because they have too much movement and tend to slip off, and then once the colors dry it is difficult to adjust your blending. Worse, all of the colors are slightly iridescent. **Beyond Color Triple Benefit Eyeshadow** *($6)* doesn't even have one benefit. It is a creamy eyeshadow you apply from a wand, it has some amount of shine that won't hide lines (it makes them more noticeable), and the color is hard to control or blend with other shades. The only real plus is that it is fairly waterproof.

☹ **EYE AND BROW SHAPER:** **Luxury Eye Lining Pencil** *($3.25)*, **Glimmerstick Brow Definer** *($4.50)*, **Perfect Wear Eye Liner** *($5.25)*, and **Glimmerstick Eye Liner** *($4.50)* are standard pencils with a soft, smooth texture; they're so much alike that it's hard to tell them apart. Stay away from the blue, green, and shiny shades. **Fine Eye Line Pen** *($6)* is a liquid eyeliner with a pen-tip applicator. It creates a line that is fairly dramatic, yet doesn't chip or smear. **Brow Shaper** *($5)* comes in a mascara container in three shades: black, brown, and clear. That doesn't cover many brow colors, but it is an option for getting brows to look fuller and neater. There are better versions of shapers like this one, but this is by far the least expensive.

☹ **Perfect Wear Liquid Eye Liner Pen** *($6)* has a stiff applicator tip that isn't the best if you want to create a controlled even line. This one goes on fairly wet, dries to a matte finish, and doesn't chip. The color can look uneven when it dries. **Brow Powder** *($6)* has shine, but of all places there should be nothing shiny there—its the color you add that creates a believable looking brow.

☺ **Hydro Liner Liquid Eye Gel Pencil** *($5.25)* is a pencil that is supposed to be 35% water, a cross between a pencil and a liquid liner. Supposedly the color is delivered to the skin like a gel. This I had to see for myself. It sounded like eye-lining was never going to be the same again. Unfortunately, this new Avon pencil has more problems than benefits, and delivers none of the advantages I was hoping for. It goes on more smoothly than most pencils, but it is rather heavy, thick, and wet, before it dries to a matte finish. If you try to smooth out the intensity it can tend to chip. Still, if you like dramatic lines this is an interesting product to check out.

☺ LIPSTICK AND LIP PENCIL: Beyond Color with SPF 12 ($6.50), Color Rich Renewable Lipstick ($5), and Continuous Color ($5), are all very emollient, mostly glossy, cream lipsticks that come in an extensive collection of colors. They do have slight stains that help keep the color around somewhat longer. Despite the differences in names between these lipsticks, they are virtually indistinguishable. Beyond Color SPF 12 does not have UVA protection. Moisture 15 Satin Smooth Lipstick with SPF 15 ($5) and Truly Translucent Gloss Stick SPF 12 ($5) are both more of a sheer gloss than lipstick, and both SPFs do not include UVA protection. Perfect Wear Double Performance Lipstick ($6.95) is Avon's version of Revlon's ColorStay. It goes on fairly creamy and wet, and takes about a minute to dry into a truly dry, ultra-matte finish. It's as good as any of the ultra-mattes. Luxury Lip Lining Pencil ($3.25) is a standard pencil that goes on slightly drier than most. Glimmerstick Lip Liner ($4.50) goes on much thicker and creamier than the Luxury Lip Lining Pencil, but is still a fairly standard pencil in a twist-up container. Perfect Wear Lip Liner ($5.25) is virtually identical to the Glimmerstick.

☺ MASCARA: Voluptuous Full-Figured Mascara ($5) is a decent mascara, but can go on spikey. Incredible Lengths ($4.25) is a thick, clumpy, do-nothing mascara. Perfect Wear Mascara ($6) is just an OK mascara. It doesn't build much length or thickness, but it also doesn't smear or smudge.

☹ Truly Sensitive ($5) claims to have been designed for sensitive eyes, but there is nothing about this product that makes it better or worse than any other mascara. What does make it truly bad is that it doesn't build any length or definition. Wash-Off Waterproof Mascara ($5) has a most confusing name! It isn't waterproof in the least, it washes off easily, and it is just an average mascara in terms of building length or thickness.

☹ BRUSHES: Avon often sells a small collection of brushes either as gift with purchase or for purchase from a sales representative for $19.95. The set comes with a blush and powder brush, a lip or eyeliner brush, a small eyeshadow brush, and an eyebrow or lash comb. The blush and powder brush is quite good, but the eyeliner brush is too thick, and the eyeshadow brush is too flimsy.

Bain de Soleil (Sun Care Only)

For more information on Bain de Soleil call (800) 543-1745.
☺ UV Sense SPF 50 ($9.89 for 3.12 ounces) and Bebe Block SPF 50 ($9.89

for 3.12 ounces) are identical despite the different names. Bebe Block is aimed at kids, but there is nothing particularly kid-oriented in the formulation. What counts for both adults and kids is the protection, and it is significant, if not a bit excessive; after all, there is only so much sunshine on any given day. Both contain titanium dioxide in a waterproof formula claiming eight hours of protection, a good option for long days out in the sun. One word of warning: Several ingredients in these products could be problematic for sensitive skin.

☺ **Mademoiselle Sunblock SPF 15** *($6.99 for 4 ounces)*, **Le Sport Sunblock SPF 15** *($6.99 for 4 ounces)*, **Le Sport Sunblock SPF 30** *($8.99 for 4 ounces)*, and **Kids Sunblock SPF 30** *($8.99 for 4 ounces)* add four more products to your options for good UVA sun protection. In part these all contain titanium dioxide. Don't worry about which one to choose; the formulations are virtually identical and work equally well to prevent sun damage. They all have a fairly light, fairly nongreasy feel.

☺ **All Day Extended Protection Sunscreen, SPF 30** *($9.19 for 4 ounces)* is a very good titanium dioxide–based sunscreen for normal to slightly dry skin. It is also waterproof.

☺ **All Day Extended Protection Sunblock, SPF 15** *($6.99 for 4 ounces)* is similar to the sunscreen above only with an SPF 15. The same review applies.

☺ **Gentle Block Sunblock, SPF 30** *($8.99 for 4 ounces)* is similar to the ones above, which makes it a good sunscreen, although there is nothing unusually gentle, hypoallergenic, or nonirritating about it.

☹ **Orange Gelee Sunscreen SPF 15** *($8.65 for 3.12 ounces)*, **Orange Gelee Sunscreen SPF 8** *($8.65 for 3.12 ounces)*, and **Orange Gelee Sunscreen SPF 4** *($8.65 for 3.12 ounces)* do not contain avobenzone, zinc oxide, or titanium dioxide, and are not recommended; considering the SPF 8 and 4 protection, why bother?

☹ **All Day Extended Protection Sunscreen SPF 8** *($6.99 for 4 ounces)*, **Mademoiselle Sunfilter SPF 4** *($6.99 for 4 ounces)*, **Mademoiselle Sunscreen SPF 8** *($6.99 for 4 ounces)*, and **Sand Resistant Oil Sunfilter SPF 2** *($5.09 for 4 ounces)* are all serious disappointments. An SPF 8 is not by anyone's definition extended protection and their SPF 4 and 2 products are unconscionable.

☺ **Sunless Tanning Spray** *($9.89 for 3.5 ounces)* comes in Dark and Very Dark, and both are worth checking out for a tan with all of the color and none of the damage.

☺ **Apres Soleil After Sun Moisture Replenishing Lotion** *($6.99 for 8 ounces)* is a good, though standard, moisturizer for dry skin, but that's about it.

☹ **Apres Soleil After Sun Revitalizing Aloe Mist** *($6.99 for 8 ounces)* claims to be alcohol-free, but it still contains benzoyl alcohol, which is a serious skin irritant and can be drying.

bare escentuals

In terms of cosmetic boutique appeal, bare escentuals is a store concept quite similar in style to Aveda. While lots of women may never have heard of bare escentuals, many women have heard of their bareMinerals loose powder eyeshadows, blushes, and face powders. That popularity is due to QVC, where bare escentuals bareMinerals products are sold as a kit. QVC reaches lots of women with its rapturous praise for everything they sell. As a result, thousands of women want to know if bareMinerals work as amazingly and purely as the spokesperson asserts. Of course, nothing ever works as well as they say in ads, though these powders are unique in their coverage, application, and simple formulation, and, depending on your point of view, they are an interesting way to apply face and eye makeup. If you are shopping QVC—(800) 345-1515—and order these products you receive the ☺ **bareMinerals Eye, Face, & Cheek Color Collection *($29.11)*,** which includes one tin of beige eyeshadow, one deep brown eyeshadow, and one cheek and one face color loose powder form. These are applied with a brush and then smoothed out. The products boast that they don't contain fragrance, oil, binders, surfactants, emulsifiers, or any otherproblematic ingredients. While that does seem to be the case according to their ingredient list (though I strongly doubt it given the number of shades from blue to red displayed in the stores, because there just aren't natural dyes available that can create this range of colors), that doesn't make these products problem-free. Bismuth oxychloride is a major ingredient in all the powder formulations and it can cause skin irritation, while the other minerals can be drying. Aside from their bogus claim about natural being good, loose powders are as messy as it gets in terms of your vanity (counter top not ego) and your makeup bag. The powder just gets all over the place! Additionally, these otherwise nicely neutral soft shades (though the ones at the bare escentuals stores come in an exotic array of colors) are extremely shiny, and make any amount of crepey skin look more so. The face powder does provide some amount of opaque coverage, but the shine and the thickness are a bit strange. The eyeshadows and blush apply in a somewhat lighter way, though they still give good coverage. If you find the loose powder concept and the shine intriguing these are an option, but I feel fairly safe in suggesting they will end up as one of those cosmetic whims that you never use more than a few times.

If you are shopping at the bare escentuals store, you'll find a huge range of products, including bath, body, skin, and aromatherapy products as well as a full line of makeup. None of this is very exciting, it's just an Aveda or Garden Botanika wannabe with a hook, though the bareMinerals is really the only good hook. For more information about bareMinerals you can call (800) 227-3990 (the $2 they charge to send out a catalog can be used as a credit against a purchase).

bare escentuals Skin Care

☹ **Rose Geranium Cleansing Lotion Normal to Dry Skin** *($18 for 5 ounces)* is mostly plant oil, thickeners, and preservatives. This is a standard wipe-off cleanser that can leave a greasy film behind on the skin.

☹ **Lavender & Wild Thyme Cleanser Normal to Oily Skin** *($18 for 5 ounces)* contains mostly water, plant oil, witch hazel, silicone, thickeners, fragrance, and tea tree oil. The plant oil and thickeners in here can clog pores and be a problem for oily skin. The amount of tea tree oil is so small it probably wouldn't be a problem for the eyes.

☺ **$$$ Tea Tree Foaming Cleanser Normal to Oily Skin** *($18 for 5 ounces)* is a standard detergent-based cleanser that can be drying for some skin types. The tea tree oil can be a problem for the eye area.

☺ **$$$ Rosewater & Lactic Acid Time Balm Normal to Dry Skin** *($29 for 2 ounces)* is a good emollient moisturizer for dry skin that contains mostly plant oil and thickeners; while it does contain lactic acid, the pH is too high for it to be an effective exfoliant.

☹ **Rose & Neroli Freshener Normal to Dry Skin** *($18 for 5 ounces)* is mostly water, witch hazel, glycerin, and fragrance. Witch hazel is an unnecessary skin irritant that can be a problem for most skin types.

☹ **Cypress & Rosemary Toner Normal to Oily Skin** *($18 for 5 ounces)* is similar to the one above and the same review applies.

☺ **$$$ Rose & Royal Jelly Anti-Oxidant Moisturizer Normal to Dry Skin** *($32 for 2 ounces)* isn't much of an antioxidant; there is only a tiny amount of vitamin E in here. This is a fairly standard but good moisturizer for dry skin that contains mostly water, glycerin, plant oils, thickeners, and preservatives.

☹ **Tea Tree & Lavender Oil Control Moisturizer Normal to Oily Skin** *($24 for 2 ounces)* includes several plant oils that would be a problem for someone with oily skin.

☹ **Tea Tree Spot Treatment Normal to Oily Skin** *($12 for 1 ounce)* contains a teeny amount of tea tree oil and a lot of plant oils, including lemon oil. Plant oils aren't best for oily skin and lemon oil is a skin irritant. Tea tree oil does not have an established track record of having any effect against breakouts.

☺ **$$$ Eye Makeup Remover** *($12 for 3 ounces)* is a standard detergent-based eye-makeup remover. Wiping off makeup is a problem for skin.

☺ **Bare Aloe Vera** *($8 for 2 ounces)* is mostly aloe, glycerin, thickeners, and preservatives. For this kind of product you would be better off going to the health food store and purchasing a huge bottle of pure Aloe Vera gel for half the price.

☺ **$$$ Papaya Enzyme Peel Mask** *($16 for 2 ounces)* is a standard clay mask with thickeners, plant extracts, and a tiny amount of papain. Papain has some exfoliating properties but is considered unstable and becomes ineffective after a short period of time.

☹ **Seaweed Clay Mask** *($16 for 2 ounces)* contains menthol, which is a skin irritant and a problem for all skin types.

☺ **Firming Eye Gel** *($14 for 1 ounce)* isn't all that firming or moisturizing, it is just a lightweight gel that contains mostly water, film former, slip agent, thickeners, plant extract, fragrance, and preservatives. It would only be OK if you weren't worried about dry skin.

☹ **Chamomile & Mallow Exfoliator** *($16 for 2 ounces)* is a fairly scratchy scrub that uses ground-up shells. This can be hard on skin.

☹ **Wisdom Glycolic Acid Multi-Vitamin SPF 15** *($20 for 2.3 ounces)* doesn't contain avobenzone, zinc oxide, or titanium dioxide, and is not recommended; moreover the pH is too high for the glycolic acid to work as an exfoliant.

bare escentuals Makeup

☺ **$$$ FOUNDATION: bareMinerals Foundation** *($24)*. See my comments in the review section above for the bare escentuals line. **liquid insurance** *($16)* is a fairly thick foundation that grabs the skin better than most, but all of the shades are shiny, and several of the eight shades are too peach or pink for most skin tones; stay away from 2, 3, 6, and 7. **A word of warning:** the salespeople I spoke to all claimed these foundations had a high SPF even though no SPF number is attributed to them. Not only is this information illegal, it is unethical: you cannot rely on any of these foundations—or any product for that matter—for sunscreen protection without an SPF rating and UVA-protecting ingredients.

☹ **CONCEALER: concealer** *($12)* comes in a tube, and all of the colors are extremely peach or pink and not recommended for any skin tone.

☺ **POWDER: bareMinerals mineral veil** *($22)* is a loose powder with a softer and lighter consistency than the bareMinerals Foundation. It has a sheer but dry powder finish, and is best for someone with normal to oily skin. **pressed mineral veil** *($24)* has a soft, sheer finish that is extremely translucent and quite nice, despite the absurd price.

☺ **BLUSH: bareMinerals blush** *($16)* has the same basic texture as the foundation, and the comments about being its being messy and hard to control are the same. There are some matte shades for this product and the application is soft and beautiful. It's hard for me to encourage this direction but I'm sure some women will love it. I would try it before buying.

☺ **pressed minerals blush** *($11)* has a limited color selection, and they are all mostly in the rose and pink color family. They do have a soft, even finish.

☺ **EYESHADOW AND EYE PENCIL: bareMinerals eyeshadow** *($11)* is similar to the blush and foundation. All of these colors are slightly shiny, though there are some great neutral shades (if you don't count the blues and the greens). I still don't get the advantage of opting for this kind of messy, flaky product, but it must be a preference issue. **a glimmer of bareMinerals** *($12)* is the same as the mineral foundation and blush except that these are ultra-shiny. This is about personal preference and style, though I don't recommend it except for evening wear. **pressed minerals eyeshadow** *($12)* is just eyeshadow with some amount of shine and a nice color selection. **signature eye pencil** *($11)* is a standard twist-up eye pencil that comes in a limited number of shades.

☺ <u>LIPSTICK AND LIP PENCIL:</u> **social security lipstick** *($14)* has a creamy, opaque, slightly emollient finish. **ice breaker lip gloss** *($12)* is a standard tube lip gloss, nice but ordinary. **signature lip pencil** *($9)* is a standard twist-up eye pencil that comes in a limited number of shades.

☹ <u>MASCARA:</u> **singled out mascara** *($13)* is a terrible mascara that builds almost no length or definition. A definite waste of money.

☺ <u>BRUSHES:</u> The brushes here range in price *(from $8 to $24)*, and for the most part these are soft and easy-to-use. The sizes offered definitely depend on your preference for application. For example there are two eyeshadow brushes, one that is rather oversized and the other that is almost too small. I would prefer two brushes in a size right between these. The Powder Brush is a great size but the Blush Brush is probably too large for most cheeks.

bareMinerals *(see bare escentuals above)*

Basis *(Skin Care Only)*

If you are looking for some good, inexpensive skin-care products, there are a handful of excellent choices in this revamped skin-care line from Basis. It is available in most drugstores across the country. For more information on Basis products call (800) 227-4703.

☹ **All Clear Bar** *($2.69 for 4 ounces)* contains a tiny amount of triclosan, an OK disinfectant, but its effectiveness is washed down the drain before it can affect the skin. It contains several ingredients that could be drying and irritating.

☹ **Cleaner Clean Face Wash** *($4.99 for 6 ounces)* is a standard, water-soluble cleanser that also contains lemon and spearmint. These can irritate and burn the eye area, and this cleanser is absolutely not recommended for anyone's face.

☺ **Comfortably Clean Face Wash** *($4.09 for 6 ounces)* is a standard, water-soluble cleanser that can be quite good for someone with normal to oily skin. This is a good water-soluble cleanser but it has a terrible taste and can be drying for some skin types.

☹ **Sensitive Skin Bar** *($2.69 for 4 ounces)* is a fairly standard bar cleanser that contains tallowate and detergent cleansing agents. Tallowate can be a skin irritant and could cause breakouts and dermatitis.

☹ **Vitamin Bar** *($1.99 for 4 ounces)* makes no sense. Even if vitamins could affect the skin, they are washed away before they have a chance. This is nothing more than a standard bar cleanser with ingredients that can dry the skin and potentially clog pores.

☺ **All Night Face Cream** *($6.55 for 2 ounces)* contains mostly water, slip agent, silicone, thickening agents, citric acid, lactic acid, more thickeners, more silicone, vitamins, more thickeners, emollient, anti-irritants, and preservatives. It is a good moisturizer for someone with normal to dry skin, but a poor AHA product.

☺ **Face the Day Lotion SPF 15** *($6.55 for 4 ounces)* is an excellent sunscreen for someone with normal to dry skin, and it meets the new qualifications for UVA and UVB protection (it contains zinc oxide), including antioxidants! It contains mostly water, silicone oil, several thickening agents, vitamins, water-binding agents, anti-irritants, and preservatives.

☺ **One Step Face Cream SPF 15** *($6.55 for 1.5 ounces)* contains mostly water, silicone, film former, slip agent, more film former, thickeners, lactic acid, glycolic acid, anti-irritant, emollient, vitamin C, thickener, vitamin D, more anti-irritant, and preservatives. This is a good moisturizing sunscreen (it contains zinc oxide), but it is a poor AHA product.

Bath & Body Works (Skin Care Only)

Over the past year many readers have asked me to review Bath & Body Works, and I want to apologize for taking so long. Actually, I almost went to print a couple of times with reviews of this compact group of skin-care products but stopped after I double-checked my facts, because products were being discontinued or new products were being launched. I'm told that the following products from Bath & Body Works are here to stay, at least for a while.

Now that Bath & Body Works has settled on their skin-care formulations, I wish I could say I like them more than I do. The price points are exceedingly attractive: everything is under $15, in relatively nice-sized containers. Also, the basic formulations are rather lightweight, and I admire the lack of hyperbole and exaggerated claims. For that alone I would love to give every product a big smiling face. Regrettably, there were problems with many of the products. I do think a couple of products are worth checking out, but if I were Bath & Body Works I would go back to the drawing board one more time. Bath & Body Works' customer service number is (800) 395-1001.

☹ **Cooling Gel Cleanser Oily Skin** *($8 for 6 ounces)* is a standard, water-soluble cleanser that lives up to its name. Unfortunately, the cooling ingredients, peppermint and pineapple, are also potentially quite irritating, especially for the eyes.

☹ **Creamy Cleanser Dry Skin** *($8 for 6 ounces)* is a greasy mess that is unquestionably not water soluble. The directions say rinse well, but all the water in the world wouldn't get this stuff off.

☺ **Foaming Face Wash Normal to Combination Skin** *($8 for 6 ounces)* is a standard, water-soluble cleanser for someone with oily skin. It can be on the drying side, so be careful if you have sensitive skin or a tendency toward dryness.

☹ **Gentle Smoothing Scrub** *($8 for 4 ounces)* has TEA-lauryl sulfate as the main detergent cleansing agent, along with papain, menthol, orange peel, and peppermint, all of which are serious potential skin irritants. This product is not recommended.

☺ **Balancing Toner Normal to Combination Skin** *($8 for 6 ounces)* contains mostly water, witch hazel, slip agents, orange extract, plant extracts, anti-irritants, and preservatives. I would prefer that this product not contain citrus, but for the most part it is a good toner for someone with normal to oily skin.

☹ **Purifying Astringent Oily Skin** *($8 for 6 ounces)* could have been a good salicylic acid product for someone with clogged pores, but it also contains alcohol and witch hazel, which make it too irritating for all skin types, and not in the least purifying.

☹ **AHA Day Lotion SPF 8 All Skin Types** *($12 for 1.75 ounces)* loses on three counts: it's SPF 8; it doesn't contain avobenzone, titanium dioxide, or zinc oxide; and there isn't enough AHA for it to work as an exfoliant. This product is not recommended.

☹ **Moisturizing Day Cream for Dry Skin** *($12 for 1.7 ounces)* doesn't contain titanium dioxide, zinc oxide, or avobenzone, and is not recommended.

☺ **Oil Free Lotion** *($8 for 4 ounces)* contains silicone, which can feel oily to some skin types. Other than that, it can be a good lightweight moisturizer for someone with slightly dry skin.

☹ **Oil Free Lotion for Oily Skin SPF 15** *($12 for 4 ounces)* doesn't contain titanium dioxide, zinc oxide, or avobenzone, and is not recommended.

☹ **Renewing Night Cream Normal to Combination Skin** *($15 for 1.5 ounces)* contains mostly water, malic acid, slip agents, plant extract, thickeners, plant oil, more thickeners, more plant oils, vitamins, plant extracts, more thickener, and preservatives. Although this product contains malic acid, a type of AHA, malic acid is not considered one of the better AHA ingredients. Even if it were, the pH of this product is too high to allow it to work as an exfoliant.

☹ **Deep Cleansing Mask All Skin Types** *($12 for 6 ounces)* contains mostly water, clay, alcohol, slip agents, witch hazel, thickeners, vitamins, plant extracts, and preservatives. For a clay mask this isn't bad, but the alcohol and witch hazel can be irritating.

☹ **Sassafras Tea Refreshing Eye Pads, for All Skin Types** *($7.50 for 30 pads)* contain eucalyptus and tea rose oil, which can be skin irritants, especially for the eye area.

☹ **Spearmint and Clay Purifying Mask, for Oily Skin** *($10 for 4 ounces)* is too irritating—the spearmint in the name speaks for itself—and this mask is not recommended.

BeautiControl

BeautiControl tries very hard to be all things to all women. The company not only gives you information about skin care and makeup application when you book a free consultation with one of its sales representatives, but they also analyze your wardrobe and tell you which colors look best on you and which clothing styles complement your body shape. Unfortunately, as always, you must depend on the expertise of the salesperson, but several of the sales representatives I met seemed to be in dire need of wardrobe counseling themselves and had little to no technical information about skin care and makeup. The color information is helpful, but it takes skill and training to translate it into a total look. For example, while there are three types of foundation, none is appropriate for someone with dry skin; one is oil-free, the second is a very thick cream-to-powder, and the third is a powder meant to be used as a foundation. That isn't a bad selection, but it's limited.

All of the colors are divided into warm and cool groups, which is helpful, but there are almost twice as many cool colors as warm. If I were an Autumn or Summer, that would be a serious shortcoming. On the other hand, a Winter or Spring might be quite pleased—though she will probably wish for a better selection.

Several of the skin-care products are rather impressive, and the average price for many of these products is under $12. As you would expect, the wrinkle products are all absurdly expensive (and unnecessary), but if you stay away from them you won't get soaked. One word of caution: The company claims that your skin type and product needs are determined by a "precise, scientific ... dermatologist-tested, proven Skin Condition Analysis." There is nothing precise or necessarily scientific about it. Little pieces of sticky paper the company calls "sensors" are stuck on different cleansed areas of your face. What comes off on these strips determines the products you are to use. Depending on the time of day I had the test done, I received different evaluations, which makes sense: my skin isn't the same in the morning as it is at the end of the day. Also, the sensors ripped off skin and left irritation and rough spots. The results aren't surprising and are often wrong. Skin isn't static: it changes with the seasons, your menstrual cycle, stress, and your environment. The idea is cute, but I wouldn't choose skin-care products based on this analysis alone.

A new addition for BeautiControl is their All Clear Acne skin care, a group of four products with one purpose in mind: combating acne. Does this line of defense work? I wish I could say yes, but BeautiControl's battle plan falls short for several reasons: there is no product to absorb excess oil, some of the products are potentially irritating, and there is no disinfectant to kill the bacteria that cause breakouts. For more information about BeautiControl call (800) BEAUTI-1 or (800) 872-0601.

BeautiControl Skin Care

☹ **Mild Rosemary Cleansing Fluide for Dry Skin** (*$13.50 for 8 ounces*) is a fairly standard mineral oil–based cleanser that must be wiped off. It also contains lanolin oil, which means this cleanser can leave a greasy film that can make dry skin look dull and cause breakouts. It also has orange, mandarin, and lemon, which are all skin irritants and can sting the eyes.

☹ **Chamomile Balancing Cleansing Lotion for Combination Skin** (*$13.50 for 8 ounces*) is a mineral oil–based cleanser that also contains some detergent cleansing agents. It can leave a greasy film but could be good for someone with dry skin. It also has orange, mandarin, and lemon, which are all skin irritants and can sting the eyes.

☹ **Purifying Cleansing Gel** (*$12 for 8 ounces*) is a standard detergent cleanser that can be good for normal to oily skin; unfortunately it also has orange, mandarin, and lemon, which are all skin irritants and can sting the eyes.

☺ **Almond Clarifying Scrub/Masque** (*$14 for 3 ounces*) is a standard clay mask that also contains apricot seeds and almond meal. It is also a scrub (and is fairly scratchy), and contains orange, mandarin, and lemon, which can be skin irritants.

☺ **Balancing Scrub for Combination Skin** (*$14 for 3 ounces*) is a standard detergent-based scrub that uses synthetic particles as the abrasive. This works as well as any scrub, although the orange, lemon, and mandarin can be irritating to skin, especially after it has been scrubbed.

☺ **Lash & Lid Bath** (*$9 for 4 ounces*) is a standard, water-soluble wipe-off eye-makeup remover. Wiping off eye makeup on a regular basis can cause the skin to sag.

☺ **Soothing Chamomile Tonic** (*$14 for 8 ounces*) contains witch hazel along with mandarin, orange, and lemon, which are all skin irritants and hardly soothing to the skin.

☹ **Balancing Tonic for Combination Skin** (*$14 for 8 ounces*) is an alcohol-based toner that can be irritating and drying for most skin types.

☹ **Clarifying Mallow Tonic** (*$14 for 8 ounces*) is an alcohol-based toner that can be quite irritating and drying for most skin types.

☺ **Herbal Hydrating Mist** (*$8 for 8 ounces*) is a good, fairly irritant-free toner that contains mostly water, water-binding agent, plant extracts, and preservatives. One of the plant extracts is arnica, which can be a skin irritant, although there isn't that much in here to be a problem for most skin types.

☺ **Essential Moisture Lotion** *($15.50 for 4.5 ounces)* is a very good emollient moisturizer for normal to dry skin. It contains mostly water, plant oil, thickener, mineral oil, more thickeners, more plant oil, vitamins, plant extracts, and preservatives. Because it doesn't contain a sunscreen, this moisturizer is best used at night. It contains the same mandarin, orange, and lemon that most of the BeautiControl products do, and they can be skin irritants.

☺ **Balancing Moisturizer** *($15.50 for 4.5 ounces)* contains mostly water, thickeners, plant oils, slip agent, water-binding agents, plant extracts, silicone, mineral oil, and preservatives. This is a good emollient moisturizer for normal to dry skin, but because it doesn't contain sunscreen it is only appropriate for use at night. The company recommends this moisturizer for someone with combination skin, but the oils in it aren't good for that skin type. It contains the same mandarin, orange, and lemon that most of the BeautiControl products do, and they can be skin irritants.

☹ **Oil-Free Moisture Supplement** *($14 for 4.5 ounces)* is supposed to be oil-absorbing, but it won't absorb oil very well. It contains mostly water, silicone, thickeners, glycerin, water-binding agents, plant extracts, and preservatives. This is a good moisturizer for someone with normal to dry skin, but it is way too emollient for someone with oily skin. Moreover, without sunscreen, this product is appropriate only for nighttime.

☺ **Oil Controller Oil Absorbing Formula** *($15.50 for 4.5 ounces)* contains mostly water, thickeners, silicone, water-binding agents, and preservatives. There is very little in this product that can control oil, and the thickening agents can clog pores.

☺ $$$ **Regeneration Face and Neck Complex** *($31 for 2 ounces)* is BeautiControl's attempt at an AHA product. It uses lactic, citric, and tartaric acid. The company won't reveal the AHA percentage of the product, but the sales reps will tell you everything from 10% to 15%. One even said it was 95% AHAs. The truth is probably closer to less than 4% for this one. It is a good moisturizer and a mild AHA product with a good pH, but it won't produce miracles. The brochure suggests that a 50-year-old woman can expect her skin become like that of a woman of 35! All that from about 4% AHAs, a percentage that can be found in a hundred different products. This is a good AHA product in an ordinary but good moisturizing base.

☺ $$$ **Regeneration 2 Face and Neck Complex** *($31 for 2 ounces)* is identical to the product above, but with about 5% AHAs, and the same review applies.

☺ $$$ **Regeneration for Oily Skin** *($31 for 2 ounces)* contains about 5% AHAs and is similar to the product above, which means it is too emollient for someone with oily skin. However, it could be good for someone with normal to dry skin who wants to try a stronger AHA product.

☺ **$$$ Regeneration 2 for Oily Skin** *($31 for 2 ounces)* contains about 6% AHAs and is similar to the product above, which means it is too emollient for someone with oily skin. However, it could be good for someone with normal to dry skin who wants to try a stronger AHA product.

☺ **$$$ Regeneration Extreme Repair** *($30 for 4 ounces)* is similar to Regeneration for Oily Skin, but with about 4% AHA. It's completely unnecessary and hardly extreme.

☺ **$$$ Regeneration Gold** *($55 for 1.8 ounces)* is AHA overkill. This one is similar to the ones above, with about a 7% AHA concentration.

☹ **Regeneration Gold Eye Repair** *($25 for 0.5 ounce)* contains about 1% AHA, an amount that makes it just a good water-binding agent, and about 0.5% BHA (salicylic acid). BHA is best for penetrating pores and not for use around the eyes.

☹ **Regeneration Blemish Duo** *($14.50 for 0.11 ounce of Blemish Gel and 0.12 ounce of Blemish Cover-Up)* is a tube with **Oil-Free Blemish Cover-Up**, which is nothing more than foundation (it comes in two colors, neither of which match most skin tones) at one end, and **Blemish Gel**, which is mostly alcohol and salicylic acid, at the other. The gel contains about 1% AHA, too little for the AHAs to be much more than water-binding agents.

☺ **$$$ Microderm Oxygenating Nighttime Line Control** *($26 for 0.81 ounce)* is a good basic moisturizer for someone with normal to dry skin. It contains mostly water, silicone, thickeners, slip agent, antioxidant, vitamin E, water-binding agent, and preservatives. The antioxidants are nice, but they won't change or prevent a wrinkle on your face, and they certainly aren't oxygenating (in fact if antioxidants did work they would be anti-oxygen—that's what antioxidant means).

☺ **$$$ Microderm Oxygenating Firming Gel** *($29.50 for 2 ounces)* is identical to the product above except without silicone, and the same review applies.

☺ **$$$ Microderm Eye-X-Cel Daily Therapy Creme** *($19 for 0.75 ounce)* contains mostly water, glycerin, a long list of thickeners, anti-irritant, plant extracts, silicone, and preservatives. This is a good, but extremely ordinary, moisturizer for someone with dry skin.

☺ **$$$ Lip Apeel** *($16 for 1.25 ounces)* is a two-part product (peel and balm) that helps peel dry skin off the lips. The peel is a bit of wax, clay, and silicate that can indeed peel off dead skin. The balm is simply a very emollient lip gloss of castor oil, petrolatum, and lanolin. It does the trick and is one of my favorite winter products for lips, but the price tag is absurd.

☺ **$$$ Corticulture Comfort Lotion** *($25 for 4 ounces)* is a good cortisone cream. Cortisone is fine for small irritations if you use it only occasionally; repeated use of cortisone can break down the skin's support structure. You can get the same effect from Lanacort and Cortaid at the drugstore.

☹ **All Clear Skin Wash** *($12 for 6 ounces)* is nothing more than a standard detergent-based water-soluble cleanser that would be great for normal to oily skin, except that it contains salicylic acid. There's no reason to risk splashing salicylic acid into the eyes, and any exfoliation potential is rinsed off and washed down the drain.

☹ **All Clear Skin Scrub** *($12.50 for 4 ounces)* contains synthetic scrub particles suspended in alcohol and grapefruit extract. Baking soda mixed with Cetaphil Gentle Skin Cleanser would be more effective and potentially less irritating.

☹ **All Clear Skin Moisture** *($12.50 for 4 ounces)* contains grapefruit extract, which may be irritating for some skin types. Someone with acne will also want to avoid this one, given that several of the thickening agents may cause breakouts, plus, the pH is too high for the salicylic acid to be an effective exfoliant.

☹ **All Clear Skin Solution** *($15 for 6 ounces)* is the most interesting of these products. It is merely 2% salicylic acid suspended in alcohol and witch hazel. It could be an option for exfoliating acne-prone skin if the alcohol weren't in here (it has a pH of 3). The exfoliation from the salicylic acid can be irritating enough for the skin without the presence of the alcohol.

☹ **Sunlogics Sun Shield Lotion SPF 15** *($13 for 4.5 ounces)* doesn't contain avobenzone, zinc oxide, or titanium dioxide, and is not recommended.

☹ **Sunlogics Tanning Mist SPF 8** *($14 for 8 ounces)* doesn't contain avobenzone, zinc oxide, or titanium dioxide, and is not recommended. The name of this product is accurate, it *is* a tanning product, because SPF 8 is not enough sun-damage protection.

☹ **Sunlogics UV Lip+Eye Stick SPF 15** *($9.50 for .06 ounce)* doesn't contain avobenzone, zinc oxide, or titanium dioxide, and is not recommended.

☹ **Sunlogics Water-Resistant Sunblock SPF 30** *($15 for 4.5 ounces)* doesn't contain avobenzone, zinc oxide, or titanium dioxide, and is not recommended.

BeautiControl Makeup

☺ <u>FOUNDATION:</u> Sheer Protection Oil-Free Liquid Foundation *($10.50)* is a lightweight foundation that provides light to medium coverage and has a soft matte finish. All of the shades are divided into cool and warm tones, but most are too pink or peach. Someone with warm skin tones should not wear a vivid peach foundation, nor should someone with cool skin tones wear a vivid pink foundation. Another caution: there are definitely ingredients in this product that could trigger breakouts and that you might want to avoid. **These are the only colors to consider:** Nude, Natural, Alabaster, Buff, Porcelain Beige, Tawny, and Mahogany. **These colors are too pink or peach:** Ivory, Bisque, Beige, Golden Honey, Peaches & Cream, Sunglow, Bronze, Desert Tan, Caramel, Nutmeg, Toffee, and Mocha.

☹ **Perfecting Creme to Powder Finish Foundation** *($11.50)* is a very thick, greasy foundation that does have a powder finish but never loses its greasy feel. Its claim to be waterproof is pretty accurate, but it is almost cleanser-proof too. It can easily clog pores if you're not careful.

☺ **Perfecting Wet/Dry Finish Foundation** *($19.50)* is a standard talc-based pressed powder that has a decent color selection and covers softly and smoothly. The texture and finish are great. It's supposed to be able to diffuse light in order to minimize lines, but it can't do that. Most of the colors in the large selection are reliable and neutral. **The only colors to avoid are:** Peaches & Cream, Bisque, Golden Honey, Sunglow, Dark, and Bronze.

☹ **Creme Sheer Protection** *($11)* is more like a creamy pancake makeup and is very greasy, containing mineral oil, heavy wax, and lanolin, which is a lot for the skin to handle. It is recommended for dry skin but it is really heavy for that skin type. The colors tend to be on the peach side.

☺ **Color Freeze Liquid Makeup SPF 12** *($19.50)* is an excellent matte-finish foundation that is great for oily skin types. The SPF 12 is decent and it does contain titanium dioxide. This is definitely an option and one of the better foundations of this type. **The only colors to avoid are:** Peaches & Cream, Bisque, Golden Honey, Sunglow, Dark, and Bronze.

☹ <u>CONCEALER:</u> Extra-Help Concealer *($5.50)* blends on easily and provides good medium coverage, but it is fairly greasy and can crease into lines around the eyes moments after being applied and continue to do so the rest of the day, while the Light and Medium shades can be too peach for most skin tones.

☹ **Color Protectors** *($10)* are standard skin-color correctors that come in three shades: Mint, Mauve, and Lilac. They can't change skin tone convincingly, cause havoc when you choose a foundation, and layer on more makeup than any woman needs.

☺ <u>POWDER:</u> Loose Perfecting Powder *($10.50)* is a standard talc-based powder that has a soft, dry texture and comes in three colors. Medium can be too peach for some skin tones. **Oil-Free Translucent Pressed Powder** *($10.50)* has a soft, somewhat dry texture. The colors are very neutral and would work well for someone with normal to oily/combination skin.

☺ **Face Feminizer Pressed Powder** *($10.50)* is a compact of either shiny pink or peach powder. It doesn't make the face any more feminine and is really just a soft shiny blush. Just don't wear it all over the face, only on the cheeks.

☺ **BLUSH:** The **Unbelievable Blush** *($12.50)* shades all have some amount of shine, but not enough to be a problem for most skin types. (Someone with oily skin may not be happy.) The colors are beautiful and the texture is soft and smooth. But be careful: the colors are fairly vivid and pastel, and there aren't many neutral shades.

☹ **EYESHADOW: Sensuous Shadows** *($12.50)* come in compacts of three shades, but some of the combinations are poor, and the colors range from somewhat shiny to very shiny; if you have any lines on your eyelids, shine will make them look worse. **Tinted Shadow Control Creme** *($6.50)* does help to keep your eyeshadow on, without creasing, for the entire day. There are four colors, but, like the eyeshadows, they are all shiny.

☺ **Color Freeze Eyeshadow Pencils** *($12)*. Although the color does "freeze" into place, sharpening the pencils isn't fun. Also, most of the colors in this group are shiny, which may be fun, but it makes wrinkles more evident.

☺ **EYE AND BROW SHAPER: Eye Defining Pencils** and **Brow Defining Pencils** *($7.50)* are standard pencils that come in a nice range of colors. They tend to be on the dry side, which makes them a little harder to apply, but they also tend to last longer. **Color Freeze Eye Liner** *($9.50)* comes in a twist-up container that does have better staying power than the Eye Defining Pencils.

☹ **Brow Control Creme** *($7.50)* comes in a squeeze tube that you apply to a mascara-like wand and then roll through the brow. I like this way of making brows look fuller, but this is a messy option. Similar products come with the brush inside, so the color is evenly distributed.

☺ **LIPSTICK AND LIP PENCIL: Lasting Lip Color** *($8)* is a very creamy, slightly greasy lipstick that doesn't last all that long, but the color selection is attractive. The colors are divided into cremes and frosts, which helps prevent the accidental purchase of an iridescent lip color if that's not what you're looking for. **Lip Control Creme** *($6.50)* is excellent. It prevents even greasy lipstick from feathering into the lines around the mouth; however, it would be better if it came in an easier-to-use applicator than having to spread it with your finger or a lipstick brush. **Lip Shaping Pencils** *($6.50)* are just standard pencils in a nice array of colors that need to be sharpened. **Color Freeze Lip Liner** *($9.50)* is a twist-up container that does have better staying power than the Lip Shaping Pencils.

☺ In the rush to compete with the new "stay-put" products, BeautiControl has brought out their own ultra-matte lipstick called **Color Freeze Lipstick *($9)***. It performs just like all the other ultra-matte lipsticks I've ever tested, only this one is so soft in the tube it smushes and deteriorates with the least amount of pressure. It isn't a bad product, just not an improvement in price or performance over Revlon ColorStay Lipstick or Maybelline Budgeproof Lip Color.

☺ <u>MASCARA:</u> **Water-Resistant Mascara *($7)*** comes off easily with water and cleanser, and it doesn't smear after a long day. It would be a great mascara if it could build long, thick lashes, but it can't. It's just OK.

☹ **Spectaculash *($7)*** and **Spectaculash Thickening *($8.50)*** are not what I would call spectacular in the least. The regular Spectaculash does build some length but it clumps terribly. The thickening version doesn't make lashes thick.

Beauty Without Cruelty (Skin Care Only)

Many companies proudly boast that they do not test their products on animals. However, it isn't always clear whether the products contain animal-derived ingredients or whether individual ingredients were ever tested on animals. Some companies, including The Body Shop, have a self-imposed five-year "grandfather clause," which means they use ingredients previously tested on animals as long as the testing took place five years prior to the date the raw ingredient was purchased. Beauty Without Cruelty is one of the few companies with a strict, rigorously defined position concerning animal testing. Its products are not tested on animals, none of its products contain animal by-products, and not one of the ingredients it uses has been tested on animals since 1965. The ethics of this company in this regard are admirable.

Of course, the company makes elaborate claims about the benefits of their plant extracts, but if you ignore that and look for the ingredients that really make a difference, you can find some very good products. They are typically distributed in health food stores and in drugstores such as PayLess and Drug Emporium. You can also order direct by calling (707) 769-5120 or (800) 227-5120.

☺ **3% Alpha Hydroxy Facial Cleanser Normal/Oily Skin Types *($7.49 for 8.5 ounces)*** is a standard detergent-based water-soluble cleanser that can be very good for someone with normal to oily skin. There isn't much AHA in here and the type isn't even delineated, so it isn't significant one way or the other.

☺ **Extra Gentle Facial Cleansing Milk Dry/Mature Skin *($7.49 for 8.5 ounces)*** contains mostly plant water, glycerin, plant oils, thickeners, aloe, more thickeners, plant oils, anti-irritant, and preservatives. This is a fairly standard wipe-off cleanser that can leave a greasy film on the skin.

☺ **Herbal Cream Facial Cleanser Normal/Dry Skin** *($7.49 for 8.5 ounces)* is a detergent-based water-soluble cleanser that also contains some plant oils. This can be a very good cleanser for someone with dry skin.

☺ **Extra Gentle Eye Makeup Remover** *($5.89 for 4 ounces)* contains mostly plant water, glycerin, detergent cleansing agents, and preservatives. This is a fairly standard eye-makeup remover, but the other cleansers in this line work well and don't irritate the eyes, so why bother with this product?

☺ **Extra Gentle Facial Smoother** *($7.49 for 4 ounces)* contains mostly plant water, glycerin, thickeners, plant extracts, more thickeners, oatmeal, almond meal, and preservatives. This can be an OK facial scrub for someone with normal to dry skin, but it isn't easy to rinse off.

☺ **Balancing Facial Toner for All Skin Types** *($7.49 for 8.5 ounces)* is a good, almost irritant-free toner that contains mostly plant water, aloe, water-binding agents, plant extracts, glycerin, plant oils, and preservatives. The plant oils can be a problem for some skin types.

☺ **Refreshing Floral Mist for All Skin Types** *($7.49 for 8.5 ounces)* is similar to the toner above, and the same basic review applies. This one contains jasmine, which can be a skin irritant.

☹ **Renewal Moisture Cream 3% Alpha Hydroxy Complex for All Skin Types** *($13.49 for 4 ounces)* doesn't contain enough AHA to or a low enough pH to make it a good AHA product.

☺ **All Day Moisturizer Normal/Dry Skin** *($12.49 for 2 ounces)* doesn't contain a sunscreen, which makes it a poor choice for all day, but it can be a very good, emollient nighttime moisturizer for someone with dry skin. It contains mostly plant water, plant oil, thickener, glycerin, more thickeners, more plant oil, water-binding agents, vitamins A and E (antioxidants), anti-irritants, anti-irritant, and preservatives.

☺ **Green Tea Nourishing Eye Gel** *($14.49 for 1 ounce)* is a very good light-weight moisturizer that can be used on the entire face. It contains mostly plant water, thickener, water-binding agents, thickener, more water-binding agents, and preservatives.

☺ **Maximum Moisture Cream Benefits Dry/Mature Skin** *($14.49 for 2 ounces)* contains plant oils, emollients, thickeners, water-binding agents, vitamins, and anti-irritants. This is a very good moisturizer for someone with very dry skin.

☺ **Oil-Free Facial Moisturizer** *($12.49 for 2 ounces)* contains mostly plant water, glycerin, aloe, thickeners, silicone, more thickeners, anti-irritant, plant oils, and preservatives. Did anyone at this company read the ingredient list before naming this product? It isn't the least bit oil-free, but it would still be a good moisturizer for someone with normal to slightly dry skin.

☺ **SPF 12 Daily Facial Lotion** *($9.49 for 4 ounces)* is a very good, emollient, titanium dioxide–based sunscreen for someone with dry skin. SPF 15 would be better, but 12 isn't bad. It contains mostly plant water, glycerin, thickener, plant oils, more thickener, more plant oils, water-binding agent, and preservatives.

☺ **Purifying Facial Mask** *($8.49 for 4 ounces)* is a standard clay mask that also contains plant water, glycerin, thickeners, water-binding agent, and preservatives. This is as good an irritant-free clay mask as any you will find.

BeneFit

What can I say about a cosmetics line that has a self-tanning product called Aruba in a Tuba; blemish products called Boo-Boo Stick and Boo-Boo Zap; eyeshadows with names like Roadkill, Guess Again, and Striptease; lipsticks called Buck Naked, Misunderstood, and Lane Change; and a wrinkle cream called Mrs. Robinson (only those of us over 40 will understand that one)? The only thing I can think of is "Cute, very cute." But what about quality? That's another story, one that takes much longer to tell.

BeneFit was developed by twins Jean Danielson and Jane Blackford, whose brief claim to fame was a stint as the Calgon twins back in the 1960s. They opened their first cosmetics store in San Francisco, circa 1976. Although they eventually branched out to three Face Place stores, they decided a little less than two years ago to establish their products as a national line. With an infusion of investment capital and a new name (one of the twins had just returned from Italy, where everything was *bene, bene*), they established their product line as BeneFit. The cleverness didn't stop with the name. Beauty can be fun, and possibly kinky, but it is assuredly successful, according to the sisters who are now in their early 50s. With brief appearances on the Home Shopping Network and mentions in fashion magazines, this line is hard to ignore, and that has helped sales soar.

Essentially, this line is a kicky version of M.A.C., with several gimmicks thrown in to grab attention. Does anyone really need seven products to take care of the lips, or Boo-Boo Sticks that contain standard acne ingredients also found in drugstore products? BeneFit's entire skin-care line is relatively straightforward, with standard products and exaggerated claims. None of the acne products contains a single ingredient or formula that isn't available a thousand times over in drugstore acne products and every cosmetics line imaginable.

BeneFit's makeup line is a little more cumbersome to describe, but it has some interesting products, including great brushes, good foundations with wonderful neutral colors, and some specialty products that are surprisingly special, or at least unique, such as Lip Smoo…ch and D'eye'namite. Shortcomings on the makeup end of things are numerous. Both foundations are matte, which leaves someone with normal to dry skin out in the cold. In contrast, almost all of the eyeshadows are shiny, so despite the fact that there are so many to choose from, with some pretty bizarre colors for those with eccentric tastes, very few are matte. Regardless of taste, shiny eyeshadow can make the eyelid look wrinkly.

BeneFit has a lot of personality going for it. Fun is a refreshing change of pace when it comes to makeup and skin care, but no matter how you slice it, wasting money on products that don't work, can't live up to their claims, or can be found cheaper and better elsewhere isn't really any fun at all. If you want to consider this line, call (800) 781-2336 for a catalog or the retail location nearest you.

BeneFit Skin Care

☺   **All Types Skin Wash** *($14 for 4 ounces)* is about as close a knockoff of Cetaphil Gentle Skin Cleanser as I've seen. At least they're on the right track for a sensitive-skin cleanser, but they're charging twice as much as Cetaphil.

☹   **Mint Souffle Facial Cleanser for Normal to Oily and Combination Skin** *($24 for 4 ounces)* is a standard detergent-based, water-soluble cleanser that contains spearmint oil, which can be a skin irritant. It also contains many ingredients that would not make someone with oily skin happy, such as shea butter (an emollient) and other plant oils.

☺   **Clean Sweep** *($14 for 4 ounces)* is a detergent-based eye-makeup remover. It will indeed wipe off your eye makeup, but why bother if water-soluble cleansers could do the job?

☹   **Honey...Snap Out of It! Scrub, For All Skin Types** *($17 for 5 ounces)* is an almond meal–based scrub with a great enticing name and an overwrought price tag. You would be better off with Cetaphil Gentle Skin Cleanser and baking soda than this mess of clay and rye flour.

☹   **Azulene Tonic** *($14 for 4 ounces)* contains mostly water, witch hazel, slip agent, citric acid, plant oil, plant extracts, and preservatives. This is a fairly standard witch hazel–based toner, and witch hazel can be an irritant for sensitive skin types. The plant oils, citric acid, and other extracts in here can also be irritants.

☹   **Rosewater Tonic** *($14 for 4 ounces)* is mostly water, witch hazel, water-binding agent, glycerin, anti-irritants, and preservatives. The witch hazel can be a skin irritant, which is a shame because the other ingredients would have made it a decent toner.

☹   **Alpha Smooth 5% AHA Toner** *($18 for 5.56 ounces)* doesn't contain a low enough pH to be an effective exfoliant.

☹   **Alpha Clean 5% AHA** *($18 for 5.56 ounces)* has AHAs, but they are wasted in a cleanser like this because the effective part is just rinsed off.

☹ **Seven % Fine Wrinkle Line Remover** *($36 for 1 ounce)* doesn't contain a low enough pH to be an effective exfoliant.

☺ **Eye Lift $$$** *($25 for 1 ounce)* contains mostly water, silicone, glycerin, plant extracts, water-binding agents, vitamins, and preservatives. This is a good, emollient moisturizer, but nothing about it will lift the eye, although at this price it should.

☺ **$$$ Hyaluronic Creme** *($22 for 2 ounces)* contains mostly water, plant oil, thickeners, water-binding agents, preservatives, vitamin E, and pollen extract. The amount of vitamin E and pollen extract in this product is at best a dusting; however, it is still a good emollient cream for someone with dry skin. Hyaluronic acid is a good water-binding agent, but no better than dozens of other such ingredients.

☺ **$$$ Very Aloe Creme, For Combo Skin** *($25 for 2 ounces)* does contain aloe as well as thickeners, silicone, water-binding agents and preservatives. This is a good lightweight moisturizer for someone with slightly dry skin.

☺ **$$$ Vita Hydrating Creme, for Sensitive/Dry Skin** *($22 for 2 ounces)* contains mostly water; vitamins E, D, and A; plant oil; slip agent; thickeners; water-binding agents; and preservatives. This is a good moisturizer for someone with dry skin, and if you want antioxidants, they're in here.

☺ **"Aruba in a Tuba" Ultra Sunless Tan** *($22 for 5 ounces)* is a sunless tanner that uses the exact same active ingredient to turn the skin brown that all other sunless tanners use: dihydroxyacetone.

☹ **In The Shade, SPF 15** *($24 for 2.5 ounces)* doesn't contain avobenzone, titanium dioxide, or zinc oxide, and is not recommended.

☹ **Out and About Tinted Moisturizer** *($18 for 2.5 ounces)* has a tint that is too peach for most skin tones.

☺ **$$$ Seaweed Mud Mask** *($19 for 2 ounces)* contains mostly water, plant oil, glycerin, lanolin, thickeners, seaweed, water-binding agents, vitamins, and preservatives. There isn't any mud in it, but if you have dry skin, this would be a good emollient mask to leave on your face for a while.

☺ **$$$ Shrink Wrap Mask, For Combo/Oily Skin** *($26 for 2 ounces)* contains mostly aloe, film former, water-binding agents, slip agents, fragrance, and preservatives. This is a good mask for most all skin types.

☹ **$$$ Boo-Boo Zap** *($16 for 0.25 ounce)* contains mostly water, two types of alcohol, salicylic acid, camphor, witch hazel, styrene (a resin), and preservative. Alcohol, camphor, and witch hazel have no effect on blemishes other than causing more irritation.

☺ **$$$ Peel and Polish** *($20 for 1 ounce)* contains mostly aloe vera, wax, petrolatum, and thickeners. Using any kind of wax on the skin can exfoliate it, and this product is no exception.

☹ **ReBalance Aromatherapy, For Combo Skin** *($30 for 1 ounce)* contains a bunch of plants that have no effect whatsoever on breakouts or skin tone.

☹ **ReEyedrate Aromatherapy, For Eyes** *($30 for 1 ounce)* includes rose and citrus, which can irritate the eye area.

☹ **RePair Aromatherapy, For Sun Damage** *($30 for 1 ounce)* contains no ingredients that can repair sun-damaged skin. This is a very misleading product that insinuates you can get sun damage and then reverse it, when you can't.

☹ **ReVitalize Aromatherapy, For Combo Skin** *($30 for 1 ounce)* may smell nice, but there are no ingredients in it that can stimulate cell generation.

☹ **Thigh Hopes** *($23 for 8 ounces)* doesn't even deserve comment. I guess most every line has to sell their version of a cellulite remover despite the fact that none of these can remove even one cell of fat.

BeneFit Makeup

☺ **FOUNDATION:** If you are looking for a truly matte foundation in a range of beautiful neutral colors, BeneFit offers **matte tint liquid foundation *($20)*.** A strong point for this foundation is its selection of light skin-tone colors. If you have very white skin, there is a color here for you, but only if you have oily skin. This matte foundation can be quite drying and not for everyone.

☺ **sheer genius** *($26)* is a standard talc-based powder meant to be used as a foundation. It comes in only four colors, which is extremely limiting. It does have a light silky texture, but it is better used as a regular powder than as a foundation.

☺ **CONCEALER: ooh la lift** *($16)* is a pink highlighting concealer/foundation in a tube. It is supposed to contain skin-tightening botanicals, but the amount of plant extracts in this product isn't enough to tighten one skin cell. (There aren't any plants that can tighten the skin, though, so the amount is actually irrelevant.) Nevertheless, this is a good highlighter and a fun makeup boost if you have time to bother with an extra step. **boi-ing** *($16)* is a rather standard cream concealer that comes in two shades, limited to say the least. It has a soft texture with minimal chance of creasing around the eyes, and provides fairly good, even coverage.

☺ **POWDER: powder tint** *($22)* is a very drying, almost chalk-like face powder that comes in seven colors. **Colors to avoid:** Coast, which is white; Chamois, which is yellow (it is meant to even out redness, but it just looks yellow on the skin); and White Lavender (I can't imagine what skin tone this one is for). **The other four are excellent neutral shades** and very good for someone with exceptionally oily skin.

☹ **get even** *($24)* is a standard pressed powder with two shades of yellow. This is supposed to invisibly get rid of shine and discoloration. Yellow powder on the face is hardly invisible; all it does is alter the color of your foundation.

☺ **$$$ <u>BLUSH:</u> benetint** *($24)* is just what it says it is: a red tint for the cheeks that you apply from a nail polish–like container and applicator. It isn't the best way to get a smooth application, but if you already have smooth skin, meaning no pores, this gives a very natural color that just melds with the skin. However, if you have pores or dry skin, you may not be happy with the results.

☺ **$$$ color wash** *($24)* is a selection of very expensive loose-powder blush colors. I find these products extremely messy to use; they make touch-ups during the day almost impossibly inconvenient.

☺ **<u>EYESHADOW:</u> lemonaid** *($16)* is an eyeshadow base that is supposed to correct lid discoloration but actually works no better than a little foundation over the lid. **eye bright** *($15)* is a pink stick concealer that turns white when you apply it. It does brighten areas you put it on, but any light concealer would do the same. **show offs** *($13)* are very loose, iridescent eyeshadow powders. This stuff is very messy and hard to control. There are plenty of pressed shiny eyeshadow colors, why make a bad idea difficult to apply?

☹ **powder eyeshadow** *($10)* comes in a huge selection of colors, but, lamentably, even though they are priced to compete with M.A.C. (they even look the same), most of the shades are slightly shiny to very shiny (while M.A.C. has an extensive range of matte colors). Moreover, BeneFit's eyeshadow colors range from the soft and beautiful to the strange and downright ugly (M.A.C. is known for its large selection of neutrals and offers few or no bizarre colors).

☺ **creaseless cream shadows** *($13)* come in small pots and apply relatively easily, for a cream eyeshadow that is. These go on smoothly and dry to a powder finish. I would suggest that it is easier to start off with a powder in the first place, but if you are interested in cream eyeshadows this is a definite option.

☺ **<u>EYE AND BROW SHAPER:</u> brow zings** *($18)* are brow colors that are a cross between a pencil and a powder: a thick waxy powder that you apply with a stiff brush. They are meant to tame brows, but they can make the brow look overdone and matted, and the hard bristles of the brush hurt the skin. If your brows need taming, there are better tricks than this one. **eye pencils** *($11)* come in a nice assortment of colors and go on smoothly. They are fairly standard but not badly priced. **babe cakes** *($14)* is a pot of eyeliner you use wet, for the dramatic eyeliner look some of us used to wear in the '70s, only these are all shiny. **she laq** *($16)* is little more than hairspray for the brows in a bottle. Not bad, but any hairspray used with a toothbrush will do the same thing for less. BeneFit also recommends that you use this product over eyeliner, but the ingredients are way too irritating to put that close to the eyes. **flash** *($11)* is a shiny beige pencil that you are supposed to place on the rim of your lower lid. Please do not place anything that near to your eye. It is not only irritating, it is unhealthy and potentially damaging to the eye.

☺ **LIPSTICK AND LIP PENCIL:** The number of lip products BeneFit offers is nothing less than amazing. Does anyone really think she needs such a makeup arsenal for her lips? Makeup addicts will think they have found heaven; I hope the rest of us will recognize some serious cosmetics puffery and foolishness when we see it. **smoo...ch** *($15)* is a lip moisturizer/gloss in a tube. It is a good emollient, but nothing out of the ordinary; lip balms by Almay and Physicians Formula (among others) are just as good and much less expensive. **lip plump** *($15)* is supposed to make your lips look large, pouty, and smooth. It has a concealer-like texture, only more waxy. I didn't see a difference when I tested this product, but it did slightly smooth out my lips, though when you place lipstick over it you get kind of a messy mixture. I can't imagine using it on a regular basis every time I apply my lipstick. If you have lipsticks you want to make lighter or darker, that's what **depth charge** *($14)* and **light switch** *($14)* are for. Basically, they are light and dark lipsticks just to the greasy side of creamy. **de-groovie** *($21)* is supposed to prevent lipstick from feathering. It does an OK job, but you can buy much better products for a lot less money, such as Coty's Stop It and Hold It.

☺ **lipstick** *($13)* comes in creams, mattes, and sheers. The creams are fairly greasy and moist, the sheers are similar to the creams but shiny, and the mattes are fairly matte but still tend to feather. **glosses** *($12)* come little pots and are exceptionally greasy and emollient. **lip liners** *($11)* come in an attractive range of colors and, although they are quite standard, go on easily and wear well.

☺ **MASCARA: masca...rah** *($12)* is just an OK mascara. It goes on nicely and tends not to smear, but it doesn't build well; if you're looking for thick lashes, this mascara is not for you.

☺ **BRUSHES:** It is always a welcome sight when a cosmetics line offers a selection of usable soft brushes. BeneFit does just that, and the 14 brushes *($7 to $22)* are impressive and not priced to blow your budget. This is a decided strong point, and by itself is worth a visit or a look through BeneFit's catalog if you need to augment your brush supply. The eyeliner and eyeshadow brushes are especially great. **get bent** *($13)* is an eyeliner brush with a bent tip claiming to be easier to use along the eye. I'm not sure I get the point, no pun intended, but the special shape doesn't really help. It is still a good eyeliner brush but it doesn't store easily in your makeup bag.

☺ **SPECIALTY PRODUCTS: high beam** *($18)* comes in a nail polish bottle and is applied to the face in a similar manner. It is just a shiny moisturizer that dries to a matte finish, leaving the shine behind. Cute, definitely cute!

Bioelements *(Skin Care Only)*

You may have seen this line of skin-care products being sold at the hair salon where you get your hair cut or nails done. It is very attractive and uses all the current buzzwords that the cosmetics industry loves to bandy about. The brochure states, "Your skin is a mirror that reflects your inner well-being. Visible surface problems like premature wrinkles, dryness, excess oil, irritation, and blemishes are often visual reflections of deeper, below-the-surface imbalances. These imbalances occur when your body is thrown out of sync by the normal everyday challenges of air pollution, chemicals, the sun, poor nutrition, or emotional upsets . . . . [This] stress[es] your system's inner balance."

That sounds great, but none of it is true. The aging process is much more complicated than this diatribe on inner peace and health lets on. The one thing they are right about is that the effects of the sun are potent, and for that they do have a good SPF 15 sunscreen. The rest of the products are on the hokey side, as are the claims that you can give extra oxygen to the skin to slow down visible signs of aging, or detoxify the skin with antioxidants. For more information on this line, call (708) 518-0900.

☺ $$$ **Decongestant Cleanser** *($18.50 for 6 ounces)* is a standard detergent-based water-soluble cleanser. It would be good for someone with oily to combination skin, but it can leave the skin feeling dry.

☺ $$$ **Moisture Positive Cleanser, If Your Skin Feels Dry** *($18.50 for 6 ounces)* is an OK cleanser for someone with dry skin. It can leave skin feeling slightly slick and does not remove makeup well without its having to be wiped off.

☹ **Twice Daily Bar Gentle Non-Soap Cleanser** *($16.50 for 5 ounces)* is one expensive bar of soap. It is indeed far more gentle than regular soap, but the detergent cleansing agents can still be drying and the ingredients that keep it in a bar form can potentially clog pores.

☹ **Makeup Dissolver, Oil-Free Formula for Your Eyes** *($15.50 for 6 ounces and a sponge)* lists witch hazel, which can irritate the eyes, as the first ingredient. (Witch hazel is about 5% alcohol.)

☺ $$$ **Measured Micrograins, Exfoliates Your Skin** *($21.50 for 2.5 ounces)* is a scrub, but the standard micrograins are just little pieces of polyethylene and the other ingredients are mostly thickeners and preservatives. It is an OK scrub, but a very expensive one, with several plant extracts thrown in to sound mysterious and healthy.

☺ $$$ **Equalizer Rebalances Your Skin** *($17.50 for 6 ounces)* contains mostly water, plant extracts, slip agents, more plant extracts, and preservatives. If the cleanser didn't unbalance your skin, you don't need to rebalance it, is my way of looking at this product. Other than that, except for a tiny amount of witch hazel, this is basically a good nonirritating toner, if you're not allergic to any of the plants here.

☹ **Quick Refiner with AlphaBlend** *($40 for 3 ounces)* is an alcohol-based AHA toner. AHAs can be irritating enough without adding further irritation from the alcohol. Not only are there cheaper AHA products available, but much less irritating ones.

☺ $$$ **Absolute Moisture Balances Combination Skin** *($29.50 for 2.5 ounces)* contains mostly water, thickeners, plant oil, more thickeners, more plant oil, water-binding agents, and preservatives. What person with combination skin wants more oil? This is a good moisturizer, but only for someone with normal to dry skin.

☹ **Beyond Hydration Moisturizes without Oil** *($29.50 for 2.5 ounces)* contains mostly water, a film former, water-binding agent, and preservatives. It also contains a small amount of peppermint, a potent skin irritant. There is never a reason to put any irritating ingredients on the skin for the sake of moisturizing.

☺ $$$ **Crucial Moisture Fortifies Your Skin with Emollients** *($29.50 for 2.5 ounces)* contains mostly water, several thickeners, silicone, plant extracts, and preservatives. There is nothing crucial or even very interesting about this product. It would be a good, though ordinary, moisturizer for someone with normal to slightly dry skin.

☹ **Everyday Protector SPF 8 Moisturizer** *($29.50 for 6 ounces)* is not recommended due to the low SPF. With the amount of sun damage possible on a daily basis, and all the wonderful SPF 15s available, there is no reason to use anything less. What a shame, because this one has both titanium dioxide and zinc oxide, which offer great UVA protection.

☹ **Eye Area with AlphaBlend** *($31.50 for 1 ounce)* contains mostly water, silicone, thickeners, lactic acid, more thickeners, more AHAs, and preservatives. The amount of AHAs and the pH of this product make it rather gentle, but it's a poor AHA exfoliating product, and that's what AHAs are supposed to do—exfoliate the skin.

☹ **Oxygen Cocktail Natural Defense Against Visible Skin Aging** *($31.50 for 1 ounce)* doesn't have enough oxygen (if any) to provide any defense for the skin or to help even one cell inhale.

☺ $$$ **Sun Diffusing Protector SPF 15 Natural Sunblock** *($29.50 for 6 ounces)* is a zinc oxide– and titanium dioxide–based sunscreen in a rather ordinary but OK base of cosmetic thickeners and minute amounts of plant extracts. But given the few zinc oxide–based sunscreens available this is a great one, just very overpriced!

☺ $$$ **Breakout Control Your Emergency Blemish Lotion** *($31.50 for 1 ounce)* contains mostly water, thickeners, 2.5% benzoyl peroxide, and preservatives. Benzoyl peroxide is a good disinfectant and can help reduce breakouts, though the standard waxy cosmetic thickeners used in this product could clog pores.

☺ $$$ **Cremetherapy Very Emollient Mask** *($23 for 2.5 ounces)* contains mostly water, plant oils, thickeners, clay, plant extracts, more plant oil, anti-irritant, and preservatives. Because there are so many emollients in this product and so little clay, it would be a fine mask for someone with dry skin.

☺ **$$$ Immediate Comfort 1% Hydrocortisone Lotion** *($22 for 1 ounce)* is a very expensive version of over-the-counter cortisone creams such as Lanacort and Cortaid. Given the similarity, the choice of whether you want to spend $3 for 1 ounce or $22 for 1 ounce is up to you.

☺ **$$$ Jet Travel Moisture Boost for Low Humidity** *($31.50 for 1 ounce)* contains mostly water-binding agent, silicone, and preservatives. This product is supposed to be worn under your moisturizer. However, if you're already using a moisturizer that contains these types of ingredients, which most moisturizers do, this becomes an unnecessary step.

☺ **$$$ Pigment Discourager** *($18.50 for 0.5 ounce)* is a standard 1% hydroquinone skin-lightening product. Hydroquinone can improve skin discolorations but not without the help of a sunscreen or a skin exfoliant, plus there are far less expensive products like this available.

☺ **$$$ Restorative Clay Active Treatment Mask** *($21.50 for 2.5 ounces)* is a standard clay mask that also contains plant oil, thickeners, plant extracts, and preservatives. If you have dry skin and want to try a clay mask, the oils in here can help soften the drying effects of the clay.

☹ **$$$ Stress Solution Calms Sensitized Skin** *($31.50 for 1 ounce)* is also similar to the Jet Travel moisturizer, except it contains tiny amounts of plant extracts and aloe vera. Aloe vera won't calm sensitive skin, although if you feel it does, it would be much cheaper to buy pure aloe vera and see how that works.

☹ **T-Zone Monitor Controls Your Oily Areas** *($31.50 for 1 ounce)* contains mostly water, horsetail extract, thickener, plant extracts, aloe vera, eucalyptus, and preservatives. There is nothing in this product that will control oil, but the eucalyptus can be a skin irritant.

☺ **$$$ Urban Detox Pollution Fighting for City Skin** *($31.50 for 1 ounce)* won't detoxify the skin, but it is an OK, extremely lightweight liquid, similar to the Jet Travel moisturizer. This one contains a good antioxidant that is considered strong but unstable. It only works to keep moisture in the skin, since antioxidants can't ward off pollution.

☹ **Instant Emollient Lip Sunscreen SPF 8 Non-PABA** *($8.50 for 0.14 ounce)* contains too low an SPF to make it adequate for reliable sun protection.

☹ **$$$ Yang Aromatherapy Oil** *($19.50 for 2 ounces)* contains a number of potentially irritating oils. If you like the way this smells that's great, just don't put it on the skin.

☹ **$$$ Yin Aromatherapy Oil** *($19.50 for 2 ounces)* contains a number of potentially irritating oils. If you like the way this smells that's great, just don't put it on the skin.

Biogime (Skin Care Only)

The name conveys a message of plants, science, and cleanliness. Although the word "Biogime" might register high on the appeal meter, the information on the ingredient list is where the consumer's focus really needs to be. Biogime's instruction booklet reads like a procedure for minor surgery. The emphasis is definitely on hygiene (don't transfer products into other containers, wash hands before starting, do not expose products to extreme heat or cold), but those warnings are true for all cosmetics. They also want you to use washcloths during the cleansing part of the routine, which can be a problem. Both the laundry-detergent residue left behind on washcloths and the terrycloth material itself can be irritating to the skin.

Two claims that Biogime lives up to beautifully are that all their products are truly fragrance-free and that they are not tested on animals. Their claim regarding the pure and natural content of the products is bogus. All the products contain their share of very unnatural preservatives, chemical emulsifiers, and synthetically derived detergent cleansing agents. That doesn't make these products bad, but it's one more example of the kind of ersatz claim the cosmetics companies love to perpetrate so the consumer never really knows what she is buying. For more information about Biogime call (800) 952-6226.

☺ **$$$ Colloidal Cleanser** *($15.95 for 6 ounces)* is a mostly standard wipe-off cleanser that contains sunflower oil instead of mineral oil. It can still leave a greasy film on the skin. Biogime's suggestion is to use this cleanser to wipe off the makeup, and then follow up with the Lathering Cleanser. I never recommend a two-step makeup-removing process. There are plenty of gentle water-soluble cleansers that can take off everything, so a wipe-off makeup remover is not necessary.

☺ **$$$ Essential Cleansing Milk** *($22.50 for 8 ounces)* is a detergent-based, water-soluble cleanser that would be good for someone with dry skin. The cleansing agent is fairly mild (not great for makeup removal). There is a little bit of oil in this product but probably not enough to be a problem.

☹ **Oil Absorbing Cleanser** *($18.95 for 6 ounces)* is a standard detergent-based, water-soluble cleanser with several irritating ingredients, including lemon oil, mandarin oil, lime oil, orange oil, and grapefruit extract, that are a problem for all skin types.

☺ **$$$ Foaming Cleanser** *($17.95 for 6 ounces)* is a standard detergent cleanser that can be drying for some skin types.

☺ **$$$ Gentle Eye Makeup Remover** *($12.95 for 2 ounces)* is just a wipe-off makeup remover that contains mostly water, sunflower oil, and some thickening agents; you could do just as well getting some sunflower oil, from your kitchen cabinet.

☹ **Gentle Facial Buff** *($17.95 for 4 ounces)* is extremely scratchy and potentially irritating to all skin types. The diatomaceous earth as the scrub may sound natural but it is incredibly rough on the skin. This product also contains spearmint oil which adds more irritation.

☹ **Oil Absorbing Citrus Scrub** *($19.95 for 4 ounces)* is even more of a problem than the one above, since while this one also contains diatomaceous earth it also uses sodium C14-16 olefin sulfate as the cleansing agent, and that is extremely drying and irritating for all skin types. This one also adds fuel to the fire with lemon oil, mandarin oil, lime oil, and orange oil.

☺ **$$$ Essential Toner** *($22.50 for 8 ounces)* is an OK, relatively irritant-free toner that could work for most skin types. It is mostly just water, slip agents, and detergent cleansing agent. It does contain some arnica and witch hazel far enough down in the ingredient listing so they probably won't be sensitizing, but be careful.

☹ **Oil Controlling Toner** *($19.95 for 6 ounces)* contains mostly witch hazel, and that can be irritating for most all skin types. One unique aspect of this product is that it contains several forms of yeast attached to a mineral base. I imagine these mineral components can do some absorbing of oil but the yeast aspect throws me. I have found no information on this and can't comment other than to say it sounds interesting. I will continue looking into it and report on what I eventually find in my newsletter.

☺ **$$$ Protective Toner** *($19.95 for 6 ounces)* is mostly water, slip agent, soothing agents, aloe vera, and preservatives. This would be a very good irritant-free toner for most skin types.

☹ **Hi PotenC Serum AHA** *($36.95 for 1 ounce)* would be a good AHA, with about an 8% concentration as stated on the label (it has a pH of 4), except that the second ingredient is witch hazel and that just adds unnecessary irritation to an otherwise good product.

☺ **$$$ Natural Conditioner** *($22.45 for 6 ounces)* contains mostly sunflower oil, thickeners, preservatives, and vitamins. This is almost identical to the Colloidal Cleanser, so the extra cost is only a marketing gimmick. It is a good moisturizer for someone with normal to dry skin. The amount of vitamins is almost negligible.

☹ **Oil-Free Gel Conditioner** *($22.95 for 4 ounces)* is indeed oil-free but the second ingredient is witch hazel, which means it isn't irritant-free.

☺ **$$$ Skin Perfection with Retinol Palmitate and Lipsosomes** *($34.95 for 4 ounces)* is almost identical to the Natural Conditioner above and Ultimate Conditioner below, only in cream form, and the same review applies. There is vitamin A in here, which is OK as an antioxidant, but little more.

☺ **$$$ Ultimate Conditioner** *($23.45 for 6 ounces)* contains mostly water, sunflower seed oil, thickeners, preservatives, and vitamins. This is almost identical to the Natural Conditioner and the same review applies.

☺ **$$$ Youthful Eye Gel** *($39.95 for 0.5 ounce)* contains mostly water, slip agents, film former, glycerin, preservatives, and plant extracts. This is mostly a plasticizer with a small amount of glycerin. It would deliver minimal moisturizing benefit for the skin, but the film former can make things look temporarily smoother. The plants are listed after the preservative, making their quantity completely insignificant.

☺ **$$$ Essential Protector SPF 15** *($30 for 2 ounces)* is a good, in-part titanium dioxide–based sunscreen that would be good for someone with normal to dry skin. By the way, this protector is virtually identical to the SPF 15 that follows, which makes its price tag a sheer marketing fantasy.

☺ **$$$ Sun Protector SPF 15** *($17.95 for 4 ounces)* is a good in-part titanium dioxide–based sunscreen. This one would be good for someone with normal to dry skin.

☺ **$$$ Self-Tanning Facial Lotion** *($19.95 for 4 ounces)* uses the same active ingredient to turn the skin brown as a $6 self-tanner found at the drugstore.

☹ **Aerobic Fitness Facial Kit** *($34.95 for 2 ounces with a small glass bowl and brush)* is supposed to rebuild tissue while tightening the 55 facial muscles. Nothing in here can rebuild tissue or tone facial muscles, although several ingredients could irritate the skin.

☺ **$$$ Bella Coola Glacial Clay Masque** *($34.95 for 6 ounces)* is just clay and preservatives. For a clay mask, this is as good as any. By the way, clay is clay, no matter what part of the world it comes from.

☹ **Blemish Relief Spot Control Formula** *($12.95 for 0.5 ounce)* contains mostly water, thickeners, aloe vera, more thickeners (including isopropyl palmitate, which can cause breakouts), plant extracts, sulfur (can be a skin irritant), and preservatives. Sulfur can be a disinfectant but it can also be a skin irritant, while several of the thickeners used in here can clog pores.

☺ **$$$ Day Essential O2** *($40 for 2 ounces)* doesn't contain enough oxygen for one breath, but even if it contained more it would go up in air before the skin could ever use it. There is no evidence that oxygen in cosmetics has one iota of benefit for skin. This product is a good moisturizer, but because it doesn't contain sunscreen there is little reason to use it for daytime.

☺ **$$$ French Botanical Masque** *($29.95 for 4 ounces)* is a fairly standard clay mask that doesn't contain French clay but does have plant extracts and vitamins. They won't feed the skin, but they sound good and that's what some women want. It contains mostly water; clay; thickeners; plant extracts (including arnica which can be a skin irritant); corn and rice starch (can be skin irritants); soothing agents; vitamins A, E, and D; and preservatives.

☺ **$$$ Night Essential O2** *($45 for 2 ounces)* is similar to the Day one above, and the same comments apply.

☺ **$$$ Retinol Palmitate** *($34.95 for 4 ounces)* contains a good amount of retinyl palmitate, and that's nice, but if you are expecting this product to behave like Retin-A or Renova you will have bought some very deceptive information. This is merely a good moisturizer for dry skin, period. The vitamin A is a good ingredient but no better then lots of other antioxidants used in cosmetics.

Biore (Skin Care Only)

New skin-care lines are usually launched with a specific gimmick to grab the consumer's attention. Biore is in this category. I have already received more letters about Biore than you can imagine. The gimmick everyone wants to know about is ☹ **Pore Perfect Deep Cleansing Strips** *($5.99 for six nose strips)*. This product is supposed to instantly clean pores. All you do is place a piece of cloth with an incredibly sticky substance on it over your nose, as you might do with a Band-Aid, wait 15 minutes for it to dry, and then rip it off. Along with some amount of skin, blackheads are supposed to stick to it and come right out of your nose. What does this miracle product contain? A lot of hair spray. The main ingredient is polyquaternium-37, a film-forming hair spray ingredient. It works little better than using regular tape over the nose. (Actually, regular tape may be less damaging to the skin because Biore can leach potentially irritating ingredients into the pores and tape can't.)

What has me most concerned about these so-called Cleansing Strips is that they are accompanied by a strong warning not to use them over any area other than the nose and not to use them over inflamed, swollen, sunburned, or excessively dry skin. It also states that if the strip is too painful to remove, you should wet it and then carefully remove it. What a warning!

You may at first be impressed with what comes off your nose. (Well, there is no question: you will be impressed.) Most people do have some oil sitting at the top of their oil glands (most of the face's oil glands are located on the nose), and whether you use these strips or a piece of tape, black dots and some skin will be removed. Is that helpful? Only momentarily, but if you use the Biore product, the plastic-forming agent can get into the pores and possibly cause breakouts and irritation.

Also, despite the warning on the package, most women will try these strips wherever they see breakouts. If I didn't know better, I know I would. The way these strips adhere, they can absolutely injure or tear skin and cause spider veins to surface. They are especially unsafe if you've been using Retin-A, Renova, AHAs, or BHA; having facial peels; or taking Accutane; or if you have naturally thin skin or any skin disorder such as rosacea, psoriasis, or seborrhea.

Biore's brochure claims this product can pull an entire blackhead plug out of the skin. It can't. If you could grab a blackhead out of the skin, your skin would be left with an empty hole (and there is nothing in this product that will close it up), but that's not what happens. Instead, just the top layer of the blackhead is removed, and then the blackhead returns because the source of the problem was never corrected. Nothing was done to reduce irritation, exfoliate skin cells, help keep oil flow normal, or close the pore. What about the rest of Biore's products? Here's my review, but clearly this line is based on these strips and little else. Biore is being sold in drugstores across the country. Call (888) BIORE-11 for more information.

☺ **Cleansing Gel, Non-Foaming** *($5.99 for 5 ounces)* is a very good water-soluble cleanser for someone with normal to dry skin, but it may not remove makeup very well. The brochure states that this cleanser and the one below use sorbitol, a natural plant extract, to dissolve dirt and remove pollutants. Didn't anyone at Biore read the ingredient lists for these products? They contain standard detergent cleansing agents, just like thousands of other water-soluble cleansers. Besides, sorbitol isn't a cleansing agent, it is a good but ordinary cosmetic thickening agent.

☺ **Foaming Cleanser** *($5.99 for 5 ounces)* is almost identical to the cleanser above, but with stronger cleansing agents and foaming agents. It can be a very good water-soluble cleanser for someone with normal to oily skin.

☹ **Pore Perfect Toner** *($4.94 for 5.5 ounces)* has three different types of alcohol in it, including the alcohol in witch hazel. What in the world were they thinking. Wait, what am I thinking, this is the company that originated the Pore Strips!

☹ **Hydrating Moisturizer** *($8.99 for 4 ounces)* contains mostly water, thickeners, plasticizing agent (a hair spray–like ingredient), silicone, more thickeners, water-binding agent, and preservatives. I concur with one reader's review of this product, that it is sticky and uncomfortable, and I would add that it's rather ineffective and ordinary.

☹ **Hydrating Moisturizer SPF 6** *($8.99 for 4 ounces)* is not recommended. SPF 6 is an embarrassingly low number, and though it may be a decent moisturizer, it doesn't contain titanium dioxide, zinc oxide, or avobenzone, which are necessary for adequate UVA protection.

☺ **Biore Mild Daily Cleansing Scrub** *($4.94 for 5 ounces)* and **Biore Self-Heating Mask** *($5.12 for six packets)* are two of the more ironic product line extensions I've ever seen. Why would a scrub to clean out pores and a mask to do the same be necessary if the Biore Strips worked? However, the scrub is just a scrub, and I wouldn't use it over Cetaphil Gentle Skin Cleanser mixed with baking soda, or the mask in place of a simple clay mask.

BioTherm

I've never done a survey, though I should, to find out how women react when they learn that the $50 Lancome product they are using is virtually identical to the

$10 product from L'Oreal. Most women seem to react with either utter shock or complete disbelief. More often than not, women just can't imagine how they fell for the advertising and marketing, not to mention the prices. From my perspective, it is easy to see how someone could get seduced into overspending, and even potentially hurting their skin. The claims and enticing product descriptions sound too good to be true, which, of course, they are.

Biotherm is owned by L'Oreal. I have a lot of respect for many L'Oreal, Lancome, Redken, Maybelline, and Biotherm products, which are all part of the L'Oreal group. I also have a lot of gripes. With Biotherm and Lancome, I am most upset about cost and claims. The other lines are the inexpensive relatives, so cost isn't as much an issue with them as their claims are.

In regard to Biotherm, despite the French accent, these products are far from unique, exotic, or specially formulated, although they do try very hard to appear exceptional and the line is so extensive it is almost mind-boggling. One ingredient Biotherm utilizes to gain your attention is something they call "biotechnological thermal plankton." For your information, plankton are microscopic plants and animals that are adrift in fresh and salt water. They come in many forms, including one-celled amoebas, tiny jellyfish, fish larvae, and some forms of algae. I imagine the thermal reference is that they were somehow heated before being stuck in some of these products. What can plankton do for your skin? That's anyone's guess. I have yet to see any research suggesting that this is the cosmetic ingredient you've been waiting for.

"Naturally purifying extracts" is another phrase Biotherm likes to use. While these products do indeed contain a handful of plant extracts, they are neither purifying nor essential. Actually, a strong point for Biotherm is that they use minimal amounts of plant extracts, which reduces the risk of allergens and irritation. Several of the products do contain decent antioxidants, including vitamin E and superoxide dismutase, and that is a benefit, but one not unusual or specific to this line.

Biotherm also has a spa gimmick—adding a group of mineral salts, including magnesium, zinc, copper, manganese, potassium chloride, and regular table salt, to their products. Minerals can't be absorbed by the skin, and they may cause irritation when left on the skin instead of being rinsed off. For more information on Biotherm, contact L'Oreal at (212) 818-1500.

BioTherm Skin Care

☺ **$$$ BioPur Pure Cleansing Gel** *($15 for 150 ml)* is a decent though truly standard detergent-based, water-soluble cleanser that would work well for most skin types. It has a small amount of copper and zinc gluconate. While these metallic powders aren't always irritating, they offer nothing much but color. The price is the only thing that might be a bit uncomfortable.

☺ $$$ **Biosensitive High Tolerance Cleansing Cream** *($20 for 125 ml)* is an incredibly overpriced cold cream–type cleanser with primarily wax, silicone, shea butter, and lots of thickening agents.

☺ $$$ **Biosensitive High Tolerance Fluid Cleansing Milk** *($20 for 150 ml)* is mostly glycerin and thickening agents. That makes it a rather ordinary wipe-off cleanser with a low-tolerance price tag.

☺ **Biosource Foaming Gel Cleanser** *($15 for 150 ml)* is a detergent-based, water-soluble cleanser that uses fairly drying cleansing agents. It also has a fairly high pH, which makes it more drying and potentially irritating than most cleansers. It is not recommended.

☹ **Biosource Instant Cleansing Foam** *($15.50 for 150 ml)* is similar to the cleanser above, and the same review applies.

☺ $$$ **Biosource Express Cleansing Fluid** *($20 for 250 ml)* is a lightweight, water-soluble cleanser that doesn't remove makeup very well, although it may be OK for someone with dry, sensitive skin.

☺ $$$ **Biosource Softening Cleansing Milk** *($19 for 250 ml)* is similar to the Cleansing Milk above, and the same review applies.

☹ **Biosource Softening Cleansing Soap** *($14 for 150 g)* is a standard tallow-based bar soap that can be quite drying for all skin types; the tallow can also clog pores.

☺ $$$ **Biosource Invigorating Cleansing Milk** *($19 for 240 ml)* is mostly mineral oil, thickening agents, fragrance, and a small amount of detergent cleansing agents. It can be an option for someone with normal to dry skin, though it can leave a greasy film.

☺ $$$ **Biosource Softening Cleansing Milk** *($19 for 240 ml)* is almost identical to the product above, and the same review applies.

☺ $$$ **Biosource Thermal Cream Wash** *($19 for 125 ml)* is a mineral oil–based wipe-off cleanser that can leave a greasy film.

☺ $$$ **Biocils Soothing Eye Make-up Remover** *($17 for 125 ml)* is a standard eye-makeup remover with slip agents and detergent cleansing agents. It can be irritating for some skin types.

☺ $$$ **Biocils Waterproof Eye Make-up Remover** *($18 for 125 ml)* is similar to the product above, but with silicone, and the same review applies.

☺ $$$ **Biosource Clarifying Exfoliating Gel** *($18 for 75 ml)* has synthetic scrubbing particles that will indeed exfoliate the skin, but baking soda and Cetaphil Gentle Skin Cleanser work far better for far less money.

☺ $$$ **Biosource Softening Exfoliating Cream** *($18 for 75 ml)* contains several emollients, thickeners, and crushed shells of small sea creatures. It works as a scrub, but as I mentioned above, this is not the best way exfoliate the skin.

☹ **BioPur Mattifying Astringent Lotion** *($20 for 250 ml)* is a lot of money for alcohol, and is not recommended.

☹ **Biolotion Pure Alcohol-Free Skin Balancing Toner** *($15 for 200 ml)* is alcohol free, but it is hardly irritant free. It contains potassium alum and thiolanediol. In 1992 the FDA stated that potassium alum has not been shown to be safe or effective in over-the-counter products. Thiolanediol is derived from phenol and can be a skin irritant. This product also contains salicylic acid, but the other ingredients negate any potential benefit.

☺ **$$$ Biosensitive Calming Thermal Spring Spray** *($20 for 150 ml)* is merely water, glycerin, preservatives, and fragrance. This just gets the ordinary toner award.

☺ **$$$ Biosource Invigorating Thermal Toner** *($19 for 250 ml)* contains mostly water, slip agent, preservatives, and fragrance, with a sprinkling of antioxidants and water-binding agents. This isn't a bad toner, but why bother?

☺ **$$$ Biosource Softening Thermal Toner** *($19 for 250 ml)* is similar to the toner above, and the same review applies.

☺ **$$$ Biojeunesse Skin Refining Day Cream** *($35 for 50 ml)* contains mostly water, glycerin, water-binding agent, silicone, a long list of thickening agents, emollient, vitamins, plant oil, fragrance, and preservatives. This is a good moisturizer for nighttime (no sunscreen means it is dangerous to use during the day). It does contain a small amount of salicylic acid, but the pH is too high for the BHA to have any exfoliating effect on the skin.

☺ **$$$ Biojeunesse Yeux Rejuvenating Eye Care** *($35 for 15 g)* contains mostly water, glycerin, vitamin, sunscreen agents (but not enough for an SPF rating), shea butter, antioxidant, water-binding agents, thickeners, film former, silicone, salicylic acid, and preservatives. This huge ingredient listing adds up to a good moisturizer for dry skin until you get to the salicylic acid. That would be a problem for the eye area, except that the pH of this product isn't low enough to let it work as an exfoliant.

☺ **$$$ Bionutrition Comfort Treatment for Dry Skin** *($34 for 50 ml)* contains mostly thickeners, sunscreen (but not enough for an SPF rating), antioxidant, silicone, petrolatum, plant oil, preservatives, and fragrance. This is a good moisturizer for dry skin.

☺ **$$$ Bionutrition Force II** *($34 for 50 ml)* contains mostly water, mineral oil, petrolatum, glycerin, thickeners, plant oil, vitamins, antioxidant, preservatives, and fragrance. This is a good emollient moisturizer for someone with dry skin.

☺ **$$$ Biosensitive Yeux Calming Eye Cream** *($35 for 15 g)* contains mostly water, plant oils, silicones, glycerin, thickeners, water-binding agents, and preservatives. This is a good emollient moisturizer for dry skin.

☺ **$$$ Fluide Biojeunesse Skin Refining Day Fluid** *($35 for 50 ml)* is identical to the moisturizer above, except this one is a lotion.

☺ **$$$ Bionuit Overnight Visibly Effective Skin Treatment** *($35 for 50 ml)* is similar to the Skin Refining Day Cream, only without the BHA, and this one contains more petrolatum. It would be a good moisturizer for someone with dry skin, but it is no more visibly effective than any other moisturizer.

☺ $$$ **Biosensitive Calming Regulating Daily Cream** *($27 for 50 ml)* contains mostly water, silicone, glycerin, plant oils, thickeners, antioxidant, preservative, and fragrance. This standard moisturizer would be good for someone with normal to dry skin.

☺ $$$ **Biosensitive Extra Comfort Cream Calming Regulating** *($27 for 50 ml)* is similar to the one above and the same review applies.

☺ $$$ **Bioregard Bi-Active Eye Contour Treatment Gel** *($32 for 15 ml)* contains mostly water, plant oil, glycerin, slip agent, thickeners, water-binding agents, caffeine, anti-irritant, preservatives, and antioxidant. This would be a good lightweight moisturizer for someone with normal to slightly dry skin. Nothing about this product makes it special for use around the eye area. Caffeine in cosmetics won't wake up the eyes; if it could, coffee compresses would be best and far cheaper too.

☺ $$$ **Hydra-Detox Daily Moisturizing Cream** *($35 for 50 ml)* can't "detox" the skin; it is merely a good moisturizer for someone with dry skin. It has one of the longest ingredient lists I've ever seen. The chances of something being in here that you could be allergic to is pretty high. It does contain salicylic acid, but the pH isn't low enough for it to work as an exfoliant.

☺ $$$ **Hydro-Detox Daily Moisturizing Lotion** *($35 for 50 ml)* is similar to the product above, only in lotion form.

☺ $$$ **Hydrologic Moisture Generator** *($34 for 50 ml)* is a good emollient moisturizer that contains mostly water, shea butter, silicone, glycerin, plant oil, slip agents, thickeners, water-binding agents, and preservatives.

☺ $$$ **Reducteur Rides Anti-Wrinkle and Firming Cream, for Very Dry Skin** *($37 for 50 ml)* is a standard mineral oil– and petrolatum–based moisturizer that would be a very good moisturizer for someone with very dry skin. It also contains thickeners and water-binding agents. It would be a very good, though overpriced, moisturizer for someone with dry skin; however, it won't firm anything or get rid of a single wrinkle.

☺ $$$ **Reducteur Rides Anti-Wrinkle and Firming Eye Creme** *($30 for 15 g)* is similar to the product above, and the same review applies.

☺ $$$ **Symbiose Daily Aging Treatment Liposome Gel** *($45 for 50 ml)* contains mostly water, glycerin, slip agent, thickener, antioxidant, water-binding agents, fragrance, and preservatives. This would be a good lightweight moisturizer for someone with normal to slightly dry skin.

☻ **Bio-Effet Instant Beauty Vials** *($13 for two 1 ml vials)* contains too much alcohol to be called beautiful. I would call it merely irritating.

☻ **BioPur Clarifying Balancing Night Gel** *($30 for 50 ml)* won't balance anyone's skin. It contains a group of standard thickening agents (several that could cause breakouts) and some clay. It also contains a small amount of salicylic acid, but the pH is too high to make this an effective exfoliant. This product is a waste of time and money.

☹ **BioPur Emergency Anti-Imperfection with AHA** *($18 for 15 ml)* contains too little AHA and BHA and doesn't have the right pH to be an effective exfoliant. It does contain several thickening agents that can cause breakouts. The second ingredient in this cream is zinc oxide and the third is clay. That makes it more like spackle than anything else.

☹ **BioPur Matte Hydrating Fluid** *($24 for 50 ml)* definitely has a matte finish because the fourth and fifth ingredients are aluminum starch octenylsuccinate and clay. This is a confused product because the oil-absorbing ingredients are negated by the silicone and thickening agents it contains. There is a small amount of BHA in here but the pH is too high for it to work as an exfoliant.

☹ **Biosource Masque Clean Skin Peel-Off** *($23 for 75 ml)* might be fun to peel off, but I can't think of a reason to put alcohol and a hair-spray ingredient on anyone's face.

☺ **$$$ Energi-Cure Smoothing Firming Mask** *($31 for 50 ml)* contains mostly water, film former, water-binding agents, antioxidant, preservatives, and fragrance. This is a lot of money for hair spray and some water-binding agents, but it is a mask and your skin will feel smooth afterwards.

☺ **$$$ Hydra-Detox Lotion** *($35 for 50 ml)* contains mostly water, silicones, alcohol, glycerin, vitamins, water-binding agents, preservatives, and fragrance. This huge ingredient list won't detox anything from your skin, it is just a good moisturizer for normal to dry skin. The alcohol in here is probably more an emulsifier than anything else and shouldn't be a problem for most skin types.

☺ **$$$ Hydra-Detox Cream** *($35 for 50 ml)* is similar to the lotion above, only in cream form.

☺ **$$$ Hydro-Cure Soothing and Moisturizing Mask** *($20 for 75 ml)* contains mostly water, glycerin, plant oils, anti-irritant, thickeners, water-binding agents, fragrance, and preservatives. It won't cure a thing and is more like a very thick moisturizer than anything else, but left on the face it can alleviate dry skin the same way any moisturizer does.

☺ **$$$ Masque BioPur Balancing Purifying Mask** *($20 for 75 ml)* contains wheat starch, which can be problematic for people prone to breakouts. Other than that, it is a basic clay mask that can't balance or purify.

☺ **$$$ Reducteur Rides Anti-Wrinkle and Firming Cream** *($37 for 50 ml)* is a good, and unexceptionally standard moisturizer for dry skin. I wouldn't count on the anti-wrinkle or firming claims; they are enticing but not true. This product contains mostly water, thickeners, silicone, petrolatum, vitamins, water-binding agents, and preservatives.

☺ **$$$ Tenseur Reducteur Rides Tensing Wrinkle and Firming Essence** *($52 for 30 ml)* contains mostly water, alcohol, glycerin, silicone, water-binding agents, vitamins, thickeners, plant oils, film former, preservatives, and fragrance. This won't firm anything, but it is a good moisturizer for someone with dry skin. The alcohol could be an irritant for some skin types.

☺ **$$$ Face Repair Soothing Balm** *($16 for 50 ml)* is just a good moisturizer for normal to dry skin; there is nothing in here that can repair skin any better than any other moisturizer. It contains mostly water, glycerin, thickeners, silicone, vitamins, petrolatum, preservatives, plant extracts, and fragrance.

☺ **$$$ Intensive Soothing After Sun Balm For Face** *($16 for 50 ml)* is merely a good moisturizer, similar to many others in this line. There are no lotions, creams, or balms that can be applied to heal skin left unprotected during the day. And, because of its emollient nature, it would be unwise to apply this over a sunburn.

☺ **$$$ Maximum Protection Lotion SPF 15** *($15 for 150 ml)* contains titanium dioxide and would be a good sunscreen for someone with dry skin.

☺ **$$$ Protective Lotion SPF 15** *($18 for 150 ml)* is an excellent sunscreen for normal to dry skin. This is definitely a Canadian or International formula, because the sunscreen base would not be allowed in the U.S.: the active ingredients include titanium dioxide and Mexoryl SX.

☺ **$$$ Soothing Repair Lotion** *($17 for 240 ml)* won't repair anyone's skin. This is merely a good moisturizer for dry skin, and a fairly standard one at that, containing mostly water, glycerin, thickeners, silicone, preservatives, water-binding agents, and a tiny amount of antioxidants. It also contains a tiny amount of AHA, but not enough and not in the right pH to make it an effective exfoliant.

☹ **Special Wrinkle Sun Block SPF 8** *($19.50 for 50 ml)* is hardly special or worth it when there are plenty of SPF 15 sunscreens available.

☺ **$$$ Special Wrinkle Sun Block SPF 15** *($19.50 for 50 ml)* is an excellent sunscreen for normal to dry skin. This is definitely a Canadian or International formula because the sunscreen base would not be allowed in the U.S., as the active ingredients include titanium dioxide, avobenzone (Parsol 1789), and Mexoryl SX.

☺ **$$$ Sun Block Lotion SPF 25** *($19.50 for 150 ml)* is an excellent sunscreen for normal to dry skin. This is definitely a Canadian or International formula because the sunscreen base would not be allowed in the U.S., as the active ingredients include titanium dioxide, avobenzone (Parsol 1789), and Mexoryl SX.

☺ **$$$ Total Intolerance Sun Block SPF 30** *($19.50 for 50 ml)* is an excellent sunscreen for normal to dry skin. This is definitely a Canadian or International formula because the sunscreen base would not be allowed in the U.S.; the active ingredients include titanium dioxide, avobenzone (Parsol 1789), and Mexoryl SX.

There is nothing about this formula that makes it preferred in any way for someone with sensitive skin.

☺ **$$$ Total Sun Block SPF 25** *($19.50 for 50 ml)* is an excellent sunscreen for normal to dry skin. This is definitely a Canadian or International formula because the sunscreen base would not be allowed in the U.S. The active ingredients include titanium dioxide, avobenzone (Parsol 1789), and Mexoryl SX.

☹ **Soin Des Levres Beautifying Lip Treatment SPF 8** *($12 for 15 ml)* has nothing beautiful to offer, the SPF is low, and it doesn't contain titanium dioxide, zinc oxide, or avobenzone. It is not recommended.

☹ **Bust Firmer** *($36 for 50 ml)*. Well, if you're even thinking of buying this product after all we've been through together, then I have a bridge I'd love to sell you in NYC!

☹ **Stomach Firmer** *($36 for 100 ml)*. See my comments above.

BioTherm Makeup

There isn't much in the way of makeup except for four foundations:

☹ **Aqua Teint Mat Long Lasting Fluide Makeup** *($26)* has a slight, but soft powder finish. It could be an option, but out of six shades three are extremely peach. The only shades to consider are: Coquillage Mat, Natural Mat, and Bronze Mat.

☹ **Climatic Tinted Treatment** *($26)* isn't much of a treatment. There are only two shades and both are exceptionally peach.

☹ **Naturel Perfection with Fruit Acids** *($26)* doesn't have much going for it. Of the four shades available only one resembles skin tone (Naturel), the other three are either too peach or too rose for most all skin tones. The fruit acids, even if they were the right kind to exfoliate the skin, aren't and don't, and the pH is too high for it to exfoliate the skin, so it loses on both counts.

☹ **BioPerfection Liposome Treatment Makeup** *($26)* comes in five shades that are all way too peach, pink, or rose for all skin tones.

Black Opal

Several cosmetics lines are courting the African-American consumer, and some are doing so with aplomb and style. Black Opal is one such line, along with Iman and Maybelline Shades of You. (Black Opal and Maybelline Shades of You are both sold at drugstores though Black Opal has been showing up in some Sears outlets, and Iman is sold at J.C. Penney.) Black Opal, to its credit, has some remarkably matte, velvety, deep shades of eyeshadow, blush, and lipstick, as well as beautiful foundation colors for a small range of darker skin tones. Actually, its color line is where Black Opal excels—what a shame there aren't more color choices. The skin-care products, although reasonably priced, have some problems. They were supposedly designed by a dermatologist, but either the dermatologist didn't do all the chemistry homework necessary to design a skin-care line or there were terrible oversights. When a skin-care line boasts about its plant extracts, I wonder exactly what a dermatologist could be thinking, given the potential for allergic reaction and the lack of evidence that these types of ingredients provide a benefit for the skin. Lastly, the designer of the skin-care line seems to think that women of color have only oily or combination skin and that darker skin tones can tolerate irritating ingredients. They can't. If anything, drying, irritating products can increase skin discolorations by causing more dead skin cells to accumulate on the surface of the skin. Still, Black Opal offers some great makeup products, and should not be overlooked by anyone with medium to very dark skin. For more information on Black Opal call (800) 554-8012.

Black Opal Skin Care

☹ **Blemish Control Complexion Bar** *($3.50 for 3.5 ounces)* contains ingredients that keep all bar cleansers in their bar form and that can exacerbate breakouts. This product is not recommended.

☹ **Blemish Control Wash** *($5.95 for 6 ounces)* has sodium lauryl sulfate, a strong skin irritant, as its detergent cleansing agent. This cleanser also contains several other serious skin irritants, including camphor, menthol, eucalyptus oil, and peppermint oil. This product is absolutely not recommended.

☺ **Oil Free Cleansing Gel** *($4.51 for 6 ounces)* is a standard detergent-based, water-soluble cleanser that can be good for someone with oily skin. It can be drying for some skin types.

☹ **Pre-Fade Complexion Bar** *($3.50 for 3.5 ounces)* contains ingredients that keep bar cleansers in their bar form, and that can exacerbate breakouts. There is nothing in this product that will help fade skin discolorations; if anything, the drying effect of the cleansing agents can make skin look more ashen. This product is not recommended.

☺ **Purifying Astringent** *($3.99 for 6 ounces)* won't purify anything, but it is a good irritant-free toner that contains mostly water, glycerin, slip agent, plant extract, anti-irritant, more plant extracts, aloe, and preservatives.

☺ **Skin Retexturizing Complex with Alpha-Hydroxy Acids** *($9.95 for 1 ounce)* contains mostly water, silicone, glycolic acid, pH balancer, film former, thickeners, plant extracts, anti-irritants, vitamin E, water-binding agents, and preservatives. This would be a very good 7% AHA product for most skin types.

☹ **Maximum Moisture Night to Day Face Creme** *($6.95 for 6 ounces)* contains mostly water, plant extracts, thickeners, glycerin, silicone, and preservatives.

Several of the plant extracts in this product, such as arnica extract, pine extract, and lemongrass oil, can cause skin irritation.

☺ **Oil Free Moisturizing Lotion** *($3.99 for 1.75 ounces)* contains mostly water, glycerin, thickeners, silicone, water-binding agent, plant extracts, and preservatives. It isn't oil-free, and some of the thickening agents aren't good for oily skin. Still, this could be a good moisturizer for someone with normal to somewhat dry skin.

☹ **Revitalizing Eye Gel with Undereye Lighteners** *($8.95 for 0.6 ounce)* contains several ingredients that can be skin irritants, and which will only make puffiness worse, including lemon, grapefruit, and witch hazel.

☺ **SPF 15 Daily Protection for Photosensitive Skin** *($3.99 for 2.25 ounces)* is a decent sunscreen for someone with normal to dry skin, but it contains aluminum starch, which could be a skin irritant, rather high up on the ingredient list.

☺ **Advanced Dual Complex Fade Gel** *($11.95 for 0.75 ounce)* is a standard hydroquinone product that also contains about 7% glycolic acid. Hydroquinone with a good percentage of AHA, like that contained in this product, can minimally help fade dark, ashy areas of the skin. But don't expect a radical difference, just a slight fading.

☹ **Advanced Dual Phase Fade Creme with Sunscreen** *($11.95 for 1.75 ounces)* doesn't contain avobenzone, zinc oxide, or titanium dioxide and can't be recommended for a sunscreen, especially in conjunction with a fade cream where sun protection is so crucial for the skin-lightening ingredients to have an effect.

☹ **Blemish Control Gel** *($5.95 for 0.35 ounce)* contains mostly water, slip agent, resorcinol (disinfectant), camphor, menthol, eucalyptus oil, and peppermint oil. These standard acne ingredients can cause many more problems than they can help. Because they can dry and irritate skin, they can cause ashy skin-tone problems for women of color.

☺ **Skin Refining Peel** *($3.99 for 1.75 ounces)* is a standard clay mask with some wax, thickeners, glycerin, silicone, and preservatives. It would be a good clay mask for someone who likes this skin-care step.

☹ **Knees and Elbows Target Treatment** *($3.99 for 2 ounces)* contains mostly water; thickener; plant oil; glycerin; plant extracts; more thickeners; silicone; water-binding agents; plant oils; vitamins E, A, and D; and preservatives. This product lists its AHA as plant extracts. That doesn't tell you what kind of extracts, but it does at least tell you it's not an acid extract, and that's the kind you need to exfoliate the skin. The product is a good moisturizer, however; you just have to get around the other claims before you can understand what you are actually getting.

Black Opal Makeup

☹ **FOUNDATION: True Color Cream Stick Foundation SPF 8** *($5.95)* comes in a stick form and looks like it will go on quite greasy, but just the opposite is the case. It goes on smooth and then dries to a soft, matte finish. It tends to stay in place once it's on, so blending can be tricky. There are only a handful of colors that for the most part are quite good, but some are too orange. Without testers, as is true for most all drugstore foundations, it's impossible to recommend the Black Opal foundations. While the SPF 8 may be a good number for darker skin tones, without UVA protection it isn't good for any skin color. **Cream-to-Powder Foundation SPF 8** *($6.82)* not only doesn't include any UVA protection, but the colors are all either too red or too peach for most skin tones.

☺ **True Color Liquid Foundation Oil-free** *($5.95)* goes on quite smooth and sheer, drying to a matte finish. It can feel very dry on the skin so it can work well for someone with oily skin. **Avoid** Simply Sienna, it is too orange for most skin tones.

☺ **POWDER: Oil Absorbing Pressed Powder** *($6.82)* is a standard talc-based powder that comes in a small assortment of colors. It has a soft, silky texture and blends easily. Café Au Lait and Cappuccino can both be too peach for most skin tones, and Tawny Bronzing Powder is too red and should be avoided.

☹ **Deluxe Finishing Powder Loose Powder** *($6.82)* has an unfriendly assortment of peach shades.

☺ **BLUSH: Natural Color Blush** *($2.85)* comes in eight beautiful matte shades that go on silky and impart rich, lasting color. These are a real find for darker skin tones.

☺ **EYESHADOW: Color Rich Eyeshadows** *($2.85)* have an exceptional matte finish and come in a small but wonderful array of colors. The shadows blend on evenly and show up well on darker skin tones. For lighter skin tones, these shades work well as eyeliners. Gold is the only shiny color in the group. There is a new group of Color Rich Eyeshadows that come in two colors, but all of these are too shiny to recommend.

☺ **EYE AND BROW SHAPER: Precision Eye Definer** *($3.27)* is a standard eye pencil that comes in a small but good selection of colors.

☺ **LIPSTICK AND LIP PENCIL: Matte Plus Moisture Lipstick** *($4.56)* isn't all that matte; if anything, it is rather creamy with an almost glossy finish. It does have a small but terrific color selection. **True Tone Vitamin Rich Lipstick** *($4.56)* is more emollient than matte, but not in the least bit greasy. This is a very good moist lipstick with a decent selection of matte shades. **Simply Sheer Lipstick with SPF 15** *($4.05)* is, as the name implies, a sheer, more glossy lipstick with a good, in-part-titanium-dioxide sunscreen. **Precision Lip Definer Pencil** *($3.27)* is a standard lip pencil with a small but good selection of colors. At this price, if you're into pencils, buy them all.

☺ **MASCARA: Lash Defining Mascara** *($4.59)* has one of the strangest brush shapes I've ever seen for mascara. It definitely doesn't aid in making lashes longer. This isn't a bad mascara, it just doesn't do much. It takes awhile to build any length or thickness. It doesn't clump or smear but there just isn't enough to give it a happy face.

Blistex (Lip Care Only)

How this small line of lip products has achieved the status of being the solution for cold sores or chapped lips eludes me. These lip products contain enough irritating ingredients to chap anyone's lips. Lots of lip products claim to be medicated, but "medicated" is a dubious term at best, with no regulated meaning. As Blistex does, these types of products often contain camphor, menthol, peppermint oil, eucalyptus, or menthol, but these are not medicines for dry lips, they make dry skin worse. Products like Blistex can include 0.5% phenol, a potent disinfectant, but phenol is strong stuff and can actually trigger some serious problems, the least of which are drying and irritation. It is not something I would recommend for anything but extremely limited use. You may have heard a rumor that lips can adapt to or get used to lip balm. It isn't possible. But if the lip balm you are using contains irritating ingredients, your lips will stay dried up. For more information about Blistex call (708) 571-2870.

☹ **Blistex Medicated Lip Ointment** *($1.50 for 0.21 ounce)* contains menthol, camphor, and phenol in a base of Vaseline. Everything but the Vaseline is too irritating for the lips, or any part of the body for that matter.

☹ **Blistex Lip Medex** *($0.86 for 0.25 ounce)* is similar to the one above, only with large quantities of the irritating ingredients.

☹ **Blistex Lip Balm SPF 10** *($0.99 for 0.15 ounce)* doesn't contain avobenzone, zinc oxide, or titanium dioxide, and is not recommended.

☹ **Blistex Daily Conditioning Treatment SPF 20** *($1.50 for 0.25 ounce)* doesn't contain avobenzone, zinc oxide, or titanium dioxide, and is not recommended.

Bobbi Brown Essentials

Bobbi Brown is a well-known New York City makeup artist who commands a consultation fee of $200, and that's just for the first hour. She has been one of the most quoted and referred-to makeup artists in fashion magazines for several years now, and her handiwork has graced the faces of countless models and celebrities. I was not surprised when she finally came out with her own cosmetics line a few years ago. What did astound me was the clamor for these products. The limited color selection and very yellow foundation choices (when the line was first launched, it included only one type of foundation that was appropriate for normal to dry skin only) didn't faze the eager women lined up at the counters when I went shopping at Bergdorf Goodman (the only store then carrying the line) in New York City. *Vogue* and *Glamour* had recently mentioned that a few of Bobbi Brown's products were the hottest thing in town, and the reaction of Manhattan's fashion police was quick and decisive. New York women were finally getting the neutral, flat look they wanted, the pale Manhattan look of the Upper East Side crowd. Women wanted those products, even though many of the eyeshadows and blushes looked suspiciously like those in the M.A.C. line.

Although I still think Brown's line is just a M.A.C. clone, it has expanded, and there are now far better options than the ultra-yellow foundation and small group of colors it started out with. The eyeshadows and blushes are still incredibly neutral and matte. The lipsticks are also fairly neutral and brown-toned; this line is not about pastels or vivids. Foundations now include an excellent oil-free version, and the overly yellow tones are yielding to more neutral shades.

At first, Brown's line sported only makeup products, but her skin-care product line has expanded too. Although many of the products are absurdly overpriced, there are some good options. Nevertheless, you just aren't truly fashionable if you haven't checked out this line, so stop by and see if your tastes match those of "the ladies who lunch." For more information about Bobbi Brown Cosmetics call (212) 980-3232.

Bobbi Brown Skin Care

☻ **Face Cleanser** *($27 for 6 ounces)* contains mostly water, thickener, glycerin, detergent cleanser, plant oil, plant extracts, and preservatives. There are some fairly irritating plant extracts in this product, including arnica, pine, kiwi, and lemon, which can all be too irritating for the eyes and for most skin types.

☻ **Gel Cleanser** *($27 for 6 ounces)* is a standard detergent-based water-soluble cleanser that contains some fairly irritating plant extracts that can be a problem for most skin types and the eye area.

☺ **$$$ Eye Makeup Remover** *($16.50 for 4 ounces)* is a fairly standard eye-makeup remover, like hundreds of others. It works as well as any.

☻ **Exfoliating Face Wash** *($18.50 for 3.5 ounces)* contains menthol, camphor, eucalyptus oil, peppermint oil, and grapefruit oil, all of which are extremely irritating and pose serious risks for the skin.

☺ **$$$ Eye Cream** *($32.50 for 0.65 ounce)* contains mostly water; plant oil; silicone; thickeners; slip agent; more plant oil; water-binding agents; vitamins E, A, and C; and preservatives. This would be a good moisturizer for someone with dry skin, but the vitamins and some of the water-binding agents barely amount to anything.

☺ **$$$ Face Cream** *($38 for 2.2 ounces)* contains mostly water, thickener, glycerin, more thickeners, silicone, water-binding agents, anti-irritant, vitamins E and A, and preservatives. This is a fairly ordinary as well as overpriced moisturizer that would be good for someone with normal to dry skin. The interesting ingredients and vitamins are too far down on the ingredient list to be more than just a dusting. By the way, the anti-irritant in here is nice, but it comes right after an irritating ingredient, lemon oil, so it's kind of a wash.

☺ $$$ Face Lotion *($38 for 2 ounces)* contains mostly water; thickener; silicone; slip agent; glycolic acid; more thickeners; plant extracts; anti-irritant; more silicone; water-binding agents; vitamins E, A, and C; and preservatives. This is about a 6% AHA product with a good pH, which would be fine for someone with normal to dry skin. However, for the money, it can't hold a candle to Pond's or Alpha Hydrox's versions at the drugstore.

☺ $$$ Hydrating Face Cream *($38 for 1.7 ounces)* contains mostly water, silicone, slip agents, thickeners, water-binding agents, vitamins, fragrance, and preservatives. This is a good but extremely ordinary moisturizer for dry skin.

☺ $$$ SPF 15 Face Lotion *($38 for 1.7 ounces)* is a good titanium dioxide–based sunscreen for dry skin. It does contain anti-irritants and vitamins, which is nice but not special.

Bobbi Brown Makeup

☺ $$$ FOUNDATION: The Foundation *($35)* is a stick that goes on slightly greasy but very sheer, and is good for someone with normal to dry skin. **These colors are great for many Caucasian skin tones:** Warm and Sand. **These colors are quite yellow:** Beige, Natural, and Honey. **These colors can turn copper:** Almond, Walnut, Chestnut, and Espresso; they might work for some darker skin tones.

☺ $$$ Oil-Free Foundation *($35)* is a rather impressive, truly matte foundation. The texture is just great and the colors, though limited, are all wonderfully neutral. One minor cautionary word: The coverage tends to be on the medium side and, like most matte foundations, it is very tricky to blend, which isn't great if you want a sheer and natural look. **Moisturizing Foundation** *($35)* is superior, with a silky, smooth texture that blends on evenly and looks polished. The only shades to watch out for are Natural and Honey, which can be too yellow; the other shades are gorgeous. ☺ $$$ Fresh Glow Cream Foundation *($35)* is definitely a creamy, emollient foundation, very reminiscent of Lancome's discontinued MaquiDouceur. There are ten colors in this group, and most are very attractive, but two of the three shades for women of color, Chestnut and Walnut, are just slightly too peachy orange for most skin tones. If you have dry skin and like the more neutral yellow-based colors Brown is known for (at least if you have lighter skin tones), you may want to give this one a try.

☺ $$$ Tinted Moisturizer SPF 15 *($35)* provides a very light, sheer hint of color with titanium dioxide as the active ingredient. That's terrific for someone with dry skin who wants a tiny bit of color, and all three shades are excellent.

☺ $$$ CONCEALER: Professional Concealer *($35)* was only recently introduced, which is a bit surprising. It comes in four great colors (only Warm Almond can go on slightly orange) and has decent coverage, but this one can crease, and keep on creasing as the day goes by.

☺ $$$ POWDER: Both the Loose Face Powder *($29)* and Pressed Powder

($26) are standard talc-based powders that have a soft, sheer, slightly dry finish. There are six colors, but three of them are extremely sallow or peach; Sunny Beige, Golden Orange, and Pale Yellow are all very yellow.

☺ $$$ <u>BLUSH:</u> The **Blush** *($19)* comes in six soft shades with a dry finish. Nothing exciting, but they are nice colors. **Cream Blush Stick** *($28)* comes only in four shades, and if one of those suits you, give it a try. I rarely recommend cream blush because it tends to be hard to control and doesn't stay well, and some just fade away. That isn't true with this one. It goes on fairly easily and evenly (you apply a swipe of color from the stick and then smooth it out with a sponge or very carefully with your fingers). You'll be surprised; I know I was. **Bronzing Stick** *($25)* is similar to the Blush Stick, but these four, nicely matte shades are a neutral range of skin tones; the only color to watch out for is Dark which can turn red. **Bronzing Powder** *($26)* shades are all soft and matte.

☺ $$$ <u>EYESHADOW:</u> **Eye Shadow** *($17)* has a nice range of colors to choose from. The selection doesn't cover as many needs as you would think, but there are some great matte neutral colors here. **Shimmering Eye Shadow** *($18)* is a group of very creamy, extremely shiny eyeshadows. One is pink, white, and gold. These are just for fun, right?

☺ $$$ <u>EYE AND BROW SHAPER:</u> The **Eye Pencils** *($15.50)* are standard pencils with a small selection of colors. They go on like almost every other pencil I've ever tested.

☺ $$$ <u>LIPSTICK AND LIP PENCIL:</u> The standard **Lip Color** *($16)* is a creamy lipstick tending slightly toward the greasy side. The **Lip Stains** *($16)* don't really stain the lips; they're just lip glosses in stick form. The **Lip Shimmer** *($18)* is like the stains only these have shine. They are OK lip products, but nothing special or unique. **Lip Gloss** *($18)* has a somewhat sticky application, but is mostly just a standard gloss. **Shimmer Lip Gloss** *($18)* is, as the name says, very shiny lip gloss. The **Lip Pencils** *($15.50)* are standard pencils with a nice selection of eight colors. They go on like almost every other pencil I've ever tested.

☹ $$$ <u>MASCARA:</u> Bobbi Brown's **Mascara** *($16)* is a decent mascara, but pricey. It doesn't clump, flake, or smear, and that's nice, but it takes awhile to build any length, and don't count on any thickness. **Thickening Mascara** *($16)* doesn't live up to its name in the least. It takes forever to build any length and the lashes never do gain any thickness. It isn't terrible; if you don't need much length or definition, it would be fine, it's just overpriced for what you get.

☺ $$$ <u>BRUSHES:</u> Most of these brushes are extremely soft and very workable. The only ones I would avoid are the **Eye Shader** *($26)*, which is too big for most women to use on their eyes, **Eye Blender** *($25)* which is too floppy to get much control of your eyeshadow placement, **Lip Liner** *($18.50)* which is so standard and ordinary that the price is embarrassing, and the **Eyeliner Brush** *($18.50)*, which is too thick to create a controlled fine line. All the other brushes are excellent, particularly the **Blush** *($19)*, **Bronzer** *($26)*, **Powder** *($29)*, **Eye Shadow** *($23.50)*, and **Brow** *($18.50)*.

The Body Shop

One of the problems in trying to do a book of this nature is giving you the most up-to-date information possible. Often that seems to be an almost impossible task. The cosmetics industry is constantly reinventing itself by adding or changing formulations, and sometimes not for the better. As this book went to press, The Body Shop was getting in a new array of products and packaging. Some of the reviews below are current but others will be changing over the next several months. I will update that information in my newsletter as the new products are launched.

I think it is interesting to note that The Body Shop is still very interested in redeeming itself from a lot of bad press it received a couple of years back that resulted in depressed stock prices. It has been doing a great job of it. What happened is that stories in the mainstream press (not fashion magazines, of course) were complaining about the minuscule amounts of natural ingredients and the presence of very unnatural ingredients in The Body Shop's products, its misleading statements about its use of animal testing, and its ad copy touting ingredients that aren't even in the products, and they caused problems for the popular British-based corporation and its founder Anita Roddick. For example, one Body Shop hair gel was described as being based on plant mixtures used by "South Ethiopian [women who] traditionally styled their hair with ochre, butter, and acacia gum." Yet not one of those ingredients is in the product. Of course, that information isn't shocking to those of you who read my newsletter and books, but it caused a sensation in the mainstream press.

Further shock resulted when The Body Shop unsuccessfully tried to block an exposé of some of its other so-called natural products. By putting legal pressure on *Vanity Fair,* the company was able to get the embarrassing story dropped. The irate reporter wanted revenge and made it his mission to get the story published anyway; to The Body Shop's woe, he did. The result was that The Body Shop received an enormous amount of unflattering news coverage, not only for using ingredients that were indeed tested on animals as recently as 1992, but also for trying to restrain freedom of the press, and consequently its stock price plummeted.

To see the results of The Body Shop's efforts to regain its standing it is worthwhile to visit one of their stores. Upon entering you are greeted by an enthusiastic sales staff wearing jeans and T-shirts that say "Cruelty-Free." Brochures describing the horrors of animal testing, the efforts of Amnesty International, the educational impact of The Body Shop in Harlem, and the beauty philosophy of the Woodabe tribe of Africa are more prominent than any information about makeup and skin care. Yet this is indeed a makeup and skin-care boutique, imported directly from England. Starting with only one small storefront in London, it has grown to hundreds of shops all over America, Europe, and Australia.

Colourings is the name of The Body Shop's color line; it has expanded considerably over the years, and there are some very interesting products to consider, such as foundation, lip products, blushes, brushes, and face powders. However, most of the powder eyeshadows are shiny, the foundation colors are limited, and the mascaras just average. The cosmetics display area in the stores is quite accessible and you are free to play with the demos all you want, which is nice, but there isn't any convenient shelving where you can put your things down, and the mirrors aren't the best. There is no sales pressure here, and the personnel are much better trained about the products than they have been in the past. For more information about The Body Shop call (800) 541-2535

The Body Shop Skin Care

☹   **Aloe Vera Face Soap** *($3.70 for 3.5 ounces)* is a standard soap that also contains aloe, but aloe can't undo the drying effect of the soap.

☺   **Balancing Cleansing Gel for Normal to Oily Skin** *($9 for 6.76 ounces)* is a standard detergent-based water-soluble cleanser that could be good for someone with normal to oily skin. It does contain a small amount of witch hazel, which may be a slight problem for some sensitive skin types.

☺   **Cucumber Cleansing Milk for Normal to Dry Skin** *($8.15 for 8.4 ounces)* contains mostly water, glycerin, mineral oil, thickeners, cucumber extract, and lanolin. It must be wiped off with either a washcloth or a tissue, and it definitely leaves a greasy residue on the skin.

☹   **Facial Cleansing Bar for Normal to Dry/Dry Skin** *($6.50 for 5 ounces)* includes ingredients that keep bar cleansers in their bar form, which can clog pores, plus the detergent cleansing agents in this bar can dry and irritate skin. There are emollients in here, but that just confuses the skin.

☹   **Facial Cleansing Bar for Normal to Oily/Oily Skin** *($6.50 for 5 ounces)* is similar to the bar above minus the emollients; instead they stuck in mint which makes it even more irritating.

☺   **Foaming Cleansing Cream for Normal to Dry Skin** *($9 for 6.7 ounces)* is a standard detergent-based water-soluble cleanser that can be very good for most skin types, not just those with normal to slightly dry skin, though it may be too drying for someone with extremely dry skin.

☹ **Glycerin & Oatmeal Facial Lather for Normal to Dry Skin** *($9.70 for 1.7 ounces)* is a potassium hydroxide–based cleanser that can be fairly drying for most skin types.

☺ **Honey Cream Cleanser for Dry Skin** *($9.70 for 3.5 ounces)* is a fairly emollient wipe-off cleanser. It can leave a greasy film on the skin.

☺ **Japanese Washing Grains for All Skin Types** *($4.75 for 1.7 ounces)* contains ground azuki beans; if that sounds like a good scrub, then these will work, but so will baking soda for far less then this.

☹ **Oil-Free Cleansing Wash for Oily Skin** *($9 for 6.76 ounces)* contains mint, which can be a skin irritant, causing problems for all skin types.

☺ **Orchid Cleansing Milk for Normal to Dry Skin** *($8.15 for 8.4 ounces)* contains mostly water, rose water, sweet almond oil, and oil of orchid. This cleanser must be wiped off with a washcloth or tissue, and it leaves a greasy residue on the skin.

☺ **Passion Fruit Cleansing Gel for Normal to Oily Skin** *($8.15 for 8.4 ounces)* is a good water-soluble cleanser that can be slightly drying to sensitive or dry skin types.

☺ **Pineapple Facial Wash for Normal to Oily Skin** *($9.70 for 3.5 ounces)* is an OK detergent-based water-soluble cleanser that can take off all the makeup, but because it contains some plant oils and problematic thickening agents that can clog pores it is not recommended for oily skin as its name implies. This product can leave a slightly greasy film on the face.

☺ **Rich Cleansing Cream for Dry Skin** *($9 for 6.7 ounces)* is basically a cold cream–type wipe-off cleanser that can leave a greasy film on the skin.

☺ **Tea Tree Oil Facial Wash** *($3 for 2 ounces)* is a standard detergent-based water-soluble cleanser with a small amount of tea tree oil. Tea tree oil has attained quite the reputation for being a wonder for the skin, when all it really turns out to be is a form of urea. That doesn't make it bad for the skin, just not a miracle. It can be an anti-irritant when there isn't much of it in a product, but if there's too much it can be a skin irritant.

☹ **Tea Tree Oil Soap** *($3.70 for 3.5 ounces)* is a standard soap with tea tree oil. Soap is drying and the ingredients that keep soap in its bar form can clog pores.

☹ **Vitamin E Cleansing Bar** *($3.50 for 3.5 ounces)* is made with ingredients that keep all bar cleansers in their bar form, which can clog pores, and the detergent cleansing agents are drying.

☺ **Chamomile Eye Make-up Remover** *($10.95 for 8.4 ounces)* is about as standard an eye-makeup remover as they come, but it does nicely remove eye makeup, though wiping off makeup can sag skin.

☹ **Conditioning Cream Scrub for Normal to Dry & Dry Skin** *($12 for 3.7 ounces)* contains mostly water, plant oil, aloe, cornstarch, lentils (as the scrub agent), thickeners, plant oils, and preservatives. It's not much of a conditioner; it can leave a greasy residue on the skin, and the cornstarch, orange oil, and orange fruit can be skin irritants.

☺ **Foaming Gel Scrub for Normal to Oily & Oily Skin** *($12 for 3.7 ounces)* is basically a detergent-based water-soluble cleanser that contains walnut shells as the scrub agent. It can be a good scrub for normal to oily skin, but it would be a problem for someone with very oily skin. Cetaphil Gentle Skin Cleanser and baking soda would be a far better scrub.

☹ **Cucumber Freshener for Normal to Oily Skin** *($8.55 for 8.4 ounces)* contains alcohol, which is an irritant and drying agent for all skin types.

☹ **Equalizing Freshener for Normal to Oily & Oily Skin** *($8 for 6.76 ounces)* is just your average water-and-witch-hazel toner. Witch hazel can be a skin irritant, and the peppermint and mint extracts in this product can be additional irritants.

☹ **Exfoliating Lotion for All Skin Types** *($9 for 6.76 ounces)* contains about 3% AHA, but it also contains alcohol and witch hazel, which irritate and redden the skin. There are better, more effective, and gentler AHA products to be found.

☹ **Honey Freshener for Dry Skin** *($8.55 for 8 ounces)* is basically just rose water (fragrance and glycerin), a truly do-nothing combination for any skin type.

☺ **Honey Water** *($5 for 4.2 ounces)* is an irritant-free toner that contains mostly rose water (that's scented glycerin) and preservatives. Pretty standard, and fine for most skin types.

☺ **Hydrating Freshener for Normal to Dry & Dry Skin** *($8 for 6.76 ounces)* is a very good irritant-free toner for most skin types. It contains mostly water, water-binding agent, slip agent, and preservatives.

☺ **Orchid Freshener for Normal to Dry Skin** *($8.55 for 8.4 ounces)* is just water and glycerin. That makes it a very ordinary but OK irritant-free toner.

☺ **Tea Tree Oil Freshener, for Oily or Blemished Skin** *($8 for 8.4 ounces)*. There is one study showing Tea Tree Oil to have some benefit similiar to benzoyl peroxide. However, this version contains witch hazel and alcohol, which can cause unecessary irritation.

☹ **Jojoba Oil for Normal to Oily Skin** *($4.95 for 1 ounce)* makes me ask, Why would someone with oily skin want to put more oil on their skin? This product designation makes no sense.

☺ **Carrot Oil for Normal to Dry Skin** *($4.95 for 1 ounce)* definitely includes carrot oil as well as other plant oils. That would be good for someone with dry skin, but it's greasy.

☺ **Evening Primrose Oil for Dry Skin** *($4.95 for 1 ounce)* is, as the name implies, a pure primrose oil with vitamin E. It would work well for dry skin but it is greasy.

☺ **Sweet Almond Oil for All Skin Types** *($4.95 for 1 ounce)* is just almond oil, which can be good for dry skin, but why would anyone want to use a pure plant oil on the skin? You could just use a bottle of almond oil you buy at the grocery store.

☹ **Tea Tree Oil** *($3.95 for 0.34 ounce)* contains alcohol and tea tree oil; this would be too irritating and drying for all skin types.

☺ **Wheat Germ Oil for All Skin Types** *($4.95 for 1 ounce)* is just wheat germ oil, as the name says. It can be good for dry skin, but why would anyone want to use a pure plant oil on the skin?

☺ **Aloe Vera Moisture Cream** *($9.50 for 1.8 ounces)* is a rich cream containing mostly water, almond oil, glycerin, cocoa butter, thickeners, and aloe vera extract. It should take good care of very dry skin.

☺ **Carrot Moisture Cream** *($9.50 for 1.8 ounces)* is a very good emollient moisturizer for someone with dry skin.

☹ **Elderflower Eye Gel** *($5.95 for 0.4 ounce)* contains mostly plant water, witch hazel, glycerin, alcohol, and preservatives. Witch hazel is a skin irritant, and so is the alcohol. This is one of the last products I would consider putting around the eye area.

☺ **Eye Supplement for All Skin Types** *($12 for 0.5 ounce)* contains mostly water, silicone oil, plant extracts, glycerin, thickeners, film former, and preservatives. It's a good lightweight moisturizer, but it doesn't add much of anything to the skin.

☺ **Hydrating Moisture Lotion for Normal to Dry Skin** *($16 for 3.38 ounces)* contains mostly water, plant oil, plant extract, thickeners, silicone, more thickeners, water-binding agent, and preservatives. This would be a very good moisturizer for someone with dry skin. There are tiny amounts of vitamins at the end of the ingredient list.

☺ **Jojoba Moisture Cream** *($9.50 for 1.6 ounces)* is only for skin types that do not break out. The second ingredient in this cream is isopropyl myristate, which can cause blackheads. Other than that, this is a rich cream that contains water, jojoba oil, wheat germ oil, thickener, and glycerin, and would be good for dry skin.

☺ **Light Moisture Lotion for Normal to Oily Skin** *($16 for 3.38 ounces)* contains mostly water, silicone, plant extract, thickeners, and preservatives. It is indeed light, but someone with oily skin isn't going to be crazy about some of the thickening agents in here. There are tiny amounts of vitamins at the end of the ingredient list, but not enough to have any effect.

☺ **Night Supplement for All Skin Types** *($14 for 1 ounce)* contains a small amount of AHA in a low enough pH to make this an exfoliant for someone with normal to dry skin.

☹ **Oil-Free Moisture Gel for Oily Skin** *($16 for 3.38 ounces)* contains peppermint, mint, and witch hazel, which are too irritating for all skin types.

☺ **Rich Moisture Cream for Dry Skin** *($16 for 3.52 ounces)* isn't all that rich but it is a good emollient moisturizer for someone with dry skin.

☺ **Rich Night Cream with Vitamin E** *($9.50 for 1.4 ounces)* is indeed a very rich moisturizer. It contains mostly water, petrolatum, mineral oil, lanolin, thickeners, preservatives, vitamin E, and fragrance. The amount of vitamin E in the cream is hardly worth mentioning, but it is a very emollient moisturizer for someone with very dry skin who doesn't have a problem with breakouts.

☹ **Tea Tree Facial Moisture Concentrate for Oily or Blemished Skin** *($6.50 for 1.7 ounces)* does contain tea tree oil but that doesn't work to help reduce oily skin or breakouts.

☺ **Tea Tree Oil Moisturizing Gel, for Oily or Blemished Skin** *($13.50 for 8.4 ounces)* is identical to the product above except that it is in gel form, and the same review applies.

☺ **Undereye Cream** *($6.05 for 0.5 ounce)*, and ☺ **Eye Supplement** *($6.05 for 0.5 ounce)* are The Body Shop's attempt to convince women they can eliminate dark circles and crepey skin in the under-eye area. Yes, keeping the area moisturized when it is dry makes a huge difference, but that's standard for any moisturizer, it doesn't require a specialty product. Changing the color of the under-eye area is limited by the thickness of the skin, natural discolorations, shadows, and existing wrinkles. They can't be changed with plants or any other ingredients. Undereye Cream is just what the name implies: a moisturizing cream. It contains mostly water, thickener, emollients, plant oil, and preservatives. Though it can be heavy for some skin types, if the skin under your eye is very dry, it can feel soothing. Undereye Gel contains mostly witch hazel, plant extract, glycerin, thickener, and preservatives. Witch hazel can be an irritant and drying, and is not best for soothing the skin under the eye. Eye Supplement contains mostly water, silicone, plant extract, rose water, thickeners, and preservative. Nothing very supplemental about this, and rose water (which is part fragrance and water) can be sensitizing for some skin types.

☺ **Vitamin E Moisture Cream** *($9.50 for 1.8 ounces)* contains mostly water, thickeners, lanolin, more thickeners, vitamin E, and preservatives. The amount of vitamin E in this cream is hardly worth mentioning, but it is a very emollient moisturizer for someone with very dry skin who doesn't have a problem with breakouts.

☺ **$$$ Facial Sun Stick SPF 30** *($6.50 for 0.6 ounce)* is a fairly expensive way to apply sunscreen, but this is a good in-part zinc oxide–based sunscreen. It does contain some thick wax ingredients that are notorious for clogging pores.

☹ **Kids Sunblock Ultra Protection, SPF 30** *($9.50 for 5.2 ounces)* does not contain avobenzone, zinc oxide, or titanium dioxide, and is not recommended.

☹ **Sun Lotion High Protection, SPF 8** *($8.50 for 5.2 ounces)* does contain zinc oxide, but calling SPF 8 high protection is an oxymoron.

☹ **Sun Block, Ultra Protection SPF 25** *($9.50 for 5.2 ounces)* does not contain avobenzone, zinc oxide, or titanium dioxide, and is not recommended.

☹ **Sun Lotion, Very High Protection SPF 15** *($8.50 for 5.2 ounces)* does not contain avobenzone, zinc oxide, or titanium dioxide, and is not recommended.

☹ **Vitamin E Lip Care SPF 15** *($2.50 for 0.15 ounce)* does not contain avobenzone, zinc oxide, or titanium dioxide, and is not recommended.

☹ **Blue Corn Scrub Mask** *($9.95 for 4.3 ounces)* is a fairly standard clay mask that uses blue corn powder as the scrub. That isn't bad, but the grapefruit, fragrances, and alcohol here can all be irritants.

☹ **Honey & Oatmeal Scrub Mask for Dry Skin** *($11.25 for 2.4 ounces)* is a standard clay mask that uses oatmeal as a scrub agent. Clay is very dehydrating for dry skin and there are no other emollients in here to offset that effect.

☺ **Intense Moisture Mask for All Skin Types** *($12 for 3.38 ounces)* contains mostly water, glycerin, film former, water-binding agent, anti-irritant, and preservative. I wouldn't call this intense moisture in the least, but it is an OK mask for someone with normal to slightly dry skin.

☹ **Sage & Comfrey Blemish Gel** *($6 for 1.5 ounces)* contains mostly alcohol (need I say more?), witch hazel, plant extracts, thickeners, and preservatives. Great—just what we need, another alcohol-based acne product.

☹ **Tea Tree Oil Blemish Stick** *($4.50)* won't help anything. Even if the tea tree oil could help breakouts, the alcohol in this product would just make a mess of things.

☹ **Warming Mineral Mask, for All Skin Types** *($12 for 5.1 ounces)* really seems warm on the skin because of the cinnamon and ginger oil, sort of like the way Red Hot candies heat up your mouth. However, they can be skin irritants, and they don't do much for the skin. This is just a standard clay mask with a gimmick that can hurt your skin.

☹ **Lip Scuff** *($5.95)* claims to rid the lips of unwanted flaky skin. To my amazement, Lip Scuff burned my lips immediately after I applied it, and the burning sensation lasted for some time afterward. To my chagrin, it was then I noticed the plastic wrapping around the product that warned, "Not recommended for use on sore or chapped lips." As natural and wonderful as the products from The Body Shop sound, this experience once again proved to me that "natural" and "good" are not the same thing (read my tingling, irritated lips). Even though my lips got rubbed the wrong way, the exfoliant action of this product is minimal.

The Body Shop Makeup

☺ <u>FOUNDATION:</u> The Body Shop has several types of foundation. Most have excellent textures and colors; sadly, the color choices are quite limited, with little to nothing for darker skin tones. What they do have is worth checking out if you have light skin. **Skin Treat SPF 8** *($15)* is a very good soft-finish foundation with a nonchemical SPF 8. The SPF number is disappointing, but I've been told they will be reformulating to a nonchemical SPF 15 soon. Wait to try this one until then.

☺ **All-in-One Face Treat SPF 15** *($15)* is a very good cream-to-powder foundation that has a soft, dry finish and a nonchemical SPF of 15. There are only four shades, which is absurdly limited, although those four are very good.

☺ **All-in-One Face Base** *($15)* can go on either wet or dry. It goes on smooth, with a slightly powdery finish. It is better used dry; trying to apply this wet can be streaky and choppy. Again, there are only four colors, and though they're all very neutral and good, that's still almost no choice at all.

☺ **Every Day Foundation** *($8.50)* goes on very creamy and light, with a smooth, soft texture. The quality is excellent, but the limited number of colors is a problem. **All of the colors are excellent;** 001 may be slightly peach for some skin tones.

☺ **Oil-Control Foundation SPF 10** *($8.50)* does contain part titanium dioxide, but the colors aren't the best and it applies somewhat choppy.

☹ **Tinted Moisturizer SPF 8** *($8)* doesn't contain avobenzone, zinc oxide, or titanium dioxide, and is not recommended.

☹ <u>CONCEALER:</u> **Every Day Concealer** *($6)* comes in a stick and goes on fairly greasy, yet it tends to crease into the lines around the eye. **Lightening Touch** *($7)* is like a tube of gloss, but the color is shiny. The consistency is a powder finish. It's an OK highlighter if you're interested, but it isn't a look I recommend.

☺ <u>POWDER:</u> **Soft Pressed Face Powder** *($10)* and **Color Balance Loose Powder** *($8.50)* have a soft, silky texture and come in three very good colors. **Tinted Bronzing Powder Compact** *($11)* is a great matte color, but that is the only color, so it isn't for everyone and works best as a blush, not as an all-over face color.

☺ <u>BLUSH:</u> **Cream Blush** *($9)* comes in only two colors, but it does have a nice texture for a cream-to-powder blush with a good matte finish. **Powder Blush** *($7.50)* has a smooth, even texture and eight very good soft shades. **Brush-on Bronze** *($13.50)* are beads of colored powders with a slight amount of shine. I find this a messy and inconvenient way to apply a product that is nothing more than blush, but it's eye-catching and fun. Speaking of fun, test the **Twist & Bronze** *($11)* and **Twist & Blush** *($10)*. These truly unique products are a two-in-one blush and brush set. The brush twists up into a layer of pressed color that you then apply to the face. It goes on rather soft and slightly shiny. It isn't my style of makeup, and I think it distributes color poorly to the brush and tends to streak, it's one of those fun splurge items I rarely encourage women to bother with, but you may want to test for yourself.

☹ <u>EYESHADOW:</u> Almost all of the regular **Eyeshadows** *($7)* are too shiny and not worth the money. How disappointing, because some of the shades are exceptional. The **Eyeshadow Pencils** *($7.15)* look more convenient to use than they are. The color glides on easily, but the tips are difficult to keep sharpened.

☺ **Continual Eye Color** *($10)* is an eyeshadow that comes in a tube; it goes on creamy and dries to a powder. There are seven colors, most rather neutral and attractive. I find this style of eyeshadow more clever than useful when it comes to blending on areas other than the lid, but it is an option. **Complete Color** *($10)* comes packaged as a thin lipstick tube in six fairly muted earth tones and is meant to be used on the eyes, lips, and cheeks. It goes on fairly creamy and dries to a soft powder. Coordinating the whole face with one color is an intriguing concept, but blending this product on the cheeks and eyes takes some skill, and the applicator isn't the best for the cheek area.

☺ **EYE AND BROW SHAPER: Eye Definer** *($5.50)* is a standard pencil with an improved array of colors. There are still a blue, green, and shiny gold to watch out for, but the rest are an option. **Brow & Lash Gel** *($7)* is a clear mascara/hair spray sort of product. It will keep brows in place and can help get a little more distance on your lashes. **Eye Liner Pen** *($10)* comes in three shades; it goes on easily with the pen applicator tip and dries smooth. This is a much improved formula from the original, but the applicator tip is stiff and hard to use against the curve of the eye. **Eye Brow Pencils** *($7)* come in three colors and are similar to the Eye Liner. **Eye Brow Powder Makeup** *($8)* is an eyeshadow that's meant for the brows. It's a bit on the dry side so the application isn't the smoothest or easy.

☺ **LIPSTICK AND LIP PENCIL: Lipstain** *($7.50)* is applied with a pen-like applicator tip. It stains the lips with deep color, then dries to almost a no-feel finish. If you don't have dry lips, Lipstain is an intriguing way to color the lips. The **Lipsticks** *($9)* are fairly glossy, in a nice range of colors. The **Lip Liners** *($5.50)* are quite good standard lip pencils, with basic soft colors and a nice, smooth texture. **No Wander** *($6.50)* is a clear lip liner that is supposed to prevent lipstick from bleeding, and guess what, it really works! **Liptint** *($6.50)* is simply a shiny gloss in a tube. It does leave a bit of a stain once it wears off, but it's too greasy-looking for daytime business wear. **Lip Shine** *($7)* is a chubby pencil that is meant to be used as a lipstick. It is fairly glossy and shiny and not any more convenient to use nor an improved texture over a lipstick. **Fragrance Colorstick** *($7)* is like the Lip Shine only in a very good matte finish. **Complete Color Lipstick** *($10)* is supposed to be a long-wearing lipstick; it doesn't last much longer than most lipsticks. You are also supposed to be able to use this product on the cheeks and eyes, but the applicator isn't the best for cheeks and it's too greasy for the eyes. Lipstick is its best use.

☹ **SPF 30 Lipstick** *($9)* and **Lip Treat SPF 20** *($9)* both do not contain UVA protection and are not recommended.

☺ **MASCARA: Every Day Mascara** *($7.50)* and **Lash Building Mascara** *($8.50)* are OK mascaras, but just OK. It takes a while to build any length, and the lashes never seem to get very thick. These don't smear or flake, so if you're not looking for much definition they are an option.

☹ <u>BRUSHES:</u> The brushes have changed and not for the better. Most are poor sizes, the hair is no longer soft, and the bristles are loosely packed so they don't control color well. **Lipstick Concealer Brush** *($6)* doesn't work well with concealer (your finger or a sponge can blend that area just fine), and it's awfully tiny for lipstick; it would take forever to get the color on. **Finishing Brush** *($7)* is a thin, fan-shaped brush whose purpose I am not quite sure of; I've never run into a professional makeup artist who used one, so it isn't necessary for you either. **Blush Powder Brush** *($8.50)* has bristles that are a little too long and too loosely packed. **Brow Brush** *($5.50)* is stiff and scratchy, which means it will irritate the skin and stroke the brow color on poorly. I also don't recommend the **Lip Brush** *($5.50)* and the **Foam Applicator Stick** *($6)*.

☺ **Foundation Contour Brush** *($7.50)* is actually the best one in the group but don't use it for foundation.

Bonne Bell

Bonne Bell isn't new, but it has been entirely revamped. It's always been aimed at the pre-adolescent looking to start experimenting with her own makeup purchases, but now not only does it have a kicky display, it also has some really cute, fun products, and even some impressive ones for females of any age. While the makeup is fun, stay away from the skin-care products, this stuff burns like crazy! It is sad for me to think that someone would formulate such irritating products for anyone, but when its directed at kids with naive notions about their skin's health, I feel angry at the company and worried about the kids. For information on Bonne Bell products please call (216) 221-0800.

Bonne Bell Skin Care

☹ **10-0-6 Medicated Deep Pore Cleanser for Acne Prone Skin** *($5.25 for 13.4 ounces)* is an alcohol-based BHA product. The irritation from this product can turn the skin red and flaky.

☹ **10-0-6 Deep Pore Cleanser Sensitive Skin** *($5.25 for 13.4 ounces)* is similar to the one above and the same review applies.

☹ **10-0-6 Deep Pore Cleanser, Normal to Oily Skin** *($4.09 for 13.4 ounces)* is similar to the one above, only this one contains resorcinol, a serious skin irritant, and one the FDA disallowed for claims in acne products in 1992. This product is not recommended.

☹ **10-0-6 Deep Cleansing Antiseptic, Original Formula for Normal to Oily Skin** *($4.09 for 13.4 ounces)* is similar to the one above and the same review applies.

☹ **No Shine Oil Control Cover** *($2.49 for 0.5 ounce)* uses a form of magnesium as the oil-absorbing ingredient. That makes this product similar to Phillips' Milk of Magnesia, which I recommend as a facial mask. Regrettably, Bonne Bell's product contains camphor and menthol, which can irritate the skin.

Bonne Bell Makeup

☺ **No Shine Oil Control Makeup** *($2.09)* comes in only four colors, but they are all excellent, neutral shades. The makeup won't necessarily control oil, but it does have a sheer, dry matte finish. For someone with oily skin, that's good, inexpensive news.

☹ **No Shine Concealer** *($3.29)* is a poor excuse for a concealer. It comes in only two shades, and both can be too peach for most skin tones; also, they easily crease into lines around the eyes.

☹ **No Shine Oil Control Powder** *($2.49)* has a smooth soft finish, but tends to go on too flaky and looks like a layer of powder on the skin.

☺ **Gel Bronze Face and Body Bronzer** *($2.09)* is a unique way to go about changing the color of skin. I generally never recommend any kind of makeup cover, but this is a lightweight gel formulation that spreads beautifully over the skin and gives it a rather natural-looking, extremely sheer tan appearance. It has no after-feel, so it works great for someone with normal to oily skin who doesn't want a feeling of makeup on the skin. One major drawback of this product is that it tints the skin, which means once in place it doesn't come off until it sloughs off along with your skin cells. **Cream Bronze Face Bronze** *($2.09)* is one of the most convincing matte colored bronzing products I've reviewed. This lotion-like formula has a believable looking tan color that blends easily into the skin leaving a slightly moist finish. Best for someone with normal to dry skin.

☺ **Powder Blush** *($2.09)* is an excellent group of matte blush shades. These are as viable an option for blush as any you'll find.

☺ **Eye Definer** and **Lip Definer** *($1.59 each)* are standard pencils with a selection of 12 shades each. Being standard pencils doesn't make them bad; quite the contrary, these are an excellent option for lining, especially for lips. The colors are diverse and wonderful. These are going in my makeup bag.

☺ Lipsticks set Bonne Bell apart from the "adult" part of the cosmetics world. They all have some kind of sweet candy-coated or berry-tasting flavor. **Lip Gear** *($2.46)* is a group of 12 lipstick shades that have a rather creamy to slightly greasy texture. They won't last long, but the coverage is good and the taste is like vanilla. **Lip Lix** *($1.59)* is a very emollient, greasy lipstick gloss, good for dry lips; **Lip Tints** *($2.46)* are small pots of creamy lip glosses; **Lip Lites** *($2.46)* are greasy tube glosses with tastes ranging from raspberry to mud pie. These all work well to keep lips moist and chap-free, but even if that isn't a concern, you have to try the mud pie—it really does taste like a brownie!

☹ **Lip Smoothers SPF 6** *($2.68)* don't have a good sunscreen despite their good taste.

☹ **Wash Off Mascara Remover Gel** *($2.49 for 2 ounces)* has warnings about not getting it in the eyes. Why would anyone make a mascara remover you can't get in your eyes? Thanks for the warning; I think we'll all stay away from this one.

Borghese

There really was a Princess Marcella Borghese; in her day she was quite a jet-setter, and she gained her title via marriage to Prince Paolo Borghese. According to information received from the company, the princess and her friendship with the late Charles Revson spawned her interest in skin care and cosmetics, and soon—*voila!*—she was in business for herself. Over the past ten years, the line has changed hands a few times (the princess is no longer involved), but it stands out as a singularly Italian flavor amidst so many French and American lines. Borghese is also one of the more expensive product lines, but then what would you expect from a cosmetics line whose namesake is a princess?

Acqua Puro Skin Care System is a new group of skin-care products from Borghese that attempts to address the needs of those with sensitive skin. While all the products do have a nice group of anti-irritants (bisabolol, glycyrrhetinic acid, and allantoin), they also have a group of fragrant oils, including rosewood oil and lavender oil, that are potential sensitizers. Those oils do smell nice but they are best left off the face. Fragrance is best applied behind the ears, at the corners of the throat, elbow bend, and behind the knees in the form of perfumes or eau de colognes, and not in skin-care products. Borghese's literature for the Acqua Puro products describes at length how the skin's "natural defenses can be compromised by pollution, UV rays, temperature extremes, and harsh chemicals and irritants found in certain skin care preparations." I agree with all of that (well maybe not the pollution part, given that there is no evidence of any kind demonstrating that people who live in a city environment have more skin-care problems then those who live in the country), but then why doesn't this group of products include a sunscreen? If UV damage is a culprit in skin damage doesn't it make sense to get in front of a problem and stop the source of damage and not behind the problem after the damage has taken place? Plus, what about the other products in Borghese's lineup that use harsh or irritating ingredients, like their cleanser and mask with peppermint, bar soap with lye, or toners with alcohol? Doesn't everyone deserve not to have their skin compromised by irritating products? That's assuredly my philosophy. While I do think the Acqua Puro products are decent formulations that can work for a variety of skin types, these come up short in some ways and they definitely cast doubts on the rest of Borghese's skin-care items.

Borghese has huge, very attractive, and inaccessible counter displays that are organized loosely into three color groupings: Oro (yellow-based), Rosso (pink-based), and Neutrale (neutral/beige). These groupings are helpful but a bit more confusing than those of some of the other cosmetics lines, which divide their colors into the traditional four color families.

Many of Borghese's skin-care products are touted as being based on the mineral content extracted from the water around the Montecatini area of Italy. This volcanic region is known for its healing waters, and Europeans flock there, as well as to other such spas around Europe and the Middle East, for a day or week of soaking up whatever restorative magic they can. Whether the spa is in France, Italy, or Israel, the boast is the same: skin-care woes are eliminated. The only research I've seen concludes that some serious skin conditions (such as eczema or psoriasis) are sometimes relieved after soaking in these high-mineral-content waters. Does that mean that if you use products that contain minerals extracted from these waters, your skin will be healed? Well, wrinkles or acne won't be healed, that's for sure. The chance that other skin disorders will be helped is also slim. There is absolutely no evidence that skin rashes can benefit from products that contain the stuff.

Mineral content is only a part of the lengthy ingredient lists covering Borghese's skin-care products. There are interesting water-binding agents, antioxidants, anti-irritants, and emollients. Of course, many of these are at the end of the ingredient list, which means you're not getting as much of the good stuff as you would hope, given the price tag. Still, there are some intriguing formulations to check out if price is no object. For more information about Borghese call (212) 572-3100.

Borghese Skin Care

☺ **$$$ Puro Fresco Gentle Fresh Cleanser** *($25 for 6.76 ounces)* is indeed a gentle cleanser, but also not very effective in getting off makeup without the help of a washcloth. It would work well if you are only wearing a minimal amount of makeup or first thing in the morning.

☺ **$$$ Puro Tonico Comforting Spray Toner** *($23 for 6.76 ounces)* is basically just water, propylene glycol, silicone, and a lightweight detergent cleansing agent. The anti-irritants are in here, but some water-binding agents would have been helpful. This is a good but ordinary irritant-free toner for most skin types.

☺ **$$$ Hydra-Puro Intensivo Moisture Renewing Creme** *($40 for 1.7 ounces)* contains mostly water, thickeners, slip agents, film former, anti-irritants, water-binding agents, fragrance, and preservatives. This is a good but extremely ordinary, overpriced moisturizer for normal to slightly dry skin.

☺ **$$$ Puro Protettivo Protective Eye Creme** *($32 for 0.5 ounce)* is almost identical to the creme above (maybe slightly more emollient, but just maybe), only the amount you get is less and the cost is more!

☺ $$$ **Hydra-Puro Moisture Renewing Oil-Free Fluide** *($35 for 1.7 ounces)* is almost identical to the one above, except in lotion form. It is a good lightweight moisturizer for someone with normal to slightly dry skin.

☺ $$$ **Puro Dolce Skin Calming Essence** *($42.50 for 1 ounce)* is similar to the Fluide above and the same review applies.

☹ $$$ **Crema Saponetta Cleansing Creme** *($28.50 for 7 ounces)* is a standard detergent-based water-soluble cleanser that can potentially dry out the skin. It can be good for some skin types.

☹ $$$ **Effetto Immediato Spa Comforting Cleanser** *($28.50 for 8.4 ounces)* is a mineral oil–based cleanser that also has a detergent cleansing agent. The long ingredient list includes all the latest water-binding agents, oils, and mineral salts, but they are too far down on the list to help the skin. Other than that, this could be a good cleanser for someone with dry skin. It can leave a greasy film on the skin.

☹ **Esfoliante Delicato Gentle Cleanser Exfoliant** *($23.50 for 2.6 ounces)* would be a lot more gentle if it didn't contain peppermint oil and two detergent cleansing agents known for being extremely irritating and drying (sodium lauryl sulfate and sodium C14-16 olefin sulfate). Did someone at Borghese check out this ingredient list before they decided to sell it?

☹ **Fango Active Mud Soap** *($18.50 for 5.3 ounces)* is a standard bar soap with lard and lye, and this one adds insults to injury by adding peppermint and menthol, two potent skin irritants.

☹ $$$ **Gel Delicato Gentle Makeup Remover** *($26.50 for 8.4 ounces)* contains mostly water, slip agent, film former, several detergent cleansers, tiny amounts of mineral salts, plant extracts, water-binding agents, and preservatives. It will definitely take off makeup, but the detergent cleansing agents can be quite drying for the eye area.

☺ $$$ **Effetto Immediato Spa-Soothing Tonic for Sensitive Skin** *($26.50 for 8.4 ounces)* contains mostly water, film former, slip agent, plant extracts, silicone, water-binding agents, mineral salts, anti-irritant, plant oils, and preservatives. This is a good toner for someone with normal to dry skin.

☹ **Tonico Minerale Stimulating Tonic** *($26.50 for 8 ounces)* is a toner that contains mostly water, alcohol, talc, slip agent, and mineral salts. This is a lot of money for alcohol and salt. It would indeed be stimulating, as well as irritating and drying, for most skin types.

☺ $$$ **Crema Correttivo Firming Eye Cream** *($35 for 0.5 ounce)* is a very good moisturizer for dry skin that contains mostly water, slip agents, thickeners, water-binding agents, plant oil, plant extracts, minute amounts of mineral salts, and preservatives.

☹ **Cura di Vita Protettivo Protective Moisturizer SPF 15** *($39.50 for 1.7 ounces)* doesn't contain avobenzone, titanium dioxide, or zinc oxide, and is not recommended.

☹ **Cura Forte Moisture Intensifier** *($65 for 1.7 ounces)* contains peppermint oil, which is an irritant not a moisture intensifier.

☹ **Cura Notte Night Therapy for Dry-to-Very Dry Skin** *($42.50 for 1.7 ounces)* contains mostly water, thickeners, slip agent, plant oils, water-binding agents, salicylic acid, silicone, lactic acid, minerals, anti-irritant, vitamins, plant extracts, and preservatives. This is about a 1% AHA and 0.5 BHA exfoliant in a very emollient moisturizing base. Salicylic acid is only appropriate for breakouts and can be too irritating for someone with this skin type, and there isn't enough AHA to work as an exfoliant.

☹ **Cura Notte Night Therapy for Normal-to-Dry Skin** *($42.50 for 1.7 ounces)* is almost identical to the product above, but without AHAs, and the same review applies.

☺ **$$$ Cura Notte Night Therapy for Normal-to-Oily Skin** *($42.50 for 1.7 ounces)* contains mostly water, film former, slip agent, silicones, salicylic acid, water-binding agents, lactic acid, vitamins, thickeners, minerals, and preservatives. Several ingredients in this product could cause problems for someone with oily skin, but it could be good for combination skin. It is a very low-percentage AHA and about a 1% BHA product. The pH is too high for it to be an effective exfoliant.

☺ **$$$ Cura Vitale Time-Defying Moisturizer for Dry-to-Very Dry Skin SPF 8** *($42.50 for 1.7 ounces)* has some sunscreen, but why bother with SPF 8 when there are so many good SPF 15s around? This one doesn't contain avobenzone, titanium dioxide, or zinc oxide, and is not recommended.

☹ **Cura Vitale Time-Defying Moisturizer for Normal-to-Dry Skin SPF 8** *($42.50 for 1.7 ounces)* is similar to the one above and the same review applies.

☹ **Cura Vitale Time-Defying Moisturizer for Normal-to-Oily Skin SPF 8** *($42.50 for 1.7 ounces)* is similar to the one above and the same review applies.

☺ **$$$ Dolce Notte ReEnergizing Night Creme** *($50 for 1.85 ounces)* contains mostly water, a long list of thickeners, silicones, petrolatum, water-binding agents, mineral salts, vitamins, plant oil, plant extracts, anti-irritants, and preservatives. This is a very good moisturizer for someone with dry skin, but the exotic ingredients are all at the end of the ingredient list, and the ordinary emollients are in the largest concentration.

☺ **$$$ Effetto Immediato Spa Lift for Eyes** *($43 for 1 ounce)* contains mostly water, thickeners, silicones, glycerin, mineral salts, several water-binding agents, plant extracts, anti-irritant, vitamin E, and preservatives. This is a good lightweight moisturizer for the eyes, but the price is likely to hurt your vision. Once again, the really interesting ingredients are far down on the ingredient list.

☺ **$$$ Energia Skin Recovery Fluid Oil-Free** *($47.50 for 1.7 ounces)* and

Energia Skin Recovery Creme *($47.50 for 1.7 ounces)*. These products are virtually identical, but the cream has more thickening agents than the fluid. Both contain water, silicone, thickeners, glycerin, plant extracts, water-binding agents, more thickeners, more plant extracts, anti-irritant, vitamins, minerals, and preservatives. These would be good moisturizers for someone with normal to dry skin. Borghese also stuck some sugarcane extract in these two products (but not much—it's at the end of the ingredient list) so they can pretend that they have natural AHA ingredients that can help cell turnover. Sugarcane can't do that, and the minuscule amount in here can't do anything else either.

☹ **Equilibrio Equalizing Restorative SPF 4** *($39.50 for 1.7 ounces)* has a SPF 4, and isn't even close to being able to protect adequately from sun damage; there is no UVA protection either.

☺ **$$$ Fluido Protettivo Advanced Spa Lift for Eyes** *($45 for 1 ounce)* is a very good moisturizer for dry skin that contains mostly water, silicones, thickeners, water-binding agents, vitamins, and preservatives.

☹ **Spa Energia Maximal Moisture Creme** *($40 for 1.4 ounces)* contains mostly water, silicone, thickeners, petrolatum, water-binding agents, vitamins, and preservatives. This product also contains peppermint, which is a skin irritant.

☹ **$$$ Spa Energia Skin Energy Source** *($40 for 1.5 ounces)* is similar to the one above and the same comments apply.

☹ **Fango Active Mud for Face and Body** *($30 for 7 ounces)* is a large jar of mud. The brochure describes it as "Fango Therapy of Montecantini." Montecantini is supposedly some kind of special volcanic clay. The product actually contains water, tallow (that's lard), detergent cleansing agent, bentonite (a white clay found in the United States), and a much smaller amount of Montecantini clay. It also contains some mineral salts and some plant oils. It does feel good when you take it off, but that's about it. The tallow can cause breakouts, and the detergent cleansing agent can dry out the skin. There are also other irritating ingredients such as peppermint oil. This is a lot of money for mud and tallow.

☺ **$$$ Botanico Eye Compresses** *($47.50 for 60 pads)* contains mostly water, witch hazel, slip agents, water-binding agents, anti-irritant, mineral salts, and preservatives. It's good that this product contains an anti-irritant, because witch hazel can act as an irritant. This is an OK, extremely lightweight moisturizing liquid for the eyes that applies in pads. It's relaxing to think of sitting back with these on your eyes, but a soft, cool washcloth, with some aromatherapy essence radiating in the background, would work just as well.

☺ **$$$ Botanico Lip Compresses** *($39.50 for 50 compresses)* are similar to the ones above, only without the witch hazel; the same basic review applies.

☺ **$$$ Crema Perfetta Perfecting Lip Conditioner** *($25 for 0.5 ounce)* is just silicone, film former, and Vaseline. It's not a great lip moisturizer nor does it do much when worn under lipstick.

☺ $$$ **Spa Mani Moisture Restoring Gloves** *($38.50)* are mitts that, while definitely a gimmicky product, are layered with a thick lining of heavy-duty silicone. Silicone comes in many different weights: in hair serums it has the consistency of an oil; in these gloves it is solid, which makes it flexible but firm. What is so impressive about silicone is its phenomenal ability to keep water in the skin and impart a silky feel to anything it touches, yet—and this is a big deal—it still allows skin to breathe. This prevents the skin from becoming too moist, which can hurt the skin's healing ability. So these Spa Mani gloves are not the same as other gloves, which tend to leave the hands feeling sweaty and damp. What these gloves do is keep the skin in contact with a substance that imparts a moisturizer all night long. If you choose to wear them to bed, you will wake up with smoother hands; it would be impossible not to.

☺ $$$ **Mani Vitale Time Defying Hand Creme** *($25 for 3 ounces)* goes along with the Spa Mani gloves. Time Defying Hand Creme won't defy anything; it is just a good basic moisturizer that contains mostly water, thickeners, plant extracts, more thickeners, vitamins, water-binding agents, preservatives, minerals, and fragrance. The brochure suggests this product will provide all-day protection, but without a sunscreen it is OK only at night. This is fairly pricey for a basic moisturizer with some plants thrown in for effect.

Borghese Makeup

FOUNDATION: Borghese has a confusing group of four different foundations, all with the same first name. The four formulations are all called Cura Naturale Time Defying Makeup, all are rated SPF 8, a disappointing number, and none of them contain titanium dioxide, zinc oxide, or avobenzone for UVA protection. Although I don't understand the thinking behind this strange and ambiguous system of identifying foundations, the four variations are for the most part very good, with great colors and worth your investigation, but you will still need an adequate sunscreen underneath.

☺ $$$ **Cura Naturale Time Defying Makeup Dual Effetto SPF 8** *($28.50)* is the least impressive of the bunch. It is just your standard talc-based pressed powder meant to be used as a foundation. It has a soft though dry finish and comes in 12 shades. **The only color to avoid** is Principessa Beige, which isn't the least bit beige (it's peach).

☺ $$$ **Cura Naturale Time Defying Makeup Oil-Free SPF 8** *($28.50)* does have a refreshingly smooth matte finish. The colors are good, with a nice range of shades, particularly for someone with fair skin. **The colors to avoid are** Cameo, Tostino, and Principessa Beige.

☺ $$$ **Cura Naturale Time Defying Makeup Normal to Dry Skin SPF 8** *($28.50)* goes on smooth and light, and should feel lovely on dry skin. **The colors to avoid** are Cameo, Crema, and Principessa Beige; the rest are terrific.

☺ $$$ **Cura Naturale Time Defying Makeup SPF 8 Creme for Very Dry Skin** *($35)* has a rich, creamy finish and blends evenly, leaving the skin looking moist and smooth. Most of the colors are great; just stay away from Cameo, Tostino, and Principessa Beige.

☺ $$$ **Molto Bella Liquid Powder Makeup** *($35)* is a wonderfully unique way to apply foundation. This is a liquid that dries to a satiny smooth powder. It has one of the most beautiful textures and isn't the least bit greasy. It is worth a stop at a Borghese counter to give this one a test drive.

☹ $$$ **Hydro Minerali** *($30)* is a sheer, light foundation with a hint of sparkle. It lists titanium dioxide on the ingredient label but has no SPF listed. It is an interesting look but I'm not sure it's all that practical for daily use. For special occasions it's easier to dust shine on the face than apply it all over in a foundation.

☹ $$$ <u>CONCEALER:</u> **Absolute Concealer** *($25)* has a soft, creamy texture but only two good colors. Ideal Light is too pink for most skin tones, but Ideal Medium is a good neutral (slightly peach) and Ideal Deep would be good on darker skin tones.

☺ $$$ <u>POWDER:</u> **Powder Milano** *($30)* is a talc-based powder that goes on very soft and smooth. All of the colors are excellent, even Terrecotte is an option (it's supposed to be a matte bronzer but works well as a powder). Candlelight is an extremely shiny dusting powder that would be for a special effects look only.

☹ **Loose Powder Milano** *($38.50)* is a standard talc-based powder. This would be a good, although expensive, powder except that all the shades are shiny. Doesn't that negate the reason for using a powder in the first place? If you want it for a special evening look that's one thing, but for regular use it isn't the best idea.

☺ $$$ <u>BLUSH:</u> **Blush Milano** *($29)* is a very satiny regular powder blush that has lovely group of colors. It feels great, but it can wear poorly on oily skin types because it is such a moist powder. **Most of the colors are superior; the only ones to avoid are:** Terracotte, Raphael, and Puccini Rosegold.

☺ $$$ <u>EYESHADOW:</u> **Shadow Milano Singles** *($16)*, **Duales** *($28.50)*, and **Trios** *($32)* have an appealing assortment of eyeshadow colors with a rich, luscious texture. Most are only slightly shiny and go on matte enough to consider them anyway. Most of the eyeshadows have a great silky texture, go on soft, and blend beautifully. **The ones to avoid because of too much shine are** Vino Nero, Marino Nero, and Espresso.

☹ $$$ <u>EYE AND BROW SHAPER:</u> The **Eye Accento Pencil** *($17.50)* and **Linea Perfetta Brow Pencil** *($18.50)* are both ordinary but good. One end of the eye pencil has a sponge tip to blend the color, and the brow pencil has a mascara wand at one end. **Shadow Liner** *($17.50)* is, just as the name implies, powder that can be used as a liner, but that's true for any powder shadow: you only need to change brushes.

☺ **$$$ Brow Milano** *($20)* is an excellent brow gel, with a fantastic brush (which is so important for getting this type of product on right). Unfortunately, the color selection is limited—there are only three shades (and no shades for ash or black eyebrows)—but what's there is superior.

☺ **$$$ LIPSTICK AND LIP PENCIL:** Borghese sells four types of lipstick in a limited selection of colors. **Lip Treatment Moisturizer SPF 15** *($18.50)* has a clear moisturizing center around a fairly greasy gloss color. It's rather ordinary for the price, but the SPF 15 is nice, and it contains part titanium dioxide for UVA protection. **Superiore State-of-the-Art** *($20)* isn't exactly state of the art, but it is a good creamy to slightly glossy lipstick. **La Moda Concentrate** *($18)* goes on in a soft matte finish which is more creamy than matte, and wears well. The package claims that the lipstick won't feather (bleed into the lines around the mouth), but it does, although not as much as some other lipsticks. **Perfetta Lip Pencil** *($18)* is a basic pencil, just like those in a dozen other lines for far less. These come in a good array of colors.

☺ **$$$ Auto-Matte Liquid Matte Lip Colour** *($22)*. The name says it all for this dispensing brush/pen lip color. You click one end of the container and it releases the color to the brush tip. Nice way to apply lip color. There are only four shades, but the application is nice and softly matte.

☹ **$$$ Gloss Conditioning** *($18)* is just a very pricey gloss easily matched and excelled by products from L'Oreal to Revlon.

☹ **$$$ Lip Wash Water Colour** *($18)* is a lip stain that you apply from a nail polish–like container and brush. This is a very watery product that bleeds quickly into lines and can slip past lips so that a lip liner must go on first in order to control it. With only two selections, the color range can only be described as limited. The stain is OK but not as lasting as Lip Ink's. It's still worth a try, but don't expect all-day lips from this product.

☹ **$$$ Lumina Lip Color** *($18)* is a group of shiny, fairly creamy/glossy lipsticks that I do not recommend, unless you're into frost.

☹ **Lip Powder Duo** *($22.50)* is a group of intensely shiny lip powders meant to be worn over or under lipstick, or alone. I remember when Cover Girl and Revlon had products like these. They didn't last very long and these won't either. They feel strange, wear off strangely, and the color selection leaves much to be desired.

☹ **MASCARA: Volumina Luxuriant Mascara** *($17)* has an unusual wand. One side is smooth with grooves, and the other has small stiff bristles. It does not lengthen lashes, and it flakes and smears as the day goes by. **State of the Art Waterproof**

Mascara *($16)* builds easily, lengthens, and thickens rather nicely without clumps; sadly, it isn't even remotely waterproof.

☺ $$$ **Maximum Mascara for Sensitive Eyes** *($17)* is an excellent mascara, but it isn't any better for sensitive eyes than any other mascara on the market. It builds beautifully and doesn't clump or smear. **Superiore State of the Art Mascara** *($16)* is also an excellent mascara that builds easily, creates great thickness, and doesn't smear or chip!

☺ $$$ <u>BRUSHES:</u> This group of brushes is pricey *($55 to $18)* and quite attractive. The texture is beautiful and soft, and though the selection is limited what they do have works well.

Cellex-C (Skin Care Only)

I'm not sure where to start with the saga of vitamin C. You wouldn't think that one nebulous little ingredient would cause so much commotion, but then we're talking about the cosmetics industry, where it only takes one ingredient to start a furor. And especially one ingredient that promises instant youth. Vitamin C is such an ingredient. I've discussed at length the research from this controversy. Dr. Sheldon Pinnell from Duke University looked at the effect of sun exposure in relation to applying L-ascorbic acid (a specific form of vitamin C) on hairless pigs. It seems the pigs with L-ascorbic acid applied did not get sunburnt. From this study it was assumed that L-ascorbic acid was an exceptional antioxidant. It was also known at the time that L-ascorbic acid was an exceptionally unstable ingredient. That's why Cellex-C, the little $70 an ounce container of L-ascorbic acid, comes in a brown bottle. When exposed to air, sun, or heat, it decomposes. Cellex-C loses its vitamin C content after just a couple of weeks.

An interesting side note is that women were experiencing smoother skin from using Cellex-C. In light of the fact that a woman would probably never notice the effect of reduced sun damage on her skin (after all, that's all we know about the effects of L-ascorbic acid; there is no clinical research about wrinkles or aging on people), how could this be? As it turns out, Cellex-C is formulated with a pH of 2.5. This highly acidic base may be stimulating some of the positive effects. Some dermatologists conjecture that a pH of 2.5 may swell the skin slightly, making it look smoother, and increase cell turnover (sort of like AHAs do). Of course, there are no studies checking this probability out, but then Cellex-C is classified as a cosmetic, and as long as women are buying it, who cares if it really works?

The story has become more complicated since I originally researched the issues surrounding vitamin C. I should mention I tried to get information from Dr. Pinnell back in 1996 when I first wrote about Cellex-C, but he never returned my calls, nor did I receive any of the documentation I requested. All the data I included in my study were obtained from other sources, including Pinnell's published research and articles.

According to information I received from Pinnell's new company, SkinCeuticals, in 1997 he stopped endorsing Cellex-C and the entire Cellex-C product line. I was also told that Cellex-C cannot use the new stabilized form of L-ascorbic acid patented to Duke University and in Pinnell's control. The new story is that Pinnell now claims to have a stabilized version of L-ascorbic acid, sold through his company Skin Ceuticals.

In the meantime, without getting into the convoluted politics between Pinnell and Cellex-C, the bottom line for this company is that the L-ascorbic acid they use is a good antioxidant, but that this form of vitamin C is one of the least desirable, because you can't get the ingredient to last. Further, regardless of what is true for any single ingredient, skin aging is more complicated than just the loss of vitamin C or any other vitamin, enzyme, protein, or fatty acid in the skin. It is the whole picture we should be concerned about, not just one small aspect. Besides, there are many other antioxidants that are as good as or even more impressive than vitamin C, including beta glucan, vitamin E, and vitamin A, to name a few.

The entire arena of antioxidants is new and there is nothing definitive to warrant the cost or tumult. They won't get rid of wrinkles or replace sunscreen, so calm down! They can offer increased sun protection, which is important, but that's it. Of course, that doesn't stop the companies selling products that contain vitamin C from making claims about reversing aging, building collagen, feeding the skin, and healing sun damage, despite the fact, as Pinnell states in his own paper published in *Les Nouvelles Esthetiques,* February 1996: "**conclusive studies of the effect of this solution [topical vitamin Cs to reduce sun damage] have not yet been conducted.**"

That's the skinny on Cellex-C. Despite Pinnell's disavowal of Cellex-C Serum and the entire line associated with it, it has quite a following. There are now over 15 more products in addition to the $70 bottle of Cellex-C.

The original question I posed some time ago is why, if the little bottle of Cellex-C is supposed to be so amazing—with mesmerizing before-and-after pictures—why do there have to be all these other products making more miraculous claims? Why would you need AHAs, toners, and other wrinkle creams if one product was doing all the work? There are some good products in this line, but the prices are stupefying, the claims are exaggerated beyond belief, and the misleading notion that a combination of several products will make a difference on the skin is farcical.

Please note that the products in the Cellex-C line that supposedly contain alpha hydroxy acid for the most part actually contain something called fruit extracts, derived from sugarcane, passion fruit, and green pea. As I've explained in other parts of this book, fruit acids don't have anything to do with alpha hydroxy acids. If you want an AHA product that exfoliates the skin (that's what AHAs do), it should have glycolic acid, lactic acid, tartaric acid, and/or citric acid, with glycolic and lactic considered to be the best. For more information about Cellex-C call (800) CELLEX-C.

☺ **$$$ Fruitaplex Active Cleanser Normal to Oily Skin** *($39 for 8 ounces)* is an exceptionally standard detergent-based water-soluble cleanser with a minimal amount of fruit extracts (which are not alpha hydroxy acids, by the way). This would be an OK cleanser for most skin types, but the price is embarrassing for what you get.

☹ **$$$ Fruitaplex Gentle Cleansing Milk** *($39 for 8 ounces)* is a plant oil–based cleanser that needs to be wiped off. It can leave a greasy film on the skin.

☹ **Fruitaplex Balancing Toner Normal to Oily Skin** *($37 for 8 ounces)* is just water, alcohol, witch hazel, fruit extracts, and preservatives. Alcohol at any price is bad for the skin, and fruit extracts are not alpha hydroxy acids.

☹ **Fruitaplex Fresh Complexion Mist** *($37 for 8 ounces)* is a new twist on the toner theme. It contains mostly rice wine, water, aloe, witch hazel, plant extracts, glycerin, anti-irritants, glycolic acid, lactic acid, tartaric acid, and preservatives. As exotic as rice wine sounds, it is just alcohol and can cause irritation and dryness. The AHAs are nice, but the 2% concentration makes them water-binding agents, not exfoliants.

☺ **$$$ Bio-Botanical Cream for Normal to Oily Skin** *($45 for 2 ounces)* contains mostly water, thickeners, mineral oil, glycerin, plant oils, water-binding agents, silicone, and preservatives. There are several ingredients in here that would not be great for someone with oily, skin but this can be an option for someone with dry skin.

☺ **$$$ Cellex-C Eye Contour Gel for Normal to Oily Skin** *($42 for 0.5 ounce)* is virtually identical to the serum below, and the same review applies.

☺ **$$$ Cellex-C High Potency Serum for Normal to Oily Skin** *($75 for 1 ounce)* is a combination of vitamin C (L-ascorbic acid), water-binding agent, zinc, and tyrosine, an amino acid. If you do decide to give it a try, just keep in mind that once you open it, it stops being effective after two weeks, or possibly even sooner depending on where you store it.

☺ **$$$ Cellex-C Skin Firming Cream Plus** *($95 for 2 ounces)* is basically just a standard moisturizer for someone with normal to dry skin. It contains mostly water, vitamin C, thickeners, slip agents, more thickeners, preservatives, silicone, plant extracts, and vitamin E. The amount of plant extracts and vitamin E is almost nonexistent. Are there really women who are willing to waste their money on this stuff?

☺ **$$$ Cellex-C Eye Contour Cream Plus for Sensitive, Dry Mature Skin** *($58 for 1 ounce)* is almost identical to the Skin Firming Cream, and the same review applies.

☺ **$$$ Fruitaplex Eye & Throat Gel for All Skin Types** *($30 for 1 ounce)* contains water, fruit extracts, glycerin, plant extract, preservatives, and thickeners. Fruit extracts do not equal AHAs, although this is a good, basic lightweight gel for someone with normal to oily skin.

☺ **$$$ Fruitaplex Line Smoother** *($48 for 1 ounce)* contains mostly water, fruit extracts, water-binding agent, plant extract, thickener, film former, and preservatives. This is a good, but extremely overpriced moisturizer for someone with normal to slightly dry skin. Fruit extracts are meaningless when it comes to identifying an AHA if you are looking for an effective exfoliant.

☺ $$$ **Fruitaplex New Complexion Cream for Normal to Oily Skin** *($48 for 2 ounces)* is mostly water, mixed fruit acids (it's unclear which ones), water-binding agent, thickeners, slip agent, plant oil, silicone, and preservatives. This doesn't have a low enough pH to be an effective exfoliant and the fruit extracts are meaningless when it comes to identifying an AHA, though this can be an OK lightweight moisturizer for slightly dry skin. Oily skin types beware: there a few thickening agents and oils in here that can cause breakouts and make skin feel oilier.

☺ $$$ **Fruitaplex Smooth Skin Complex for Normal to Dry Skin** *($48 for 2 ounces)* is similar to the Eye Contour Cream, and the same review applies.

☺ $$$ **G.L.A. Dry Skin Cream for Dry Skin** *($48 for 2 ounces)* adds another miracle ingredient to the Cellex-C stable. Now the big cure for wrinkles is gamma linolenic acid (GLA). While linolenic acid is a good fatty acid, it isn't going to cure wrinkles any more than L-ascorbic acid can. Again, it seems bizarre that L-ascorbic acid is supposed to be such a miracle ingredient, yet the skin needs more miracles to get results. This ends up being a very good emollient moisturizer for dry skin; it contains mostly water, thickeners, plant oils, vitamins, petrolatum, water-binding agents, silicone, and preservatives. It does contain a tiny amount of lemon oil which can be a problem for sensitive skin types.

☺ $$$ **G.L.A. Extra Moist Cream for Excessively Dry Skin** *($55 for 2 ounces)* contains mostly water, glycerin, thickeners, mineral oil, plant oil, water-binding agent, preservatives, and vitamins, and the same comments about GLA described above apply here.

☺ $$$ **G.L.A. Eye Balm for Dry Skin** *($44 for 1 ounce)* is very good moisturizer for dry skin that contains mostly water, glycerin, water-binding agents (fatty acids), plant oils, vitamins, petrolatum, plant extract, silicone, and preservatives. The same comments about GLA described above apply here. This product contains a small amount of lemon oil which can be a problem for around the eyes for sensitive skin types.

☺ $$$ **Hydra 5 B-Complex Moisture Enhancing Gel for All Skin Types** *($55 for 1 ounce)* contains mostly water, water-binding agents, and preservatives. It also contains vitamin B, and that's a good antioxidant, but it's not anything essential for skin care or this kind of price. This is a good lightweight moisturizer, but the price could cause your hair to stand on end.

☺ $$$ **Seline-E Cream, for Normal Skin** *($48 for 2 ounces)* contains mostly water, mineral oil, thickeners, vitamins, silicone, preservatives, and selenium. Selenium is a good antioxidant but the amount in here is barely noticeable. This is a good moisturizer for dry skin but that's about it.

☺ **$$$ AlphaShade SPF 8 for All Skin Types** *($55 for 2 ounces)* includes both titanium dioxide and zinc oxide as the active sunscreen ingredients, but the low SPF number is absurd from a line claiming to know so much about skin care. How come they don't know the American Academy of Dermatology and the Skin Care Institute both recommend at least an SPF 15?

☺ **$$$ Fruitaplex Purifying Clay Mask for All Skin Types** *($33 for 2 ounces)* is just an OK clay mask; it won't purify anything.

☺ **$$$ Salicea Gel for All Skin Types** *($45 for 1 ounce)* is a lightweight gel that contains mostly water, water-binding agents, plant extracts, and preservatives. It would be a good lightweight moisturizer for normal to slightly dry skin.

Cetaphil (Skin Care Only)

Galderma is the company that manufactures Cetaphil Gentle Skin Cleanser. Those of you who have been familiar with my work from the beginning know that Cetaphil Gentle Skin Cleanser is a facial cleanser I have been impressed with for quite some time. In 1983, when I first discovered this obscure little cleanser, I was almost alone in recommending it, because no one else knew about it. Back then there were very few good products available for women to clean their faces with. Until recently, the only options were cold cream or cold cream–like products, which had to be wiped off and left the face greasy, and bar cleansers or soaps, which left the face dried out and irritated. Cetaphil Gentle Skin Cleanser was one of the only water-soluble cleansers available that cleaned the face without drying it out or leaving it feeling greasy. Times have changed, of course, and there are now many more alternatives for cleaning the face, but Cetaphil Gentle Skin Cleanser remains a primary option for women with dry, sensitive skin who don't wear much makeup. Unfortunately, Cetaphil Gentle Skin Cleanser is not very good for removing makeup, but it is dynamite in the morning or if you wear minimal makeup, and now they have Cetaphil Oily Skin Cleanser that can be used to remove makeup, regardless of skin type. For more information about Cetaphil products call (800) 582-8225.

☺ **Cetaphil Gentle Skin Cleanser** *($8.31 for 16 ounces)* is a very good cleanser for someone with dry, sensitive skin. It is a simple formulation containing thickeners and a detergent cleasing agent. One word of warning: it doesn't remove makeup very well, so it is best for daytime or at night if you use minimal to no foundation.

☺ **Cetaphil Oily Skin Cleanser** *($5.50 for 2 ounces)*. Finally Cetaphil has an oily skin version, although it is really an all-skin cleanser. It removes makeup nicely, far better than the original Cetaphil Gentle Skin Cleanser, and doesn't irritate the eyes or dry out the skin. The price and amount are hard to understand, but you don't need very much when you use it.

☹ **Cetaphil Gentle Cleansing Bar for Dry, Sensitive Skin** *($3.29 for 4.5 ounces)* is a standard bar cleanser that uses a detergent cleansing agent. It does contain tallow, which can cause breakouts. It is best used from the neck down.

☺ **Cetaphil Moisturizing Lotion** *($7.49 for 16 ounces)* contains mostly water, glycerin, thickeners, plant oil, silicone, more thickeners, and preservatives. This is a good moisturizer for someone with sensitive normal to dry skin.

Chanel

Ah, Chanel. The very name summons images of everything from urban sophistication to suburban chic and more. Those intertwining Cs are an icon for fashion at its best. At least, that's the intended effect, and it is a powerful one. Far be it from me to burst anyone's bubble, but Chanel hasn't swept me off my feet in quite a while. Their shiny eyeshadows, poor concealer, and overpriced skin-care products offer little to extol. Even their display has a strong hands-off, inaccessible appearance. Chanel has some great foundation textures and decent colors, but their SPFs are disappointing and very few have UVA protection. Their lipsticks are wonderful, but lots of lines have wonderful lipsticks for far less. Their powders have an excellent texture, yet some of the colors are strange and the loose powders in both matte and dry skin formulas are iridescent. Most of the eyeshadows are shiny and exceptionally overpriced, while the pencils very standard and commonplace. In general, there is little about this line that warrants the price tag. All of the products have far less expensive counterparts that easily outperform Chanel's, and that is particularly true when it comes to skin care, eyshadows, blushes, lipsticks, and foundations.

The salespeople dress in Chanel uniforms and are very enthusiastic about the fact that Chanel originated in France (never mind that not one of the products seems to be manufactured there). As far as Chanel's skin-care products are concerned, the very length of their ingredient lists makes this company stand out—although I've never seen any research that equates expansive content with a superior cosmetic. Nevertheless, if you want to make sure you don't miss out on any exceptional or inexplicable ingredients for the skin, including everything from amniotic fluid to seashells, Chanel may be the line for you: you'll probably find every single ingredient you've ever thought of in just one of Chanel's skin-care products. However, a great number of Chanel's products are stunningly basic, with the same standard thickening agents, emollients, oils, and sunscreens that everyone else uses. The only difference for Chanel is the price tag. For more information about Chanel call (212) 688-5055.

Chanel Skin Care

☺ **$$$ Foaming Gel Cleanser** *($32.50 for 6.8 ounces)* is a standard detergent-based water-soluble cleanser that can be drying for some skin types. It also contains a tiny amount of animal protein and a water-binding agent, far down on the ingredient list, along with some plant oils, which are listed after the preservatives. Those are interesting ingredients, but the amounts are too tiny to matter.

☺ $$$ **Gentle Cleansing Bar** *($25 for 4 ounces)* is a detergent-based bar cleanser that contains tallow and a small amount of water-binding agents. It can be quite drying for some skin types, and the tallow may cause breakouts.

☺ $$$ **Gentle Exfoliating Cleanser** *($32.50 for 2.5 ounces)* is a mineral oil–based cleanser that uses shells for the scrub particles. This rather overpriced, but indeed gentle, scrub also contains some water-binding agents and vitamins far down on the ingredient list, which means they're barely there. Anyway, in a cleanser, their effectiveness is washed away. This product can leave a greasy film on the skin.

☹ **Oil Relief Purifying Bar** *($25 for 3.6 ounces)* won't relieve oily skin but it can be drying, and the ingredients that keep the bar in its bar form can clog pores.

☺ $$$ **Total Cleansing Milk** *($32.50 for 6.8 ounces)* is a standard mineral oil–based cleanser that contains some water-binding agents and vitamins, but again, they are far down on the ingredient list, and even if they did have an effect on the skin, they would be wiped away before that could happen. This product can leave a greasy film on the skin.

☺ $$$ **Dual Phase Eye Makeup Remover** *($23.50 for 3.4 ounces)* contains mostly water, silicone, slip agents, film former, and preservatives. This will take off eye makeup, but the ingredient list is incredibly ordinary for the money.

☺ $$$ **Gentle Eye Makeup Remover** *($23.50 for 3.4 ounces)* is just silicone and mineral oil with some preservatives and a tiny amount of anti-irritant. Pure mineral oil can give you the same results for much less.

☺ $$$ **Firming Freshener** *($32.50 for 6.8 ounces)* contains mostly water, slip agents, lanolin oil, plant extract, more slip agents, water-binding agents, anti-irritant, fragrance, and preservatives. This won't firm anything, but it is a good emollient toner for someone with dry skin. The lanolin oil can be a problem for some skin types.

☹ **Refining Toner** *($32.50 for 6.8 ounces)* is alcohol-based and won't refine anything, but it will irritate and dry the skin.

☺ $$$ **Complexe Intensif Night Lift Cream** *($31 for 1 ounce)* contains mostly water, thickeners, slip agents, plant oils, water-binding agents, plant extracts, preservatives, vitamins, and fragrance. This huge ingredient list has everything but the kitchen sink, but that still just makes it a very good moisturizer for dry skin.

☺ $$$ **Creme No. 1 Skin Recovery Cream** *($95 for 1 ounce)* is $95 for an ounce, and should help you recover something, yet it is just a good emollient moisturizer for dry skin. The collagen in here won't replace your collagen, and the cream offers nothing you can't get elsewhere, and for less.

☺ **$$$ Creme No. 1 Skin Recovery Eye Cream** *($70 for 0.5 ounce)* contains mostly water, thickeners, mineral oil, water-binding agents, lanolin, plant oils, anti-irritant, silicone, a teeny amount of lactic acid, and preservatives. This is a good, emollient moisturizer for dry skin, but surprisingly basic. It's the price tag that's anything but basic.

☹ **Day Lift Plus Multi-Hydroxy Refining Cream SPF 8** *($48.50 for 1 ounce)* doesn't contain avobenzone, zinc oxide, or titanium dioxide, and is not recommended.

☹ **Day Lift Plus Oil-Free Multi-Hydroxy Refining Lotion SPF 8** *($48.50 for 1 ounce)* doesn't contain avobenzone, zinc oxide, or titanium dioxide, and is not recommended.

☹ **Emulsion No. 1, Skin Recovery Emulsion SPF 8** *($58.50 for 1 ounce)* doesn't contain avobenzone, zinc oxide, or titanium dioxide, and is not recommended.

☹ **Eye Lift Intense** *($48 for 0.5 ounce)* has one of the longest ingredient lists I've ever seen. But the third ingredient is witch hazel, and that can be too intense for the eyes, and there are also some potentially sensitizing plant extracts in here as well.

☹ **Eye Protection Total Defense Eye Defense SPF 8** *($45 for 0.5 ounce)*. If Chanel believes SPF 8 for casual daytime wear is just fine, I disagree, as do the American Academy of Dermatology and American Cancer Society, with whom I strongly concur. While this is a nonchemical (titanium dioxide)–based SPF 8, SPF 8 isn't as reliable as an SPF 15.

☺ **$$$ Firming Eye Cream** *($50 for 0.5 ounce)* contains mostly water, rose water, plant oils, water-binding agent, thickeners, slip agents, plant extract, anti-irritant, more water-binding agents, and preservatives. This would be a good moisturizer for someone with dry skin, but it won't firm anything.

☹ **Formule Intensive Day Lift Plus Multi-Hydroxy Refining Lotion SPF 8** *($48.50 for 1 ounce)* doesn't contain avobenzone, zinc oxide, or titanium dioxide, and is not recommended.

☹ **Formule Intensive Day Lift Refining Complex, Multi-Hydroxy Refining Lotion SPF 8** *($48.50 for 1 ounce)* doesn't contain avobenzone, zinc oxide, or titanium dioxide, and is not recommended.

☺ **$$$ Hydra Serum Multi-Vitamin Moisture Supplement** *($50 for 1 ounce)* contains mostly water, alcohol, silicone, water-binding agents, film former, vitamins, fragrance, and preservatives. Alcohol can be an irritant, but in this product it is probably more an emulsifying agent than anything else. This is a good lightweight moisturizer for someone with normal to slightly dry skin.

☹ **Hydra System Levres, Maximum Moisture Lip Treatment SPF 8** *($25 for 0.12 ounce)* is little more than an emollient lip balm with wax thickeners, lanolin, and petrolatum, but for daytime the SPF 8 isn't great and it doesn't contain avobenzone, zinc oxide, or titanium dioxide.

☹ **Hydra-Systeme Maximum Moisture Cream SPF 8** *($52.50 for 1.7 ounces)* doesn't contain avobenzone, zinc oxide, or titanium dioxide, and is not recommended.

☹ **Hydra-Systeme Maximum Moisture Lotion SPF 8** *($50 for 1.7 ounces)* doesn't contain avobenzone, zinc oxide, or titanium dioxide, and is not recommended.

☺ **$$$ Lift Serum Extreme Advanced Corrective Complex** *($56 for 1 ounce)* contains mostly water, water-binding agents, thickeners, vitamins, silicones, plant extracts, anti-irritant, and preservatives. This is a good moisturizing lotion for someone with dry skin, and it does contain a host of interesting water-binding agents, but it won't lift your skin anywhere.

☺ **$$$ Source Extreme** *($65 for 1.7 ounces)* is not all that extreme, though it can be a very good moisturizer for someone with normal to dry skin. It contains mostly water, several thickeners, slip agent, vitamins, water-binding agents, plant extracts, more water-binding agents, silicone, mineral oil, and preservatives. The plants and vitamins are standard ingredients put in to help make the consumer think she is getting more than she really is, but the water-binding agents are rather impressive.

☺ **$$$ Night Lift Plus, Multi-Hydroxy Overnight Refining Treatment** *($68.50 for 1.7 ounces)* is about a 4% AHA and .05% BHA moisturizer but does not have a low enough pH to work as an exfoliant. It contains several thickening agents, plant oils, silicones, vitamins, water-binding agents, and preservatives. This has the most amazing list of water-binding agents you may ever see anywhere. Of course, the product contains only a token amount of almost all of them, but if you're afraid of missing out on some special ingredient, it's probably in here.

☹ **Protection Totale Total Defense Moisture Lotion SPF 15** *($48.50 for 1.7 ounces)* doesn't contain avobenzone, zinc oxide, or titanium dioxide, and is not recommended.

☹ **Protection Totale Total Defense Oil Control Moisture Lotion SPF 15** *($48.50 for 1.7 ounces)* doesn't contain avobenzone, zinc oxide, or titanium dioxide, and is not recommended.

☹ **Pure Response Firming Control Gel** *($50 for 1.7 ounces)* contains, as the second ingredient, aluminum starch—yes, the same ingredient you find in deodorants. It doesn't firm the skin, but it can irritate.

☹ **Bronzage Automatique Perfect Color Self-Tanning Lotion SPF 8** *($27 for 3.5 ounces)* is fine as a self-tanner using the same active ingredient, dihydroxyacetone, as all other self-tanners do. However, it doesn't contain avobenzone, zinc oxide, or titanium dioxide and is not recommended, at least not for outdoor use.

☹ **Bronzage Douceur Oil-Free Protective Bronzing Mist, SPF 10** *($28.50 for 3.5 ounces)* doesn't contain avobenzone, zinc oxide, or titanium dioxide, and is not recommended.

☹ **Protection Intense Oil-Free Sun Shelter, SPF 23** *($25 for 2.5 ounces)* doesn't contain avobenzone, zinc oxide, or titanium dioxide, and is not recommended.

☺ $$$ **Gentle Cleansing Mask** *($42 for 2.5 ounces)* is a basic clay mask that contains mostly clay, witch hazel, slip agents, thickeners, and preservatives. It can be drying for some skin types.

☺ $$$ **Natural Exfoliating Mask** *($42 for 2.5 ounces)* contains mostly water, petrolatum, lanolin, thickeners, and preservatives. This is a very ordinary, but very emollient, mask for someone with dry skin. It is also a lot of money for Vaseline and some lanolin, though.

Chanel Makeup

☹ <u>FOUNDATION:</u> **Teint Pur Matte SPF 8** *($47.50)* is not a foundation you can rely on for sun protection; the SPF 8 isn't the best, and this one doesn't have any UVA protection.

☻ $$$ **Teint Naturel SPF 8** *($50)* has a sheer, moist finish and would be excellent for someone with normal to dry skin. What a shame the SPF is so low and there's no UVA protection in this foundation. **Teint Exact Colour Reflector** *($50)* is a selection of five colors, four for medium to darker skin tones and a very white shade of white. This is a logical way for Chanel to extend its color range for the Teint Naturel foundation, which has been sorely lacking in darker and very white skin tones. The idea is that these five colors can be blended with Teint Naturel to create the color you want.

☻ $$$ **Teint Lift Eclat SPF 8** *($50)* is a resounding disappointment if you are hoping to hide a few wrinkles behind your foundation. It doesn't diminish wrinkles in the least, and the SPF 8 is not the best (though it is titanium dioxide–based); an SPF 15 would be far better. If wrinkles aren't your problem, this is a good, soft, matte, slightly powdery finish foundation with good light to medium coverage; it's good for someone with oily to combination skin, but a problem for someone with dry skin or sun damaged skin. From my perspective, this pricey foundation made every wrinkle on my face seem more evident.

☺ $$$ **Teint Perfecting Compact Makeup** *($40)* is a cream-to-powder foundation that has a very silky feel and goes on very sheer, although it's somewhat creamy for someone with combination to oily skin, which is how it is recommended. It is best for someone with normal to slightly oily or slightly dry skin. It does dry to a soft, creamy powder finish. This is a wonderful product, and **the color selection is excellent**.

☺ $$$ **Double Perfection Makeup** *($42)* is a powder-type foundation and has a satiny smooth finish, with a slightly dry texture. There are nine shades, of which only two may be unusable for most skin tones. **Avoid** Tender Bisque (can turn pink) and Sable (which can be too ash). This type of foundation is often recommended to be used with a wet application, but that tends to make it look streaked and choppy.

☺ **$$$ Teint Extreme Lumiere with Non-Chemical SPF 8** *($50)* contains mostly water, talc, and silicone, has a nice, silky texture, and is best for someone with normal to dry skin. The SPF 8 is unimpressive, although it is a nonchemical sunscreen base. **All of the colors are excellent.** It comes in an attractive, innovative pump container that pushes the color up from the bottom and prevents waste—which is nice, because at this price, wasting even a drop is expensive.

☺ **$$$ Teint Lumiere Creme with Non-Chemical SPF 8** *($55)* has a great creamy texture (it is a mineral oil–based foundation) that would be appropriate only for someone with dry skin. The titanium dioxide SPF 8 is just OK, at least for UVA protection; the SPF would be much more appealing as a 15. As it is, this is only OK for limited sun exposure. **These are the best colors:** Alabaster, Fawn, Porcelain Ivory, Soft Bisque, Beige Naturel, Beige Intense, and Golden Beige. **These colors are too be avoided:** Porcelain and Tawny Beige.

☺ **$$$ Teint Caresse Naturel** *($42)* is an extremely lightweight foundation that blends on smooth and even, providing sheer coverage, but it doesn't erase lines or perfect skin. It's just a good, light foundation. By the way, Teint Caresse is another one of those foundations that claims to diffuse light to make skin look flawless and natural. If you're hoping the effect will be something like a soft-focus photograph, think again. Where this foundation fails is that it comes in only eight shades. All of the nine colors are excellent.

☹ <u>CONCEALER:</u> Chanel's under-eye **Estompe Corrective Concealer** *($27)* has a slightly greasy texture, and the colors are not as good as they could be: Professional is too blue/green and combines poorly with the foundation; Light is slightly pink, but may be acceptable for some skin tones; Medium can turn slightly rosy. Also, this concealer can crease. **Extreme Estompe Cover Up** *($30)* has a beautiful creamy texture and the colors, Light, Medium, and Deep, are quite good. What a shame it creases so easily into the lines around the eyes and continues to do so all day long.

☺ **$$$ Quick Cover Concealer** *($32.50)* has four great shades, blends on easily, and actually holds up pretty well. It is relatively waterproof and is the best of the concealers Chanel has to offer.

☺ **$$$ Eyeshadow Base** *($25)* is a standard, matte-finish base that does help eyeshadows stay on better, although if you were wearing a matte-finish foundation that would work all by itself over the lid and this base would be unnecessary. But if you are wearing an emollient foundation this may be an option.

☺ **$$$** <u>POWDER:</u> **Perfecting Pressed Powder** *($38.50)* tends to go on very dry in spite of its lovely silky texture. It is just a standard talc– and mineral oil–based powder for an unusually high price tag. **All of the colors are excellent. Luxury Powder Compact** *($100)* is a stunning gold compact that would be worth the money if it were a necklace, but it's not. The compact is refillable and the colors for it are slightly shiny.

☹ **Perfecting Loose Powder** *($42)* comes in three shades that are supposed to have "light-reflecting properties," but they are just shiny powders; the shine sort of negates the purpose of using a finishing powder, doesn't it? For an evening look it can be fine but the sparkles on your face in daylight just look too noticeable. **Matte Loose Powder** *($42)* shades are all shiny, which isn't really the definition of matte now is it? There are also shades of pink and green, which are shiny. These are supposed to be professional colors but they just add a strange color to the skin. **Perfecting Bronzing Powder** *($38.50)* comes in two shades; Golden Bronze is very shiny and Deep Bronze is matte but can turn red.

☺ **$$$** **Matte Pressed Powder** *($38.50)* has four shades that are all extremely translucent and have a dry finish. Unfortunately, two of the four aren't the best; Medium can turn pink/peach and Banana is a strange shade of yellow.

☺ **$$$** <u>BLUSH:</u> **Powder Blush** *($36)* goes on very smoothly and the color selection is rather attractive, but a bigger plus is that the shades are mostly matte. **Contour Colour Blush** *($36)* is somehow supposed to be different from the Powder Blush, but it is essentially the same texture and the colors are pastel and attractive. There is nothing contouring about these shades. The only difference is that the colors are applied with a thin, fan-like brush. They have only a slight amount of shine. **Cheek Rouge** *($36)* is a liquid-to-powder blush that dries to a soft powder finish. It blends on beautifully and would be a great option except that almost all the colors are shiny.

☹ <u>EYESHADOW:</u> Chanel has a thing for shiny eyeshadows. Haven't they noticed how well other lines are doing with matte shadows? What is the fascination with having the eyes glitter? The only matte, **Quadra Eyeshadow** *($50),* is a group of four colors in one compact, and the only matte shades are Les Mats Neutrals, Sables, and Fauves. The rest are too shiny to recommend though the texture is quite lovely and smooth. **Eye Essentials** *($52)* are three products in one: an eyeliner, eyeshadow, and cake mascara all in the same color. It isn't in the least essential; in fact, it is impractical and overpriced for what you get. The eyeliner is very standard, and the cake mascara, well, who wants to bother with that. Even the salesperson behind the Chanel counter encouraged me not to bother with this one. **Shadow Lights Double Effect Eye Color** *($25 each)* are single eyeshadow colors. Most of these shades are shiny, so their primary effect will be to make wrinkles look more prominent. They

The Reviews C

do go on wet or dry and the wet effect is interesting, but the shine tends to flake all over. **Basic Eye Color** *($40)* are three shadows in a compact, one meant for color, the other for shading, and the third for highlighting. Nice thought, but only two of these are matte, and the combinations for most of the sets are rather unworkable. **Satin Eye Color** *($30)* is more shine for the eyes, this time in a wand-type liquid applicator. It is waterproof—well, at least it will hold up under a few dunks into the water—but why you would chose this one is definitely a matter of personal taste.

☺ $$$ <u>EYE AND BROW SHAPER:</u> **Precision Eye Definers** *($25.50)* are simply very expensive standard pencils that have a slightly dry finish, with a smudge tip on one end. **Eye Color Stick** *($21.50)* is just a twist-up eyeliner, radically overpriced for this very standard product. **Professional Eyeliner** *($45)* isn't all that professional. It is just a powder that can go on dry or wet. It comes in three choices of two colors each. The color combinations are a bit strange; you would be better off buying one deep-colored (not shiny) eyeshadow and lining your eyes with it. **Instant Eyeliner** *($25)* is a black liquid in a pot; it goes on very severe and will remind you of Twiggy lashes (if you're old enough). **Double Effect Eye Pencil** *($23.50)* is an interesting way to do a dramatic line—the double effect in the name means that these pencils can create a liquid-liner look by simply wetting the pencil point. But the four colors are a meager selection: one is black, two are intensely blue, and the fourth is a burgundy. If you need a liquid liner, for the money, and so you don't have to worry about sharpening, I would stay with a liquid liner. Besides, as pencils, these are very standard and ordinary. **Precision Brow Definer** *($28)* goes on rather dry, which means it doesn't look so greasy, but it still tends to make defined lines. One end of the pencil is a mascara wand, which can help soften the line you draw on. **Sculpting Brow Pencil** *($25.50)* is similar to the Precision Brow, only slightly drier, and this one has a stiff brush at one end to use to try to undo the drawn-on brow look.

☹ **Perfect Brows** *($60)* is not only absurdly expensive, it is useless. One set of three different shades of powder—light tan, deep brown, and dark brown—is all well and good, but if you have dark brown to black eyebrows, what are you supposed to do with the tan shade? If you have blonde brows, what are you supposed to do with the dark brown tone? The concept has merit. No one's brows are a solid color. But stroking on three different shades takes a great deal of skill and patience, and these three shades are too disparate to work together as a unit. Perfect Brows comes with teeny-weeny tweezers that are too small to use and a teeny-tiny brush that is awkward to use. For $60, everything should be full-size and the colors more coordinated for varying shades of brows. Someone with blonde brows looking to build a "perfect" brow could use three closely related shades of tan, but not light brown to almost black.

☺ **$$$ Brow Shaper** *($28.50)* is a brow gel with a small color selection: Soft Brown, Taupe, Black, and Clear. There are no shades for brunettes, blondes, or redheads, but brows definitely stay in place and the gel goes on easily, without smearing, which is very important for this type of product.

☺ **$$$ LIPSTICK AND LIP PENCIL: Creme Lipstick** *($20)* is a good creamy lipstick. **Sheer Lipstick** *($20)* is, as the name implies, more sheer gloss than lipstick. It's nice but standard. **Matte Finish Lipstick** *($20)* is not all that matte, but rather creamy. **Extreme Lip Color** *($25)* is not in the least extreme but it is a good creamy lipstick with a slightly more matte finish than the other Chanel Lipsticks. By no means is this a matte lipstick. **Super Hydrating Lipstick** *($22.50)* is just a fairly emollient creamy lipstick, with rich, opaque coverage. Avoid it if you have any problems with feathering; this one moves into the lines around the mouth almost the minute you put it on. **Lip Intensities** *($47.50)* is a compact of lip color divided into four sections. The four quadrants all have the same shade, but with different textures. One-quarter of the compact has a creamy consistency; the others are matte, glossy, and sheer. It's hardly convenient. It is far easier to use a lipstick tube and quickly sweep color across the lips instead of having to use a brush. Although it sounds nice to have the texture of your choice, most women prefer one over the others. If you have a problem with lipstick feathering, the gloss and the sheer will slide into the lines around your mouth. If your lips have a tendency to be dry, the matte isn't great. The creamy lipstick may be fine, but then the other three are a waste. On the other hand, if you like variation, this is one of the more interesting ways to get it. **Precision Lip Definer** *($25.50)* resembles dozens of other lip pencils. This one happens to have a lip brush on one end, which is convenient, but it doesn't warrant the steep price tag. Everyone from Max Factor to Revlon has their version for far less, but with identical quality. **Lip Color Stick** *($21.50)* is just a twist-up lip liner, radically overpriced for this very standard product.

☺ **$$$ Triple Colour Crayon** *($35)* is an oversized, fat, crayon type pencil that can be used over the eyes, lips, or cheeks. It is a fun application that goes on rather shiny but can blend out fairly sheer over cheeks and eyes. It isn't very practical and there are lots better lipstick-type pencils than this one. Triple Colour Crayon is billed as being waterproof, but it is no more waterproof than any other pencil. If you want similar fun at a far more reasonable price, check out the Jane One-For-All product reviewed below. **High Gloss SPF 8** *($25)* doesn't have UVA protection but it is a richly colored, very greasy gloss. **Crystal Lip Gloss** *($28.50)* is a set of two very slippery and glossy lip glosses in one compact. But I couldn't tell much difference between this one and the lip glosses for $3 from Bonne Bell or M Professional at the drugstore. **Lip Glow** *($47.50)* is a compact with four fairly standard though extremely shiny lip glosses.

The Reviews C

☺ $$$ <u>MASCARA:</u> **Instant Lash Mascara** *($20)* builds long, thick lashes fairly fast, so the name is apropro, and you'll get the length and thickness with minimal clumping and no smudging or smearing. **Instant Waterproof Mascara** *($20)* goes on great, builds quickly with no clumps, and holds up beautifully under water!

☹ $$$ **Sculpting Mascara Extreme Length** *($20)* and ☺ $$$ **Extreme Length Fine Lashes** *($20)* consist of a single mascara formula that comes packaged with two different brush options. The Extreme Length Fine Lashes version has a very small, tiny-thin brush that built extremely long, thick lashes with no clumping. The Extreme Length mascara has a full, round brush that was far less impressive for building long lashes.

☺ $$$ <u>BRUSHES:</u> Chanel has an attractive, satiny, fairly useful group of brushes. **Powder Dome Brush** *($40)* and **Blush Brush** *($37.50)* are full and soft but perhaps a bit too loosely packed for optimum control, and at these prices they should be perfect. The **Eye Liner Brush** *($20)*, **Contour Eyeshadow Brush** *($21)*, **Touch Up Brush** *($26)*, and three **Eyeshadow Brushes** *($21)* are all very good.

Chantal Ethocyn (Skin Care Only)

Ethocyn has had quite a history. In ads, a side of a woman's face treated with Ethocyn is smooth and practically line-free, while the other side, without Ethocyn, is a mass of wrinkles. The reason for that improvement, according to the company, is that Ethocyn can produce elastin. No other before-and-afters were ever used, just this one woman for several years in a row.

Dr. John Bailey, director of the FDA's Office of Cosmetics and Colors, says, "The intense marketing campaign for this product reminds me of what happened with thigh creams two years ago." The Cosmetic, Toiletry, and Fragrance Association (CTFA) lists Ethocyn as nothing more than a "skin-conditioning agent." Nonetheless, the product line is being endorsed by a Richard Strick, M.D., from the UCLA School of Medicine. On the surface, that endorsement is extremely impressive. However, I interviewed several dermatologists and medical researchers, including two doctors who had worked with Dr. Strick at UCLA, and not one was familiar with his work on Ethocyn (work that he has been involved with since at least 1986), nor were any of them willing to say that he had discovered anything significant or worthwhile. In fact, Dr. Richard Reisner, past head of dermatology at UCLA, who has done research on Ethocyn with Chantal Burnison (the creator and owner of Ethocyn), said he had no information about what this ingredient does, and he doubted that it could do much of anything.

Several dermatologists told me that because data on Ethocyn has never been published in any medical journal or been subject to peer review, it isn't anything they would be interested in. I was told repeatedly that building elastin might be helpful for the skin; however, without at the same time building collagen, which is the major support structure of the skin, it may look interesting in the laboratory under a microscope, but it won't help remove a wrinkle. (According to the Ethocyn patent, Dr. Strick claims that his product builds elastin but *decreases* collagen, because collagen gets hard with age, so you don't want it around.)

My intense skepticism was boosted by a personal letter from Dr. Strick that accompanied the package of information I received from the Chantal Pharmaceutical Corporation (formerly called Chantal Cosmetics, but that doesn't sound quite so scientific, does it?). The letter states that "[Ethocyn] has been around for about 15 years or so from the time it was first discovered . . . [but] this is the company's first product to actually be sold to the general public." That simply isn't true. Chantal Ethocyn, under the name Elasyn, was retailed to the public at Saks and Bloomingdale's back in 1986, while the patent was still pending. It was also advertised in *Vogue, Harpers Bazaar,* and *Elle* magazines. It failed and was removed from the market.

It turns out that Ethocyn is not exactly a natural molecule, at least not the kind of "natural" the consumer is hoping for. According to the *International Cosmetic Ingredient Dictionary,* it is a by-product of ether and alcohol that functions as a skin-conditioning agent. Ethocyn, in essence, is little more than an emollient, and a rather average one at that.

Ethocyn has limited distribution in drugstores across the country, but can be mail ordered by calling (800) 227-2085.

☹ **Gel Cleanser** *($23 for 6.7 ounces)* contains mostly water, alcohol, slip agents, plant oils, thickeners, and preservatives. The alcohol is a possible skin irritant and not something you should use near your eyes; other than that, this is a fairly ordinary skin cleanser.

☺ **$$$ Ethocyn Eye Cream** *($30 for 0.5 ounce)* contains mostly water, witch hazel, thickeners, plant oil, Ethocyn, thickeners, and preservatives. The witch hazel is a possible skin irritant that can plump lines and cause dryness.

☺ **$$$ Ethocyn Hydrating Complex Moisturizer** *($40 for 2 ounces)* contains mostly water, silicones, several thickeners, slip agents, algae extract, Ethocyn, several water-binding agents, and preservatives. This would be a good moisturizer for someone with normal to dry skin. The algae is a nice gimmick, but it has little to no value for the skin.

☺ **$$$ Ethocyn Essence Vials** *($50 for 0.23 ounce)* contain mostly water, several standard slip agents, thickeners, Ethocyn, plant oil, and preservatives. This would be a good lightweight moisturizer for someone with dry skin, but it's incredibly expensive and not all that different from any of the other products in this line that contain Ethocyn.

☺ **$$$ Revitalizing Mask** *($25 for 2 ounces)* is a standard clay mask with a tiny amount of plant oils. Clay is a potential irritant for some skin types.

Charles of the Ritz

Charles of the Ritz is in desperate need of a face-lift. Is no one tending to this line or are they just letting it die a slow death? There have been almost no changes since I last reviewed these products two years ago; if anything, the color options have decreased. The foundation colors are terrible, the eyeshadows limited, and the powders have barely acceptable colors. Also, the display unit is a bit confusing, but only because there is so little to it. The eyeshadows and blush are the only two saving graces for this line. Other than that, Charles of the Ritz has become a real "Why bother?" For more information about Charles of the Ritz call (800) 473-8566.

Charles of the Ritz Skin Care

☺ $$$ **Biochange Cleanser** *($19 for 6.5 ounces)* contains nothing that's changed. It needs to be wiped off, and several ingredients high on the ingredient list can cause breakouts.

☺ $$$ **Revenescence Feather Touch Cleanser** *($22.50 for 12 ounces)* couldn't be further from a "feather touch" if it were a ton of bricks. It contains mostly mineral oil, water, lanolin, petrolatum, heavy thickeners, slip agent, and preservatives. This is a very emollient wipe-off cold cream. Does anybody really use this kind of stuff anymore?

☺ $$$ **Revenescence Moisture Cream Cleanser** *($20 for 4 ounces)* is actually more lightweight than the cleanser above, but it is still a standard mineral oil–based wipe-off cleanser that can leave a greasy film on the skin.

☹ **Revenescence Liquid** *($40 for 6 ounces)* is a detergent cleanser that includes sodium lauryl sulfate high up on the ingredient list. This cleansing agent is acceptable in only the tiniest amounts because it a strong skin irritant.

☺ $$$ **Revenescence Softening Lotion 100% Alcohol Free for Dry or Sensitive Skin** *($18.50 for 8 ounces)* contains mostly water, water-binding agents, slip agent, anti-irritant, plant extracts, plant oil, and preservatives. It is a very good anti-irritant toner for someone with dry skin.

☺ $$$ **Any Age Self Protection for Eyes** *($30 for 0.4 ounce)* contains mostly water, silicone oil, glycerin, thickeners, more silicone, slip agent, more thickeners, water-binding agents, plant extracts, anti-irritant, vitamin E, more water-binding agents, vitamin A, plant oils, antioxidant, thickeners, and preservatives. This is a very long ingredient list that adds up to a good moisturizer for dry skin. The specialty ingredients are too far down in the ingredient list to add much benefit for the skin.

☺ $$$ **Any Age Self Protection for Face SPF 15** *($25 for 1.8 ounces)* contains mostly water, silicone, several thickeners, water-binding agents, plant extracts, vitamin A, plant oils, vitamin E, more water-binding agents, thickeners, and preservatives.

This is a very good moisturizing sunscreen for someone with dry skin, but the price is completely excessive for an otherwise basic, in-part titanium dioxide SPF 15.

☺ $$$ **Moisture Balancing Day Care Skin Soother** *($18.50 for 2 ounces)* contains mostly water, mineral oil, slip agent, plant oil, thickeners, anti-irritant, petrolatum, lanolin, and preservatives. It's a very emollient moisturizer for someone with extremely dry skin.

☺ $$$ **Revenescence Brightening Face and Eye Hydrating Cream** *($20 for 1 ounce)* contains mostly water, thickeners, water-binding agents, petrolatum, slip agents, vitamins, silicone, anti-irritant, fragrance, and preservatives. It won't brighten anything but it is a very good moisturizer for dry skin.

☺ $$$ **Revenescence Cream** *($42.50 for 4.4 ounces)* contains mostly water, glycerin, mineral oil, lanolin, heavy thickeners, and preservatives. This is a very heavy, ordinary moisturizer for someone with extremely dry skin, but the price tag is inane. It is almost identical to Revenescence Feather Touch Cleanser; you could use that product as your moisturizer and pocket the change.

☺ $$$ **Special Formula Emollient** *($28.50 for 4 ounces)* is almost identical to Revenescence Cream above, only thicker and heavier, and the same basic review applies.

☺ $$$ **Revenescence Moist Environment Night Treatment** *($42.50 for 2.2 ounces)* contains mostly water, thickeners, petrolatum, more thickeners, a tiny amount of water-binding agent, and preservatives. This is an overly expensive, very ordinary emollient moisturizer for someone with extremely dry skin.

☹ **Timeless Difference Day Recovery Lotion SPF 6** *($30 for 2 ounces)* is not recommended. SPF 6 doesn't provide adequate sun protection, just as any sunscreen that doesn't contain avobenzone, zinc oxide, or titanium dioxide for UVA protection, and it is not recommended.

☺ $$$ **Timeless Difference Night Recovery Cream** *($35 for 1.7 ounces)* contains mostly water, water-binding agents, slip agents, mineral oil, a long list of thickeners, vitamin E, plant oils (fragrance), and preservatives. This won't help skin recover from anything, but it is a good moisturizer for someone with dry skin.

☺ $$$ **Biochange Replacement Therapy Serum for Changing Skin** *($30 for 1.9 ounces)* contains mostly water, silicone, slip agents, thickeners, film former, soothing agent, vitamins, a long list of water-binding agents, plant extracts, and preservatives. This is a very good moisturizer, but it won't stop aging.

☹ **Disaster Cream** *($15 for 0.5 ounce)* is, to my way of thinking, a disastrous product. It contains mostly water, zinc oxide, cornstarch, clay, and preservatives. Not one of these ingredients is the least bit helpful for getting rid of blemishes or helping skin in any way. Also, cornstarch can be an irritant and may cause breakouts. How's that for a disaster?

☹ **Revenescence Firmescence 770 Wrinkle Lotion** *($30 for 2 ounces)* contains mostly water, glycerin, alcohol, slip agents, lemon oil, and preservatives. If the term "wrinkle lotion" means this product can *cause* wrinkles, then it's close to accurate. Alcohol and lemon oil can irritate and dry skin. Nothing in this lotion is appropriate for wrinkles.

☺ **$$$ Timeless Difference Eye Recovery Cream** *($25 for 0.5 ounce)* contains mostly water, water-binding agent, thickeners, plant oil, slip agent, vitamins, anti-irritants, silicone, and preservatives. This would be a very good moisturizer for dry skin.

☹ **T-Zone Controller, Skin & Color Corrector** *($17.50 for 2 ounces)* contains mostly water, alcohol, slip agent, thickeners, salicylic acid, and preservatives. Alcohol is an irritant and won't help control anything.

☺ **$$$ Line Refine for Eyes** *($15 for 0.5 ounce)* contains mostly water, silicones, glycerin, a long list of thickeners, and preservatives. This won't refine anything, but it is an OK lightweight moisturizer for slightly dry skin. One of the emulsifying ingredients is sodium lauryl sulfate, an unnecessarily irritating ingredient in an eye product.

☺ **$$$ Line Refine for Lips** *($15 for 0.5 ounce)* is just talc, thickeners, and a water-binding agent. It doesn't make much sense for the lips.

☺ **$$$ Moisture Intensive Facial** *($20 for 4 ounces)* contains mostly water, thickeners, slip agent, plant oil, several water-binding agents, anti-irritants, plant oils, and preservatives. This is a good emollient facial mask for someone with dry skin.

Charles of the Ritz Makeup

☺ <u>FOUNDATION:</u> **Superior Moisture Foundation for Normal to Dry Skin** *($20)* provides medium coverage and has a smooth, moist finish. **These colors are very good:** Natural Ivory, Soft Beige, New Beige, and Bronzed Beige. **These colors should be avoided:** Beige Sand, Deep Beige, Beige Blush, and Tender Beige.

☹ **Superior Foundation 100% Oil-Free for Normal to Oily Skin** *($20)* has a limited range of colors and they are all too peach or pink to recommend.

☹ **Perfect Finish Solid Powder Foundation** *($22.50)* is a pressed-powder foundation that has a very choppy, uneven finish; the colors are all too pink or peach to recommend.

☺ **Complete Cover Makeup SPF 10** *($21)* tends to go on rather thick, but it does blend out relatively sheer, though it almost sticks to the skin like a stain and is extremely difficult to get off regardless of the cleanser used. If you want long-lasting makeup, this is one of the few that will hold up under almost any condition. The SPF is nonchemical and the sun protection is good, though an SPF 15 would be better. **Only two colors are acceptable:** Light Cameo and Soft Cameo. **The rest are all too peach or pink to even consider.**

☺ **Moistureful Line Defying Makeup SPF 20** *($26.50)* is a very creamy, emollient foundation for someone with dry skin. The SPF is part titanium dioxide, so this would provide excellent coverage. This foundation has the best color choices of any of the Ritz foundations, but of the colors to consider there are none for very light skin tones or very dark skin tones either. **The colors to avoid** are Smooth Bisque, Smooth Blush, and Smooth Sand.

☹ **Revenescence Moisture Reservoir Liquid Makeup** *($26.50)* has a terrible assortment of pink or peach shades of foundation.

☹ <u>CONCEALER:</u> **Complete Cover Concealer** *($14)* comes in a pot and goes on rather thick and dry, and then continues to crease all day long.

☹ <u>POWDER:</u> **Translucent Pressed Powder** *($20)* is a standard talc-based powder that is quite silky and sheer and that comes in three good shades, though all have a slight amount of shine, which negates the effect of dusting down shine on the face.

☺ <u>BLUSH:</u> **Moistureful Cheek Color** *($17.50)* comes in ten good color choices that are quite soft and have a silky, sheer texture, and blend on smooth and slightly matte.

☺ <u>EYESHADOW:</u> **Moistureful Eye Color Duets** *($17)* come only in sets of two shadows. The color combinations are quite impressive, with very compatible and surprisingly neutral shades. These are mostly matte, and only a few have minimal shine. These are slightly shiny, but they don't appear shiny on the eye. My only hesitation is that the colors blend on almost too soft and sheer. None of these shades would be appropriate if you want a dramatic look or have a darker skin tone.

☺ <u>EYE AND BROW SHAPER:</u> **Classic Liners for Eyes** *($11)* are fairly standard pencils that have a slightly greasy texture. There aren't many colors, but most are just fine.

☺ <u>LIPSTICK AND LIP PENCIL:</u> **LipSTICK** *($14)* is Charles of the Ritz's version of Revlon's ColorStay, which isn't surprising, since Revlon owns Charles of the Ritz. It is an excellent, very matte lipstick that doesn't bleed, and it wears just as smooth as the new ColorStay. There are only a handful of colors, though, so it doesn't even begin to compete with its kissing cousin in that regard. **Moistureful Lip Color** *($14.50)* has a creamy consistency that is a bit on the greasy side, and several of the colors are shiny. The "maximum wear" claim on these lipsticks is a fair one; they have a stain that helps keep them around longer. **Classic Liners for Lips** *($11)* are fairly standard pencils that have a smooth texture, but only four colors. **Perfect Lip Color** *($10)* is not perfect, but it is very shiny and glossy.

☺ <u>MASCARA:</u> **Perfect Finish Lash** *($12)* is an excellent mascara with great lengthening ability, but it does have a slight tendency to smudge by the end of the day.

☹ **Every Last Lash Mascara** *($13.50)* takes forever to build what length it can, which isn't much, and it tends to smear.

Christian Dior

Dior is a great name when it comes to fashion, but it seems to have lost its footing in the world of makeup. There is nothing particularly outstanding in this line. For the most part, the eyeshadows are all extremely shiny and the color combinations highly contrasting and hard to use, at least for daytime. Dior is one of the few lines with a five-color eyeshadow set, but the colors are almost all too shiny to recommend other than for evening wear. The foundations come in a very limited selection of colors, and although I like some of the textures and coverage very much, most of the colors are too pink, peach, or orange. The lipsticks are fairly creamy and have a good texture, and the mascaras are still excellent, which is nice but still not much to get excited about. The counter displays are attractive enough, though none of the products are accessible without asking for them first, and the colors aren't organized by color families (they actually aren't organized at all), which can make finding your color range difficult. Dior's one claim to fame is a large selection of hair mascaras. They were the first line out with this new cosmetic twist and it clearly has done well for them, as is evident, although I'd like to see a wider range of colors. For more information about Christian Dior call (212) 759-1840.

Christian Dior Skin Care

☺ $$$ **Equite Gentle Gel Face Wash** *($27.50 for 4.2 ounces)* is a mineral oil–based cleanser that can leave a greasy residue on the skin. It may indeed be gentle, but it is also a remarkably ordinary wipe-off cleanser.

☺ $$$ **Equite Purifying Facewash** *($27.50 for 6.8 ounces)* is a standard detergent-based water-soluble cleanser. It can be good for someone with normal to oily skin.

☺ $$$ **Equite Wash-off Cleansing Foam** *($27.50 for 6.8 ounces)* is similar to the one above and the same comment applies.

☹ **Equite Wash Off Cleansing Gel** *($27.50 for 6.8 ounces)* is a standard detergent-based, water-soluble cleanser that uses sodium C14-16 olefin sulfate as the cleansing agent, one which is exceptionally drying and irritating for the skin.

☺ $$$ **Equite Clear Eye Makeup Remover** *($21 for 3.4 ounces)* is an average makeup remover that contains slip agents and a few emulsifiers, standard cosmetic ingredients that can cut through oil and makeup. Most eye-makeup removers contain the same ingredients, and this one is no exception.

☺ $$$ **Equite Face and Eye Makeup Remover** *($27.50 for 6.8 ounces)* contains mostly water, mineral oil, thickeners, plant extract, glycerin, more thickeners, preservatives, and fragrance. This is a lot of money for mineral oil; it will wipe off makeup but may leave a greasy film on the skin.

☺ $$$ **Equite Very Gentle Makeup Remover for the Face, for Dry Skin** *($27.50

for 5 ounces) contains mostly water, mineral oil, and thickeners. It is gentle, but it's also boring and overpriced and not that different from the one above.

☺ **$$$ Equite Waterproof Eye Makeup Remover Lotion** *($21 for 3.4 ounces)* contains mostly water, slip agent, thickeners, and preservatives, which will take off waterproof makeup just like all the ones above.

☺ **$$$ Equite Exfoliant Rose Exfoliating Gel** *($30 for 3.6 ounces)* is just thickeners, mineral oil, and scrub particles. This can exfoliate, but you may get a film left behind, and it won't work better than Cetaphil Gentle Skin Cleanser mixed with baking soda.

☺ **$$$ Equite Exfoliating Gel** *($30 for 3.6 ounces)* contains mostly water, glycerin, thickeners, mineral oil, fragrance, and preservatives. This is a gentle exfoliator, but it's not worth the money; it uses the same standard synthetic exfoliating agent (polyethylene) as most scrubs of this nature (most of which are considerably cheaper). The mineral oil can leave skin feeling greasy.

☹ **Equite Extra Exfoliating Scrub** *($32 for 3.1 ounces)* has an extra part, but it's more abrasive, strong detergent cleansing agents, and menthol. The extra in this product means extra irritating.

☹ **Equite Alcohol-Free Skin-Soothing Lotion for Dry Skin** *($27.50 for 6.8 ounces)* contains mostly water, thickeners, glycerin, fragrance, film former, preservatives, alcohol (so it's obviously not alcohol-free), water-binding agent, and more preservatives. It contains some emollients, but nothing of special interest. It also contains a minute amount of anti-irritant, but hardly enough to affect the skin at all. There isn't enough alcohol in this product to be an irritant for most skin types, so why add it at all and why call it alcohol-free when it's not?

☹ **Equite Alcohol-Free Softening Lotion for Dry Skin** *($27.50 for 6.8 ounces)* is almost identical to the lotion above, and the same review applies.

☺ **$$$ Equite Alcohol-Free Softening Toner** *($27.50 for 6.8 ounces)* is a good, but ordinary, irritant-free toner containing mostly water, slip agents, water-binding agent, silicone, and preservatives. Finally, this one really is irritant-free.

☹ **Equite Purifying Toner, for Oily Skin** *($27.50 for 6.8 ounces)* contains enough irritants to hurt, including alcohol, camphor, and menthol.

☹ **Equite Stimulating Toner for Normal & Combination Skin** *($27.50 for 6.8 ounces)* is an alcohol-based toner that also contains menthol and camphor (somewhat less than in the one above), but you wouldn't call this one stimulating; "irritating" and "drying" would be more accurate.

☺ **$$$ Capture Essential Time-Fighting Serum with Pure Micro-Proteins** *($70 for 1.7 ounces)* contains mostly water, slip agents, thickeners, water-binding agents, fragrance, and preservatives. This is a lot of money for just an OK moisturizer for dry skin.

The Reviews C

☺ **$$$ Capture Eyes Contour Gel** *($45 for 0.5 ounce)* contains mostly water, glycerin, thickeners, plant extract, film former, preservatives, fragrance, water-binding agents, and anti-irritant. Many of the more interesting ingredients are listed after the preservatives and fragrance, meaning they are present only in minute amounts. This is a good, but rather average, moisturizer for the eye area.

☺ **$$$ Capture Lift Complexe Liposomes** *($62 for 1 ounce)* is a good but rather ordinary moisturizer for dry skin. It contains mostly water, glycerin, water-binding agents, vitamins, thickeners, and preservatives.

☺ **$$$ Capture Lift Firming Night Treatment for the Face** *($58 for 1 ounce)* contains mostly water, water-binding agents, thickener, and preservatives. Minuscule amounts of vitamins and other water-binding agents also appear on the ingredient list way after the preservatives, which means they don't count for much. There is also a tiny amount of film former, which can temporarily make the skin look smooth. This is a good, but extremely average, moisturizer for normal to dry skin, but to call this "firming" or a "treatment" is almost funny.

☹ **Capture Rides Fluide Multi-Action Wrinkle Lotion SPF 8 with cyclic AHA** *($45 for 1 ounce)* has a SPF 8, but that isn't enough and this product doesn't contain avobenzone, zinc oxide, or titanium dioxide, and is not recommended.

☹ **Capture Rides Multi-Action Wrinkle Creme SPF 8** *($45 for 1 ounce)* is similar to the one above and the same review applies.

☺ **$$$ Capture Rides Wrinkle Creme for Eyes** *($45 for 0.5 ounce)* contains mostly water, film former, slip agents, thickeners, water-binding agents, vitamins, silicone, preservatives, and fragrance. This is a good moisturizer for dry skin.

☺ **$$$ Hydra-Star Moisture Creme for Dry Skin** *($46 for 1.7 ounces)* contains mostly water, film former, a long list of thickening agents, silicone, vitamin E, plant extract, a long list of water-binding agents, fragrance, and preservatives. This would be a very good moisturizer for someone with dry skin, but a lot of the interesting ingredients are at the end of a very long list.

☺ **$$$ Hydra-Star Night Treatment Creme for Dry Skin** *($56 for 1.7 ounces)* is similar to Hydra-Star Moisture Creme above except for texture differences, and the same review applies.

☺ **$$$ Hydra-Star Moisture Creme Emulsion for Dry Skin** *($46 for 1.7 ounces)* is identical to the product above except for texture differences, and the same review applies.

☹ **Hydra-Star Moisture Creme, for Normal and Combination Skin** *($46 for 1.7 ounces)* is similar to Hydra-Star Moisture Creme for Dry Skin but is unacceptable for someone with combination skin.

☺ **$$$ Hydra-Star Moisture Emulsion for Dry Skin** *($46 for 1.7 ounces)* is similar to Hydra-Star Moisture Creme for Dry Skin except for texture differences, and the same review applies.

☺ **Hydra-Star Moisture Emulsion for Normal and Combination Skin** *($46 for 1.7 ounces)* is similar to Hydra-Star Moisture Creme for Dry Skin and is unacceptable for someone with combination skin.

☺ **Hydra-Star Moisture Fluide for Normal to Combination Skin** *($46 for 1.7 ounces)* is a very lightweight moisturizer that contains water, thickeners, vitamin E, water-binding agents, silicone, film former, and preservatives. It would be a good moisturizer with antioxidant for normal to slightly dry or combination skin, but is not in the least appropriate for someone with combination skin.

☺ **$$$ Hydra-Star Night Treatment Creme, for Normal to Combination Skin** *($56 for 1.7 ounces)* is similar to Hydra-Star Moisture Creme for Dry Skin except for texture differences, and the same review applies.

☹ **$$$ Icone Hypersensitive Skin Emulsion for the Face** *($58 for 1 ounce)* contains mostly water, thickeners, glycerin, silicone, slip agent, water-binding agents, anti-irritant, film former, preservative, and fragrance. Additional interesting water-binding agents are listed after the preservative, but there's not enough of them to count for anything. This would be a good moisturizer for someone with normal to dry skin, but nothing about it makes it more suitable for sensitive skin.

☺ **$$$ Icone Principe Regulateur for All Types of Dryness** *($70 for 1.7 ounce)* contains mostly water, plant oil, thickener, glycerin, more thickeners, water-binding agents, silicone, preservative, and fragrance. This is a good though exceptionally overpriced moisturizer for someone with dry skin, and it won't regulate your skin in any way, shape, or form.

☹ **$$$ Equite Instant Radiance Purifying Mask** *($35 for 2.5 ounces)* comes in two parts: a "purifying gel," which contains water, glycerin, slip agent, thickeners, plant extract, and preservatives; and a "radiance gel," which contains almost the same ingredients. For the money, this is an incredibly boring list of ingredients. This mask won't purify anything, but it would be OK for someone with normal to slightly dry skin.

☹ **$$$ Equite Instant Radiance Relaxing Mask** *($35 for 2.5 ounces)* comes in two parts: a creamy "moisturizing emulsion," which contains mostly water, plant oil, thickeners, lanolin, silicone, anti-irritant, fragrance, and preservatives; and a "radiance gel," which contains mostly water, glycerin, slip agent, thickeners, preservatives, water-binding agent, and more preservatives. This would be a good mask for someone with dry skin.

☺ **Equite Purifying Cleansing Mask for Oily Skin** *($27.50 for 2.1 ounces)* is a standard clay mask with the addition of several skin-irritating ingredients including menthol and camphor.

☺ **$$$ Icone Sebum Control Treatment, Oil-Free Fluid** (*$44 for 1 ounce*) contains mostly water, glycerin, water-binding agents, oil absorber, and preservatives. It would be OK as an extremely lightweight moisturizer, but I wouldn't recommend using it to control oil because the product is not all that absorbent.

☹ **Ultra-Mat Perfect Matte-Finish** (*$32 for 0.5 ounce*) is basically an expensive version of the milk of magnesia I recommend as a facial mask. It works to help keep oil in check but, because of the alcohol, the irritation it can cause makes it impossible to recommend.

☹ **Svelte Cellulite Control Complex** (*$51 for 6.8 ounces*). I couldn't stop myself—I had to review this for you anyway, even though it has nothing to do with the face. It contains mostly alcohol, water, thickeners, plant extracts, anti-irritant, and preservatives. If you want to believe that rubbing alcohol and plant extracts on your thighs can do anything but swell and irritate the skin (the same as any astringent), it's up to you. However, you would be better off rubbing the $49 you spent on this product on your thighs, because at least that won't dry out your skin.

Christian Dior Makeup

☺ **$$$ FOUNDATION: Teint Dior Eclat Mat Demi-Mat** (*$42.50*) has a great soft texture and provides light coverage. It blends on evenly, giving the face a smooth, slightly matte appearance. It is minimally matte, which makes it only appropriate for someone with normal to dry skin. What a shame the color selection is so poor for this foundation. **Only these colors are worth trying:** Soft Beige, Medium Beige, and Beige. **These colors are too pink, peach, or orange for almost all skin tones:** Soft Golden, Light Golden, Medium Golden, Dore Golden, Soft Rose, and Light Rose.

☹ **Teint Ideal Mat** (*$42.50*) is hardly ideal; most of the colors are utterly terrible, ranging from very peach to orange, or too pink for most all skin tones.

☺ **$$$ Teint Dior Eclat Satin** (*$42.50*) is a light, soft foundation designed for normal to dry skin, and this one has a decent group of acceptable colors. **All these colors are excellent:** Light Golden Beige, Barely Beige, Medium Beige, and Soft Beige. **Avoid these colors:** Tres Claire Beige, Natural Golden Beige, Beige, and Soft Rose.

☺ **$$$ Teint Dior Actuel** (*$42.50*) supposedly softens lines. Don't count on it, but this thicker, moist, creamy foundation would work nicely for someone with extremely dry skin. It blends better than you would think from the look of it. **All these colors are beautiful:** Soft Golden Beige, Soft Beige, Medium Beige, and Beige. **These colors are too peach or pink for most skin tones:** Tender Rose Beige, Delicate Rose Beige, Rose Beige, Golden Beige, and True Golden Beige.

☺ **$$$ Teint Dior Dual Poudre Foundation** (*$42.50*) is a talc-based pressed powder that is more powder than foundation. It is slightly heavier than some pressed powders, but has a slightly dry, silky finish. It is meant to be used either as an all-over foundation or as a powder. **All nine colors are excellent.**

☺ $$$ **Teint Dior Light SPF 10** *($38.50)* is an exceptionally sheer, smooth, soft, matte-finish foundation with a decent part titanium dioxide–based sunscreen. The color selection here is small and not all that varied, but most of the colors are excellent. The only ones to avoid are 202 and 203.

☹ **Basic Teint SPF 15** *($26)* is a sheer tint foundation with a part titanium dioxide–based sunscreen. The colors are a bit strange, but I was told they are meant to be worn under makeup. I don't see the point; it would only turn the makeup a strange shade. Here, 001 is white, 003 is pink, 004 is peach, 005 is peach, and 007 is bronze. The only color that is a normal skin tone is 008.

☺ $$$ **Teint Dior Compact Lisse SPF 15 (titanium dioxide–based SPF)** *($38.50)* has a soft and powdery finish, with no moist or greasy after-feel. While it claims to be oil-free, it does have waxy thickening agents that can be a problem for blemish-prone or oily skin. Though this foundation feels matte when you first put it on, it doesn't hold up well during the day if you have oily to combination skin. A word of warning, though: Even though the nonchemical sunscreen in these foundations is impressive, the sheer powdery finish makes me skeptical of how well the sunscreen actually covers the skin and therefore how well it protects, so be cautious. Dior Teint Compact Lisse comes in nine colors of which most are fairly peach or pink, and there are definitely no darker shades to choose from. **Avoid these colors:** Soft Golden, Light Golden, Deep Golden, Light Rose, Soft Rose, and Medium Rose; all of these can be too peach for most skin tones.

☺ $$$ <u>CONCEALER:</u> **Hydrating Concealer** *($19.50)* comes in a squeeze tube with a decent range of colors. It provides good coverage and has a smooth, soft finish. You can also count on minimal to no creasing. The only color to watch out for is Light Rose, which can be too pink for most skin tones.

☹ **Stick Concealer** *($18.50)* has a dry, thick texture that tends to crease into the lines around the eyes and comes in only two colors. It is recommended to be used over blemishes, but that will just contrast with your foundation color and look strange.

☺ $$$ <u>POWDER:</u> The powder selection for Dior is at best described as complicated, and as many times as I tried to grasp the differences between the products I was still left wondering. Overall the powders have a wonderful soft texture. There is a good selection of **Pressed Powder** *($35)* and **Loose Powder** *($42.50),* which come in identical shades with much improved colors. The powders have a soft dry finish and a great group of colors. **Dior Light Oil-Free Pressed Powder** *($35)* is a standard talc-based powder with a dry, silky finish.

☺ $$$ **Sun Powders Terra Bella** *($31)* are bronzers and, refreshingly, two kinds are beautifully matte though they are a bit on the peach side instead of tan; if that's what you're looking for, they're perfect. There are also two shiny ones, but you can just ignore those.

☹ **Dior Light Oil-Free Loose Powder** *($42.50)* has three shades, all with some shine. I assume that someone looking for an oil-free formulation wants to achieve a matte finish, and the iridescence in this one would negate that effect.

☺ $$$ **BLUSH: Blush Final** *($32)* has a wonderfully silky consistency and texture, although it is slightly shiny. The colors are mostly beautiful. **Powder Blush Trio** *($35)* is an interesting option, but not one to get too excited about. Of the three colors in each set, one is shiny (for highlighting), one is a brown tone (for contouring), and one is for blushing. They still have a great texture, and the options for defining are interesting, but only for special occasions; this isn't something you would want to bother with every day.

☹ **EYESHADOW:** All of Dior's eyeshadow **Singles** *($20)* and **Duos** *($30)* are fairly shiny. Plus the Duo set is arranged in such a way that it makes keeping the colors separate fairly difficult to do. The **Five Couleurs Eyeshadow Compact** *($49.50)* is very pretty to look at but not great to use. All the colors are shiny, and the combinations are too contrasting for a soft, defined look. There is also a compact of four eyeshadow colors with an accompanying eyeliner color *($49.50)*.

☺ $$$ **Powder Eyeshadow and Eyeliner Palette** *($49.50)* are four different sets of matte (well, fairly matte) colors with five shades each, and one dark powder eyeliner color. This product is actually quite good, with a wonderful silky texture, but the color combinations are a bit strange. Six colors might seem like a deal, but the amounts you are get almost negligible. **Eye Liner Compact** *($19.50)* is a set of two eyeliner colors that can be applied dry or wet. The combinations are extreme: one is white and navy and the other brown and green, not the most usable combinations of shades I can think of.

☺ $$$ **EYE AND BROW SHAPER:** The **Eye Pencil** *($19.50)* is standard fare, and like dozens of other cosmetics pencils. One end has a foam tip to soften the liner. **Kohl Pencil** *($19.50)* is a creamy finish pencil in three shades, one of which is blue. These can be a smeary mess by day's end. **Brow Pencils** *($19.50)* come in six shades; each has a rather dry texture and a brush at one end. Even though I don't care to use a pencil on the brow, this one isn't bad, although any pencil with a similar texture and a separate brow brush could function as well.

☺ $$$ **LIPSTICK AND LIP PENCIL: Rouge a Levres (Cream)** *($20)* feels very moist and creamy, almost luscious, and there are some great colors, but watch out for the frosted ones. **Rouge Accent (Matte)** *($20)* is a small collection of lipsticks that aren't all that matte, but they do go on thick, and come in more vivid colors.

Rouge Brilliant (Sheers) *($18)* is a fairly standard lip gloss that comes in a tube. **Diorific** *($20)* is just a good creamy lipstick. The **Lip Liner Pencil** *($19.50)* is a fairly standard, creamy-finish lip liner that comes in a nice array of colors and has a lipstick brush at one end. It's exceptionally overpriced for what you get.

☹ $$$ **Dior Rouge Incorruptible** *($22.50)* is one of the worst ultra-matte lipsticks I've ever tested. The clever packaging is nice: the lip color is dispensed onto a brush with two clicks of the handle and then painted on. It dries to a solid matte finish that then proceeds to pill, roll off, peel in clumps, and shred. This does not make for a pretty picture.

☺ $$$ <u>MASCARA:</u> **Fascination Mascara** *($19)* is an excellent mascara. It builds thick, ultra-long lashes in just a few coats and it holds up the entire day. While that might not be fascinating, it is good news. **Lengthening Mascara with Cashmere** *($19)* has no benefit for the lashes, as nice as cashmere sounds. Still, it's a very good mascara that builds good length without any clumping and stays all day. It also comes in colors appropriate for redheads. **Mascara Parfait** *($18)* goes on great, building beautiful thick lashes without clumping; unfortunately, it can smear by the end of the day. **Mascara Flash Highlights for Hair** *($19.50)* is nothing less than delightful hair-makeup fun! A large range of opalescent colors ranging from white to violet and lots in between go on the hair in much the same way you apply mascara to the eyelashes. What a great effect! These clever (though way too expensive) colors can create either a subtle highlight on the hair or place streaks of white, violet, or gold for a more avant garde appearance. For me, the brown shade went on only slightly shiny but the coverage nicely helped hide some gray that was peeking through due to a long-overdue date with my hairdresser. Apply the Mascara Flash where you want it (it is not safe for use on the eyes, hair only), let it dry, and then brush it through. It is only slightly stiff and sticky but completely brushable and totally water soluble.

☹ **Dioromatic Waterproof Mascara with Cashmere** *($19)* builds decent length and thickness, but it tends to clump and get thick, and then it gets really clumpy when wet.

☺ $$$ <u>BRUSHES:</u> Dior has a great range of brushes that are worth taking a look at.

Circle of Beauty

Probably the first thing you think of when you hear the name Sears is washing machines, power tools, lawnmowers, or even vacuum cleaners. Call me a snob, but even though Sears sells some impressive cosmetics lines (including Iman and Color Me Beautiful), I wouldn't exactly encourage anyone to go there for fashion inspiration. When I heard that Sears was introducing a new line of skin-care and makeup products, and that Sears had also created and developed the line, I was eager to take a look, but also very skeptical. (Actually, I'm always skeptical, no matter who makes the products or where they're sold, but Sears isn't fashion headquarters despite their advertising slogans.)

Circle of Beauty is a huge line, with more than 600 items, retailed in a very inviting, very user-friendly display. (Appropriately, the counters form a complete circle with the products on the outside.) You can play to your heart's content, with easy access to every single product, but you'll never get to all of them.

The good news is that ColorWorks, Circle of Beauty's makeup line, offers some remarkable, reasonably priced products. A significant strong point is that color choices are available for a wide range of skin tones, from the very light to the very dark. Of four foundation types, two are superior in terms of application and texture, but the SPF is a disappointing SPF 8 and includes no UVA protection. However, when it comes to blushes, both the powder and the cream-to-powder are excellent. The line also has good eye pencils, a superior cream/matte lipstick in 49 shades, and a great concealer. The eyeshadows have improved greatly, and though there aren't many matte ones, those that are work quite well.

The bad news is that the line falls abysmally on its face with the cream-to-powder foundation, a sticky, dry mess that stains the skin and comes in a limited selection of very dark orange colors. Even more bad news is Skinplicity, Circle of Beauty's skin-care line. There are five "circles" of products for five different skin types: oily, combination/oily, combination/dry, dry, and dehydrated. That's 25 products, plus an array of specialty products. There isn't much of a difference between related products in the different groupings, and often every product in a group has the same shortcomings. This can be confusing for both the consumer and the salespeople. Despite this, some products are very impressive; of course, there are some products you should absolutely ignore.

One particularly striking aspect of the skin-care line is that almost every product contains three anti-irritants known for their skin-soothing properties: bisabolol, kola nut extract, and green tea extract. Circle of Beauty refers to this as its exclusive "Trisoothal Irritation Shield." These anti-irritants are often rather high on the ingredient list. Unfortunately, many of the products also contain a batch of "essential" oils that can be skin irritants. Ylang ylang oil, lemon oil, lavender oil, geranium oil, and bergamot oil are all well-known skin sensitizers. These ingredients are really more of a nuisance than a help, although the consumer usually thinks that the "naturalness" of these oils means they are good for the skin.

Depending on what you are looking for, there are definite finds at Sears' Circle of Beauty, and when you're done you can check out the appliance department or buy a set of screwdrivers. For more information about Circle of Beauty call (212) 598-4400.

Circle of Beauty Skin Care

☹ **Come Clean Cleanser Oily Type 1** *($8.50 for 6 ounces)* is a standard deter-gent-based water-soluble cleanser that uses TEA-lauryl sulfate, which is fairly drying and can be too irritating for most skin types, as the cleansing agent. Several anti-irritants in the product will help the irritation, but not the dryness. This cleanser also contains several plant oils, especially lemon and lavender, that can be sensitizing, particularly around the eyes.

☹ **Come Clean Cleanser Combination Oily Type 2** *($8.50 for 6 ounces)* is almost identical to the Type 1 cleanser, and the same review applies. However, the Type 2 cleanser also contains sodium hydroxide (lye), which can be more drying and irritating for the skin, high on the ingredient list.

☹ **Come Clean Cleanser Combination Dry Type 3** *($8.50 for 6 ounces)* is almost identical to the Type 1 cleanser, and the same review applies.

☹ **Come Clean Cleanser Dry Type 4** *($8.50 for 6 ounces)* is more a wipe-off cleanser than a water-soluble one. It contains several thickeners, plant oil, anti-irritants, more plant oils, and preservatives. It could be good for someone with dry skin, although the plant oils can be skin sensitizers and could cause problems in the eye area.

☹ **Come Clean Cleanser Dehydrated Type 5** *($8.50 for 6 ounces)* is similar to the Type 4 cleanser, and the same review applies.

☺ **Be Delicate Dual Phase Eye Make-up Remover** *($12.50 for 4 ounces)* is a silicone-based eye-makeup remover with some anti-irritants. It can feel good on the skin though I don't recommend wiping off makeup.

☺ **Easy Go Eye Make-up Remover** *($8.50 for 6 ounces)* is a standard deter-gent-based makeup remover. It will take off makeup but wiping off makeup isn't the best idea.

☹ **Be Smooth Face and Body Exfoliator** *($10 for 4 ounces)* is a standard deter-gent-based water-soluble cleanser that uses TEA-lauryl sulfate, which is fairly drying and can be too irritating for most skin types, as the cleansing agent. The abrasive in this product is also unnecessarily harsh.

☹ **Skin Refiner Oily Type 1** *($8.50 for 8 ounces)* is an alcohol-based toner that is too irritating and drying for all skin types. Alcohol can cause problems for the skin.

☹ **Skin Refiner Combination Oily Type 2** *($8.50 for 8 ounces)* is almost iden-tical to the Type 1 refiner, and the same review applies.

☹ **Skin Refiner Combination Dry Type 3** *($8.50 for 8 ounces)* is very similar to the Type 1 refiner, and the same review applies.

☺ **Skin Refiner Dry Type 4** *($8.50 for 8 ounces)* contains mostly water, slip agent, anti-irritants, water-binding agent, vitamin E, several plant oils, and preserva-tives. Some of the plant oils can be skin sensitizers and irritating for the skin.

☺ **Skin Refiner Dehydrated Type 5** *($8.50 for 8 ounces)* is similar to the Type 4 refiner, and the same review applies.

☺ **All Even AHA Skin Serum Oily Type 1, 2, 3, 4, 5** *($15 for 1 ounce)* do contain lactic acid, but the pH here isn't low enough to permit it to work as an exfoliant.

☹ **Action + Moisture Cream Oily Type 1, SPF 8** *($16 for 4 ounces)* is a disappointment with its low SPF 8; it doesn't contain avobenzone, zinc oxide, or titanium dioxide and is not recommended.

☹ **Action + Moisture Cream Combination Oily Type 2, SPF 8** *($16 for 4 ounces)* is a disappointment with its low SPF 8; it doesn't contain avobenzone, zinc oxide, or titanium dioxide, and is not recommended.

☹ **Action + Moisture Cream Combination Dry Type 3, SPF 8** *($16 for 4 ounces)* is a disappointment with its low SPF 8; it doesn't contain avobenzone, zinc oxide, or titanium dioxide, and is not recommended.

☹ **Action + Moisture Cream Dry Type 4, SPF 8** *($16 for 4 ounces)* is a disappointment with its low SPF 8; it doesn't contain avobenzone, zinc oxide, or titanium dioxide, and is not recommended.

☹ **Action + Moisture Cream Dehydrated Type 5, SPF 8** *($16 for 4 ounces)* is a disappointment with its low SPF 8; it doesn't contain avobenzone, zinc oxide, or titanium dioxide, and is not recommended.

☹ **Action + Moisture Lotion Oily Type 1, SPF 8** *($16 for 4 ounces)* is a disappointment with its low SPF 8; it doesn't contain avobenzone, zinc oxide, or titanium dioxide, and is not recommended.

☹ **Action + Moisture Lotion Combination Oily Type 2, SPF 8** *($16.50 for 4 ounces)* is a disappointment with its low SPF 8; it doesn't contain avobenzone, zinc oxide, or titanium dioxide, and is not recommended.

☹ **Action + Moisture Lotion Combination Dry Type 3, SPF 8** *($16.50 for 4 ounces)* is a disappointment with its low SPF 8; it doesn't contain avobenzone, zinc oxide, or titanium dioxide, and is not recommended.

☹ **Action + Moisture Lotion Dry Type 4, SPF 8** *($16.50 for 4 ounces)* is a disappointment with its low SPF 8; it doesn't contain avobenzone, zinc oxide, or titanium dioxide, and is not recommended.

☹ **Action + Moisture Lotion Dehydrated Type 5, SPF 8** *($16.50 for 4 ounces)* is a disappointment with its low SPF 8; it doesn't contain avobenzone, zinc oxide, or titanium dioxide, and is not recommended.

☺ **Lighten It Eye Cream** *($8.50 for 0.6 ounce)* is just a mineral oil–based moisturizer with titanium dioxide that leaves a slight white layer behind on the skin. This can be good for dry skin, but it isn't really lightening anything.

☺ **Overnight Eye Treatment** *($15 for 0.6 ounce)* contains mostly water, thickener, mineral oil, more thickeners, anti-irritants, more thickeners, and preservatives.

This isn't much of a treatment, but it is emollient, and the anti-irritants could be good for the eye area.

☹ **Moisture Wrap Peel Off Mask** *($8.50 for 5.5 ounces)* contains mostly plastic, alcohol, anti-irritants, plant oils, and preservatives. Alcohol and plastic won't moisturize anyone's skin, and the anti-irritants can't stop the irritation caused by the alcohol.

☹ **Over and Out Blemish Cream** *($8.50 for 0.5 ounce)* contains zinc oxide and cornstarch high up on the ingredient list and both of those can clog pores, not great for a blemish product.

☺ **Pore Purge Clay Mask** *($10.50 for 8 ounces)* is a standard clay mask with the same anti-irritants and plant oils as the rest of the Skinplicity line. It would be good for someone with normal to oily skin, but it can't empty pores any better than any other clay mask, which is to say, it won't do much.

☹ **Smooth Off Lip Buffer** *($8.50 for 0.12 ounce)* is too abrasive (with its ground walnut shells) for the lips, and the peppermint extract will burn them.

Circle of Beauty Makeup

☹ <u>FOUNDATION:</u> **Skin Image Soft Matte Makeup SPF 8** *($11.50)* has an excellent shine-free finish and provides medium coverage, while **Skin Image Dewy Moist Makeup SPF 8** *($11.50)* has a sheer, moist texture. But for both of these, the low SPF is a problem and there are no UVA protecting ingredients.

☺ **Skin Image Wet or Dry Makeup** *($12.50)* is a standard talc-based powder that you can apply wet or dry. It is a decent alternative for a light layer of makeup, but do not try to apply this wet, it will only streak and look choppy. The colors also tend to be on the peach side, so be very careful testing this one; be sure to check it out in bright daylight.

☹ **Skin Image Cream to Powder Makeup** *($12.50)* feels thick and sticky, blends poorly, stains the skin, and the color choices are poor to awful. Most of the colors are too orange, too peach, or too yellow. **Skin Image Primer** *($10)* is a color corrector that comes only in green. I don't recommend color correctors under makeup anyway, so don't worry about the fact that the only skin color this line thought needed correcting was red. Foundation should be all the skin needs to correct any uneven skin tones. **Skin Image Highlighter** *($10)* is a shiny pink liquid. I wouldn't recommend using it even if I could explain how to wear it.

☺ <u>CONCEALER:</u> **Out of Sight Sponge-on Concealer** *($7)* comes in six shades that are just borderline OK; these aren't the best for most skin tones.

☺ **No Flaw Maximum Cover Concealer** *($7)* is outstanding. **The color selection is great,** the texture is soft, it doesn't crease, and, best of all, it covers well without being heavy or thick.

☺ <u>POWDER:</u> **Natural Finish Press Powder** *($9)* is a standard talc-based pow-
der with a good color selection and a sheer, soft texture. The only problem is that it
tends to be on the dry side. It would be appropriate only for someone with normal to
oily skin. **Natural Finish Loose Powder** *($12)* has a soft, light texture with good
colors, though it too is slightly on the dry side.

☺ <u>BLUSH:</u> **Blush Lightly** *($10)* has a soft texture and a nice array of colors for
a wide range of skin tones, but some of the colors can grab the skin, meaning they go
on stronger than they appear in the container, or they tend to go on choppy, so test
them before buying. **Sun Pretender Powder** *($10)* is a bronzing powder; two shades
are shiny, but one is surprisingly matte and an option if you are into this sort of
thing. Of course, no one thinks a colored powder dusted over the face looks like a
real tan, unless you're already tan, which you shouldn't be, right?

☺ **Blush Creamy Cream-to-Powder** *($10)* has a soft, silky-sheer texture and
application. The color selection is small but beautiful.

☺ <u>EYESHADOW:</u> Both the **Eyeshadow Singles** *($8)* and **Duos** *($11.50)* have
greatly improved since I last reviewed them. The matte shades go on smoothly and
evenly and have decent staying power. But for the most part the other colors are not
only shiny, they are strange shades that seem dated and unusable.

☺ <u>EYE AND BROW SHAPER:</u> **Stroke Up Brow Pencil** *($7)* is a twist-up
pencil that comes in four colors and has a soft, easy-to-use texture. "Twist-up" means
no sharpening required, which I appreciate. **Eye Defining Pencil** *($7)* is also a twist-
up, and has a texture identical to the Brow Pencil. **Color Up Brow Cake** *($8)* is a
powder for the brow; it works well, and the color selections are great. The little stiff
brush this comes packaged with is best thrown out; buy a softer professional-sized
brush that can effectively fill in the brows without hurting the skin. **Groom Up
Brow Gel** *($8)* is simply hair-spray ingredients in a clear gel. It will softly keep your
brows in place.

☺ <u>LIPSTICK AND LIP PENCIL:</u> I love to find a good lipstick that doesn't
bleed, since most lipsticks run into the lines around my mouth. **Satin Matte Lipstick**
($8.50) is wonderful, and with 49 colors to choose from, you are likely to find one
you like. **Rich Lasting Cream Lipstick** *($8.50)* is more greasy than creamy. It does
have a stain that makes the color last longer than usual. **Crystal Cream** *($6)* is a pot
of gloss that comes in four colors; they are all extremely iridescent, with sparkle that
doesn't quit. **Lip Comfort** *($8.50)* is a very emollient, lipstick-applicator lip gloss
that can help keep lips moist and prevent chapping.

☹ **Sheer Treat Lipstick** *($8.50)* is just a sheer translucent hint of color that
claims to have a sunscreen, but no SPF is indicated and no active ingredients are listed,
so do not rely on this claim. **Smooth-Off Lip Buffer** *($8.50)* is just a gloss with some
walnut shells in it; it doesn't do much for the lips and is a waste of time and effort.

☹   <u>MASCARA:</u> Your lashes won't be able to tell the difference between the **Long and Silky Mascara** *($8)* and the **Velvety Lashes Mascara** *($8)*. Neither comes close to living up to most of the claims in the package insert. They don't build well, especially Velvety Lashes, which clumps, and it takes a long time to get any thickness or length.

☺   **Waterplay Lashes** *($8)* builds nice length but it does tend to clump. At least it does end up being fairly waterproof. **Hair Glazer** *($8.50)* is a hair mascara that works as well as any, but the three colors are a limitation.

☺   <u>BRUSHES:</u> This line has a small but attractive group of brushes you might want to check out. The **Eyeshadow Brush** *($6.50)*, **Blush Brush** *($9.50)*, and **Face Brush** *($13.50)* are all soft, have a good amount of density, and are easy to use.

Clarins

Clarins offers an imposing procession of skin-care products. Besides their standout red-and-white packaging and French breeding, Clarins is also capitalizing heavily on the "botanical" craze of the '90s. The ingredient lists, full of usual and unusual herbs, flowers, and vegetables, are a veritable jungle, and the labels make the far-out promises that usually accompany these ingredients. Like Aveda, Origins, The Body Shop, and dozens of other lines, Clarins wants you to believe that a little herb concentrate can do wonders for your skin. However, according to *Rodale's Illustrated Encyclopedia of Herbs*, many of the extracts used in Clarins' products (as well as other botanical-type lines) are potentially irritating. For example, according to this encyclopedia, coltsfoot is potentially carcinogenic, and sage and horsetail extracts can cause skin irritation. Always keep in mind that "natural" and "good" are not the same thing; many natural things in the environment are bad for the skin.

One of Clarins' brochures says, "Clarins promises no miracles, only effective results [from] time-proven natural extracts." Yet claim after claim sounds like a miracle. This line even has "bust-firming" products. Doesn't that sound like a miracle? (It would be for me.) Other claims that sound fairly miraculous to me include "maintains firm facial features," "takes advantage of the beneficial toning action of facial expressions while helping to reduce apparent slackening," and "refines skin texture, firms skin tone." "Proven" is obviously a relative term.

One shocking piece of misinformation can be found on page 36 of the Clarins brochure, which claims "dermatologists state that more than 75% of skin aging results from wide-ranging temperature and humidity changes…" That simply isn't true. You couldn't find a dermatologist who would say that. Every published dermatological paper over the past ten years reiterates that sun is the major cause of aging, followed by (a close second) the fact that we do get old. But the sun is the worst culprit of all.

Clarins' foundation shades have improved, but there are still some fairly peach and pink shades to avoid. The eyeshadows have become more matte, and that's great, and the blushes have a soft, silky texture with some great soft tones. The counter display is now divided into five color groupings—Corals, Red, Plum, Pink, and Brown—which is helpful. For more information about Clarins call (212) 980-1800.

Clarins Skin Care

☹ **Cleansing Milk with Alpine Herbs Dry or Normal Skin** *($25 for 8.6 ounces)* is recommended for people with dry to normal skin, according to its label, but the alpine herbs (mint, arnica, and pine) can cause skin irritation and drying, which makes it a poor product for this skin type. Other than that, this is a standard cleanser that doesn't rinse off very well and can leave a film on the skin.

☹ **Cleansing Milk with Gentian Oily/Combination Skin** *($25 for 8.6 ounces)* is almost identical to the cleanser above except that the herbs are different, and they have no effect on oily skin.

☺ **$$$ Extra-Comfort Cleansing Cream with Bio-Ecolia Very Dry or Sensitized Skin** *($30 for 7 ounces)* contains mostly water, plant oil, several thickeners, silicone, and preservatives. This rather ordinary cleanser needs to be wiped off and can leave a greasy film. I am always skeptical when a product with fragrance claims to be good for sensitive skin.

☹ **Gentle Foaming Cleanser** *($19 for 4.4 ounces)* is a very drying water-soluble cleanser for any skin type. It contains strong detergent cleansing agents and potassium hydroxide rather high up on the ingredient list.

☺ **$$$ Oil-Control Cleansing Gel Oily Skin with Breakout Tendencies** *($18 for 4.4 ounces)* is a standard detergent-based water-soluble cleanser that can be drying for some skin types. It won't control oil, but it will clean the skin.

☺ **$$$ Gentle Eye Make-Up Remover Cream-Gel** *($16.50 for 2.7 ounces)* isn't exactly gentle. It will take off eye makeup, but the third ingredient is fairly alkaline and can be a skin irritant.

☺ **$$$ Gentle Eye Make-Up Remover Lotion** *($16.50 for 3.4 ounces)* is mostly rose water (glycerin and water), plant extract, slip agents, and preservatives. It's gentle enough, but pretty ordinary, and unnecessary if the other cleansers in this line worked.

☺ **$$$ Gentle Exfoliating Refiner for Face** *($21 for 1.7 ounces)* contains mostly water, several thickeners, plant extract, and preservatives. The exfoliating fibers are synthetic pieces of nylon, not all that harsh, but gentle is a relative term.

☺ **$$$ Extra-Comfort Toning Lotion Very Dry or Sensitized Skin** *($25 for 8.8 ounces)* contains mostly water, aloe, silicone, slip agents, plant extracts, film formers, fragrance, and preservatives. Plenty of ingredients in this product can be problematic for sensitive skin, but it could be a good irritant-free toner for dry skin.

☺ **$$$ Toning Lotion for Dry to Normal Skin** *($21 for 8.4 ounces)* contains mostly water, slip agents, plant extract, fragrance, and preservatives. This is a fairly good irritant-free toner.

☹ **Toning Lotion for Oily/Combination Skin** *($21 for 8.4 ounces)* is an alcohol-free toner that contains water, aloe, plant extracts, slip agents, witch hazel, and preservatives. Several of the plant extracts (orris root and guava) as well as the witch hazel are possible irritants and provide no benefit for oily skin.

☹ **Balancing Night Gel for Oily Skin with Breakout Tendencies** *($25 for 1 ounce)* contains water, film former, slip agents, plant extracts, fragrance, and preservative. Several of the plant extracts can be skin irritants.

☺ **$$$ Extra-Firming Day Cream All Skin Types** *($50 for 1.7 ounces)* is a good emollient moisturizer for someone with dry skin, but there is nothing in here that will firm skin. It contains mostly water, plant oil, thickeners, film former, silicone, water-binding agents, and preservatives. The emollients and thickeners in here are not appropriate for all skin types.

☺ **$$$ Extra-Firming Day Cream for Dry Skin** *($50 for 1.7 ounces)* is, like the one above, not great for daytime because it lacks sunscreen, but it is a good emollient moisturizer for very dry skin, similar to the one above.

☺ **$$$ Extra-Firming Night Cream All Skin Types** *($60 for 1.7 ounces)* contains mostly water, mineral oil, thickeners, water-binding agent, slip agent, plant oils, plant extracts, anti-irritant, glycerin, fragrance, thickeners, water-binding agents, and preservatives. This is a good moisturizer for someone with normal to dry skin, but the claims about being extra-firming stretch what these standard cosmetic ingredients can really do.

☺ **$$$ Face Treatment Plant Cream "Blue Orchid" for Dehydrated Skin** *($29 for 1.7 ounces)* is a good standard mineral oil–based moisturizer for dry skin. It contains mostly water, mineral oil, plant oil, thickeners, silicone, lanolin oil, plant extracts, fragrance, and preservatives.

☹ **Face Treatment Plant Cream "Lotus" for Combination Skin Prone to Oiliness** *($29 for 1.7 ounces)* is virtually identical to the cream above (but minus the lanolin) and so is still completely inappropriate for someone with combination or oily skin. Plus, several of the ingredients in here, including lemon and grapefruit, can be irritants.

☺ **$$$ Face Treatment Cream for Dry or Reddened Skin** *($29 for 1.7 ounces)* is a good, emollient moisturizer that contains mostly water, mineral oil, vegetable oils, thickeners, rice bran oil, a small amount of sunscreen (not enough to protect the skin), lanolin oil, water-binding agents, preservatives, and herb extracts. There is nothing about this product special for reddened skin.

☺ **$$$ Face Treatment Plant Cream "Santal" for Dry or Extra Dry Skin** *($29 for 1.7 ounces)* is almost identical to the cream above, and the same review applies.

☺ **$$$ Firming Neck Cream For A Youthful Neck** *($50 for 1.7 ounces)* is said to be for the neck and not the face, but why is anyone's guess: there is nothing in here that will lift the neck. This is an incredibly ordinary moisturizer containing water, silicone, thickeners, plant oil, and preservatives. It is a good moisturizer for slightly dry skin.

☺ $$$ **Gentle Day Cream for Sensitive Skin** *($39 for 1.7 ounces)* contains mostly water, mineral oil, several thickeners, silicone, more thickeners, anti-irritants, and preservatives. This is a very good but rather ordinary mineral oil–based moisturizer for dry skin. Because it contains no sunscreen, it isn't best for daytime wear, unless your foundation contains one.

☺ $$$ **Gentle Night Cream for Sensitive Skin** *($49 for 1.7 ounces)* is almost identical to the cream above, and the same review applies. Vitamins are present in this cream, but only in negligible quantities. Why this product is more expensive than the one above is a complete mystery.

☺ $$$ **Hydration-Plus Moisture Lotion for All Skin Types** *($30 for 1.7 ounces)* contains mostly water, slip agent, thickener, silicone, film former, more thickeners, water-binding agents, plant extracts, more slip agents, vitamin E, and preservatives. This is a good lightweight moisturizer for someone with normal to somewhat dry skin.

☺ $$$ **Hydration-Plus Moisture Lotion SPF 15 for All Skin Types** *($30 for 1.7 ounces)* is similar to the Hydration-Plus above, only with sunscreen (part titanium dioxide). Now this is a daytime sunscreen your skin can live with, although the price isn't warranted for what you get.

☹ **Moisturizing Tint SPF 6 with Plant Marine "Cell Extracts"** *($27 for 1.7 ounces)* has a SPF 6, but that's not a number you should count on despite the fact this is a titanium dioxide–based sunscreen.

☺ $$$ **Multi-Active Day Cream for All Skin Types** *($45 for 1.7 ounces)* is a good though extremely ordinary moisturizer for normal to dry skin that contains mostly water, thickeners, aloe, silicone, plant oils, fragrance, anti-irritants, and preservatives.

☺ $$$ **Multi-Active Day Cream "Speciale" for Very Dry Skin** *($45 for 1.7 ounces)* isn't all that special or all that different from the cream above, and the same review applies. It is slightly more emollient, but only slightly.

☺ $$$ **Multi-Active Night Lotion for All Skin Types** *($50 for 1.7 ounces)* contains mostly water, thickeners, plant oil, film former, more thickeners, plant extracts, more thickeners, more film formers, more plant oils, and preservatives. This is a good moisturizer for someone with dry skin, but other skin types will find the oil and thickening agents too emollient. It does contain a tiny amount of vitamins, but not enough to help your skin at all.

☺ $$$ **Multi-Active Night Lotion Very Dry Skin** *($50 for 1.7 ounces)* is almost identical to the lotion above, and the same review applies.

☹ **Multi-Tenseur Skin Firming Concentrate** *($47.50 for 1 ounce)* contains mostly water, aloe, plant extracts, water-binding agent, slip agents, preservatives, and fragrance—rather ordinary ingredients for this kind of money. However, if you believe condurango extract (from the bark of the condurango tree—the third ingredient in this product) can firm the skin, you probably should get your money back on my book right now!

☹ **Oil Control Moisture Lotion** *($25 for 1.06 ounces)* contains little that will control oil, but some ingredients could be problematic for someone with oily skin. The main ingredients are water, silicone, several thickeners, plant extracts, fragrance, and preservatives.

☺ **$$$ Revitalizing Moisture Cream with Plant Marine "Cell Extract"** *($50 for 1.7 ounces)* contains boring ingredients, in contrast to its long, beguiling name. It contains mostly water, mineral oil, several thickeners, glycerin, petrolatum, more thickeners, water-binding agents, a tiny amount of plant extracts, fragrance, and preservatives. The amount of plant marine extract is so minuscule as to make the company look silly for putting it in the name of the product. This is a good, but exceedingly overpriced, moisturizer for someone with dry skin.

☺ **$$$ Revitalizing Moisture Base with Plant Marine "Cell Extract" for All Skin Types** *($30 for 1.1 ounces)* is similar to the one above, only in a more lotion-like form.

☺ **$$$ Self Tanning Gel without Sunscreen** *($21 for 4.4 ounces)*, as all self-tanners do, uses a form of dihydroxyacetone to turn the skin brown.

☺ **$$$ Self Tanning Milk SPF 6** *($21 for 4.4 ounces)* contains less than an SPF 15 and is not recommended for outdoor use, but as a self-tanner it works just fine.

☹ **Sun Care Gel Intensive Tanning SPF 3** *($18.50 for 4.4 ounces)* contains far less than SPF 15 and is not recommended. Doesn't it seem ironic that a skin-care company selling so many anti-wrinkling products would sell a sunscreen encouraging tanning? Isn't that like a lung cancer specialist selling cigarettes?

☹ **Sun Care Oil Intensive Tanning, SPF 3** *($18.50 for 5.8 ounces)* contains far less than SPF 15 and is not recommended. The same comments apply as for the product above.

☹ **Sun Care Milk Advanced Tanning SPF 6** *($18.50 for 4.4 ounces)* contains less than an SPF 15 and is not recommended.

☹ **Sun Care Milk High Protection SPF 10** *($18.50 for 4.4 ounces)* contains less than an SPF 15 and is not recommended.

☺ **$$$ Sun Block SPF 25 Ultra Protection for Face/Sensitive Areas** *($19.50 for 2.7 ounces)* is a good in-part titanium dioxide–based sunscreen for dry skin, but there is nothing about this formula that would make it better for sensitive skin. For sensitive skin a pure titanium dioxide or pure zinc oxide base sunscreen would be best.

☺ **$$$ Sun Block Stick SPF 19 Sensitive Areas** *($16.50 for 0.17 ounce)* is a good in-part titanium dioxide–based sunscreen for very dry skin. But much like the SPF 25 above, this one is not in any way preferred for someone with sensitive skin.

☺ **Sun Care Cream SPF 15** *($18.50 for 4.4 ounces)* is a partly nonchemical sunscreen that contains thickeners, silicone, film former, plant oil, water-binding agents, and preservatives. This is a good sunscreen for someone with dry skin.

☹ **Sun Care Gel SPF 15** *($18.50 for 4.3 ounces)* doesn't contain avobenzone, zinc oxide, or titanium dioxide, and is not recommended.

☺ **$$$ Sun Care Milk SPF 19** *($18.50 for 2.7 ounces)* is a very good in-part titanium dioxide–based sunscreen and would be good for someone with dry skin.

☹ **Sun Wrinkle Control Cream SPF 15** *($19.50 for 2.7 ounces)* doesn't contain avobenzone, zinc oxide, or titanium dioxide, and is not recommended.

☺ **$$$ After Sun Gel Ultra Soothing** *($20 for 5.3 ounces)* is a good, ordinary, extremely lightweight gel moisturizer that contains mostly water, silicone, aloe, slip agents, and thickeners.

☺ **$$$ After Sun Moisturizer** *($20 for 5.3 ounces)* is a good emollient moisturizer that contains mostly water, mineral oil, thickeners, emollients, fragrance, preservatives, and vitamins.

☺ **$$$ After Sun Moisturizer with Self Tanning Action** *($20 for 5.3 ounces)*, like all self-tanners, uses the ingredient dihydroxyacetone to turn the skin brown. This one works as well as any.

☺ **$$$ After Sun Skin Conditioner with Plant Extracts** *($22.50 for 1.4 ounces)* is a good moisturizer that contains mostly water, thickeners, emollient, silicone, plant oils, water-binding agents, anti-irritants, and preservatives.

☹ **Absorbent Mask Oily Skin with Breakout Tendencies** *($19 for 1.7 ounces)* is a very standard clay mask that contains mostly water, clay, thickeners, plant extracts, and preservatives. It will absorb oil, but there are irritating ingredients in here that can be a problem for the skin.

☹ **Beauty Flash Balm** *($30 for 1.7 ounces)* is an extremely average moisturizer that contains mostly water, slip agent, several thickeners, witch hazel, plant extract, water-binding agent, anti-irritant, and preservatives. Witch hazel and rice starch can be problematic for most skin types.

☺ **$$$ Bio-Ecolia Perfecting Creme-Mask with Controlled Fruit Acids** *($39 for 1.7 ounces)* supposedly contains "controlled fruit acids." There are no such things as controlled (or uncontrolled) alpha hydroxy acids. This mask contains a tiny amount of AHAs, probably not more than a 2% concentration. Otherwise, it is an OK mask for someone with normal to slightly dry skin. All of the ingredients are fairly standard cosmetic thickeners and water-binding agents. Some amino acids show up at the end of the ingredient list; they could be interesting water-binding agents, but that's about it.

☺ **$$$ Blemish Gel** *($14 for 0.53 ounce)* contains water, slip agent, glycerin, plant extracts, zinc sulfate, preservatives, tea tree oil, and witch hazel, in a tiny bottle. Zinc sulfate, orris root, and witch hazel can prove irritating and won't do much for blemishes. The amount of tea tree oil is too minuscule to do much good, and there is no evidence it has a positive effect on breakouts.

☺ **$$$ Double Serum 38 Extra Firming Skin Supplement** *($65 for 0.5 ounce)* is a mixture of several plant oils ranging from hazelnut to apricot, sesame, and avocado. There are a handful of cosmetic thickening agents thrown in and some vitamins, but for the most part this is oil straight out of your kitchen cabinet. This can be great for dry skin, but the price is absurd for what you get. You could get the exact same effect by mixing your own plant oils together (non-fragrance types like the ones I've mentioned, to reduce the risk of irritation), or just use pure sesame oil at night over excessively dry areas of your face or body.

☺ **$$$ Double Serum Total Skin Supplement, Plant Based Concentrate Hydro Serum and Lipo Serum** *($70 for two 0.5-ounce bottles)* claims to control the appearance of aging, but mixing these two liquids together does little to control aging or anything else. Together they contain mostly water, rose water, silicones, plant oils, mineral oil, water-binding agents, film former, slip agents, plant extracts, and preservatives. Vitamins, plant extracts, and oyster extracts are also present, in amounts so tiny they are essentially nonexistent. This would be a good lightweight moisturizer for most skin types, but the claims are absurd. Of course, one should wonder, if any of the other multitude of antiwrinkle products in this line worked, why would you need this overpriced stuff?

☺ **$$$ Eye Contour Balm** *($30 for 0.7 ounce)* contains water, thickeners, water-binding agent, film former, and preservatives. This would be an OK but ordinary moisturizer for dry skin.

☺ **$$$ Eye Contour Balm "Special" for Very Dry Skin** *($30 for 0.7 ounce)* contains mostly water, thickeners, mineral oil, plant oil, more thickeners, water-binding agent, anti-irritant, silicone, plant extracts, and preservatives. This isn't special—it's actually quite typical—but it would be a good moisturizer for someone with dry skin.

☺ **$$$ Eye Contour Gel** *($30 for 0.7 ounce)* is mostly water, plant extracts, more plant extracts, thickeners, film former, and preservatives. This is an OK lightweight moisturizer for slightly dry skin.

☹ **Face Treatment Oil "Blue Orchid" for Dehydrated Skin** *($33 for 1.4 ounces)* contains hazelnut oil, patchouli oil (mint), rosewood oil, fragrance, and orchid extract. The patchouli oil and fragrance can be irritating to the skin.

☹ **Face Treatment Oil "Santal" for Dry or Reddened Skin** *($33 for 1.4 ounces)* contains hazelnut, sandalwood, cardamom, parsley seed, hayflower, and lavender oils. Sandalwood, parsley, and lavender oils can all cause skin irritation, which isn't great for someone with reddened skin.

☹ **Face Treatment Oil "Lotus" for Combination Skin/Prone to Oiliness** *($33 for 1.4 ounces)* contains hazelnut oil, geranium oil, fragrance, rosemary oil, lotus extract, chamomile oil, and sage oil. This product is supposed to help "balance" surface oils. What it does is place more oils on the skin, and the chamomile, rosemary, and sage oils can be irritants. Someone with oily skin could end up with oilier, more irritated skin.

☹ **$$$ Face Treatment Oil "Santal" Dry or Extra Dry Skin** *($33 for 1.4 ounces)* is mostly hazelnut oil, along with some fragrant oils of cardamom and lavender. The fragrance can be irritating and you can get hazelnut oil at the grocery store for far less and with no risk of allergic reaction.

☹ **$$$ Gentle Facial Peeling** *($25 for 1.4 ounces)* will exfoliate the skin, something that happens any time you rub wax or clay over the skin, which is what you would be doing with this product. That isn't bad, but rubbing can be hard on the skin. There are easier ways to exfoliate.

☺ **$$$ Purifying Plant Facial Mask** *($23.50 for 1.7 ounces)* contains mostly water, talc, mineral oil, thickeners, clay, plant extracts, film former, fragrance, and preservatives. It won't purify anything, but it is a good mask for someone with dry skin.

☺ **$$$ Revitalizing Moisture Mask with Plant Marine "Cell Extract" for All Skin Types** *($28 for 1.7 ounces)* is mostly water, thickeners, glycerin, plant extracts, water-binding agents, fragrance, and preservatives. This is a good mask for someone with dry skin, but "cell extract" must be in quotation marks because it has no meaning.

☹ **Skin Beauty Repair Concentrate** *($42 for 0.5 ounce)* includes some plant oils, particularly peppermint and lavender oil, that can cause skin damage via the irritation they cause.

☹ **$$$ Skin-Smoothing Eye Mask with Plant Extracts** *($35 for 1.05 ounces)* is an OK emollient moisturizer for dry skin, nothing less, nothing more. The third ingredient is rice starch, which can be a skin sensitizer for some skin types.

☺ **$$$ Lip Beauty Multi-Treatment** *($16.50 for 0.09 ounce)* is a standard emollient lip gloss with standard thickeners, castor oil, emollients, and plant oils. It is good for dry lips, but to spend this kind of money on such an ordinary "gloss" is almost embarrassing.

☹ **"Cellulite" Control Gel** *($41.50 for 5.3 ounces).* I wasn't going to review products like these and the "bust" products that follow, but I couldn't help myself. The quotation marks around the word cellulite are a way for Clarins to get around the truth-in-advertising laws. Quotes allow a great deal of leeway in how a word is legally defined. In this case, what the company legally means by "cellulite" is totally different from what they want you to think they mean. You think they are referring to the bumpy fat in your thighs, but what they legally mean is only the surface texture of the skin (the appearance of cellulite). Because of the quotation marks, the interpretation is vague enough that truth-in-advertising laws haven't been breached. The second ingredient in this product is alcohol, which irritates and swells the skin. This irritation may reduce the appearance of bumps on the surface of the skin for a few minutes. Of course, you could buy a bottle of rubbing alcohol and get the same results for 89 cents. Aside from all that, you cannot burn or beat up fat from the outside in, so save your money.

☹ **Plant Milk for Bust Beauty Tightening and Toning** *($35 for 1.7 ounces)* doesn't deserve an explanation, but for those of you who wonder what could possibly be in a product that claims to "tighten" and "tone" your breasts, the ingredients are water; mineral oil; thickeners; fragrance; more thickeners; hop, fennel, and lemon extracts (which can all cause skin sensitivities); and preservatives.

☹ **Bust Firming Gel** *($42 for 1.7 ounces)* contains water, fish protein (skin cells from a dead fish), algae extract (seaweed juice), plant extracts, and thickeners. If you believe this product can work, I have a bridge you may be interested in.

Clarins Makeup

☹ <u>FOUNDATION:</u> **Satin Finish Foundation** *($29.50)* has a lightweight texture, but it isn't particularly satiny. The squeeze tube makes it difficult to control the amount that comes out, so a lot will get wasted if you aren't careful. Most of the colors are way too pink or peach to recommend.

☺ **$$$ Matte Finish Foundation** *($29.50)* is a fairly matte foundation that goes on light and does have a nice soft, matte finish. Of the ten shades available, only Beige Sable, Soft Beige, and Golden Honey are too peach or pink for most skin tones.

☺ **$$$ Oil-free Ultra Matte Foundation** *($29.50)* is a good matte foundation with a disappointing range of colors. Of the eight shades available, four are too peach. **Colors to avoid:** Cool Beige, Warm Beige, Honey Beige, and Subtle Beige.

☺ **$$$ Compact Powder Foundation** *($29.50)* isn't all that different from the Pressed Powder below. It goes on soft and sheer, with a lovely satin finish. All of the colors are rather good, with only Natural Sand and Soft Beige to be cautious about; they can be slightly too peach for some skin tones.

☹ **Color Veil** *($27)* is supposed to correct the skin's color, but these four mostly peach and orange shades, and one shiny white color, will only cause more pigment problems.

☹ **Moisturizing Tint Foundation SPF 6** *($28.50)* has four poor shades, a dismal SPF, and no UVA protection.

☺ <u>CONCEALER:</u> **Concealer** *($14.50)* comes in three shades: Light, which is too pink for most skin tones; Medium, which is darker than what I would call medium but still a good color; and Dark, which isn't all that dark but is also OK. It has a dry finish and it tends not to crease, but the color choices leave much to be desired.

☹ <u>POWDER:</u> The **Powder Compact Pressed Powder** *($24)* has a lovely texture but comes in a poor color selection.

☺ $$$ **Bronzing Duo** *($24)* is a single compact with two shades of brown; both are matte. One is slightly peach, so try it on before you buy it (though it could make for a good blush color).

☺ $$$ <u>BLUSH:</u> **Powder Blush** *($21)* has a beautiful soft texture and great colors. Most of the colors are fairly matte and worth checking out.

☺ $$$ <u>EYESHADOW:</u> **Duo Eyeshadow Sets** *($23)* have some amount of shine, but of all the colors there are several that are fairly matte and blend on quite soft and sheer for a soft, subtle look (you won't get drama out of these colors). The combinations are actually quite workable; take a closer look at Biscuit/Sable, Toast/Mocha, Nude/Plum, and Wine/Malt.

☺ $$$ **Soft Shimmer Eye Colour Singles** *($15)* are a group of very soft, light pastel, and very shiny eyeshadows. I'm sure there is a reason to consider these, I just can't think of one.

☺ $$$ <u>EYE AND BROW SHAPER:</u> The **Eye Liner Pencil** *($13.50)* is a standard pencil that has a soft texture and comes in a nice array of colors. The consistency can be a bit creamy, so watch out for smearing. One end of the pencil has a sponge tip for softening the line. The **Brow Pencil** *($14)* has a firm texture and comes in a small but good group of colors. One end is a brush, which is a nice touch for softening the effect of the pencil.

☺ $$$ <u>LIPSTICK AND LIP PENCIL:</u> Clarins has one of the more impressive selections of red lip colors to be found anywhere. You can rouge up your lips to your heart's content. **Sheer Lipstick** *($16)* is more gloss than lipstick and has minimal staying power. **Cream Lipstick** *($16)* has a soft texture and a slight tint, which helps it stay around for a while. **Shimmer Lipstick** *($16)* is a slightly shiny, glossy lipstick. The **Lip Liner Pencil** *($13.50)* is a standard pencil that has a good, easy-to-apply texture and an attractive color selection. One end is a lipstick brush, which is convenient.

☹ $$$ <u>MASCARA:</u> **Lengthening Mascara** *($15.50)* doesn't build much length or thickness, especially not in comparison to Clarins' Volumizing mascara, but if you don't need much length or thickness, this would be an option, because it doesn't flake or smear during the day.

☺ $$$ **Volumizing Mascara** *($15.50)* is rather impressive. It just builds long thick lashes with no clumping and it lasts all day.

☹ $$$ <u>BRUSHES:</u> Clarins has a collection of brushes that aren't the best. The bristles are soft enough but the **Powder Brush** *($25)* is too large for most applications and face sizes, while the **Blush Brush** *($22)* is way to small to get an even application of blush over the cheek. The **Angle Brush** *($17.50)* is rather stiff, while the **Eyeshadow Brush** *($17.50)* is an interesting shape and may be useful, though it isn't for everyone.

Clean & Clear by Johnson & Johnson
(Skin Care Only)

For more information about Johnson & Johnson products call (800) 526-3967.

☹ **Clean & Clear Bar & Buff** *($2.69 for 3 ounces)* contains sodium tallowate (can cause blackheads and irritation), water, glycerin, alcohol, thickeners, detergent cleansers, slip agent, preservatives, and coloring agents. It's a standard bar soap, although the alcohol can make it particularly drying.

☹ **Clean & Clear Bar Regular** *($2.19 for 3.75 ounces)* contains ingredients similar to those in the Bar & Buff, but it has a mild antiseptic and no alcohol. It is drying to the skin.

☹ **Clean & Clear Deep Action Cream Cleanser** *($3.85 for 6.5 ounces)* contains mostly thickeners, salicylic acid, fragrance, menthol, and preservatives. The menthol can be a skin irritant, and salicylic acid in a cleanser is a problem for the eyes. Also, because it contains a BHA ingredient (salicylic acid), it could be too irritating if you use another BHA or AHA product afterwards.

☹ **Clean & Clear Foaming Facial Cleanser** *($2.65 for 8 ounces)* is a standard detergent-based, water-soluble cleanser. The cleansing agent is sodium lauryl sulfate, which can be drying and irritating for most skin types.

☺ **Clean & Clear Sensitive Skin Foaming Facial Cleanser** *($3.79 for 8 ounces)* may be a good detergent-based, water-soluble cleanser for someone with normal to oily skin. It is definitely more gentle than the cleanser above.

☹ **Clean & Clear Blemish Fighting Pads** *($3.69 for 50 pads)* contains salicylic acid (skin irritant and peeling agent); preservative; camphor, clove oil, eucalyptus oil, and peppermint oil (all skin irritants); alcohol; and water. This won't fight anything, but it will cause irritation.

☹ **Clean & Clear Blemish Fighting Stick** *($3.99 for 1 ounce)* contains the same ingredients as the pads, and the same warning applies.

☹ **Clean & Clear Sensitive Skin Invisible Blemish Treatment** *($3.85 for 0.75 ounce)* is a 5% salicylic acid product that also contains thickener and alcohol. The combination of alcohol and salicylic acid makes this product too irritating for most skin types.

☹ **Clean & Clear Oil Controlling Astringent** *($3.79 for 8 ounces)* contains water, alcohol, eucalyptus oil, camphor, peppermint oil, clove oil, and salicylic acid. If you don't have red, dry, irritated skin before using this product, you will after. This product cannot control oil; in fact, the irritation it causes can make oily skin more oily.

☹ **Clean & Clear Sensitive Skin Oil Controlling Astringent** *($3.79 for 8 ounces)* is almost identical to the astringent above, but with slightly less alcohol. It could be a disaster for someone with sensitive skin.

☺ **Clean & Clear Extra Strength Persa-Gel 5% Benzoyl Peroxide Dr. Prescribed Acne Medication Combination Skin Formulation** *($3.92 for 1 ounce)* is a very good 5% benzoyl peroxide gel. If you want to try a benzoyl peroxide product, this one would be just fine.

☺ **Clean & Clear Maximum Strength Persa-Gel 10% Benzoyl Peroxide Dr. Prescribed Acne Medication** *($4.99 for 1 ounce)* is a very good 10% benzoyl peroxide liquid. If you want to try a stronger benzoyl peroxide product this one would be just fine.

☺ **Clean & Clear Sensitive Skin Balancing Moisturizer** *($3.79 for 4 ounces)* contains mostly water, thickeners, silicone oil, more thickeners, salicylic acid and preservatives. This can be a good BHA product for someone with normal to dry skin who tends to break out.

☺ **Clean & Clear Skin Balancing Moisturizer** *($3.79 for 4 ounces)* is virtually identical to the moisturizer above, and the same review applies.

☺ **Clean & Clear Dual Action Moisturizer** *($3.79 for 4 ounces)* is similar to the one above and the same review applies.

Clearasil (Skin Care Only)

Clearasil has been around as a teenage acne product for decades! Has it cured anyone's acne? Not that I've seen. The products leave much to be desired when it comes to texture, color, and irritation. From what I remember, these products didn't work for anyone when I was a kid and they still don't. For more information about Clearasil call (800) 543-1745.

☹ **Clearasil Adult Care Acne Medication Cream** *($3.69 for 0.6 ounce)* contains mostly water, alcohol, clay, sulfur, resorcinol, thickeners, silicone oil, and preservatives. Both resorcinol and sulfur are potent disinfectants that can be extremely irritating. Resorcinol is no longer approved by the FDA for disinfecting and preventing acne. Also, one of the thickeners is isopropyl myristate, which can cause breakouts. Aside from being very drying and irritating, this product may also clog pores.

☹ **Clearasil Antibacterial Soap** *($1.91 for 3.25 ounces)* is a standard tallow-based soap with a detergent cleansing agent. It contains the disinfectant triclosan, but its effects are washed away in a soap, and the tallow can cause blackheads.

☺ **Clearasil Daily Face Wash** *($4.99 for 6.5 ounces)* is a standard detergent-based, water-soluble cleanser that may be OK for someone with oily skin, though it can be drying. It contains the disinfectant triclosan, but its effects are washed away in a soap.

☹ **Clearasil Medicated Deep Cleanser** *($7.50 for 7.75 ounces)* is misnamed. There's nothing deep about this cleanser, and it can be irritating. It contains mostly water, aloe, menthol, soothing agent, thickeners, fragrance, water-binding agents, and preservatives. The amount of water-binding agents is too small to be significant. In addition, menthol is a skin irritant, and salicylic acid is wasted in a cleanser and increases the risk of irritation if you use other BHA products afterwards.

☹ **Clearasil Double Textured Pads Maximum Strength** *($4.19 for 40 pads)* is mostly alcohol and salicylic acid. This product would be too drying and irritating for most skin types.

☹ **Clearasil Double Textured Pads Regular Strength with Skin Soothers** *($4.19 for 40 pads)* contains a small amount of aloe vera, but it won't counteract the irritation of the alcohol and salicylic acid.

☹ **Clearasil Ultra Pads, Maximum Strength** *($3.47 for 40 pads)* is similar to the ones above only with 2% salicylic acid. The alcohol makes it too irritating for all skin types.

☺ **Clearasil Moisturizer** *($6 for 3 ounces)* contains mostly water, thickeners, water-binding agent, more thickeners, mineral oil, silicone oil, salicylic acid (2%), and preservatives. This could be an option if you want a moisturizer-based BHA product, but mineral oil and silicone oil can cause problems for oily skin.

☹ **Clearasil Tinted Cream Maximum Strength** *($6 for 1 ounce)* is a 10% benzoyl peroxide product with a tint, but few people have skin the color of this tint. You can find similar products without tints that won't look strange on your skin.

☹ **Clearasil Vanishing Cream Maximum Strength** *($6 for 1 ounce)* is unlikely to cause anything to vanish. It is a 10% benzoyl peroxide product that also contains clay and thickeners. One of the thickeners is isopropyl myristate, which can cause breakouts.

☺ **Clearasil Vanishing Lotion Maximum Strength** *($5.69 for 1 ounce)* is similar to the cream above, minus the isopropyl myristate. It could be an option for someone looking for a minimally moisturizer-based benzoyl peroxide product.

☹ **Clearasil Clearstick Maximum Strength** *($5.19 for 1.2 ounces)* is mostly alcohol, aloe, menthol, and salicylic acid. Menthol is a skin irritant, and you already know about salicylic acid. No one needs the alcohol or menthol.

☹ **Clearasil Clearstick Regular Strength** *($5.79 for 1.2 ounces)* is almost identical to the Clearstick above, and the same review applies.

☹ **Clearasil Clearstick Sensitive Skin Maximum Strength** *($6 for 1.2 ounces)* is the same as the maximum-strength Clearstick above, minus the menthol, and the same review applies.

Clear LogiX (Skin Care Only)

This line of acne products is neither logical nor effective, though it can be terribly irritating. How disappointing! For more information about Clear LogiX call (800) 966-6960.

☹ **Oil Free Medicated Acne Wash** *($5.99 for 8 ounces)* uses sodium C14-16 olefin sulfate as the main detergent cleansing agent; I don't even recommend this ingredient for hair-care products. It also contains AHA and BHA, which are wasted in a cleanser, and eucalyptus, which serves no purpose for the skin except to burn the eyes and irritate the skin.

☹ **Acne Night Treatment Serum** *($6.99 for 2 ounces)* does contain salicylic acid, but it also contains lots of alcohol and eucalyptus and is therefore not recommended.

☹ **Acne Spot Treatment** *($5.99 for 0.75 ounce)* has the same problems as the product above, and is not recommended.

☹ **Acne Spot Treatment Tinted Formula** *($5.25 for 0.75 ounce)* has the same ingredients as the product above, but it is tinted a strange shade of peach.

☹ **Deep Cleansing Acne Treatment Pads** *($4.27 for 75 pads)* has the same problems as the other products, plus this one also contains ammonium xylenesulfonate, an ingredient used as nail polish solvent!

☹ **Oil Absorbent Acne Mask** *($6.14 for 4 ounces)* is a fairly standard clay mask with sulfur and eucalyptus. Sulfur can be an effective disinfectant for breakouts, but combined with the eucalyptus it is just too irritating to recommend.

Clientele (Skin Care Only)

Hunter Tylo from the soap opera *The Bold and the Beautiful* is once again busy endorsing a skin-care line, namely Clientele's new group of products called Elastology. I last encountered Tylo on the *Vicki Lawrence Show* (a since-discontinued afternoon talk show), where she was busy endorsing Neways's cellulite-reducing cream. This extremely thin, scantily clad, young, gorgeous woman looked me right in the eye and said this thigh product really worked for her, except, of course, she didn't have much cellulite to begin with and she was dieting and exercising. When I asked her how she knew it was the cream working on her cellulite and not the dieting and exercising, she just smiled and said she didn't, but she loved the product anyway. Of course her smile and endorsement on the actual taping of the show wasn't that honest.

Now Tylo is done with Neways, and wants you to believe that Elastology makes her skin feel "soft and firm." Apart from Tylo's believability, I am curious how Clientele rationalizes adding a new group of products to their already antiwrinkle list of products. Why do all their other antiwrinkle products need additional help?

According to Clientele's brochure (before they added Elastology) their products have "proven effects" and "miraculous antioxidant properties." Further, Clientele was the "first to identify 'free-radicals' as a key factor aging the skin and use antioxidants to help slow the process." If that's true it isn't documented in any research I've ever seen, and the company couldn't produce any either (vitamin E, the classic antioxidant, has been around in cosmetics for many years). Nevertheless, this company believes it is a forerunner in the world of antioxidants, and they do include several, such as superoxide dismutase, beta glucan, selenium, vitamin C, and vitamin E, in several of their products. This is just one of many lines that sell antioxidant lotions and potions for wrinkle relief. What you the consumer must decide is whether you want to believe in the unproven benefits of antioxidants when it comes to preventing skin from aging. If you decide to swallow any of this, the next question is, Which company should you believe? As it turns out, because none of these ingredients are specialized or unique, there are lots and lots of products that contain antioxidants, actually more do than don't. Of course, all lines want you to believe their mix of ingredients is the best.

The question that never quite gets answered by the companies selling these products is, Given the presence of air all around us, how can you prevent air from affecting the skin? Antioxidants are anti-air, meaning they keep air molecules away from the skin cells. Free-radical damage is a chain reaction caused by the presence of air, and it doesn't take much air for it to kick into action. How can you keep air constantly away from the skin, and how much antioxidant does it take to accomplish that? Nevertheless, this line has more vitamins and antioxidant ingredients than most, so if you are a believer in this concept this line excels.

Clientele also sells vitamin supplements. An interesting sideline for a cosmetics company, but one growing in popularity. I am all for healthy eating, but suggesting that these vitamins will improve your skin, nails, and hair is a stretch of the imagination.

Clientele also has a new line of products called Time Therapy Sacred Lotus Seed. I guess the other Clientele ingredients didn't work, so they had to create new products with this sacred plant so now you can get really get rid of wrinkles. Catch my drift? Which is it, Clientele, Elastology? Activator? Wrinkle Treatment? Or the Lotus Seed? From my point of view the answer is none of the above. For more information about Clientele, call (800) 327-4660.

☹ **Gentle Cleansing Bar for Normal to Dry Skin Sensitive Skin Formula** (*$16 for 4 ounces*) is a standard detergent-based bar cleanser that also contains some plant oils, including lemon oil, which can be irritating for all skin types.

☹ **Gentle Cleansing Bar for Normal to Oily Problem Skin** *($16 for 4 ounces)* is a sulfur-based bar cleanser that also contains lime oil. Sulfur is a disinfectant but in a soap its effects are rinsed off before it has a chance, and besides there are more gentle ways to disinfect skin. Lime does nothing for the skin other than cause irritation.

☺ **$$$ Oil-Free Eye Makeup Remover** *($14 for 2 ounces)* is a standard detergent-based eye-makeup remover. It will take off eye makeup, but these are some of the most common ingredients for an absurd amount of money.

☹ **Surface Refining Lotion Normal to Dry Skin Sensitive Formula, 40 Strength** *($30 for 8 ounces)* contains mostly alcohol, water, witch hazel, acetone, glycerin, and menthol. Thirty dollars for alcohol and acetone (that's nail polish remover)? They've got to be kidding. What kind of insanity depicts these ingredients as being good for sensitive skin?

☹ **Surface Refining Lotion Normal to Oily, Problem Skin Formula, 60 Strength** *($30 for 8 ounces)* is similar to the product above, and the same review applies.

☹ **Moisture Concentrate Oil-Free** *($40 for 4 ounces)* contains mostly water, thickeners, and preservatives. This is indeed oil-free, but it contains isopropyl palmitate, which is known for causing breakouts.

☹ **Daytime Moisture Concentrate with SPF 6** *($40 for 4 ounces)* has an SPF of 6, which is not enough to protect from the sun. This product is absolutely not recommended. The comment in the brochure says this product protects but allows you to tan. That's like a cancer specialist offering you a cigarette, and is completely unethical for any skin line to offer.

☺ **$$$ Nourishing Night Oils** *($100 for 10 vials)* contains plenty of oil, including sunflower, corn, and olive oil, as well as vitamins. This won't feed the skin, and the price is obnoxious for what you get. Yes, the oils would be great for someone with dry skin, but you could mix this up on your own for a fraction of the price (some sunflower oil with a capsule of vitamin E oil would do it).

☺ **$$$ Preventative Age Treatment** *($50 for 2 ounces)* contains mostly water, plant oils, thickeners, silicone, glycerin, thickeners, vitamins, more thickeners, water-binding agents, vitamin C, and preservatives. This is a good emollient moisturizer for someone with dry skin, but that's about it. There aren't enough antioxidants in here to be of any benefit to the skin.

☺ **$$$ Time Therapy** *($75 for 1.1 ounces)* contains mostly water, plant extract, silicone, vitamin E, thickeners, shea butter, more thickeners, water-binding agents, more plant extracts, antioxidants, and preservatives. This is a good emollient moisturizer for someone with dry skin. Like the previous product, this one contains antioxidants, but they're less than 1% of the product. If you're going to spend this much money on a product that claims to combat free radicals with antioxidants, shouldn't it be more than 1% of the product?

☺ **$$$ Wrinkle Treatment** *($75 for 1.1 ounces)* contains mostly water, plant oil, aloe, mineral oil, several thickeners, more plant oils, silicone, antioxidant, vitamins, and preservatives. This is a good emollient moisturizer for someone with dry skin, nothing more. Plus, if this product is for wrinkles what are all these other expensive products for?

☺ **$$$ Preventative Age Solar Block SPF 25** *($42 for 4 ounces)* contains mostly water, plant extracts, several thickeners, plant oil, vitamin E, glycerin, plasticizing agent (hair spray), more thickeners, pH balancer, more vitamins, more plant extracts, and preservatives. This is a good, partly titanium dioxide–based sunscreen. It would be best for someone with dry skin, but there are hundreds of sunscreens equal to or better than this for a lot less money.

☹ **Activator for Normal to Dry Skin with SPF 10** *($50 for 60 packets/90 grams)* doesn't contain avobenzone, zinc oxide, or titanium dioxide, and is not recommended. For all their carrying on about latest formulations, how did Clientele miss on this one?

☹ **Activator for Problem Skin Normal to Oily Skin with SPF 10** *($50 for 60 packets/90 grams)* contains plenty of ingredients that would make oily skin more oily, but it doesn't contain avobenzone, zinc oxide, or titanium dioxide, and is absolutely not recommended.

☺ **$$$ Elastology Builder with Triple Alpha Hydroxys** *($65 for 1.1 ounce)* is a lot of money for an AHA product. This one does contain AHAs and some vitamins, but the pH isn't low enough for the AHAs to work as exfoliants.

☹ **Elastology 50 Restorative Complex** *($100 for 0.5 ounce)* is a good emollient moisturizer with lots of plant oils and vitamins; it even contains progesterone for those worried about menopause (though I do not recommend creams with plant hormones unless a doctor is consulted first—plant hormones do not automatically minimize risks of cancer if you are in a high-risk group). Those ingredients may all be fine and good, but this product also contains cortisone. Using cortisone on a regular basis can destroy the collagen in your skin. This product is not recommended.

☺ **$$$ Elastology Firming Eye Cream** *($45 for 0.5 ounce)* contains about 4% AHA in an emollient base along with plenty of vitamins. The pH isn't low enough for it to be an exfoliant, but it can be an OK moisturizer.

☺ **$$$ Elastology Firming Night Cream for Normal/Dry, Sensitive Skin** *($95 for 1.1 ounce)* contains mostly water, plant oils, thickeners, water-binding agents, vitamins, plant extracts, and preservatives. This is a good emollient moisturizer. The vitamins won't alter a wrinkle but they are good for the skin nevertheless.

☺ **$$$ Elastology Firming Target Treatment Roll-On** *($40 for 0.35 ounce)* is a good lightweight moisturizer for slightly dry skin. It has its share of vitamins and AHA, but the pH isn't low enough for the AHAs to work as an exfoliant and the vitamin content for this absurd amount of money is up to you.

☺ $$$ Elastology Oil-Free Firming Night Cream for Normal/Oily Skin *($95 for 1.1 ounce)* is a good lightweight moisturizer for dry skin, never for oily skin. It contains water, thickeners, vitamins, and preservatives.

☺ $$$ Elastology Age Blocker with SPF 25 *($95 for 1.1 ounces)* is a good, partly titanium dioxide–based moisturizer with a high SPF. That's great, but because sunscreens are supposed to be used liberally and then reapplied after exercise don't expect this product to last for more than a week or two at best.

☹ Elastology Lip Treatment Duo Conditioner & Lipstick Sealer *($19 for 0.15 ounce)* is a two-in-one product that is disappointing. The Conditioner isn't all that conditioning. It leaves a film over the lips that can help prevent lipstick from bleeding, but it can also make dry lips drier. The Lip Sealer is mostly alcohol and hairspray, and that just doesn't feel great on the lips.

☹ Facial Masque Oily Problem Skin Formula *($45 for six 6-ounce packets)* contains mostly clay, alcohol, acetone (that's nail polish remover) and menthol. This product is amazingly irritating for all skin types.

☹ Facial Masque Normal/Dry Sensitive Skin Formula *($45 for six packets = 30 treatments, 6 ounces)* is almost identical to the one above and is absolutely not recommended.

Clientele's Time Therapy Sacred Lotus Seed

Please note that these products are not sold separately. The cost is $89.95 for all ten products, or $49.95 for three products and $10 for each additional product. I would not encourage anyone to use all of the products that come in these kits. As is true with any skin-care line, you have to pick and choose depending on your skin-care needs and the formulation of the products. This line is sold exclusively by phone-order (800) 327-4660. By the way, these are way too many AHA products for one face.

☺ $$$ Alpha Hydroxy Face Wash for Normal/Dry, Sensitive Skin *(8 ounces)* is a standard detergent-based water-soluble cleanser that contains about 2% AHA, not enough to be a problem for the eyes.

☹ Alpha Hydroxy Face Wash for Normal/Oily Skin *(8 ounces)* is a standard detergent-based water-soluble cleanser that includes witch hazel, AHA, and BHA. The AHA isn't enough to be a problem but the other two ingredients are unnecessary irritants for the eyes or face.

☹ Alpha Hydroxy Roll-On Rinse for Normal/Dry, Sensitive Skin *(1 ounce)* does contain about 8% AHA (glycolic acid) but the pH is around 5, and that means it isn't an effective exfoliant. The high pH might make it better for sensitive skin, but it makes a poor AHA product.

☺ **$$$ Alpha Hydroxy Roll-On Rinse for Normal/Oily Skin** *(1 ounce)* is similar to the one above, only without any emollients and with a pH of 3, which means it is definitely an option for a good AHA lotion.

☹ **Wrinkle Alpha Hydroxy Roll-On Regular Strength** *(0.35 ounce)* does contain about 8% AHA (glycolic acid) but the pH is around 5, and that means it isn't an effective exfoliant. That might make it better for sensitive skin, but it makes a poor AHA product.

☺ **$$$ Day Serum SPF 25, for Normal/Dry, Sensitive Skin** *(1 ounce)* is a good, part titanium dioxide–based sunscreen, but the amount you get is absurdly small. Given how much you are supposed to use to obtain maximum sun protection, this won't last more than a week or two. It does have a good emollient base for dry skin but that's about it.

☺ **$$$ Day Serum SPF 25 for Normal/Oily Skin** *(1 ounce)* is a good partly titanium dioxide–based sunscreen, but the amount you get makes it one of the most expensive ways to protect the skin from sun damage. It is in a good lightweight base for someone with normal to oily skin.

☹ **Instant Age Eraser Duo** *(includes both products* **Wrinkle Eye Cream** *0.15 ounce and* **Treatment Conceal** *0.15 ounce).* The cream is a good emollient moisturizer for dry skin, with plant oils and water-binding agents. The concealer is a fairly greasy one that can crease into the lines around the eyes. Only part of this product is worth it, and the cream part is so tiny why bother when there are so many other good moisturizers to be found?

☺ **$$$ Night Serum for Normal/Dry, Sensitive Skin** *(1 ounce)* is a good moisturizer for someone with dry skin. It contains mostly water, plant extract, plant oils, thickeners, antioxidants, water-binding agents, silicones, fragrance, and preservatives. There are some very interesting water-binding agents and antioxidants in this product but don't count on them erasing or stopping a wrinkle.

☹ **Night Serum, for Normal/Oily Skin** *(1 ounce)* is almost identical to the serum above, just without some of the plant oils, though there are still plenty of ingredients that make it inappropriate for someone with oily skin.

☺ **$$$ Wrinkle Serum** *(1 ounce)* contains mostly water, plant oils, thickeners, vitamins, anti-irritant, and preservatives. This is a good moisturizer for someone with dry skin.

☹ **Acne Blemish Roll-On for Normal/Dry, Sensitive Skin** *(0.35 ounce)* contains sulfur, and that can be an irritant for many skin types. There are ways to disinfect blemishes that are easier on the skin, especially for someone with sensitive skin.

☹ **Acne Blemish Roll-On for Normal/Oily Skin** *(0.35 ounce)* is similar to the one above except that this one includes resorcinol, alcohol, and witch hazel. Resorcinol is a serious skin irritant, and one the FDA disallowed for claims in acne products back in 1992. The other two ingredients are just drying and irritating.

The Reviews C

☺ **$$$ Spot Lightening Roll-On** *(0.35 ounce)* is a good hydroquinone-based skin lightening product. It can work, but there are other far less expensive versions of this available.

Clinique

Clinique has assembled a huge line of products over the years. Myriad foundations, eyeshadows, lipsticks, pencils, powders, and skin-care items make its counters almost overwhelmingly alive with choices. Strangely, despite the growth in product selection, this is still a strictly Caucasian line, with few to no choices for women of color. The foundation colors do not include deep brown to ebony skin tones; the eyeshadows and blushes go on too softly to work on darker skin; and the lipstick shades are all fairly soft and light, also not adequate for darker skin tones.

Clinique's products, particularly those for skin care, are aimed at oily or combination skin types, which is probably why Clinique attracts a young clientele. And the makeup line includes products and colors geared toward younger tastes, such as color rubs and tints for the cheek (best for flawless, unlined faces), very sheer blushes and eyeshadows, and a variety of clever eye pencils (more gimmicky than useful). Unfortunately, many of the pencils, eyeshadows, and color rubs are extremely shiny and not the best for daytime or on over-thirtysomething skin, or for a professional look at any age, for that matter. Clinique does seem to be expanding its potential market somewhat with a new selection of matte shades, exquisite blush colors, impressive foundations, and matte lipsticks that are less greasy than the other lipsticks in the line.

Many women, regardless of age, are faithful Clinique customers, probably because they believe the products are hypoallergenic and better for their skin (they aren't). The salespeople, dressed in white lab coats, reinforce this belief (they were the first to have this quasi-professional attire). There are several counter displays available, but most of the products can be tested only with the help of a salesperson. The color products are arranged into four groupings: Nudes/Naturels (which are not all that nude), Tawnies/Corals, Pinks/Roses, and Violets/Berries. It's a little confusing, but can be helpful if you know what color groups you look best in. One plus is that the products are by far more affordable than those of numerous other lines. You also get great service at the Clinique counters; there always seem to be four to six white-jacketed women dashing around behind those counters. For more information about Clinique call (212) 572-3800.

Clinique Skin Care

☺ **Crystal Clear Cleansing Oil** *($12.50 for 6 ounces)* is just mineral oil with some vitamins; you would be just fine with plain mineral oil from the drugstore for a fraction of the price. But either way you would be wiping off your makeup, and that's not best for skin.

☺ **Extremely Gentle Cleansing Cream** *($19.50 for 10 ounces)* is a traditional cold-cream product (that is, it requires wiping off) that contains mostly mineral oil, water, beeswax, petrolatum, thickeners, and preservatives. Wiping off makeup is not good for the skin.

☹ **Wash-Away Gel Cleanser** *($15.50 for 6 ounces)* contains several ingredients that can burn skin and eyes, including lemon and eucalyptus.

☺ **Water-Dissolve Cream Cleanser** *($15.50 for 5 ounces)* leaves a greasy film on the skin and doesn't take off all the makeup without the help of a washcloth.

☹ **Facial Soap Extra Mild** *($8.50 for 6 ounces)* is standard-issue bar soap, meaning it is mostly lard and lye. This is a lot of money for your average, everyday bar of soap.

☹ **Facial Soap Mild** *($8.50 for 6 ounces)* is similar to the soap above, and the same review applies.

☹ **Facial Soap Extra-Strength** *($8.50 for 6 ounces)* is similar to Facial Soap Extra Mild, and the same review applies.

☺ **Rinse-Off Foaming Cleanser** *($15.50 for 5 ounces)* is a standard detergent-based water-soluble cleanser that can be fairly drying for most skin types.

☺ **Extremely Gentle Eye Makeup Remover** *($9.50 for 2 ounces)* contains mostly mineral oil, thickeners, lanolin, plant oil, and preservatives. It is gentle, but it is also just good old-fashioned cold cream.

☺ **Rinse-Off Eye Makeup Solvent** *($12 for 4 ounces)* contains mostly water, detergent cleanser, and slip agents. It is a standard detergent-based eye-makeup remover.

☺ **Take The Day Off Makeup Remover, for Lids, Lashes and Lips** *($14.50 for 4.2 ounces)* is a silicone- and detergent-based makeup remover. It works, but it needs to be wiped off, and that's not great for any part of the face, especially the eyes.

☺ **7 Day Scrub Cream** *($15 for 3.5 ounces)* contains mostly mineral oil, water, beeswax, sodium borate (antiseptic), and thickeners. This very thick, heavy product can cause the same problems it's trying to eliminate, because beeswax and ozokerite (one of the thickening agents) can cause skin to break out.

☺ **7 Day Scrub Cream Rinse Off Formula** *($14 for 3.4 ounces)* rinses off better than the one above but not by much. It can still leave a greasy film on the skin and contains several pore-clogging ingredients.

☹ **Exfoliating Scrub** *($13.50 for 3 ounces)* was probably added to the Clinique line because the other two scrubs make such a greasy mess. This detergent-cleanser scrub definitely rinses better than the two above but it contains menthol which is unnecessarily irritating for skin.

☺ **Gentle Exfoliator Rinse-Off Formula** *($13.50 for 3 ounces)* contains mostly water, mineral oil, a long list of thickeners, a long list of plant extracts, anti-irritant, vitamin E, more thickeners, and preservatives. This is a gentle exfoliant with very little abrasive, but I wouldn't call it rinseable. The mineral oil leaves a residue on the skin.

☹ **Clarifying Lotions 1, 2, 3, and 4** *($15.50 for 12 ounces)* all contain varying degrees of alcohol, benzalkonium chloride, and menthol, which are all extremely irritating, and none are recommended unless you are looking for red, irritated, dry, and flaky skin. The best thing I can say is that at least Clinique finally took the acetone out of these formulations.

☺ **Mild Clarifying Lotion** *($15.50 for 12 ounces)* contains about a 0.5% concentration of BHA, recommended for dry, sensitive skin. The pH of this toner is about 4, which isn't the best, but BHA is only appropriate for blemish-prone skin because of its ability to penetrate the pore. This can be an option for someone with breakouts, but a pH of 3 would make it more effective.

☺ **$$$ Advanced Cream Self Repair System** *($32.50 for 1 ounce)* contains mostly water, slip agent, plant oil, thickener, glycerin, mineral oil, plant oils, several more thickeners, algae extract, vitamins A and E (antioxidants), silicone, and preservatives. This overpriced but extremely emollient moisturizer for someone with dry skin won't repair anything, but it will help keep dryness away.

☺ **$$$ All About Eyes** *($25 for 0.5 ounce)* feels silky when you rub this light lotion into your skin, primarily from the silicone base; silicones are the first two ingredients on the list. That's not bad, but these ingredients aren't about eyes in particular, and this is just a good lightweight moisturizer that can feel soothing anywhere on the face. It contains mostly silicones, water, thickener, slip agents, water-binding agents, plant extracts, anti-irritant, vitamins, more thickeners, petrolatum, more silicones, and preservative. It is a good lightweight moisturizer for dry skin.

☺ **$$$ Daily Eye Benefits** *($25 for 0.5 ounce)* contains mostly water, slip agent, thickeners, plant oil, plant extracts, more thickeners, water-binding agents, anti-irritant, aloe vera, silicone, vitamin A, petrolatum, and preservatives. The plant extracts are supposed to reduce puffiness around the eyes, but it's unlikely your skin would notice. This is a good emollient moisturizer with an incredibly high price tag. Slice up a cucumber and see if that can get rid of puffy eyes before investing in this product at $1,200 a pound.

☺ **$$$ Daily Eye Saver** *($25 for 0.5 ounce)* contains mostly water, slip agent, aloe, plant oil, thickener, glycerin, plant extracts, water-binding agents, vitamin E, and preservatives. Although the price is unwarranted, this is a good lightweight moisturizer that won't save eyes from anything.

☺ **Dramatically Different Moisturizing Lotion** *($10.50 for 2 ounces, $19.50 for 4 ounces)* contains mostly water, mineral oil, sesame oil, water-binding agent, thickeners, petrolatum, lanolin, and preservatives. This is a good, basic moisturizer for dry skin, although it isn't "dramatically different" from other emollient moisturizers on the market.

☺ $$$ **Moisture In Control** *($30 for 1.7 ounces)* won't control anything. There is no way a product can put moisturizing ingredients in a dry area on the face, but keep them off the face in other areas and instead apply ingredients that absorb oil. That's impossible. Basically, this product contains water, slip agent, aloe (which is mostly water), thickeners (including potato starch, which can be a problem for breakouts), more slip agents, several good water-binding agents, a small amount of lactic acid (not enough to be an exfoliant, just a water-binding agent), vitamins, silicone, silica (can be absorbent, but only minimally in this amount, so mostly it will absorb the oils in the product, not oil on the skin), thickeners, and preservatives.

☺ $$$ **Moisture On-Call** *($30 for 1.6 ounces)* is supposed to help skin cells "remember" how to produce their own moisture barrier. The company calls this memory-booster effect "mnemonic." In fact, you can achieve the same effect with the daily use of *any* moisturizer, which is the only claim Clinique is really making. This product contains mostly water, jojoba oil, thickener, humectant, shea butter, silicone, water-binding agents, plant extracts, more water-binding agents, vitamin E, more thickeners, and preservatives. It is a very good emollient moisturizer for someone with dry skin, but no more special than hundreds of other moisturizers.

☺ $$$ **Moisture On Line** *($30 for 1.7 ounces)* is almost identical to Moisture on Call, and supposedly can reeducate the skin. There are no moisturizing ingredients anywhere in the world that can change the nature of skin and make skin remember anything. But skin cells can look better if you faithfully reapply the moisturizer every day, which is exactly what the instructions on this moisturizer tell you to do. Separated from the hype, it is a good moisturizer for someone with normal to dry skin. It contains mostly water, silicone, glycerin, slip agents, thickeners, lactic acid, plant extracts, water-binding agents, more water-binding agents, vitamin E, petrolatum, and preservatives. The lactic acid in this product works more as a water-binding agent than as an exfoliant, given that there is only about a 2% to 3% concentration of it.

☺ **Moisture Stick** *($12.50 for 0.13 ounce)* is more like a lip gloss than anything else. It is definitely emollient and extremely greasy. Several of its ingredients can cause breakouts.

☺ **Moisture Surge Treatment Formula** *($32.50 for 2 ounces)* contains mostly water, several water-binding agents, vitamins A and E, more water-binding agent, plant extracts, thickeners, and preservatives. This is a very good lightweight moisturizer with a nice quantity of water-binding agents and antioxidants.

☺ **Skin Texture Lotion Oil Free Formula** *($19.50 for 1.25 ounces)* contains mostly water, slip agents, thickeners, water-binding agent, vitamins A and E, more thickeners, and preservatives. Don't be mislead by the term oil-free, there are still thickening agents in here that could cause breakouts and that would be a problem for someone with oily skin. It is a good lightweight moisturizer for normal to slightly dry skin.

☺ **Turnaround Cream** *($27.50 for 2 ounces)* has a great name; it sounds as if this cream can turn your skin back to a younger time, but it can't. It contains mostly water, several thickeners, salicylic acid, silicone, anti-irritant, vitamin E, and preservatives. Salicylic acid (a BHA) is an effective exfoliant, but only at a pH of 3 in a concentration of 1% to 2%. There is no information about concentration for any of the Turnaround products, but even if there were, the pH is 5, which makes them ineffective as exfoliants. This is a fairly matte, lightweight moisturizer for normal to slightly dry skin, and that's about it.

☺ $$$ **Turnaround Cream for Dry Skin** *($27.50 for 2 ounces)* is much more emollient than the cream above and would definitely be good for someone with dry skin, but the same review applies.

☺ **Turnaround Lotion Oil-Free** *($23.50 for 1.7 ounces)* contains mostly water, silicone, film former, thickeners, salicylic acid, water-binding agents, anti-irritant, vitamin E, more thickeners, and preservatives. If you have normal to slightly oily skin, this can be a good lightweight moisturizer, but it is a poor BHA product.

☺ $$$ **Weather Everything SPF 15** *($37.50 for 1.7 ounces)* is an overpriced, titanium dioxide–based sunscreen containing mostly water, silicones, thickeners, anti-irritant, water-binding agents, vitamins, more thickeners, and preservatives. It would provide impressive protection for someone with dry skin, but I wouldn't recommend it for oily or combination skin. I wish Clinique had brought out a daily sun-care product years ago, but better late than never.

☺ $$$ **City Block Oil-Free Daily Protector SPF 15** *($13.50 for 1.4 ounces)* is a good nonchemical sunscreen for someone with dry skin. There are several ingredients in here, including the titanium dioxide (the nonchemical sunscreen agent) that can be a problem for someone with oily or blemish-prone skin.

☹ **Face Zone Sun Block SPF 30** *($13.50 for 1.7 ounces)* doesn't contain avobenzone, zinc oxide, or titanium dioxide, and is not recommended.

☹ **Full-Service Sun Block SPF 15** *($12.50 for 3 ounces)* doesn't contain avobenzone, zinc oxide, or titanium dioxide, and is not recommended.

☹ **Full-Service Sun Block SPF 20** *($12.50 for 3 ounces)* doesn't contain avobenzone, zinc oxide, or titanium dioxide, and is not recommended.

☺ **Special Defense Sun Block SPF 25** *($13.50 for 3 ounces)* is a good nonchemical sunscreen with emollients, water-binding agents, and minimal amounts of antioxidants.

☺ **Total Cover Sun Block SPF 30** *($12.50 for 3 ounces)* doesn't contain avobenzone, zinc oxide, or titanium dioxide, and is not recommended.

☺ **Lip Block SPF 15** *($7.50 for 0.15 ounce)* is a good, standard, petrolatum-based lip gloss with a good sunblock. This can nicely ward off dry lips and protect from sun damage.

☹ **Oil-Free Sun Block SPF 15** *($12.50 for 4 ounces)* doesn't contain avobenzone, zinc oxide, or titanium dioxide, and is not recommended.

☺ **$$$ Self-Tanning Face Formula Skin Types I and II** *($14.50 for 1.7 ounces)* is a good standard dihydroxyacetone-based self-tanner and this one works as well as any of them.

☺ **$$$ Self-Tanning Face Formula Skin Types III and IV** *($14.50 for 1.7 ounces)* is the same as the one above and the same comments apply.

☹ **Anti Acne Spot Treatment** *($11 for 0.5 ounce)* is just alcohol, slip agents, and salicylic acid. Didn't we get enough alcohol and salicylic acid with the Clinique toners and Turnaround moisturizers? This is overkill by almost anyone's standard and the alcohol just adds fuel to the fire.

☹ **Deep Cleansing Emergency Masque** *($18.50 for 3.4 ounces)* contains more salicylic acid, this time in a standard clay mask. Between this, the Turnaround creams, and the toners, it would be a wonder if you had any skin left when you're done.

☹ **Sheer Matteness T-Zone Shine Control** *($12.50 for 0.5 ounce)* is supposed to help skin look less oily. Given its ingredient listing I suspect it can do that for a brief period of time, after all the second ingredient is alcohol, which can degrease just about anything. Of course, what you are supposed to do with the resulting dryness and irritation isn't mentioned. This product also contains silicone (I suspect that's to soothe the effect of the alcohol but it can be a problem for very oily skin types), film former, slip agent, witch hazel, and BHA. There isn't enough BHA here to be effective for exfoliation, but the irritating ingredients make this a problem for any skin type.

☺ **$$$ Exceptionally Soothing Cream for Upset Skin, Anti-Itch Cream** *($30 for 1.7 ounces)* and **Exceptionally Soothing Lotion for Upset Skin** *($30 for 1.7 ounces)* both contain hydrocortisone acetate, which can indeed soothe irritated skin. For years I have been recommending Lanacort and Cortaid, both found in the drugstore for less than $5 for an ounce, to deal with minor skin problems. What is potentially distressing about finding hydrocortisone in a cosmetic is that continuous use of hydrocortisone over time can actually cause skin damage by thinning the skin and breaking down the skin's support structure. If you are aware of this very serious shortcoming and plan only occasional use, there are many reasons why you may prefer Clinique's two new products to Lanacort or Cortaid. Even though the active ingredient in these products is the same, the moisturizing base in both Clinique products is exceptional. In the long run, the base shouldn't make that much difference, because you will only be using it for the short run.

☺ **$$$ Skin Calming Moisture Mask** *($18.50 for 3.4 ounces)* contains mostly water, aloe, thickeners, plant oils, slip agents, water-binding agents, anti-irritants, film former, and preservatives. This is a good moisturizing mask for dry skin.

☹ **All About Lips** *($20 for 0.5 ounce)* contains a long list of thickening agents, anti-irritants, water-binding agents, and a small amount of salicylic acid. That can help exfoliate the lips but it's not what I would recommend for daily lip care. Salicylic acid is just too strong an exfoliant for the lips.

Clinique Makeup

✓☺ FOUNDATION: **Almost Makeup SPF 15** *($16.50)* comes in **five great light colors**, which is pretty slim pickings, but it's an excellent sheer to lightweight foundation with a nonchemical sunscreen.

☺ **City Base Compact Foundation SPF 15** *($20)* is simply a cream-to-powder foundation with a nonchemical, titanium dioxide–based sunscreen. It has a silky feel, drying to a somewhat creamy finish. The powder part of this foundation can be drying for someone with dry skin, and the cream part can be greasy for someone with combination to oily skin, so that makes it best for someone with normal to slightly dry or slightly oily skin. City Base comes in ten very attractive colors that would work for a wide range of skin tones, from light to dark, but not for someone with very light or very dark skin.

☹ **Workout Makeup SPF 6** *($18.50)* is a puzzle. I'm not sure where you're supposed to "work out" with this minimal sun protection except indoors, but regardless, the color selection is poor and this product pales when compared to the other Clinique foundations with SPF. It's supposed to be water-resistant, but it leaves something to be desired when sweating. If you work out and don't sweat, it will stay on, but that's about it.

✓☺ **Stay True Oil-Free** *($14.50)* is a great oil-free liquid foundation with a semi-matte finish and **all the color choices are great.**

☺ **Balanced Makeup Base** *($13.50)* is for normal to dry skin, and is also a very good liquid foundation; most of the 12 colors are excellent. **Colors to avoid because they are too peach:** Natural Glow, Creamy Peach, and Warmer.

☺ **Super Powder Double Face Powder Foundation** *($15.50)* is a pressed powder that contains talc and mineral oil; it can be used as an all-over sheer foundation or as a finishing powder, and the colors are so sheer it's like wearing no makeup at all. **All of the colors are excellent** although there are only five shades to choose from. It is often recommended to wear this type of foundation wet. Don't—it only makes it look thick, streaky, and choppy.

☺ **Continuous Coverage Makeup SPF 11 (nonchemical)** *($14.50)* is a very thick, opaque, oil-based foundation intended for those who want to cover scarring.

It should not be used as an everyday makeup unless you need heavy coverage. **The six colors are all excellent**, and it is one of the better foundations of this type.

☺ **Soft Finish Makeup** *($18.50)* is worth checking out if you have normal to dry skin. This good lightweight foundation has a smooth, even texture and blends on easily. How does it compare to Clinique's Balanced Makeup? Well, it's similar and perhaps slightly more sheer, but only slightly. **All of the colors are excellent.**

☺ **Extra Help** *($18.50)* makeup has a nice consistency and would be good for extremely dry skin. The color selection has been reformulated, and **all the colors except one are wonderful.** Avoid Fawn Beige, which is too rose for almost all skin tones.

☹ **Pore Minimizer** *($13.50)* contains mostly alcohol with talc. The alcohol is irritating, and the talc provides little to no coverage and tends to go on dry and flaky. I am almost shocked that this is still available, but as this book went to press it was obvious Clinique was about to phase it out.

☺ **$$$ Super Balanced Makeup** *($16.50)* claims to be oil-free, but it isn't: it contains silicone. It also claims to contain sponge-like ingredients that will absorb oil in oily areas but still moisturize dry areas of your face. It ends up doing neither very well. After less than two hours, it showed shine in areas of my face that never get shiny, and the areas of my face that do struggle with being too oily looked that way shortly after I put it on. There is no way for any product to recognize the difference between the oil on your skin and the emollients in the product. The so-called sponges will absorb any oil or emollients they come in contact with, leaving your dry side unhappy; and the moisturizing ingredients will get deposited over areas you don't want to be greasy. What that adds up to is a foundation that is best for someone with normal to slightly dry skin. Someone with any amount of oil would not be happy with the finish nor with how it wears during the day. Furthering my disappointment, the colors for the Super Balanced Makeup are astonishingly poor, especially for lighter skin tones. Clinique usually has a first-class line of foundation colors in neutral shades for a wide range of skin tones, but not this time. Although the darker shades are actually some of the best around, many of the lighter colors are strongly peach to orange! **Avoid all of the following colors:** Petal, Fair, Ivory, Cream Chamois, Neutral, Linen, Porcelain Beige, Sunny, Warmer, and Honeyed Beige. **Colors to consider:** Vanilla, Porcelain, Sand, Wheat, Golden, Amber, Toffee, Clove, and Cocoa.

☺ **CONCEALER: Quick Corrector** *($9.50)* comes in a tube with a wand applicator. Of the four shades, only medium is too pink for most skin tones; the others are excellent for light or medium skin tones. The texture is smooth without being greasy, but it can be too drying and matte for some skin types. It stays on well with only minimal creasing. **Soft Concealer Corrector** *($10.50)* has excellent colors. It has a great consistency and goes on well with only a slight tendency to crease.

☺ **City Cover Compact Concealer SPF 15** *($12.50)* has a great SPF, but this very creamy concealer only works if you have no lines around the eye, because it does tend to crease and crease and crease. Other than that it is a decent concealer with excellent colors for lighter skin tones.

☺ **Advanced Concealer** *($10.50)* comes in a squeeze tube and goes on like a liquid but dries to a powder. It comes in two shades, Light and Medium; both are excellent. But beware: This product works only if the skin under your eyes is smooth; any dry or rough skin will look worse when this type of concealer is placed over it.

☹ **Anti-Acne Control Formula Concealer** *($11.50)* is very thick and heavy. It comes in two shades, Light and Medium, and both are poor color choices. The anti-acne parts of the formula are colloidal sulfur and salicylic acid. BHA is an option for exfoliation but it isn't necessary in makeup, and sulfur is too much of an irritant. There are more gentle ways to disinfect without causing irritation. **Concealing Stick** *($11.50)* comes in just one color, which means it might work if you happen to have just the right skin tone. It can be greasy, and it creases easily.

☺ <u>POWDER:</u> **Soft Finish Pressed Powder** *($15.50)* is a talc-based powder that goes on soft and slightly more satiny than the Matte version. This one comes in four great shades. **Stay Matte Sheer Pressed Powder** *($15.50)* is an oil-free talc-based powder that goes on very sheer and soft and the ten color choices are excellent. **Blended Face Powder with Brush** *($15.50)* is a loose, talc-based powder with a soft texture and a good selection of colors. Only Transparency 2 may be slightly pink; and Transparency Bronze is fairly iridescent.

☺ <u>BLUSH:</u> **Beyond Blusher** *($15)* has an exquisite selection of soft colors, all with a soft, light texture and application, though you can build color definition. **Soft Pressed Powder Blusher** *($14.50)* is somewhat shiny but not terrible and the colors are all very attractive and blend on soft for a sheer finish. **Bronze Doubles** *($14.50)* have no shine and can be great contour colors, but be careful not to end up having your face look shades darker than your neck. One of these shades is more peach than tan, and better as a blush than an all-over color.

☺ $$$ **BlushWear** *($15)* is Clinique's version of a cream-to-powder blush with an unusually dry finish. Even the salesperson warned me that it is helpful if you apply a moisturizer first to help it spread more easily. How to work that out when you're wearing foundation wasn't explained. It is tricky though, and given the mode of application, not that much easier to use than Almay's Amazing Lasting Blush *($7.59)* or Revlon's ColorStay Cheek Color *($7.89)*.

☺ <u>EYESHADOW:</u> **Stay the Day Eyeshadows** *($11)* consist of 20 shades that aren't supposed to crease. They stay on just fine, but the application can be quite sheer, and have problems clinging evenly. Plus most of the shades have some amount of shine, not bad, just not great. **Pair of Shades Eyeshadow Duo** *($13)* color pairs are attractive and mostly neutral, with a small but soft selection of browns and grays, but, alas, they all have some amount of shine. They apply almost identically to the Stay the Day version above. **Touch Base for Eyes** *($11)* is a cream-to-powder shadow that comes in a small group of colors, all with a slight sheen. The major problem is that this product tends to dry out in the container and then it is almost impossible to use. **Smudgesicles** *($12.50)* are a cloyingly cute name for eight shades of stick eyeshadow that has a cream-to-powder finish. They are all shiny and they are all an option for a fast application if you don't want to have to bother with blending, but they are tricky to use when trying to blend shades together.

☺ <u>EYE AND BROW SHAPER:</u> **Water Resistant Eyeliner** *($13.50)* is an old-fashioned cake liner that comes in two colors and can be used wet or dry. It isn't all that water-resistant, but it does create a dramatic line. **Quick Eyes** *($14.50)* are an eye pencil at one end of the stick and a powdered eyeshadow section with a sponge-tip applicator at the other. The eyeshadow is released into the sponge tip when you shake it. If the eyeshadows weren't so shiny, I would recommend this gimmicky product as a convenient tool for doing a fast eye design.

☺ **$$$ Quick Liner for Eyes** *($13.50)* are merely standard pencils that you twist up rather than sharpen. That makes application easier, and not having to sharpen is quicker; but Almay, Revlon, and lots of other cosmetics companies have pencils like these for less. **Eye Shaping Pencils** *($10)* are standard pencils in a good range of colors (avoid the shiny ones) that go on soft, without feeling greasy. **Brow Shaper** *($12)* is a powder meant to be used for the brows. It works quite well, but an eyeshadow that matches your brow color would do just as well. The brush that accompanies this compact is too hard and scratchy.

☹ **Touch Liner** *($11.50)* is a liquid liner in a tube. All three colors are shiny.

☺ <u>LIPSTICK AND LIP PENCIL:</u> Clinique's lipsticks come in an excellent color selection for lighter and medium skin tones. **Sun Buffer Lipstick** *($10.50)* is more gloss than lipstick but it does have a reliable SPF 15. **Almost Lipstick** *($12.50)* is extremely similar to the Sun Buffer, only its a gloss in a tube. Talk about redundancy. **Different Lipstick** *($10.50)* is slightly more creamy than the Sun Buffer, but only slightly. It does have a slight stain, which means it can last somewhat longer on the lips. **Long Lasting Lipstick** *($12.50)* is an excellent semi-matte lipstick, even though they call it a matte. It has a beautiful consistency and tends not to bleed. **Long Lasting Soft Shine Lipstick** *($12.50)* is similar to the regular Long Lasting Lipstick, only this one has a little bit of shine and a little more gloss to it. Clinique's **Superlast Cream Lipstick** *($13.50)* is an impressive, ultra-matte lipstick. It performs similarly to Revlon ColorStay (their reformulation, not the original version), Almay Amazing Lasting, et al. Clinique's lipstick goes on with a damp, smooth finish and dries to a solid but smooth covering. It won't rub off on your coffee cup, and it tends not to chip or roll off. **Lip Shaping Pencils** *($10)* have a soft, smooth texture and come in an excellent array of colors. **Quick Liner for Lips** *($12.50)* are merely standard pencils that you twist up rather than sharpen. That makes application easier, and not having to sharpen is quicker; but Almay, Revlon, and lots of other cosmetics companies have pencils like this for less.

☺ **$$$ Chubby Stick** *($12.50)* is an oversized (at least in width, not in height) lip pencil that is supposed to double as a lip liner and lipstick. To some extent, that's exactly what it does, but not very well. Like all chubby lip pencils, these are difficult to sharpen. The color part is so soft that it is impossible to keep a tip on the end, so you can never create a smooth, even line around the mouth, and that means you have to sharpen often because the tip keeps disappearing, and the lipstick part is, well, just a slightly glossy lipstick.

☹ **Gloss Wear SPF 8** *($11.50)* is too a low an SPF and it doesn't have UVA protection.

☺ **MASCARA: Naturally Glossy Mascara** *($11)* is an OK mascara but not great. It goes on quickly and builds some length and thickness, just not very much. If you want a more natural look for your lashes this one is it. **Full Potential Mascara** *($11)* is a fairly great mascara. It definitely makes the lashes look thicker and longer, but it has a slight (but only slight) tendency to smudge and clump. **Super Mascara** *($11)* is worth a consideration. It does take some effort to get length and definition, but it does get someplace eventually. Faster would be better, but this is a decent mascara with no clumping or smearing.

☺ **Gentle Waterproof Mascara** *($11.50)* is an excellent mascara. It builds length fast and easily and thickens without clumping, and, best of all, it holds up well when wet!

Club Monaco (Makeup Only)

Hoping to be another Canadian cosmetic success story like M.A.C., Club Monaco Cosmetics, out of Toronto, has launched in a handful of cities across the United States and Canada. It is supposed to be a reasonably priced line of professional makeup products that embraces "everyday wearable colour and the *hottest look* of the moment."

To give this line a bit of New York élan (after all, Canada doesn't quite have the panache of the Big Apple, despite M.A.C.'s origins), it is being represented by Denice Markey, a New York makeup artist. With or without Markey's fashion magazine credentials the question I always want to know is, How do these products hold up for everyday use? Even trendy makeup products have to go on evenly without streaking, clumping, or fading.

One interesting concept of this line I was very curious to check out was their claim that many of the color products were formulated with less pigment or decreased pigment concentrations to create a more sheer look and prevent the colors from grabbing on the skin. According to Markey, "Many cosmetic products 'take' as soon as you apply them and then you have to live with the outcome. Our products are the complete opposite. That way women are able to avoid mistakes like heavy edges around the jaw or hair line." Interesting notion. Eyeshadows and blushes or lipsticks that have a grainy, wet texture (M.A.C. is one line like this I've warned about) do tend to grab quickly and make blending difficult or make the color look more prominent than you may want. However, the problem with colors that go on too softly, like Clinique shadows and blushes for example, is getting them to last or build any intensity.

How does Club Monaco fit into this picture of color application and price? In some ways quite well. It is definitely a fun counter, and nicely organized, and the prices are, for the most part, under $15 each, and that's not bad for a department-store line. Backlit counters have a clean, white-frosted and metal look, with only the colors of the shadows and products peeking out from the glare. Displays are easily accessible and you can play to your heart's content. There are only two types of foundation, but the colors are some of the most beautifully neutral around, with some great shades for very light to medium dark skin tones as well. There is a range of matte (well, only slightly shiny) to very shiny eyeshadows that do indeed go on softly; they also don't fade. The handsome array of blush colors go on softly and blend on easily too. Even the concealer gets high points; it didn't crease, and the colors are some of the best around.

The only real disappointment here is that the Oil-Free Makeup and the Liquid Makeup are indistinguishable, with the oil-free foundation turning slick within less than two hours. The Wet/Dry Powder has a poor color selection, with all the shades leaning toward the peach side. Strange colors, when all the other face products are so neutral. Another surprise are the overpriced brushes. Although they are quite nice and soft, the prices are steep given the other price points.

If you live in a city where this line is found (Toronto, Chicago, Seattle, San Francisco, or New York), it's worth a visit. For more information about Club Monaco call (800) 281-3395.

☺ **FOUNDATION: Oil-Free Foundation** *($18)* has excellent colors. These are some of the most beautiful neutral shades around. It also goes on very sheer and even. What a shame it is a terrible foundation for someone with oily skin. This will show shine in no time, even if you don't have oily skin, but if you have normal to dry skin this is one to try. **Liquid Makeup** *($18)* is quite similar to the oil-free; you won't really be able to tell much of a difference. This is slightly more moist than the oil-free, but only slightly.

☺ **Wet/Dry Powder** *($21)* comes in a poor group of colors that lean toward the peach side, plus the application is very choppy. It's the only real mistake in the bunch.

☺ **CONCEALER:** With 11 mostly terrific shades and a creamy smooth texture that doesn't crease I would give Club Monaco's **Concealer** *($10)* a test spin if you happen by their counter. It is really excellent.

☺ **POWDER: Pressed Powder** *($16)* is an average powder with some great colors and a soft, silky texture. It goes on rather translucent and smooth. Even the **Bronzers** (part of the pressed powders) *($16)* have believable tan colors with minimal shine. **Loose Powder** *($18)* has a soft, dry finish in four very usable shades.

☺ **BLUSH:** Blush *($16)* goes on very silky and soft. The array of colors is beautiful and interesting, and these are not your average blush colors either.

☺ **EYESHADOW:** Eyeshadow *($11)* have three versions that describe them to a T: Matte (well, it is slightly shiny, but only slightly, it doesn't show when blended on), Satin (a little bit more shiny), and Frost (very shiny). The color selection is attractive, and these shades blend on quite softly. It's hard to build a dramatic look with these colors but they do create an easy-to-apply sheer design.

☺ **$$$ Shimmer** *($15)* are small vials of loose, shiny, colored powders. I'm sure there is a very hot, trendy reason to use these, but if you want shine there are plenty of pressed powders around that can give the same performance without the mess and flaking.

☹ **Eye Grease** *($13)* is, just as the name implies, a very greasy cream eyeshadow. Three of the colors are very dark, in shades of navy, brown, and black. The other three colors are pale shiny colors of gray, white, and gold. I'm sure this creates some kind of hot look but putting on eyeshadows that I know are going to smear and crease on purpose is a look I suggest passing on.

☺ **$$$ EYE AND BROW SHAPER:** The **Eye** and **Brow Pencils** *($10)* are almost indistinguishable. They both have very dry finishes and good range of colors.

☺ **$$$ LIPSTICK AND LIP PENCIL:** All of the **Lipsticks** *($13)* have a great feel, and the color range is attractive and not as trendy as I was expecting. The Matte shades aren't all that matte, though they do have a nice creamy consistency. It is hard to discern any difference between the Cream lipsticks for this line and the Matte ones, while the Cream Frosts are just slightly more glossy than the Cream version. **Lip Gloss** *($13)* is a very standard sheer gloss and is as good as any, and very overpriced. I wouldn't give up my $2 Bonne Bell pot gloss for this one, that's for sure. **Lip Pencil** *($10)* is just a very standard pencil in a nice range of colors, and has an almost too dry application. There still isn't a reason to spend more than $4 on any lip or eye pencil.

☺ **$$$ MASCARA:** *($12)* is a fairly good mascara that builds length quickly with minimal clumping. It does tend to smear slightly during the day, but only slightly, though I wouldn't give up Cover Girl Professional Advanced Mascara for this one.

☺ $$$ <u>BRUSHES:</u> Club Monaco has an attractive set of brushes that range in price from $12 to $38. The hair isn't the softest, but these are still quite usable and the shapes are adaptable to most size faces and eyes. There are less expensive brushes to be found but these are a viable option.

Color Me Beautiful

Carole Jackson hasn't owned this line for some time. The Color Me Beautiful public relations department told me it would probably be best to remove her name from this introduction. Somehow that seems like sacrilege. Carole Jackson introduced the art of wearing the right colors for your skin type to an entire generation of women via her "seasons" theory, which explained what colors work best with a particular skin tone and hair color. Once a woman knew whether she was a Spring (blonde hair and pink skin tones; requires pastel colors with a yellow undertone), Summer (blonde hair and sallow skin tones; requires pastel colors with a blue undertone), Autumn (red hair and pink skin tones; requires yellow-based earth tones), or Winter (brunette or black hair and any skin color; requires vivid blue-toned pastels), she could find colors that enhanced her skin tone instead of draining the color from it. This philosophy has clearly changed the way women shop for clothing and makeup colors.

Ms. Jackson created this makeup line in response to the demand for her color expertise. Sadly, with or without her, the line doesn't deliver the color organization you may be looking for. The color trays are divided into the appropriate seasons, but many of the colors overlap and not all of the appropriate color swatches are represented. Some colors are in both the Winter drawer and the Spring drawer, which doesn't make any sense given Jackson's beliefs about color. Also, most of the eyeshadows and some of the blushes are just too shiny; there is only one type of foundation (which is incredibly limiting); and there is only one pressed powder color. Finally, the foundation colors are divided into the four seasons groupings, but, because the shades overlap, there are really only two color groupings, not four. Although I agree wholeheartedly with the idea of using color to complement and enhance skin tone, all foundations should be neutral, with no pink or peach. Dividing these foundations into color groupings doesn't make sense. Just because a woman's skin has pink tones doesn't mean she needs a pink foundation. Her underlying skin color is still neutral. Adding pink to already pink skin only makes the skin look more pink and artificial. And there is never a reason to buy a peach-colored foundation. In fact, when I asked the salespeople if they sold much of the peach-colored foundations, they said no, none at all. What a surprise! For more information about Color Me Beautiful call (800) 533-5503.

The Reviews C

Color Me Beautiful Skin Care

☹ **Creamy Cleanser for Dry Skin** *($15.50 for 6 ounces)* is a very greasy mineral oil–based wipe-off cleanser. It is more a cold cream than anything, which isn't great for skin, but what is really terrible for skin are the lemon, orange, grapefruit, and lime oils in this product, which are all seriously irritating.

☹ **Lathering Cleanser for Normal/Dry Skin** *($15.50 for 4.5 ounces)* is a standard detergent-based, water-soluble cleanser that includes even more irritating plant oils than the cleanser above, including peppermint and spearmint.

☹ **Foaming Cleanser for Normal/Oily Skin** *($15.50 for 4.5 ounces)* is very similar to the cleanser above, and the same review applies.

☹ **Makeup Remover Gel** *($13 for 2 ounces)* contains pine and lemon extracts that can irritate the skin, especially the eye area.

☹ **Balancing Toner for All Skin Types** *($12 for 6 ounces)* contains grapefruit, citronella, and witch hazel, which are too irritating for all skin types.

☹ **Refining Toner for All Skin Types Except Very Oily** *($13 for 6 ounces)* contains a host of irritating plant oils, including lemon, orange, lime, and grapefruit.

☺ **$$$ Visible Results Glycolic Skin Conditioner for All Skin Types I** *($18.50 for 1 ounce)* contains mostly water, glycolic acid, thickeners, slip agent, vitamins E and A, water-binding agents, plant extracts, and preservatives. This is a very good 8% AHA product for normal to dry skin.

☺ **$$$ Visible Results Glycolic Skin Conditioner for All Skin Types II** *($18.50 for 1 ounce)* is similar to the one above, but has only about 6% AHA.

☹ **Multi-Action Booster Vitasome Energizing Treatment** *($22.50 for 1 ounce)* is supposed to "fight time with a vitamin-and-mineral-packed anti-wrinkle serum." What it can primarily do for the skin is cause irritation due to the plant extracts and oil of lemon, pine, grapefruit, mandarin, and citronella it contains.

☹ **Thirst Aid Anti-Wrinkle Serum for Dehydrated/Mature Skin** *($24.50 for 1.1 ounces)* contains too many irritating plant extracts and oils to recommend. See the list of them in the product above.

☹ **Thirst Aid Intensive Night Treatment for Normal/Dry Skin** *($24.50 for 2 ounces)* is similar to the one above and the same review applies.

☺ **Thirst Aid Intensive Hydrating Mask for All Skin Types** *($16.50 for 2 ounces)* is a BHA mask that contains several ingredients that are problematic for all kinds of skin types. Someone with dry, sensitive skin shouldn't be using a BHA product, nor should someone with oily, blemish-prone skin be using some of the plant oils and thickeners in here.

☹ **Daily Defense Light SPF 15 for Normal/Combination Skin** *($17.50 for 1.6 ounces)* doesn't contain avobenzone, zinc oxide, or titanium dioxide, and is not recommended.

☺ **Daily Defense Oil-Free SPF 15 for Oily Skin** *($17.50 for 1.6 ounces)* doesn't contain avobenzone, zinc oxide, or titanium dioxide, and is not recommended.

☹ **Daily Defense Rich SPF 15 for Dry Skin** *($17.50 for 1.6 ounces)* doesn't contain avobenzone, zinc oxide, or titanium dioxide, and is not recommended.

☺ **$$$ Triple Action Eye Cream, all Skin Types** *($18.50 for 0.5 ounce)* contains mostly water, slip agent, thickeners, plant extract, a long list of thickeners, plant oil, silicone oil, plant extract, water-binding agents, vitamins and preservatives. This is a very good moisturizer for dry skin.

☺ **$$$ Endless Tan Self-Tanning Lotion** *($15 for 8 ounces)* uses the same active ingredient, dihydroxyacetone, as all self-tanners, and this one is as good as any, and reasonably priced!

☺ **$$$ Fade Away for All Skin Types** *($15 for 1.9 ounces)* is a standard 2% hydroquinone-based moisturizer that can be helpful to lighten dark skin patches, but only when used in conjunction with a good sunscreen.

☹ **Instant Result Mask for All Skin Types** *($16.50 for 4 ounces)* contains mostly aloe, plant water, wax, synthetic scrub particles, thickeners, plant oil, cleansing agent, AHAs, a BHA, anti-irritant, and preservatives. There aren't enough AHAs here to count as exfoliants, but combining scrub particles with a BHA is too irritating for many skin types.

☺ **$$$ Conditioning Lip Balm** *($9.50)* is a good emollient lip balm.

Color Me Beautiful Makeup

☺ FOUNDATION: **Liquid Foundation** *($18)* is quite good and light with a soft creamy texture, but only for someone with normal to dry skin. Some of the colors are quite good but the ones that are bad are really bad. **These colors are too intensely peach or pink:** Beige Blush, Cool Beige, Peach Blush, Warm Beige, Country Blush, and Mahogany.

☹ **Soft Focus Skin Perfecting Oil-Free Foundation SPF 8** *($19.50)* has a poor SPF and doesn't have UVA protection. It is not recommended.

☺ **Illusion Age Defying Foundation SPF 15** *($20)* is a very creamy, soft, cream-to-powder foundation. It has an excellent SPF and is part titanium dioxide. There is every reason to give this one a try if you have normal to slightly dry skin. **The colors to avoid are** Sand, Cool Beige, Porcelain, Ecru, and Ivory.

☺ **Perfection Microfine Powder Foundation** *($20)* is a pressed powder–type foundation. It has a great, dry, but soft texture and wonderful colors. **These colors are excellent:** Ivory, Tabasco Beige, Creamy Beige, Whisper Beige, Sepia Beige, Toasty Beige, Fawn Beige, Cameo Beige, Cocoa Beige, Golden Glow, and Golden Sand. **These colors are too pink:** Rose Glow and Pink Sand.

☹   **Color Adjuster** *($15)* is a light mint green foundation meant to reduce pink skin tones. I dislike color correctors in general, and this one is like all the others: an extra, unnecessary step that can leave a strange hue on the face.

☹   **Eyeshadow Base** *($18)* is applied like a concealer over the eye area. It dries to a sticky powder finish, but it doesn't hold eyeshadow any better than using nothing. Plus, the one color it comes in is slightly pink, and won't work for most skin tones, and will change the color of the eyeshadow you are applying.

☹   <u>CONCEALER:</u> **Cover Stick** *($9.50)* comes in four shades: Light, which is too pink, and Medium, Medium/Deep, and Deep, which are great. The texture isn't the best (it tends to be greasy), but it blends easily. Unfortunately, the color slips into the lines around the eye.

☺   <u>POWDER:</u> **Translucent Loose Powder** *($13.50)* has a smooth, dry finish. It comes in three shades, and all are great.

☺   <u>BLUSH:</u> **Powder Blush** *($12)* comes in a nice array of colors with a smooth application. There are shiny ones to avoid, but there are decent matte ones to check out. Some of the colors go on strongly, so they work well for darker skin tones.

☺   <u>EYESHADOW:</u> Most of the **Eyeshadows** *($9)* have improved texture though many are too shiny. There are a handful of mattes that are worth looking into. **The colors to consider are:** Fog, Camel, Haze, Fawn, Taupe, Wheat, Malted Milk, BlusHHH, Parchment, and Auburn.

☺   <u>EYE AND BROW SHAPER:</u> **Smudgeliner** *($9.50)* is a standard pencil with one end having a sponge tip. **Brow Color** *($12)* is a dry eyeshadow for the brows. It is a great way to apply brow color, although any eyeshadow that matches your brows would work just as well. **Brow Fixative** *($9)* is a clear gel meant to keep eyebrows in place. It works well, but no better than hair spray on a toothbrush brushed through the brow.

☺   <u>LIPSTICK AND LIP PENCIL:</u> **Satin Lipstick** *($9.50),* which comes in a wide range of colors, is very creamy, and even the soft colors have decent staying power. **More Than Matte Lipstick** *($9.50)* is a superior matte lipstick that has good staying power and doesn't bleed. This isn't ultra-matte (it does have some creamy movement), but it is indeed matte without being the least bit drying. **Lip Pencil** *($8)* is just a standard lip pencil with only a handful of colors to choose from.

☺   **Color Fix Lipstick** *($10)* is an interesting product make up of alcohol and a film former. This places a layer of hair spray over the lips, which can feel strange—but it does hold lipstick in place.

☺   <u>MASCARA:</u> **Lush Lash** *($9.50)* is an excellent mascara. It goes on easily, doesn't smudge, and builds long, relatively thick lashes.

☺   **Sensitive Eyes Mascara** *($9.50)* doesn't go on as well as the Lush Lash and takes a long time to build any length and thickness. It may or may not be better for sensitive eyes—there doesn't seem to be much difference in the ingredient lists—but it isn't better for defining lashes.

Complex 15 (Skin Care Only)

☺ **Complex 15 Cream** *($5.18 for 2.5 ounces)* and **Complex 15 Lotion** *($6.99 for 8 ounces)* are simple, rather ordinary moisturizers that have been around for a long time. They get recommended by dermatologists a lot, which is the primary reason they stay on the market, but I wonder if any dermatologist has checked out the ingredient labels. Both contain mostly water, thickeners, glycerin, silicone, and preservatives. None of that is bad, just boring. There are far more elegant and interesting formulations out there. Also, without sunscreen, these are only an option for nighttime. For more information about Complex 15 write Schering-Plough at Schering-Plough HealthCare Products, Inc., P.O. Box 377, Memphis, TN 38151.

Coppertone (Sun Care Only)

Coppertone makes one of the most disappointing groups of sunscreen products around. Except for their new **Shade UVA Guard SPF 30** (the first avobenzone-based sunscreen that is now under the Coppertone label), all the other sunscreens in their lineup have no real UVA protection. No titanium dioxide, zinc oxide, or avobenzone in any of them. Word of caution: for some reason Coppertone also has a product called **Shade SPF 45** that does not contain avobenzone or any other UVA-protection ingredients and that sounds a lot like their **Shade UVA Guard SPF 30**. Coppertone also boasts that their sunscreens for kids are the ones recommended most by pediatricians. If that's true, be sure you find another pediatrician. It would mean your doctor doesn't have the latest information on sun damage from UVA rays, and I would worry about what else he or she wasn't up to date on. For more information on Coppertone call (973) 822-7000.

☹ **Bug & Sun Sunscreen with Insect Repellent Adult Formula SPF 15** *($6.99 for 4 ounces, $8.59 for 8 ounces)* might get rid of bugs, but this product doesn't contain avobenzone, zinc oxide, or titanium dioxide, and is not recommended.

☹ **Bug & Sun Sunscreen with Insect Repellent, Kids Formula, SPF 30** *($6.99 for 4 ounces, $8.59 for 8 ounces)* might get rid of bugs, but this product doesn't contain avobenzone, zinc oxide, or titanium dioxide, and is not recommended.

☹ **Coppertone Gold Dark Tanning Exotic Oil Spray, with Vitamin E & Aloe** *($5.29 for 8 ounces)* makes me angry. There's something about a skin-care line that offers sun protection as well as products that encourage tanning that's just plain unconscionable. None of these "tanning" products are recommended; that would be like recommending skin cancer!

☻ **Coppertone Gold SPF 2 Dark Tanning Dry Oil, with Vitamin E & Aloe** *($5.29 for 8 ounces)* gets the same review as the one above.

☻ **Coppertone Gold SPF 4 Dark Tanning Oil, with Vitamin E & Aloe** *($5.29 for 8 ounces)* gets the same review as the one above.

☻ **Coppertone Gold SPF 2 Dark Tanning Exotic Lotion, with Vitamin E & Aloe** *($5.29 for 8 ounces)* gets the same review as the one above.

☻ **Coppertone Gold Tan Magnifier Intensive Oil with Vitamin E & Aloe** *($5.29 for 8 ounces)* gets the same review as the one above.

☻ **Coppertone Gold Tan Magnifier Solar Gel with Vitamin E & Aloe** *($5.29 for 8 ounces)* gets the same review as the one above.

☹ **Coppertone Kids SPF 40 6 Hour Waterproof Sunblock Lotion** *($6.99 for 4 ounces, $8.59 for 8 ounces)* doesn't contain avobenzone, zinc oxide, or titanium dioxide, and is not recommended.

☹ **Coppertone Oil-Free Waterproof Sunblock SPF 15** *($6.99 for 4 ounces, $8.59 for 8 ounces)* doesn't contain avobenzone, zinc oxide, or titanium dioxide, and is not recommended.

☹ **Coppertone Oil-Free Waterproof Sunblock Lotion SPF 30** *($6.99 for 4 ounces, $8.59 for 8 ounces)* doesn't contain avobenzone, zinc oxide, or titanium dioxide, and is not recommended.

☹ **Coppertone Oil-Free Waterproof Sunscreen Lotion, SPF 8** *($6.99 for 4 ounces)* doesn't contain avobenzone, zinc oxide, or titanium dioxide, and is not recommended.

☹ **Coppertone Shade Oil-Free Gel SPF 30 UVA/UVB Protection** *($6.99 for 4 ounces)* doesn't contain avobenzone, zinc oxide, or titanium dioxide, and is not recommended. Many products make claims about UVA protection that are truly misleading. Without the three UVA protecting ingredients above, that cover about 80% to 90% UVA radiation, other formulations only protect you from about 20% UVA radiation.

☹ **Coppertone Shade Sunblock Lotion SPF 45 UVA/UVB Protection** *($6.99 for 4 ounces)* doesn't contain avobenzone, zinc oxide, or titanium dioxide, and is not recommended.

☹ **Coppertone Sport All Day Protection SPF 48 UVA/UVB Sunblock** *($6.99 for 6 ounces)* doesn't contain avobenzone, zinc oxide, or titanium dioxide, and is not recommended.

☹ **Coppertone 4 Waterproof UVA/UVB Protection PABA Free Moisturizing Suntan Lotion** *($4.79 for 4 ounces)* doesn't contain avobenzone, zinc oxide, or titanium dioxide, and is not recommended; moreover, the SPF 4 is damaging and misleading when it comes to sun protection.

☹ **Coppertone 8 Waterproof UVA/UVB Protection Ultra Moisturizing with**

Aloe & Vitamin E Sunscreen Lotion *($4.79 for 4 ounces)* doesn't contain avobenzone, zinc oxide, or titanium dioxide, and is not recommended; and the SPF 4 is damaging and misleading when it comes to sun protection.

☹ **Coppertone Waterproof Ultra-Moisturizing SPF 15 with Aloe & Vitamin E** *($4.97 for 4 ounces, $6.97 for 10.64 ounces)* doesn't contain avobenzone, zinc oxide, or titanium dioxide, and is not recommended.

☹ **Coppertone Waterproof Ultra-Moisturizing SPF 30 with Aloe & Vitamin E** *($6.97 for 10.64 ounces)* doesn't contain avobenzone, zinc oxide, or titanium dioxide, and is not recommended.

☹ **Coppertone Waterproof Ultra-Moisturizing SPF 45 with Aloe & Vitamin E** *($5.97 for 4 ounces, $7.58 for 8 ounces)* doesn't contain avobenzone, zinc oxide, or titanium dioxide, and is not recommended.

☹ **Kids Colorblock Disappearing Purple Sunblock Waterproof SPF 40 6 Hour** *($6.99 for 4 ounces, $8.59 for 8 ounces)* doesn't contain avobenzone, zinc oxide, or titanium dioxide, and is not recommended.

☹ **Water Babies UVA/UVB Sunblock Lotion SPF 30** *($6.99 for 4 ounces, $8.59 for 8 ounces)* doesn't contain avobenzone, zinc oxide, or titanium dioxide, and is not recommended.

☹ **Water Babies UVA/UVB Sunblock Lotion SPF 45** *($6.99 for 4 ounces, $8.59 for 8 ounces)* doesn't contain avobenzone, zinc oxide, or titanium dioxide, and is not recommended.

☺ **Shade UVA Guard SPF 15** *($9.99 for 4 ounces)* is a very good avobenzone-based sunscreen for someone with normal to dry skin.

☺ **Shade UVA Guard SPF 30** *($9.99 for 4 ounces)* is a very good avobenzone-based sunscreen for someone with normal to dry skin.

☺ **Coppertone After Sun Aloe & Vitamin E Moisturizing Lotion** *($4.79 for 16 ounces)* is a very good emollient moisturizer for dry skin; it includes water, slip agent, mineral oil, thickeners, cocoa butter, lanolin, fragrance, silicone, and preservatives.

☺ **Coppertone Gold After Sun Cool Gel, with Vitamin E & Aloe** *($5.29 for 12 ounces)* is a very lightweight gel containing mostly water, aloe, and glycerin. It's actually quite good for just a soothing feel on the skin, but it is minimally moisturizing.

Corn Silk (Makeup Only)

I remember Corn Silk from when I was teenager. Yes, it's been around that long. At that time Corn Silk was synonymous with not having to worry about looking like an oil slick by midday. Corn Silk was supposed to be the oil-absorbing powder to end all powders. I recall buying it at several different junctures way back when, hoping it would work miracles on my sludge-laden skin.

Sad to say, it didn't work wonders back then and it still can't today. In fact, there is nothing about ☹ **Corn Silk Loose Powder** *($3.99)* or **Corn Silk Pressed Powder** *($3.99)* that I can recommend. The packaging doesn't allow you to see the colors; the colors themselves are OK, but most are slightly pink or peach; the new darker shades and all the loose powders all have shine (what were they thinking with that twist; powder is supposed to eliminate shine, not add it); and the fragrance is so sickly sweet that I could barely tolerate reviewing them. Yes, Corn Silk powders have a soft, dry texture and they do go on very sheer and soft, but the serious limitations don't make up for the decent application.

By the way, ☹ **Corn Silk Liquid Concealer** *($3.75)* and **Enriched Cover Stick** *($3.75)* come in shades that are peachy, green, or yellow; they all crease, and they have poor staying power. ☹ **Corn Silk Liquid Makeup** *($3.75)* has some nice shades, but it too has a sickly sweet fragrance and is just awful. For more information about CornSilk call (800) 745-2429.

Coty (Makeup Only)

Hiding in a corner of most drugstores is the perennial but sparse cosmetic line called Coty. Although this line doesn't have much I'd recommend, you shouldn't overlook it completely. Yes, the foundations lack testers (one of them is even packaged so you can't see the color in the container). And yes, most of the pressed- and loose-powder colors are hidden by the powder puff, so you can't begin to guess which color is best for you. But where Coty excels is in its varied collection of lip products. This line has some of the most innovative lipsticks around. If your lipsticks tend to bleed into the lines around your lips, Coty can save you. Also, the small selection of eye and lip pencils, though fairly standard, are every bit as good as a hundred other pencils on the scene, only cheaper. Coty has a handful of skin-care products that are not widely distributed, but that isn't necessarily bad news, because they aren't much to get excited about. For more information about Coty call (212) 850-2300.

✍ ☺ <u>FOUNDATION:</u> The **Line Minimizing Makeup** *($6.77)* is a soft, talc-based powder; it doesn't minimize lines, but it does go on rather soft and silky and comes in some excellent shades. Like most powder-foundations, this one is more powder than foundation. Still, it goes on smoothly and provides light, sheer coverage. Warning: It is also highly fragranced and not for everyone's nose.

☹ **Chronology Hydrating Creme Makeup** *($6.02)* has no testers at the counter, and there is no way to see even a hint of the color, given its black tube. **Airspun Powderessence Liquid Matte Makeup** *($6.02)* has a terrible selection of very pink and peach shades.

☹ <u>POWDER:</u> **Correctives Pressed Powder with Natural Astringents** *($4.81)* is one of those products that make me angry enough to yell. This is supposed to be for someone with oily skin, and the label carries on about "oil-free" and "oil-absorb-ing" and "translucent," but what they don't tell you is that the powder is *iridescent*. That's right, it has shine. What a joke! In trying to get rid of shine, you add more. Coty, wake up and smell the coffee.

☺ **LIPSTICK AND LIP PENCIL: Lip Doctor Color Therapy Stick with AHA** *($3.95)* is a very emollient lip gloss in a tube that can be good for chapped lips. It does contain a small amount of menthol, which doesn't doctor the lips and can be an irritant for some skin types. It also contains about 1% AHAs, which makes them good water-binding agents in terms of moisturizing, but it won't exfoliate or help reduce lines. **Sheer to Stay 6 Hour Lip Color** *($3.20)* is a rich emollient gloss that goes on smoothly, but to suggest it lasts six hours is stretching the truth by a few hours. It contains a small amount of tint, so it tends to stay a little better than an ordinary gloss, but not that much better. **Self-Sealing Lip Makeup** *($3.73)* is applied with a wand and goes on like a gloss, but it dries to a soft, matte, powdery texture. It is actually quite nice, and an interesting twist on the ultra-matte look. The color selection is extremely limited, but what is available is worth checking out. **'24' Hour Creme Lipstick** *($4.63)* is a matte lipstick with just enough "slip" to feel somewhat pleasant when you rub your lips together during the day. This lipstick doesn't bleed and stays on incredibly well. Like all truly matte lipsticks, it tends to cake, but this one doesn't dry out the lips. **Stop It Anti-Feathering Stick for Lips** *($3.57)* and **Hold It Wear Extending Base for Lips***($4.16)* are two of the absolute best on the market. No lipstick, not even reds, can bleed past these two clear lipstick bases. And they don't dry out the lips, cake, or peel. What a find! **Lip Writer Stayput Lipstick** *($4.50)* is another amazing lip product. It is an ultra-matte lipstick in a stick form, like a thick eye pencil. It goes on incredibly smoothly, and it absolutely doesn't budge. In fact, this one is hard to get off. Worth checking out!

☹ **Silkstick Lipstick** *($2.08)* is a fairly greasy cream lipstick that feels almost too slick. It's more gloss than silk, that's for sure.

Cover Girl (Makeup Only)

There is a part of me that is just amazed at Cover Girl's continued looming presence at the drugstore. It had one of the largest displays in most every store I visited, yet this line has some of the absolute worst color products in the industry. The foundations are the most awful shades of pink, peach, and rose imaginable. The powders are unidentifiable, blocked by sponge applicators that don't allow you to see the color. But don't worry, even if you could see the color you wouldn't be impressed, these are as peach and pink as the foundations, not to mention the fragrance, which is literally overwhelming. But as terrible as the foundations and powders are, they can't compete with the unpleasant textures and shades of Cover Girl's concealers.

The Reviews C

Another shortcoming is that Cover Girl hasn't updated its color selection for quite some time. The blush shades are leftovers from the late '80s, with vivid pinks, roses, and corals, nary a natural tan or earth tone in the bunch. Cover Girl's eyeshadows are still more shiny than matte, and the matte shades, while not terrible, don't adhere well and tend to go on choppy. Perhaps it's the attraction Cover Girl holds for the teenage consumer who doesn't know what to avoid or how to select colors for herself that keeps the line's popularity unchallenged. Other lines such as Bonne Bell and Jane are starting to make inroads but only slightly.

One strength for this line are Cover Girl's mascaras and lipsticks. There are some good choices with excellent prices to consider. For more information about Cover Girl call (800) 543-1745.

☹   FOUNDATION: Unfortunately, testers for Cover Girl foundations are still not available at the counters, but even if they were, almost all of the 12 different types of foundations have unbearable, unnatural shades of pink, peach, and rose. They are also so overly fragranced the fumes will knock your socks off.

☹   MoistureWear ($3.69) has terrible colors and an even worse fragrance. Clarifying Acne Treatment ($3.69) contains menthol and camphor, which can cause irritation; the fragrance is intolerable; and the colors have no relation to skin tone. Fresh Complexion ($3.69) is similar to the one above and is not recommended for any skin type. Clean Makeup ($3.69) contains camphor, menthol, clove, and eucalyptus, which are extremely irritating, but it also contains isopropyl myristate, which can trigger breakouts, and mineral oil which can feel greasy. This foundation is a mistake waiting to happen. Replenishing Liquid to Powder Makeup ($5.49) has the most obnoxious colors you are likely to run into anywhere. Every one of them is glaringly pink, peach, or rose. Simply Powder Foundation ($4.95) goes on thick and heavy and easily cakes on the skin. It isn't simply powder, it is a messy layer over the skin.

☺   Ultimate Finish Liquid Powder Makeup ($5.49) has a small but good color selection and decent textures, but it also contains aluminum starch (a skin irritant) as the second item on the ingredient list, as well as isopropyl myristate, which can aggravate breakouts. It may be OK for some skin types, but definitely not someone with oily or blemish-prone skin. It also has a tendency to exaggerate every dry skin cell you have your on your face.

☺   Balanced Complexion for Combination Skin Makeup ($5.49) has better colors than many of the other foundations in this group. It goes on light, smooth, and matte, and stays that way for most of the day. It also doesn't slip into lines. What a shame there aren't testers so you could try this one out. Sometimes they do sell little samples for $1, though, so you can test products before buying a full-size container. Most of the colors are surprisingly good; the color to avoid is Natural Beige.

☺   ContinuousWear Natural Makeup ($6.29), unlike most of Cover Girl's foundations, has very wearable colors that blend on smoothly and look great for someone with normal to dry skin. Unfortunately you can't tell the color from the container (the exterior is opaque), preventing any chance of identifying a color match! What a shame.

☺ CONCEALER: Clarifying Concealer *($3.69)* and Replenishing Concealer *($3.05)* all have the worst color selections I've ever seen. Almost all of the colors are too peach or pink, and the textures streak and crease easily. MoistureWear Concealer *($3.45)* has a terrible range of colors and it easily creases into the lines around the eyes.

☺ Invisible Concealer *($3.69)* is a surprisingly excellent concealer. The six colors are great for lighter to medium skin tones, and it goes on smooth and even without creasing! This is one to try.

☺ POWDER: The Cover Girl line offers several types of pressed powder, but you can't see the color you're buying through the packaging. How strange and inconvenient! And why package a pressed powder with a puff when it should be applied with a brush anyway? The Clarifying Pressed Powder *($3.24)*, Clarifying Loose Powder *($3.79)*, and Professional Translucent Powder *($3.76)* all contain eucalyptus and camphor, which can be skin irritants, and the fragrance is dreadful. At any rate, regardless of the irritating ingredients and smell, I can't recommend any of these pressed powders because you can't see the color you'd be buying. Clean Fragrance-Free Pressed Powder *($3.25)* clears the air, but you still can't see the color you're considering, and the same is true for Moisture Wear Pressed Powder *($3.05)* and Balanced Complexion Pressed Powder *($3.05)*.

☺ BLUSH: Continuous Color Moisture Enriched Blush *($3.09)*, Instant Cheekbones *($3.23)*, Cheekers *($2.85)*, Professional Color Match Blush Duo *($3.04)*, and Classic Color Brush-On Blush *($3.22)* are the range of Cover Girl blushes. The colors for these haven't been updated for some time. They are all rather pastel and intense, which may be OK for darker skin tones, but there aren't any subtle colors in the bunch. All of the colors go on easily without streaking. Most of the blush colors are slightly shiny, but not terribly, and can be an option for some skin types; but if you have oily skin, you will look shiny even before the oil starts coming through. One continuing problem for these blushes is the sickeningly sweet fragrance they all have.

☺ EYESHADOW: The eyeshadows come in lots of shades, including a few matte shades, but mostly the selections are abundantly shiny. NonStop Eye Color *($3.79)* contains three eyeshadows, one of which is shiny, and an eyeshadow base. The base is on the greasy side and doesn't hold eyeshadow any better than a foundation, and the shiny eyeshadow is a waste of money. Professional Color Match *($4.25)* and Professional Eye Enhancers *($4.25 for sets of eight colors, $3.25 for Trios, and*

$3.25 for Quads), **Pro Colors Singles** *($1.81)*, and **Professional Eye Enhancers Singles** *($1.81)* are labeled as matte or perle, but most are very shiny to slightly shiny (yes, even the matte ones have a small amount of shine). Some of the matte shades are worth checking out, but they tend to blend on choppy or unevenly. In the multicolor sets, the color combinations are poor; in others, one or more of the shades are shiny and they tend to apply choppy and cling poorly.

☺ <u>EYE AND BROW SHAPER:</u> **Perfect Blend Eye Pencil** *($2.84)* is a fairly standard pencil that goes on slightly more dry than most and has decent staying power. **Perfect Point Plus** *($3.53)* is a self-sharpening pencil that glides on easily without being greasy and does have a great, consistent point.

☹ **Brow Enhancer** *($1.63)* is a standard pencil that goes on exceptionally thick and heavy, which is not great when it comes to creating a natural look. **Liquid Pencil Soft Precision Liner** *($3.60)* is a traditional liquid liner dispensed in what looks like a soft felt-tip pen. The colors are poor, and the dispensing streaky and messy. What a shame, because it doesn't chip or flake during the day and it stays and stays, but the application and poor color choice are hard to get around. **Soft Radiants** *($1.39)* is a standard eye pencil that goes on fairly greasy and most of the colors are shiny.

☺ <u>LIPSTICK AND LIP PENCIL:</u> Cover Girl makes several very impressive lipsticks with an excellent selection of attractive bright and muted colors. **Continuous Color Self Renewing Lipstick** *($3.73)* claims that all you have to do is press your lips together to refresh the color. Now, for what lipstick (besides the ultra-mattes which rub off when you press your lips together) *isn't* that true? How silly. Nevertheless, this is a somewhat greasy, lightweight lipstick. I strongly suggest staying away from the frosted colors, but if you prefer a lip gloss application for your lipsticks this is an option. **Marathon Lipcolor** *($4.32)* is an excellent addition to the lineup of ultra-matte lipsticks; it is as good an option as any of them. **In Condition Lip Blush** *($2.55)* is Cover Girl's version of a "mood" lipstick. It goes on as a sheer gloss, and in a minute or two it tints your lips in a way that is supposed to enhance your own lip color. This is a very good emollient gloss with a tint that is supposed to be activated by skin temperature, but I didn't notice any color change when I put it on, maybe I wasn't in a mood.

☺ **LipSlicks LipGloss** *($2.99)* is a fairly standard, emollient lip gloss with some fairly shiny shades in packaging that makes getting it on the lips evenly tricky for someone with thin lips. There is an SPF indicated on the display, but if it's not on the label do not count on any SPF protection.

☺ **Luminesse Lipstick** *($3.04)* is an average, rather greasy, shiny, and frosted cream lipstick. However, if you want frost there is no reason not to consider this one. **Remarkable Lip Definer Lip Pencil** *($2.53)* is a good twist-up/no-sharpen lip pencil that comes in five good but limited colors. It's only slightly more greasy than most.

The package lists the Cover Girl lipstick colors that coordinate with that pencil color—nice touch. **Continuous Color Lip Definer** *($2.99)* is fairly greasy and the color range is rather small.

☺ **MASCARA:** **Long 'N Lush** *($3.87)* is indeed long and lush and a wonderful mascara to consider trying. **Curved Brush Professional Advanced Mascara** *($3.05)* builds good length and thickness, though I find the curved brush incredibly awkward to use, while the **Straight Brush Professional Advanced Mascara** *($3.05)* is excellent, and both hold up well during the day. No clumps, no smears, and long thick lashes! **Super Thick Lash** *($4.76)* is a great mascara. It builds thick, long lashes with only a slight tendency to clump. If you don't like any clumping, though, stay away from this one. **Natural Lash Darkener** *($3.95)* is advertised as making the lashes naturally darker, with no artificial lengthening or thickening. Well, you might not get any thickening, but you do get decent length.

☺ **Marathon Waterproof Mascara** *($3.68)* goes on poorly, making lashes look spiked, and takes forever to build any length or thickness. However this stuff will stay on underwater all day. **Remarkable Washable Waterproof Mascara** *($3.87)* has a confusing name, but that can be forgiven because it goes on well, builds length easily, and doesn't smear. However it isn't at all waterproof. What were the Cover Girl executives thinking when they named this product! **Extension Waterproof Mascara** *($3.24)* builds well, making lashes look full with no clumping, but it smudges when wet.

☹ **BRUSHES:** Cover Girl has two blush/powder brushes that are not the best. The **Large Blush Brush** *($4.79)* and the **Medium Blush Brush** *($4.50)* are just OK. The bristles are not as soft as some and are too sparse to provide the best control.

Decleor Paris (Skin Care Only)

Decleor is a high-end skin-care line with prices steep enough to upset most people's investment portfolios, yet these are some of the most standard basic formulations I've seen anywhere. None of them are nearly as impressive or as current as, say, some of the products from Estee Lauder, L'Oreal/Lancome, Alpha Hydrox, Neutrogena, Eucerin, or Avon. What can I say about a line whose average product costs about $50 and whose typical recommended skin-care routine ranges from $250 to $400 (and that doesn't include sunscreen)? What I really want to know is how women can be so misled into believing that exceptionally expensive lines have something to offer that other lines don't. Do they think that these elegant European lines have a roomful of elite scientists using special formulas that will finally erase those wrinkles and bumps that every other product they purchased promised to eliminate but evidently didn't? They don't. Basically, I've found nothing special or exclusive about the products offered by Decleor, except for the prices. If you are one of those women who feel better spending excessive amounts of money on skin care, there is every reason to consider Decleor. It isn't a bad line as such, just a regular one with some plant extracts to make it look exotic. Do be aware that this line consists of an incredibly redundant multitude of moisturizers, a sad display of sun protection, mediocre AHA products, no BHA product, and problematic cleansers. Of course, Decleor's brochure tries hard to convince you that every product they sell will bring nirvana to your face, but these formulations fall far short of the ad copy, and in more ways than one. If you want more information about Decleor, call (800) 722-2219.

☺ **$$$ Cleansing Lotion for the Eyes with Plant Extract** *($18 for 4.2 ounces)* contains mostly water, detergent cleansing agents, slip agents, plant extracts, and preservatives. This very standard eye makeup remover is boringly ordinary.

☹ **Cleansing Oil for the Face and Eyes with Sweet Almond Oil** *($31 for 8.4 ounces)* is a lot of money for almond oil that you could easily pull out of the cupboard. It will remove makeup, but you'll have to wipe it off (a no-no) and it leaves skin feeling greasy.

☹ **Gentle Facial Cleanser with Plant Extracts** *($24 for 5 ounces)* is a detergent-based, water-soluble cleanser with mineral oil and emollients. This cleanser can leave a greasy residue on the face and really needs to be wiped off (bad) instead of rinsed off (good).

☹ **Purifying Cleansing Bar with Essential Oils for Combination Skins** *($16 for 3.5 ounces)* is a standard bar cleanser that contains sodium lauryl sulfate (SLS), a detergent cleanser known for its extremely irritating properties. It also contains tallow, which can clog pores and cause skin irritation.

☹ **Regulating Cleansing Gel with Plant Extracts** *($22 for 5 ounces)* is a water-soluble cleanser that uses sodium C14-16 olefin sulfate as the detergent cleansing agent. This ingredient is extremely irritating and drying for all skin types.

☺ **$$$ Velvet Cleansing Milk with Plant Extracts** *($24 for 8.4 ounces)* is a cold cream–like cleanser with basic thickening agents and plant oil. It needs to be wiped off and is embarrassingly overpriced for what you get.

☺ **$$$ Prolagene Gel for Face and Body for All Skin Types** *($26 for 1.69 ounces)* has a very fancy name for a stunningly bland product. It contains mostly water, slip agent, thickener, preservatives, and fragrant oil. There is little this product can provide for the skin, though it probably won't hurt anyone either.

☹ **Regulating Tonic Lotion with Plant Extracts for Combination and Oily Skins** *($30 for 13.5 ounces)* contains several irritating ingredients that are a problem for most skin types, including orris root, zinc sulfonate, and chlorhexidine. All of these are known for their sensitizing potential. I can't imagine what they are doing in any skin-care product, let alone one for someone with oily skin.

☹ **S.O.S. Regulating Gel with Plant Extracts and Essential Oil for Combi-**

nation Skins *($25 for 0.5 ounce)* contains mostly water, rice starch, talc, pH balancer, glycolic acid, thickener, lactic acid, alcohol, hair styling agent, thickener, water-binding agent, tea tree oil, orris root, and preservatives. While this is an OK AHA product in terms of pH and concentration, it falls short in several other areas. First, AHAs aren't the best way to deal with oily or blemish-prone skin; BHA is. Orris root is an irritant, and rice starch and paraffin (one of the first thickening agents) can clog pores. This product is not recommended.

☹ **Face Peel, with Plant Extracts and Essential Oils for All Skin Types** *($31 for 1.69 ounces)* contains mostly water, thickeners, pH balancer, slip agent, clay, more thickeners, plant oils, plant extracts, and preservatives. The second ingredient is paraffin, which can clog pores. It also contains lemon oil and lavender oil, which can be skin sensitizers. The clay can exfoliate the skin, but why stick in all these other ingredients that can cause problems?

☺ **$$$ Contour Firming Serum for the Eyes with Plant Extracts, for All Skin Types** *($36 for 0.5 ounce)* contains mostly water, water-binding agents, plant extract, glycerin, slip agents, and preservative. This rather standard, lightweight moisturizer has minimal plant extracts, but could be an OK lightweight moisturizer for normal to slightly dry skin.

☺ **$$$ Day Alpha Hydrating Cream with Plant Extracts and Alpha-Hydroxy Acids, SPF 12, for All Skin Types** *($42 for 1.69 ounces)* is a decent sunscreen that contains titanium dioxide, and it does have about a 6% concentration of AHAs in an appropriate pH. This is an option for a two-in-one product, but a slightly higher concentration of AHAs would be better for exfoliation.

☺ **$$$ Day Hydrating Cream with Plant Extracts** *($56 for 1.69 ounces)* doesn't contain a sunscreen, which makes it a very poor daytime moisturizer, though it can be good for dry skin at night.

☺ **$$$ Eternance Cream with Plant Extracts, for Mature Skins** *($53 for 1.69 ounces)* contains mostly water, thickeners, plant oil, plant extract, more thickeners, and preservatives. This is a very ordinary, dated moisturizing formula. It would be good for someone with dry skin, but for the money there are more interesting and unique formulas out there.

☺ **$$$ Eye Contour Gel with Plant Extracts, for All Skin Types** *($27 for 0.5 ounce)* contains mostly water, plant extract, slip agent, thickener, plant extracts, pH balancer, and preservatives. This standard gel formulation contains minimal plant extracts. It can be OK for someone with oily skin who wants the most minimal amount of moisturizer possible.

☺ **$$$ Firming Face and Neck Lotion with Plant Extracts, for Mature Skins** *($60 for 1 ounce)* contains mostly water, plant extract, slip agents, more plant extracts, fragrance, and preservatives. Are they serious? Slip agents and plant extracts for *$60?* This is little more than tea water with some waxy thickeners. It isn't bad, but why bother?

☺ **$$$ Firming Neck Gel with Plant Extract for Mature Skins** (*$48 for 1.69 ounces*) contains water, slip agent, water-binding agents, plant extracts, thickeners, fragrance, and preservatives. I guess if the product above didn't firm you up, you might want to try this one and be disappointed all over again.

☺ **$$$ Instant Beauty Booster, with Plant Extracts for All Skin Types** (*$42 for 1.69 ounces*) contains mostly water, water-binding agent, slip agent, plant oils, thickeners, fragrance, vitamin E, and preservatives. This would be an OK, light-weight moisturizer for someone with normal to slightly dry skin. Expecting anything in the way of instant beauty is great marketing, but is just not possible.

☺ **$$$ Moisturizing Face Cream with Plant Extracts and Essential Wax for Normal Skins** (*$50 for 1.69 ounces*) contains mostly water, plant oil, thickener, slip agent, water-binding agent, more thickeners, fragrance, and preservatives. It's a good lightweight moisturizer for someone with normal to slightly dry skin. The idea of essential waxes is an interesting slant, but I prefer mine in candles; that way they won't have a chance of clogging pores.

☺ **$$$ Moisturizing Face Cream with Plant Extracts and Essential Waxes, for Dry Skins** (*$50 for 1.69 ounces*) contains mostly water, silicone, plant oils, thickeners, glycerin, plant extracts, fragrance, and preservatives. This would be a good moisturizer for someone with dry skin.

☺ **$$$ Moisturizer Day Cream with Plant Extracts, for Normal Skins** (*$29 for 1.69 ounces*) contains mostly water, water-binding agent, slip agent, plant oils, several thickeners, plant extracts, fragrance, and preservatives. This would be a good moisturizer for someone with dry skin (not normal skin), although, because it doesn't contain sunscreen, it would be appropriate for nighttime only.

☺ **$$$ Stimulating Concentrate with Plant Extracts and Essential Oils, for Mature Skins** (*$70 for 0.5 ounce*) contains mostly plant oils, slip agent, more plant oils, vitamin E, and plant extract. This is a group of very standard grocery store–type oils and fragrant oils. The fragrant oils—musk, clove, and cinnamon—can all be potential irritants, while the grocery-store oils are just fine for the skin. The only thing this will stimulate is Decleor's bottom line.

☹ **$$$ Soothing Anti Redness Day Cream, with Plant Extracts and Essential Oils** (*$58 for 1.69 ounces*) contains mostly water, thickeners, emollient, water-binding agent, plant extract, more thickeners, plant oils, preservatives, vitamin E, and more preservatives. Some of the plants and oils in here can be skin sensitizers, so the claim about reducing redness is bogus, and without a sunscreen this is useless as a daytime moisturizer.

☺ **$$$ Soothing Night Cream with Plant Extracts and Essential Oils, for**

Normal Skins *($35 for 1.69 ounces)* contains mostly water, thickeners, plant oil, more thickeners, glycerin, silicone, more plant oils, vitamin E, and preservatives. This would be a good moisturizer for someone with normal to dry skin.

☺ $$$ **Soothing Serum with Plant Extracts and Essential Oils** *($69 for 1 ounce)* contains mostly water, thickener, water-binding agent, plant extract, glycerin, plant oils, silicone, more water-binding agents, preservatives, vitamin E, and more plant oils. This is a good lightweight moisturizer for someone with dry skin, but several of the plant oils here are fragrant and can cause skin irritation.

☹ $$$ **Timecare Cream with Plant Extracts, Fruit Acids and Aromatic Essences, for Mature Skins** *($70 for 1.69 ounces)* contains mostly water, plant extract, thickeners, plant oils, emollient, glycerin, more thickeners, water-binding agent, several more plant extracts, preservatives, and fragrance. Nothing in this cream will have any effect on aging skin, and there are no fruit acids (meaning AHAs), just plant extracts, which have nothing to do with effective exfoliation. Several of the plant oils in here are fragrant and can cause skin irritation.

☹ $$$ **Timecare Serum with Plant Extracts, Fruit Acids, and Aromatic Essences, for Mature Skins** *($72 for 1 ounce)* makes the same claims as the cream above, but the formulations are completely different! This lightweight moisturizer does not contain fruit acids (or AHAs) and cannot change mature skin. Several of the plant oils in here are fragrant and can cause skin irritation.

☹ **Tinted Skin Care Cream with Plant Extracts** *($21 for 1.75 ounces)* is a lightweight slightly tinted moisturizer that could be an option for daytime except that it does not contain any protection against UVA rays. It is not recommended.

☹ $$$ **Super Lifting Excellence Firming Face and Neck Lotion with Plant Extracts for Mature Skins** *($60 for 1 ounce)* contains mostly water, slip agent, film-forming agent, plant extracts, fragrance, and preservatives. The film-forming agent, a standard hairstyling-type ingredient, can make the face feel somewhat tighter, but it isn't unique to this product. This one isn't excellent but it is an OK moisturizer for normal to slightly dry skin.

☺ $$$ **Vitalite Nourishing and Firming Face Cream with Plant Extracts and Essential Oils** *($56 for 1.69 ounces)* contains mostly water, thickener, emollient, plant oils, more thickeners, water-binding agents, silicone, more plant oils, fragrance, more water-binding agents, vitamins, and preservatives. This would be a very good moisturizer for someone with dry skin, but it won't nourish the skin.

☺ $$$ **Vitarome Cream with Plant Extracts and Essential Oils, for Dry Skins** *($39 for 1 ounce)* contains mostly water, plant extract, plant oils, thickeners, preservatives, vitamins, emollients, and preservatives. This is a very good moisturizer for someone with dry skin, although it contains several fragrant oils that can cause skin irritation.

☺ $$$ **Contour Mask for Eyes and Lips with Plant Extracts for All Skin**

Types *($31 for 1 ounce)* contains mostly water, glycerin, water-binding agents, film-forming agent, slip agent, plant oil, thickeners, and preservative. This is a standard mask that places a layer of hairstyling-type ingredients over the face. It can't "contour" anything, but your skin will feel temporarily smoother when you take it off.

☺ $$$ **Corrective Care with Plant Extracts for Sensitive Skins** *($19 for 0.5 ounce)* contains mostly water, mineral oil, thickeners, glycerin, lanolin, anti-irritant, plant extracts, more thickener, and preservatives. This is a good moisturizer for someone with dry skin, but lanolin is hardly the ingredient to put in a product for someone with sensitive skin.

☹ $$$ **Essential Face Balm 100% Natural Aromatic Product for Combination Skins** *($52 for 1 ounce)* has nothing essential in it, but it does contain plant oils and car wax (yes, car wax). Some of the oils are fragrant and can irritate the skin; car wax can clog pores.

☹ $$$ **Essential Harmony with Plant Extracts and Essential Oils for All Skin Types** *($57 for 1.69 ounces)* is supposed to calm sensitive skin, but it contains too many sensitizing plant oils and extracts to be good for most skin types, let alone sensitive skin.

☺ $$$ **Moisturizing Creamy Face Mask with Plant Extracts for All Skin Types** *($32 for 1.69 ounces)* contains a bunch of moisturizing ingredients, similar to those found in all Decleor products, along with a film-forming agent. It is definitely creamy, and it could be a good mask, but the claims in the brochure have nothing to do with reality.

☺ $$$ **Regulating Face Mask with Plant Extracts and Natural Aromatic Essences for Combination Skins** *($26 for 1.69 ounces)* is a standard clay mask that also contains some emollients, thickeners, water-binding agents, plant oils, and preservatives.

☹ **Regulating Gel for Local Imperfections with Plant Extracts and Aromatic Essences, for Combination Skins** *($27 for 1.69 ounces)* contains way too many irritating ingredients for any skin type. This won't improve imperfections, but it can cause them. This product contains alcohol, orris extract, lemon oil, and bitter orange oil, all highly sensitizing ingredients.

☺ $$$ **Timecare Mask with Plant Extracts and Aromatic Essences** *($34 for 1.69 ounces)* contains mostly water, film former, thickeners, water-binding agents, plant oils, thickeners, fragrance, and preservatives. It's fine for a mask, but the miracles it's supposed to accomplish, from toning skin to erasing years off the face, don't hold water.

☹ **Sea and Mountain Sun Protection Cream Sun Tan Care with Plant Extracts SPF 20** *($21 for 2.5 ounces)* can't protect skin from UVA rays and is not recommended.

☹ **Self Tanning Cream, Sun Tan Care with Plant Extracts SPF 4** *($21 for 4.2 ounces)* can't protect skin from UVA rays, and the SPF is so low as to encourage the risk of skin cancer and wrinkles. This product is absolutely not recommended.

☹ **Sensitive Zone Stick, Sun Tan Care with Plant Extracts SPF 15** *($15 for 0.26 ounce)* can't protect skin from UVA rays and is not recommended.

☹ **Tan Accelerator, Sun Tan Care with Plant Extracts** *($17 for 2.5 ounces)* is as unethical a skin-care product as I can imagine. It is one thing to sell creams that don't protect skin from sun damage; it is another thing to sell a product that encourages women to tan. Why doesn't this line hand out cigarettes too?

☺ **$$$ Aromatic Harmony Balm 100% Natural Aromatic Product for Sensitive Skins** *($52 for 1 ounce)* contains mostly plant oils that you could find in a grocery store, plus emollients and fragrant oils. This would be good for someone with dry skin, but the fragrant oils can cause problems for sensitive skin.

☺ **$$$ Eye and Lip Precious Contour Balm with Plant Extracts for Mature Skins** *($34 for 0.5 ounce)* contains mostly water, plant oil, aloe, film former, slip agent, thickeners, anti-irritant, and preservatives. This would be a good moisturizer for someone with dry skin.

☺ **$$$ Natural Face Oil with 100% Natural Aromatic Essence for Normal and Sensitive Skins** *($55 for 0.5 ounce)* is plant oil (mostly hazelnut and avocado) with some wax thrown in. That's good for dry skin, but the orange oil makes it a problem for sensitive skin.

☺ **$$$ Natural Face Oil Ylang Ylang with 100% Natural Aromatic Essences, for Combination Skins** *($55 for 0.5 ounce)* contains a group of oils that are primarily fragrant, feel greasy on the skin, and are known sensitizers.

☺ **$$$ Natural Face Oil Angelique with 100% Natural Aromatic Essences for Dry Skins** *($55 for 0.5 ounce)* contains a group of oils that can be found on the grocery shelf and a handful of fragrant oils. The basic oils are great for dry skin, but it would be much cheaper to buy and mix them together yourself, and that way you won't be slathering your face with fragrant oils, which can cause negative reactions.

☹ **Skin Care Gel for Pigmentation Marks with Plant Extracts for Mature Skins** *($29 for 1.69 ounces)* contains no hydroquinone, kojic acid, AHAs, or BHA, the only ingredients from the world of cosmetics that can have a positive effect on skin discolorations.

Dermablend

Dermablend is a small line of products designed to help women with major skin problems they want to cover up. For those women, Dermablend's offer is hard to ignore. The question is how well the products work and whether they are good for the skin. The **Cover Creme Foundation** *($18)*, **Leg & Body Cover** *($13.50)*, **Quick Fix** (cover stick) *($15)*, **Setting Loose Powder** *($15)*, and **Setting Pressed Powder** *($15)* are supposed to provide complete, opaque coverage that hides any kind of scarring or birthmarks (no matter how severe) and spider veins on the legs. These are not lightweight products that magically place a camouflaging film over the face and legs. Not surprisingly, each product has an unusually thick texture that can blend out to thin but opaque coverage. Basically, this is heavy-duty stuff.

All of the colors are actually quite good and natural. If you spread an even layer of the foundation, bodycover, or cover stick over your face or legs, you can be assured of a good deal of coverage that, depending on the depth of discoloration, will hide your problem from view. The deeper the discoloration, the less likely you will be able to hide it. The question is, Do you really want that much coverage? What you get in place of the discoloration is a noticeable layer of foundation. Even if you spread it on as thinly as possible, it still has a heavy texture. Plus, the thinner you blend it on, the less coverage you get. There is no way that these products can look natural, but they can cover. Also, the Leg & Body Cover can be a problem to use, because even though it is waterproof and won't come off in the rain, it will rub off, and there's nothing you can do to prevent that. The Setting Powder, a white talc powder that looks very pasty on the skin, should not be used at all. Almost any neutral pressed or loose powder will work just as well.

It's difficult for me to recommend this product line, yet I know that many women have strong feelings about their facial discolorations. I may think the heavy look of the foundation is no better than the discoloration itself, but the problem isn't on my face. Emotions are strong when it comes to issues like this, so **testing the products yourself is probably the only way to make a decision, which is why I've left out face ratings for these products.**

Dermablend introduced **Active Cover Creme Foundation SPF 15** *($18.50),* a very thick and creamy foundation that offers medium to heavy coverage. It offers an excellent SPF 15 with titanium dioxide, and isn't as heavy as the original Cover Creme Foundation. That can be a definite plus if you are looking for good coverage that isn't as thick and greasy as the original. Most of the eight shades are exceptionally neutral, although Ivory is slightly pink and Bare is slightly peach.

Recently Dermablend extended their small group of skin-care products. For more information about Dermablend call (800) 631-2158.

Dermablend Skin Care

☹ **Cleanser** *($12.50 for 6.3 ounces)* is a detergent-based, water-soluble cleanser. The second item on the ingredient list is TEA-lauryl sulfate, a very drying and potentially irritating cleansing agent.

☹ **Maximum Moisturizer SPF 15 PABA-Free** *($22.50 for 2 ounces)* doesn't contain avobenzone, zinc oxide, or titanium dioxide, and is not recommended.

☹ **Advanced Chromatone Plus with Alpha-Hydroxy, Fade Cream with Sun-**

screen *($14 for 1.7 ounces)* is a good 2% hydroquinone-based moisturizer that can help lighten brown skin discolorations. Unfortunately the sunscreen is woefully inadequate, and does not contain any UVA protection. Also, their are no AHAs in this Alpha Hydroxy product.

☹ **Chromatone Plus Fade Creme with Sunscreen** *($15 for 3.75 ounces)* is similar to the one above and the same review applies.

Dermalogica (Skin Care Only)

Image is a major factor in most women's decisions about buying products. Image can convey the value of a company's products through an appeal to emotions. A beautiful model, a charismatic actress, or a distinctive brochure and packaging can be all the impetus necessary to persuade unwary consumers to make a purchase. What other consideration is there for buying a cosmetic product—particularly a skin-care product? If a cream promises to firm the skin or protect it from environmental damage, we have very little to go on other than the impression we get from the advertising and the packaging (and, of course, the salesperson).

With that in mind, I have always been most intrigued by cosmetics lines that choose to create a scientific image instead of a glamorous image. Dermalogica has honed its image to a tee. The name implies a relationship to dermatology, which sounds as if you are getting serious skin care. The subtitle on Dermalogica's products is even more commanding: "A Skin Care System Researched and Developed by the International Dermal Institute." But what is the International Dermal Institute? Are there any dermatologists there? Apparently not: The International Dermal Institute is a school for facialists who want an education beyond what is required for their cosmetology license, and the classes are taught by facialists. (If you're going to get a facial, although I would not suggest you spend your hard-earned money on one, it is best to go to someone who has training from somewhere other than just a cosmetology licensing school. In that regard, the International Dermal Institute provides a good, albeit expensive, service.)

Does the professional atmosphere of the school associated with Dermalogica mean better products? The proof is in the pudding, and this pudding is just Jell-O, not chocolate mousse. The company's literature expounds at length on the ingredients the products *don't* contain, such as mineral oil (because it's greasy and sits on the skin, although the same could be said of many of the plant oils and water-binding agents that the products do contain). But some of the products contain petrolatum, from which mineral oil is derived, so even if mineral oil were a culprit in skin-care products (it isn't), this line's claim that it doesn't contain any is misleading.

Dermalogica products also don't contain isopropyl myristate, lanolin, or coal tar–based dyes, because, as the brochure explains, they can cause breakouts. That is true, but Dermalogica's products do contain ceresin, beeswax, forms of acrylate, and other ingredients that can potentially clog pores, drying and irritating cleansing agents, and extremely sensitizing plants.

Another misleading statement is the claim that the products don't contain formaldehyde, a preservative that can cause problems for the skin. In fact, many of the products contain diazolidinyl urea, a preservative that can release formaldehyde. The products also claim to be fragrance-free, but many of the plant extracts and oils used in the products indeed provide fragrance. Fragrance, regardless of its origin, can be irritating to the skin. I could go on, but I'll let the products and their ingredient lists speak for themselves. For more information about Dermalogica you can call (800) 831-5150.

☹ **Anti-Bac Skin Wash** *($34 for 16 ounces)* is an extremely drying detergent cleanser, and between the sodium C14-15 olefin sulfate, mint, menthol, and camphor it contains, this product is too irritating for words.

☹ **Essential Cleansing Solution** *($34 for 16 ounces)* contains mostly water, plant oil, thickeners, ceresin, beeswax, and more thickeners. It can leave skin feeling greasy, and ceresin and beeswax can clog pores.

☹ **Dermal Clay Cleanser** *($34 for 16 ounces)* contains menthol, mint, lemon, and arnica, all of which are too irritating for all skin types.

☹ **Special Cleansing Gel** *($34 for 16 ounces)* is a standard detergent-based, water-soluble cleanser that can be OK for someone with oily or combination skin. It contains balm mint, which can be irritating for some skin types.

☺ **Soothing Eye Makeup Remover** *($15 for 2 ounces)* is a standard detergent-based eye-makeup remover.

☹ **Gentle Cream Exfoliant** *($27.50 for 2.5 ounces)* contains several seriously irritating ingredients, including papain, sulfur, lemon, and orange, that make it about as far from gentle as you can imagine.

☺ **$$$ Skin Prep Scrub** *($22 for 2.5 ounces)* is a detergent-based, water-soluble cleanser that uses cornmeal as the scrub. It would probably be better to just use cornmeal from the grocery store if you want a cornmeal scrub, but this one shouldn't be a problem and at least it doesn't contain all the irritating additives the other cleansers in this line do.

☹ **Multi-Active Toner** *($21.50 for 8 ounces)* contains mint and lavender, which are too irritating for all skin types.

☺ **Active Moist** *($38.50 for 3.5 ounces)* would be a good emollient moisturizer for someone with dry skin.

☹ **Active Firming Booster** *($41 for 1 ounce)* contains too many irritating plant extracts for all skin types, including lemon, pine, and orange. This won't firm except for a little swelling.

☺ **$$$ Gentle Soothing Booster** *($41 for 1 ounce)* contains mostly water, red raspberry juice, standard water-binding agent, and preservatives. Raspberry juice can be irritating for some skin types and may cause allergic reactions. Besides, there is no benefit in putting raspberries on the skin, especially not at $41 an ounce.

☺ **$$$ Intensive Eye Repair** *($35 for 0.5 ounce)* is a good emollient moisturizer for dry skin, but it won't repair anything. It does contain some good emollients, water-binding agents, and vitamins that feel good on the skin, but that won't repair damage, and then you have to reapply it again the next day. If things got repaired you wouldn't need to buy this product again, right? One word of warning: there is a small amount of arnica in here that can cause irritation especially around the eyes for some sensitive skin types.

☺ **$$$ Intensive Moisture Balance** *($31 for 1.75 ounces)* is similar to the product above only somewhat less emollient. It would be good for someone with normal to dry skin.

☺ **$$$ Intensive Moisture Concentrate** *($45 for 1 ounce)*, like many moisturizers, uses a film former as the main ingredient. It places an imperceptible layer of plastic over the skin that helps the skin temporarily look smoother. It is just a good lightweight moisturizer for slightly dry skin.

☺ **$$$ Specific Skin Concentrate** *($45 for 1 ounce)* is similar to the moisturizer above, and the same review applies.

☹ **Intensive Oil Replacement** *($31.50 for 0.5 ounce)* contains several plant oils, including lavender oil, which can cause problems upon sun exposure; eucalyptus oil, which can be a skin irritant; and sandalwood, which can cause an allergic reaction in sensitive skin types.

☹ **Oil Control Lotion** *($27 for 1.7 ounces)* contains mint, camphor and menthol, which won't control oil in the least, but will cause redness, dryness, and irritation.

☺ **$$$ Skin Smoothing Cream** *($42 for 3.5 ounces)* is a good emollient moisturizer for someone with dry skin. It contains all the appropriate emollients, plant oils, vitamins, and water-binding agents.

☺ **$$$ Special Clearing Booster** *($37 for 1 ounce)* is a fairly expensive 5% benzoyl peroxide–based product. There are much cheaper benzoyl peroxides available at the drugstore, and I would recommend starting with 3% hydrogen peroxide or 2.5% benzoyl peroxide for acne before jumping to 5% benzoyl peroxide.

☹ **Skin Renewal Booster** *($41 for 1 ounce)* is a 10% AHA product that also contains sulfur and salicylic acid. The pH of this product isn't low enough for the AHA to be an effective exfoliant, and the sulfur is unnecessarily irritating.

☺ **$$$ Total Eye Care** *($31.50 for 0.75 ounce)* makes me wonder, if this product is total eye care, what is the Intensive Eye Repair product above for? Nonetheless, it is a good lightweight moisturizer that contains lactic acid, though the product doesn't have a low enough pH for it to work as an exfoliant.

☹ **Full Spectrum Block, SPF 15** *($23 for 4 ounces)* doesn't contain avobenzone, zinc oxide, or titanium dioxide, and is not recommended.

☺ **$$$ Protective Self-Tan SPF 15** *($24 for 4 ounces)* doesn't contain avobenzone, zinc oxide, or titanium dioxide, and is not recommended for outdoor use; as a self-tanner it should work just fine.

☺ **$$$ Solar Defense Booster SPF 30** *($30 for 1 ounce)* does contain avobenzone, so this one has good UVA protection! However for someone reason this line is big on mint and lemon in their product, which just isn't the best for skin. This one even has lavender oil, a known photosensitizer (meaning sun exposure can trigger a reaction). What's that doing in a sunscreen?

☹ **Solar Shield SPF 15 (stick)** *($9.50 for 0.28 ounce)* doesn't contain avobenzone, zinc oxide, or titanium dioxide, and is not recommended.

☹ **Sunswipes SPF 15** *($28 per carton)* don't contain avobenzone, zinc oxide, or titanium dioxide, and are not recommended.

☺ **$$$ Ultra Sensitive Bodyblock SPF 15** *($22 for 4 ounces)* is a pure titanium dioxide–based sunscreen but, like many other products in this line, it contains mint, lemon, grapefruit, and lavender, which have no place in a product for sensitive skin.

☺ **$$$ Ultra Sensitive Face Block SPF 25** *($22 for 1.75 ounces)* is similar to the one above and the same concerns apply.

☹ **Pigment Relief SPF 15** *($45 for 1.7 ounces)* doesn't contain avobenzone, zinc oxide, or titanium dioxide, and is not recommended.

☺ **$$$ Intensive Moisture Masque** *($32.50 for 2 ounces)* contains mostly water, plant oil, thickeners, plant extracts, silicone, vitamins, and preservatives. This would be a good moisturizing mask for someone with dry skin, although a good emollient moisturizer left on the skin a little thicker and a little longer than usual can have the same effect.

☺ **$$$ Skin Hydrating Masque** *($28.50 for 2.5 ounces)* contains mostly water, plant extracts, thickener, several water-binding agents, and preservatives. This would be a good moisturizing mask for someone with dry skin, although a good emollient moisturizer left on the skin a little thicker and a little longer than usual can have the same effect.

☺ **$$$ Skin Refining Masque** *($27.50 for 2.5 ounces)* is a standard clay mask that contains little else besides clay. It would be a good mask to absorb oil, but not as good as plain Phillips' Milk of Magnesia you can find at the drugstore.

☹ **$$$ Skin Purifying Wipes** *($25 for 36 towelettes)* contain camphor and mint, and all I can say is ouch!

Derma Wand

This is the first "anti-aging machine" I've seen that comes with a warning. It clearly states, "Do not use Derma Wand on skin which is prone to excessive amounts of broken capillaries or on skin which is prone to rosacea." As forthright and valid as that warning is, that includes about 75% of the female American population. Almost all Caucasian women are prone to broken, surfaced capillaries. It doesn't take much to hurt delicate capillaries and produce a red, spiraling network across the face. And rosacea probably occurs in about 15% of the Caucasian population. That excludes a lot of women from using the Derma Wand, and we haven't even begun to discuss the claims.

The Derma Wand emits an electrical charge that supposedly generates some amount of ozone—that is, supercharged oxygen. It works sort of like a miniature stroke of lightning, and the user feels a slight sting, like a rubber-band snap, which isn't surprising given the electricity being generated. The zapping and the ozone production are supposed to help with the penetration of anti-aging creams and lotions. Naturally that assumes the anti-aging creams and lotions work in the first place, and will work even better if they penetrate the skin. Neither is the case, and anyway, oxygen can't help creams penetrate better, because the skin can't handle more oxygen than is already in the air. Even if it could, the possibility of damage from the electrical charge isn't worth it. The Derma Wand is also supposed to zap zits, because pure oxygen can kill the bacteria causing the blemish. The theory is sound, but skin cells are also destroyed by pure oxygen, and how the wand gets around this dilemma isn't explained. For more information about the Derma Wand call (800) 704-1209.

DHC USA (Skin Care Only)

I've been perplexed by the number of e-mails I've received lately asking me about a line of skin-care products called DHC USA. Then to my further amazement I received a sort of invitation from the president of the company asking me to consider taking a closer look. It was one of the most unusual cosmetic mailers I've ever received. The mailer describes how the president of the company, back in 1993, while river-rafting in Colorado, was introduced by a fellow traveler to a soap that would completely change the way she looked at skin care. The letter from her says "It was unlike anything I'd ever tried—simple, pure and amazingly effective. Created by a Japanese company called DHC, it was only available overseas. I knew right away that American women needed this soap. DHC is unique because our products suit your skin, and your lifestyle, instantly. They never contain perfumes, dyes, or anything else that might clog or irritate your skin."

Well, I'm not sure what skin-care products this woman was using before, but the soap is not unique in the least: it is a standard tallow-based bar soap. Tallow can cause problems for the skin. It is great that these products don't contain dyes or fragrance. However, I would suggest that there are still problematic formulations and potentially irritating ingredients in some of the products. There are lots of good moisturizers, and many make claims about firming and getting rid of wrinkles, yet how many of these products will it take before they live up to their claim and do get rid of wrinkles? My eternal question is, If one antiwrinkle product works, why would you need the others? Still, this line is great about sending samples of all their products, so you might want to take advantage of that. For more information about DHC USA call 1-800-DHC-CARE.

☹ **Mild Soap** *($12 for 3.1 ounces)* is a standard tallow-based bar soap made of lard and lye, just like any other soap. It does have an attractive appearance, but the lard can clog pores and the cleansing agent can be too drying for most skin types.

☹ **Gentle Cleansing Foam for Normal Skin** *($14 for 4.9 ounces)* is a fairly alkaline cleanser that can be too drying for most skin types. It contains potassium hydroxide fairly high up on the ingredient listing, and that make it a problem for some skin types.

☺ **$$$ Mild Cleansing Cream for Drier Skin** *($14 for 4.9 ounces)* is a standard mineral oil–based wipe-off cleanser. This is just pricey cold cream with lots of ordinary thickening agents that don't rinse off the face.

☺ **$$$ Facial Wash for Oilier Skin** *($18 for 6.7 ounces)* is a standard detergent-based water-soluble cleanser. The main cleansing agent is disodium lauryl sulfosuccinate, which can be too drying for some skin types.

☺ **$$$ Oil-Free Makeup Remover** *($15 for 3.3 ounces)* is a very standard, typical, detergent-based makeup remover, as good as any other.

☺ **Deep Cleansing Oil** *($14 for 5 ounces)* actually doesn't contain much oil at all, it is mostly standard thickening agents. This is just an emollient wipe-off cleanser with a tiny bit of vitamin E for effect and rosemary oil for scent. The recommendation is to use this product with another cleanser in the line, and you would have to do that to get this stuff off the face.

☺ **Facial Scrub** *($14 for 4.9 ounces)* uses apricot seeds as the exfoliant. That and some thickeners along with a detergent cleansing agent makes this a standard, OK exfoliant for someone with normal to dry skin.

☺ **Balancing Lotion for Normal Skin** *($12 for 6 ounces)* is a good irritant-free toner that contains mostly water, glycerin, water-binding agents, AHA, and preservatives. There isn't enough AHA in here for it to act as anything other than a water-binding agent. That's not bad, just maybe not what you were expecting. One of the water-binding agents in here is placental protein. That one just always gets me.

☺ **Soothing Lotion for Drier Skin** *($12 for 6 ounces)* is similar to the one above and the same comments apply. At least this one doesn't contain placenta.

☹ **Clean Finish Lotion for Oilier Skin** *($12 for 6 ounces)* is mostly alcohol and that's bad for skin.

☺ **$$$ Rich Moisture for Normal to Drier Skin** *($24 for 3.3 ounces)* contains mostly water, plant oil, water-binding agents, thickeners, vitamin E, and preservatives. This is a good emollient moisturizer for dry skin.

☺ **$$$ Light Moisture for Normal to Oilier Skin** *($24 for 3.3 ounces)* is similar to the one above, only in lotion form. The second ingredient is olive oil, and some of the water-binding agents like collagen, which is good for dry skin, aren't the best for oily skin. This is a good moisturizer for normal to slightly dry skin, just don't use it over oily areas.

☺ **$$$ Oil-Free Hydrator for Oilier Skin** *($22 for 3.3 ounces)* contains mostly water, glycerin, and a tiny amount of water-binding agents. This could be a good moisturizer for slightly dry skin, but again, keep it off the oily areas.

☺ **$$$ Extra Nighttime Moisture** *($30 for 1.5 ounces)* is a good emollient moisturizer for dry skin. It is similar to the Rich Moisturizer above and the same basic comments apply.

☺ **$$$ Hydrating Nighttime Moisture** *($28 for 1 ounce)* contains mostly water, water-binding agents, and preservatives. This is a good lightweight moisturizer for someone with slightly dry skin.

☺ **$$$ Collagen Eye Stick** *($29 for 0.12 ounce)* is a very emollient, clear, lip gloss–type moisturizer for the eyes. It is very emollient and good for very dry skin, but don't expect the collagen to do anything special, it's just a water-binding agent, nothing more. It can't help shore up your own collagen. If only it were that easy, given how long collagen has been around as a skin-care ingredient, none of us would have wrinkles.

☹ **Soothing Eye Gel** *($24 for 0.7 ounce)* would just be a pretty do-nothing eye gel except this one contains orange peel and lemon, which can irritate the skin around the eyes.

☺ **$$$ Pure Squalane** *($25 for 1 ounce)* is indeed pure squalane, a plant oil. There are lots of plant oils in the world you can use for far less cost than this one. It is a good moisturizer addition, but no more so than safflower or sunflower oil from the grocery store.

☺ **$$$ Advanced Collagen Treatment** *($40 for 1 ounce)* definitely contains collagen, but other than being a good moisturizer, this won't do anything else for skin. The collagen won't penetrate or affect the collagen in your skin in any way, shape, or form. I thought collagen as a miracle skin-care ingredient died in the late '80s.

☺ **$$$ Nourishing Mist** *($35 for 6 ounces)* is just water, glycerin, and some cucumber juice. $35 for this is a bit shocking. It can be a good, ordinary toner, but there isn't much reason to spray this on yourself. It's supposed to help with jet lag but I wouldn't use this over melatonin.

The Reviews D

☺ **$$$ Skin Conditioning Oil** *($30 for 1 ounce)* is just olive oil and some fragrance oils of lavender and rosemary. You don't need the fragrance, so all that counts is the olive oil. You can find much better olive oil than this at your drugstore and still have enough left over for many months' worth of Caesar salad.

☺ **$$$ Dual Defense SPF 25** *($24 for 3.5 ounces)* is a good, partly titanium–dioxide–based sunscreen for someone with dry skin. What is most disappointing about this line are all the moisturizers claiming to fight wrinkles, yet there's only one sunscreen, and it isn't for everyone as the copy claims, because someone with normal to oily skin would not be happy with this product.

☹ **Hydrating Facial Mask** *($16 for 3.5 ounces)* is a standard clay mask with some film former and thickening agents. It is exceptionally ordinary, but as a mask it won't hurt.

☹ **$$$ Deep Cleansing Facial Mask** *($24 for 2.1 ounces)* is a standard clay mask, period. It can absorb oil, and this one doesn't really contain anything that can hurt so skin, so it may be fun to try.

☹ **$$$ Firming Kelp Facial Mask** *($30 for 0.6 ounce liquid and 3.5 ounce gel)* comes in steps. Step 1 is a toner that you place on the skin before you apply the mask, which is Step 2. The toner is just water and some water-binding agents. The DNA in here won't affect your own DNA, and you wouldn't want it to! The mask is mostly film former (hair spray), so you peel this one off. That can help skin feel smooth and soft, just as any peel-off mask does.

Donna Karan New York (Skin Care Only)

Donna Karan has gone from designing clothing and accessories to wear from the neck down to designing products for the neck up. As a rule, it is hard to know what input designers have on the products that bear their names. Yves St. Laurent and Calvin Klein have their names on more than 800 products each, most of which they've probably never even seen. But designers' names convey a certain status, and people believe that designer products are inherently better than products with names they don't recognize. Nevertheless, for skin care and cosmetics, what counts isn't who designs the products but how the products work. Donna Karan's stuff is no exception.

This line is based on the concept of simplicity—much like Ms. Karan's line of clothing, I imagine. Unbelievably, a mere four products comprise the line. Wouldn't it be great if skin care could really be that simple? To some extent it is, but not with these four products. First, no one group of four products can work for all skin types. Plus, the sunscreens in this line are inadequate, and what happens if you have breakouts or need a gentler cleanser? You would be out of luck. The prices of these four unimpressive items tell more about who the originators of this line expect to impress with the designer angle than they do about good skin care. For more information call (800) 647-7474.

☺   **$$$ Formula for Clean Skin** *($25 for 5 ounces)* is a fairly standard detergent cleanser with some castor oil, which might make rinsing a bit of a problem. This would be a good cleanser for someone with normal to slightly dry skin.

☹   **Formula for Facial Moisture SPF 20** *($45 for 1.5 ounces)* doesn't contain avobenzone, zinc oxide, or titanium dioxide, and is not recommended.

☹   **SPF 20 Sheer Color Moisturizer All Shades** (ranging from Light to Dark) *($45 for 1.5 ounces)* doesn't contain avobenzone, zinc oxide, or titanium dioxide, and is not recommended.

☹   **Formula for Renewed Skin Exfoliating Mask and After Mask Skin Conditioner** *($55 for two 1-ounce containers)* is a two-part facial mask system that is supposed to be used once a week. The Exfoliating Mask contains witch hazel, cornstarch, aloe vera, clay, papaya enzyme, and preservatives. Witch hazel, papaya, and cornstarch can all cause skin irritation, and papaya is an unstable exfoliating agent. The After Mask Skin Conditioner is a witch hazel–based toner, which makes it a possible skin irritant; also, it's just too expensive for what you get.

Dove (Skin Care Only)

For more information about Dove products, call (800) 451-6679.

☹   **Beauty Bar** *($1.99 for two 4.75-ounce bars)* is a standard tallow-based bar cleanser that contains some emollients to cut the irritation and dryness caused by the detergent cleansing agents. It is still quite drying, and although it is technically not soap, the ingredients can clog pores. It is probably just fine for most skin types from the neck down, but not from the neck up.

☹   **Beauty Bar (Unscented)** *($1.99 for two 4.75-ounce bars)* is similar to the bar above, and the same review applies.

☹   **Sensitive Skin Beauty Bar New Milder Formula** *($1.99 for two 4.25-ounce bars)* is similar to the bar above and I don't really see any difference that makes it new or more mild.

eb5 (Skin Care Only)

You're supposed to believe that this pharmacist-developed line has secrets for stopping aging. It doesn't. In fact, these are some of the most unimpressive skin-care products around and it's a bit shocking that they are still around and still so amazingly overpriced. For more information about eb5 call (800) 454-4747.

☺   **Cleansing Formula with Dernex** *($14 for 6 ounces)* is a fairly gentle cleanser that contains a small amount of detergent cleansing agents, and would be best for someone with normal to dry skin, though it doesn't do a very good job of taking off makeup.

☹ **Toning Formula with DermaFirm** *($14 for 8 ounces)* contains a few too many irritating ingredients to recommend, including arnica and witch hazel.

☺ **$$$ Facial Cream for Younger-Looking Skin** *($35 for 4 ounces)* contains mostly water, slip agent, mineral oil, thickeners, vitamins, and preservatives. This very ordinary, almost boring moisturizer would be good for someone with dry skin, but it's not worth this price.

☺ **$$$ Age Spot Formula** *($25 for 6 ounces)* is a standard 2% hydroquinone fade cream. It also contains fruit extracts, but these are not the kind of AHAs that can exfoliate the skin and help lighten brown spots, plus the sunscreen here is inadequate and doesn't contain any reliable UVA protection.

Elizabeth Arden

As this book went to press Arden only had two sunscreen products in their line. I was told all the others were being reformulated. That is just shocking to me. How can a line of this size and reputation not have even one well-formulated sunscreen (of the three they have, one is a mere SPF 4 and the other two that are an SPF 15 have no UVA protecting ingredients). To make all the claims about repairing and healing skin without a good sunscreen in sight just seems so misleading. It is dangerous for the skin not to have a reliable sunscreen, and all of Arden's ceramides can't change that.

Now that I've gotten that out, speaking of ceramides, that ingredient is a big issue at Arden. Arden's ceramide line of products is quite popular. It started out with one product and has expanded to many others. From the consumer's point of view, one should ask why the one ceramide product wasn't enough, warranting more and more. Whether or not a multitude of ceramide products is necessary, it turns out this ingredient is a rather impressive water-binding agent that the skin has a good affinity for, but it isn't the best one, just a good one.

Arden's counters are very accessible and easy to test. Several of the foundations have decent SPF 10s with titanium dioxide, some of the colors are quite excellent and the textures smooth and satiny. Although many of the eyeshadows are too shiny, many have a great smooth matte finish and should be checked. The blush colors are attractive—with some lovely soft shades! For information about Elizabeth Arden products call (212) 261-1000.

Elizabeth Arden Skin Care

☺ **$$$ Millennium Hydrating Cleanser** *($25.50 for 4.4 ounces)* is an OK water-soluble cleanser that leaves a slightly greasy film on the skin. It also may not remove all traces of makeup.

☹ **Millennium Revitalizing Tonic** *($24.50 for 5 ounces)* contains mostly water and alcohol. This is too irritating for most skin types.

☺ **$$$ Millennium Day Renewal Emulsion** *($54.50 for 2.6 ounces)* contains mostly water, plant oil, slip agent, silicone, thickeners, lanolin oil, and preservatives. This very rich, emollient moisturizer should be used only for very dry skin. However, if you tend to break out, stay away from it; also, without sunscreen, it's a poor choice for daytime.

☺ **$$$ Millennium Eye Renewal Cream** *($39.50 for 0.5 ounce)* is a very rich, thick, ordinary moisturizer that contains mostly water, mineral oil, lanolin, thickeners, and preservatives. It will indeed take care of dry skin but is incredibly overpriced.

☺ **$$$ Millennium Night Renewal Creme** *($82 for 1.7 ounces)* is similar to the product above, and the same review applies, except it's a night cream.

☺ **$$$ Millennium Hydra-Exfoliating Mask** *($29.50 for 2.65 ounces)* is a clay mask that also contains some oil, wax, and a silicate (like sand). Because of the oil, it isn't as drying as most clay masks, but it is still just another clay mask.

☺ **$$$ Visible Difference Deep Cleansing Lotion** *($18.50 for 6.7 ounces)* is a good water-soluble cleanser that lathers and rinses well. However, it can be drying and may burn your eyes. Also, the third item on the ingredient list is isopropyl myristate, which can clog pores.

☹ **Visible Difference One Great Soap** *($12.50 for 5.3 ounces)* has ingredients that keep bar cleansers in their bar form, which can clog pores, and the cleansing agents are too drying for most all skin types.

☺ **Visible Difference Gentle Scrub Creme for the Face** *($17.50 for 3.5 ounces)* leaves a somewhat greasy film on the face (the second item on the ingredient list is petrolatum). It uses standard synthetic scrub particles, which are gentle enough, so this may feel good to someone with extremely dry, parched skin.

☹ **Visible Difference Refining Toner** *($15 for 6.7 ounces)* contains mostly water, witch hazel, alcohol, glycerin, and preservative. The alcohol and witch hazel make it too irritating for most skin types.

☺ **$$$ Visible Difference Eyecare Concentrate** *($30 for 0.5 ounce)* is an ordinary but good moisturizer for dry skin; it contains mostly water, mineral oil, silicone, thickeners, plant oil, more thickeners, and preservatives.

☺ **$$$ Visible Difference Perpetual Moisture** *($38 for 1 ounce)* contains mostly water, glycerin, silicones, thickeners, water-binding agents, emollient, vitamins, fragrance, film former, and preservatives. This is a very good moisturizer for dry skin.

☹ **Visible Difference Refining Moisture Lotion SPF 4** *($28.50 for 1.35 ounces)* has an SPF 4, and that's bad enough, but this product also doesn't contain avobenzone, zinc oxide, or titanium dioxide for UVA protection.

☺ **$$$ Visible Difference Refining Moisturizer Creme Complex** *($47.50 for 2.5 ounces)* contains mostly water, thickener, glycerin, more thickeners (including isopropyl myristate, which can cause blackheads), plant oil, beeswax, and preservatives. This is a somewhat heavy, though ordinary, moisturizer for someone with very dry skin.

☺ $$$ **Ceramide Purifying Cleansing Cream** *($19.50 for 4.2 ounces)* won't purify anything. It is a fairly standard mineral oil–based wipe-off cleanser with ordinary thickening agents to give it a creamy appearance, and it can leave a greasy film on the skin.

☹ **Ceramide Purifying Toner** *($18.50 for 6.7 ounces)* is a very expensive alcohol-based toner. Alcohol doesn't purify the skin, but it can cause irritation.

☺ $$$ **Ceramide Eyes Time Complex Capsules** *($37.50 for 0.35 ounce, includes 60 capsules)* contain mostly silicone, thickener, witch hazel (can be a skin irritant, particularly around the eyes), plant oils, water-binding agents, and vitamins. This would be a good lightweight oil to put around the eyes if your skin doesn't have a problem with the witch hazel—and if you can get over the $1,700-per-pound price tag.

☺ $$$ **Ceramide Firm Lift Intensive Lotion for Face and Throat** *($45 for 1 ounce)* contains mostly water, silicone, thickeners, water-binding agents, vitamins, film former, and preservatives. This is a good moisturizer for someone with normal to dry skin, but there is nothing startling or particularly interesting about this product. If you already own one of Arden's Ceramide products, there is no reason to add this to your arsenal.

☺ $$$ **Ceramide Night Intensive Repair Creme** *($45 for 1 ounce)* contains mostly water, glycerin, several thickeners, emollient, water-binding agents, vitamins, fragrance, and preservatives. The ingredient list is surprisingly ordinary; the only interesting item is almost at the end of the list and barely amounts to anything. The second ingredient is a neutralized form of salicylic acid, which means the product won't exfoliate the skin. This is just a good emollient moisturizer for dry skin.

☺ $$$ **Ceramide Time Complex Moisture Cream** *($45 for 1.7 ounces)* contains mostly water, silicones, several thickeners, slip agents, water-binding agents, vitamins, fragrance, and preservatives. This is a good moisturizer for too much money for someone with dry skin.

☺ $$$ **Ceramide Advanced Time Complex Capsules** *($55 for 0.97 ounce, includes 60 capsules)* are the most popular product Arden sells, yet these tiny gelatin capsules contain some fairly ordinary stuff: silicones, plant oil, water-binding agent (including ceramide), and vitamins. This is a good lightweight, soothing moisturizer for the face, but that's about it. What is particularly nice about this product is no preservatives; due to the encapsulation there is no need for them.

☹ **Ceramide Time Complex Moisture Cream SPF 15** *($45 for 1.7 ounces)* doesn't contain avobenzone, zinc oxide, or titanium dioxide, and is not recommended.

☺ **$$$ Modern Skin Care 2-in-1 Cleanser** *($17.50 for 4.2 ounces)* is a very good, detergent-based, water-soluble cleanser for someone with normal to oily skin. It doesn't do anything to "minimize the appearance of pores," and it can be drying for some skin types despite what the brochure claims. It claims to contain antioxidants, but they aren't evident in the ingredient list. Even if the plant extracts in here are supposed to do that job, the effect would be washed down the drain.

☹ **Modern Skin Care Daily Moisture SPF 15** *($32.50 for 1.7 ounces)* doesn't contain zinc oxide, titanium dioxide, or avobenzone, and is not recommended.

☺ **$$$ Skin Illuminating Complex** *($42.50 for 1 ounce)* contains mostly water, silicones, a form of salicylic acid (beta hydroxy acid), slip agent, thickeners, vitamins, water-binding agents, and preservatives. How illuminating is this lightweight lotion? Not very. The form of salicylic acid used in this product is not effective for exfoliating the skin. Arden makes much ado about their patent-pending formula that includes retinyl linoleate, which is just a good thickening/emollient agent. They claim it contains a "skin identical molecule." At an infinitesimally small microscopic level there are billions and billions of varying molecular structures, and finding one that that looks like a component of skin isn't all that difficult. And what does that have to do with the health of the skin anyway? They left that piece of information out, but you're still supposed to believe that this molecular similarity will allow this lotion to somehow merge with the molecules of your skin in some way and improve it. Did I forget to mention the antioxidant vitamins? They're here, but they are standard in skin care these days and don't mean much for the skin. To shed some final light on the subject, Skin Illuminating Complex is a good lightweight lotion.

☹ **$$$ Skin Basics Deep Milky Cleanser** *($18.50 for 6.7 ounces)* is a mineral oil–based wipe-off cleanser. This isn't milky, it's greasy, and it needs to be wiped off.

☹ **Skin Basics Skin Lotion** *($16 for 6.7 ounces)* is a water- and alcohol-based toner that is too drying for most skin types.

☺ **$$$ Skin Basics Beauty Sleep** *($32.50 for 2.5 ounces)* is a basic, but extremely emollient, moisturizer that contains mostly water, mineral oil, lanolin oil, thickeners (one is isopropyl myristate, which can cause blackheads), lanolin, more thickeners, and preservatives. Only for very, very dry skin.

☺ **$$$ Skin Basics Velva Moisture Film** *($38.50 for 6.7 ounces)* contains mostly water, lanolin oil, thickeners, and preservatives. This is a very emollient, rich moisturizer for very dry skin.

☺ **$$$ Eight Hour Cream** *($20 for 4 ounces)*, one of the original products in the Arden skin-care arsenal, contains mostly water, petrolatum, lanolin, mineral oil, fragrance, salicylic acid, preservatives, plant oils, vitamin E, and preservatives. Salicylic acid isn't best for dry skin, but the pH in here doesn't make it work great as an exfoliant, so this is just a good very emollient moisturizer for dry skin.

☺ **$$$ Micro 2000 Stressed-Skin Concentrate** *($42.50 for 0.85 ounce)* contains mostly silicones, thickeners, water, plant oil, minerals, water-binding agents, vitamins, and preservatives. This won't help stressed skin any more than any other moisturizer. The ingredients are just average—nothing special—but the product would be good for dry skin.

☹ **$$$ Eye-Fix Primer** *($15.50 for 0.25 ounce)* is just moisturizing ingredients with talc. That won't work any better than a foundation to hold eyeshadow in place.

☹ **Velva Cream Mask** *($20 for 3.5 ounces)* contains mostly water, thickener, zinc oxide, phenol, and preservative. This mostly zinc oxide mask won't do anything for the skin. Phenol is one of the first preservatives on the ingredient list, and it is most definitely a skin irritant.

☹ **Eight Hour Lip Protectant Stick SPF 15** *($12.50 for 0.13 ounce)* doesn't contain avobenzone, zinc oxide, or titanium dioxide, and is not recommended.

☹ **Conditioning Waterproof Eye Makeup Remover** *($13.50 for 4 ounces)* isn't conditioning in the least; it is simply a silicone-based wipe-off cleanser that also contains a small amount of detergent cleansing agents. It will wipe off eye makeup, but you wouldn't have to bother with this step if all the other cleansers in this line worked.

☹ **Visible Difference Pore Fix-C** *($12.50 for 10 strips)* are strips that come with the same warnings as the Biore strips, meaning they can rip skin. Just like the Biore strips, these Arden knock-offs have a hair spray–type ingredient that can't pull blackheads from the surface of the nose. The minuscule amount of vitamin C used on these strips is actually a problem. The form of vitamin C is ascorbic acid, considered to be more of an irritant than a help for skin.

Elizabeth Arden Makeup

☺ **$$$ FOUNDATION: Flawless Finish Hydro Light Foundation SPF 10** *($30)* is a soft-textured cream foundation that smoothes on evenly, providing medium coverage. Most of the colors are superior, and the effect is excellent for someone with dry skin. Though an SPF 15 would be better, it still provides reliable titanium dioxide–based protection. **These colors are the best:** Mocha, Buff, Ivory, Vanilla, Sable, and Chestnut. **These colors can be too peach or orange for most skin tones:** Honey, Fawn, Bronze, Bisque, Cameo, and Cream.

☺ **$$$ Flawless Finish Every Day Makeup SPF 10** *($25)* is a lightweight liquid foundation that goes on even and sheer, leaving a soft feel on the skin, and SPF 10, while not great, isn't terrible either, and this one is also titanium dioxide–based. This is best for someone with normal to dry skin; it is actually quite similar to the Matte Makeup below. **The only colors to avoid are:** Cream, Cameo, and Fawn.

☺ **$$$ Flawless Finish Complete Control Matte Makeup SPF 10** *($25)* is a liquid foundation that won't control oil, and though it does go on smoothly and only slightly matte, it just doesn't hold up matte during the day; do expect shine after a few hours. It has an even, soft finish and is best for someone with normal to dry skin. The SPF 10 titanium dioxide–based protection would be better at SPF 15, but this isn't bad for casual wear. It provides medium coverage. **The only colors to avoid are:** Bisque, Ivory, Cream, and Cameo.

☺ **$$$ Flawless Finish Dual Perfection Makeup** *($25)* is a pressed powder meant to be used wet or dry as a foundation, though wet can be really choppy and streaky. It is a standard talc-based powder that has a silky feel. This type of foundation works best for someone with normal to slight dry or slightly oily skin. **Most of the colors are excellent.** The only ones that may be a problem are Cream and Cameo, which may be too peach for most skin tones.

☺ **$$$ Flawless Finish Sponge-On Cream Makeup** *($25)* is fairly thick and somewhat greasy cream compact makeup. This is only good for someone with very dry skin who wants medium coverage. For the money and texture, I would check out Lauder's Impeccable, which at least has a nonchemical SPF 20, but if you do want to try this type of finish **stay away from all these colors:** Toast Rose, Warm Beige, Porcelain Beige, Bronzed Beige, and Honey.

☹ **$$$ Flawless Finish Mousse Makeup** *($25)* comes out like a foam and covers the face with a light, sheer, though fairly dry finish. The color selection is OK, but it can take a while to master the application technique. I tend to prefer traditional foundation consistencies; this one is a bit too gimmicky. **These colors are too orange, rose, yellow, peach, or pink for most skin tones:** Champagne, Natural, Melba, and Ginger.

☺ **$$$ Flawless Finish Control Matte Powder Makeup** *($25)* is a talc-based pressed powder that Arden recommends for use by itself as a foundation. It comes in a good range of colors, but the texture is rather on the dry side for use all over the face. It can be used as a regular pressed powder.

☹ **$$$ CONCEALER: Perfecting Cover Concealer** *($14)* comes in a traditional tube and has a good smooth consistency. The five shades are quite good, but they tend to crease, and keep on creasing during the day.

☹ **$$$ POWDER: Flawless Finish Pressed Powder** *($22.50)* isn't all that flawless. It is just a standard, soft, pressed powder that comes in five fairly translucent soft shades. Only Medium can be too peach for some skin tones. **Flawless Finish Loose Powder** *($22.50)* has a fairly powdery, dry finish. Be careful how you apply this one, it can go somewhat thick and it grabs so you can see it lying on the face.

☺ **$$$ BLUSH: Cheek Color** *($20)* has some beautiful soft colors to check out. There are 12 excellent shades with a sheer application, which means these only work for lighter skin tones.

☺ $$$ <u>EYESHADOW:</u> **Single Eyeshadows** *($13.50)* have a small but excellent group of soft matte shades that work best for lighter skin tones. The shiny ones are a problem, but they are still attractive colors. But let me warn you, despite the low price, the amount of eyeshadow you get is shockingly small. **All of these shades are wonderful:** Wisteria, Camel, Mahogany, Teak, Melon, Wheat, Mist, Vanilla, Espresso, Slate, Fawn, Mushroom, Blossom, Driftwood, Pebble, Cinnamon, Flannel, Bamboo, Cedar, and Linen.

☺ $$$ <u>EYE AND BROW SHAPER:</u> Arden has a large array of both eye and lip pencil colors. **Smooth Lining Eye Pencils** *($13.50)* are standard pencils that go on smooth and soft, with very little slip or greasy feel. **Smoky Eyes Powder Pencil** *($15)* is not in the least powdery; in fact, it goes on much like any standard pencil. One end of the pencil has a smudge tip that can help soften the line. **Great Color Brow Makeup** *($15)* comes in five excellent colors. Using powder instead of pencil is the way to go, and these are as good as any. **Dual Perfection Brow Shaper and Eye Liner** *($15)* is a standard pencil with a slightly drier texture than most; it comes in five very good colors, and has a soft matte finish, but it's still just one more pencil.

☺ $$$ <u>LIPSTICK AND LIP PENCIL:</u> Both types of lipstick are easily accessible for testing and are divided into extremely helpful color groupings of Plum, Pink, Coral, and Red. **Luxury Moisturizing Lipstick** *($15)* goes on sheer and fairly glossy and bleeds easily. **Lip Spa** *($15)* is not all that different from the Luxury Moisturizing Lipsticks. It is very greasy, without much staying power, although for a glossy lipstick it's fine. **Exceptional Lipstick** *($16)* from Arden is not all that exceptional; it is just another lipstick with a fairly glossy finish. **Lip Talkers** *($12.50)* is Arden's attempt at a pencil/lipstick. Of all these chubby lipstick pencils available from Maybelline Lip Express to Prescriptives Matte Lip Crayon, I think Arden's is great. It is more matte than most, and has a slight stain, so it has great staying power; actually, it's a bit difficult to get off. Give this one a try next time you are at the cosmetics counters. **Lip Definer** *($12.50)* comes in a very attractive array of colors. It is just an ordinary pencil, but it goes on soft without being too greasy or dry.

☹ $$$ **Lip Fix Creme** *($17.50)* is supposed to prevent lipstick from feathering. It works well for most but not all lipsticks, but I don't care for the squeeze-tube applicator. It goes on like a moisturizer and must dry before you put on your lipstick. It is less than convenient for touch-ups during the day. I prefer anti-feathering products that come in lipstick form with no waiting between applications. The ones by Coty are some of the best and least expensive.

☺ $$$ <u>MASCARA:</u> When it comes to mascara, Arden has its act together; these mascaras are very good. **Twice as Thick Two Brush Mascara** *($15)*, **Two Brush Mascara Regular** *($15)*, and **Defining Mascara** *($15)* build long lashes with minimal thickness, but no clumping. The only problem with the Two Brush Mascara is the two brushes. The idea sounds good—one brush for applying the mascara, the other for lengthening and separating—but I didn't notice a real difference between the two. **Natural Volume Mascara** *($16)* is a very good mascara that goes on easily and builds long lashes without clumping. It also doesn't smear or flake. That's great but not necessarily worth the expense, given the number of great inexpensive mascaras found at the drugstore. **Two Brush Waterproof Mascara** *($17)* builds quickly, but it can clump slightly if you overdo it, although it does hold up wonderfully under water.

English Ideas—Lip Last (Makeup Only)

You may have heard about this line from fashion magazines as being an amazing solution to keep lipstick on for hours. Or you may have seen it displayed on a counter at Nordstrom or Macy's. Regardless of how you heard about it, what is most important is, Does it work? Who doesn't want their lipstick to last all day? Is this another promise made in vain, one of thousands claiming to keep lipstick on, or will your lips look luscious from morn to night without touch-ups? I bet you've answered the question. Yes, it would be a great idea if these products worked, but alas, don't count on leaving your lipstick at home, you will need touch-ups with these products, almost as many as you normally would without. For more information about English Ideas call (800) LIP-LAST.

☺ **$$$ Lip Last** *($17.50)* is said to be a patented technological breakthrough that is supposed to solve the problem of keeping lipstick on the lips. All this tiny little bottle contains is a film-forming ingredient that burns when you apply it to the lips. If you apply an even layer, you definitely get a great covering over your lipstick that creates a matte seal. It does prevent transferring and bleeding, yet it ends up being quite similar to products like Revlon ColorStay. It does last for a good length of time but it tends to chip and roll off the lips and the lipstick does come off, though definitely not as easily as usual. That is, this isn't impervious, and lunch with any oil content will take it right off. It is tricky to apply, and the irritation from the burning can be a problem. It does help prevent lipstick from bleeding but there are easier ways to do that than with this pricey little liquid.

☺ **$$$ Lip Definer & Foundation** *($15)* is just a rose shade of pencil. It's amazing how you can describe a standard, ordinary lip pencil and somehow make it sound special. This is nice enough, just not different in any way. If you apply any lip pencil all over the lips it can work as a "foundation"; you don't need this pencil to do that.

☹ **Lip Balms SPF 18** *($9)* are just very sheer glosses that leave your lips out to dry when it comes to UVA protection. The Concealer shade is supposed to hide cold sores, but it simply doesn't work; no concealer can hide a full-blown cold sore. It contains tea tree oil which is supposed to help heal cold sores and blemishes, and there is no evidence that it can do that, either.

☹ **Kolour Creme SPF 15** *($15)* is just a fairly glossy lipstick, and though it boasts to be the first lipstick to contain ceramide, a better brag would be that the SPF 18 included UVA protection which it doesn't.

☺ **$$$ Kolour Crayon Lip Pencil** *($12)* is just a standard lip pencil, available in six shades, and is way overpriced for such a basic product.

☺ **$$$ Lip Hi-Lites** *($22.50)* is a very shiny, slightly powdery finish lipstick applied from a self-dispensing sponge tip. It's just extra shine, and that can create an interesting evening look, but any shiny powder over a favorite lipstick can do the same thing for less.

☹ **Lip Refine** *($32 for 0.5 ounces)* is a lotion that contains AHAs and is supposed to exfoliate the lips. I would be concerned about AHAs on the lips because of the delicate nature of the skin in that area, but this product doesn't have a low enough pH to create any exfoliation. Even if it did, there are far less expensive and far more effective AHA products available.

☺ **$$$ Lip Makeup Remover** *($10)* uses plant oil to cut through their Lip Last. It works, but any oil would do the same thing. Of course, this product makes much ado about not containing mineral oil or petroleum-based ingredients as if they were somehow evil; they aren't. In fact, because mineral oil doesn't turn rancid like plant oils it is in many ways better for the skin.

☺ **$$$ Lip Brush** *($25)* is just a very standard lip brush for way too much money and the **Duo Brush** *($35)* is just a two-sided brush; one end is a lip brush, the other a thin eyeliner brush. If that sounds convenient, I guess it's worth the money, but I prefer standard retractable lip brushes that keep the lipstick brush neatly tucked away from making a mess or having to be capped, which often wrecks the bristles.

Erno Laszlo

Erno Laszlo's continued following is beyond me. I made a bet years ago, when the products first came out at upper-end department stores, that this line wouldn't last. I believed women would never pay $14 (that was in the first edition of this book), then $23 (for the second edition) and now an astounding $30 (for this fourth edition) for a bar of soap. I was wrong. It is still around, and it still has a following.

According to the company's brochure, "Erno Laszlo has been the authority in advanced skin care for over 50 years. No one blended the art of cosmetology with the science of dermatology before Dr. Laszlo's time." Great copy, except that Erno Laszlo was never licensed to practice medicine in this country, and some say he was never a medical doctor in Eastern Europe, where he was from, although the brochure makes it sound as if he was a dermatologist. In his time, Dr. Laszlo's claim to fame was prescribing skin-care regimes for wealthy women who could afford to visit his clinic and spa. What he was truly best-known for was his belief in using old-fashioned bar soap (he had women with dry skin cover their face in oil before using soap), then splashing the face 30 times with a basin full of the soapy rinse water, then splashing the face 30 times with scalding hot water. When that was done, his patients would finish by soaking their skin with apple cider vinegar. Dr. Laszlo claimed that nothing cleaned better than hot water and soap, but because soap's alkaline content destroyed the skin's pH level, apple cider vinegar was needed to restore it. As one reader described it, "Much of the Laszlo line was ruined each time it traded owners in the last years. The whole point was simplicity and only a few products were needed by anyone. Slowly the line began to include more and more cremes and treatments—separate for the eyes, throat, etc. I am disgusted."

(I should mention that I totally disagree with this skin-care regime, although I have to admit I admire its originality and concept. Hot water is too damaging to the skin, irritating it and causing capillaries to surface as small spider veins. I also feel that bar soap is too drying and irritating for the skin. We just aren't that dirty; this intense twice-a-day cleansing can cause more problems than it helps. The notion of restoring the skin's pH level after soap has stripped it off is a good idea, but if you clean the face gently, without destroying the pH balance in the first place, you won't need to restore it.)

In 1966 Laszlo sold the right for Chesebrough-Pond's to use his name and retail his products. Now, some 30 years after Laszlo's death, are the current products in alignment with Laszlo's original skin-care theories? For the most part, the skin-care routines still include the bar soap and splashing first with soapy hot water and then with clean hot water. The rest of the routine is only loosely based on the "doctor's" concepts. The toners are all alcohol-based, just like many other toners on the market. The line includes a few token makeup products, mostly foundations; they are overpriced but much improved from my last review. For information about Erno Laszlo products you can call (800) 865-3222.

Erno Laszlo Skin Care

☺ $$$ Active pHelityl Oil Pre-Cleansing Oil for Dry to Slightly Oily Skin *($30 for 6.8 ounces)* is supposed to be used before you use the soaps below, to protect the skin and help remove makeup. But why buy two products when all you need is one cleanser that doesn't dry out your skin and doesn't need help? All this product contains is mineral oil, plant oil, fragrance, and preservatives. This is some of the most expensive mineral oil you're likely to find anywhere.

☹ Active pHelityl Soap for Dry and Slightly Dry Skin *($23 for 6 ounces)* is a standard tallow-based bar of soap, with the same ingredients found in all soaps. This one does contain some plant oil, but that won't help the dryness caused by the other ingredients. This is a lot of money for a very ordinary bar of soap.

☺ **$$$ HydrapHel Cleansing Bar for Extremely Dry Skin** *($24 for 6 ounces)* doesn't contain any tallow, but it has all the other detergent cleansing agents that can cause dry skin. This is a standard bar cleanser with a tiny amount of emollients, and it's not the best for dry skin.

☺ **$$$ HydrapHel Cleansing Treatment Liquid Cleanser for Extremely Dry Skin** *($25 for 4.3 ounces)* is mostly Vaseline and thickening agents. This is little more than an expensive cold cream.

☹ **Sea Mud Soap for Normal, Slightly Oily, and Oily Skin** *($23 for 6 ounces)* contains the standard soap ingredients of tallow and sodium cocoate, with a little sea mud thrown in. It's still soap, and the mud makes it more drying and leaves a slight film on the skin. Also, tallow can cause breakouts.

☹ **Special Skin Soap for Oily and Extremely Oily Skin** *($23 for 6 ounces)* contains the standard soap ingredients of tallow and sodium cocoate, along with the detergent cleanser sodium lauryl sulfate, which is very drying and irritating. This is a fairly drying, average bar soap, and the tallow can cause breakouts.

☺ **$$$ Multi-pHase Eye Makeup Remover for All Skin Types** *($25 for 4 ounces)* is basically just silicone and plant extracts. It will allow you to wipe off eye makeup, and silicone does feel great on skin, but this is a very expensive way to go about it and wiping off makeup is just not best for the face.

☺ **$$$ pHelitone Gentle Eye Makeup Remover** *($18 for 3 ounces)* does remove eye makeup, but it contains just a standard detergent cleansing agent and some slip agents.

☹ **Conditioning Preparation for Oily to Extremely Oily Skin** *($26 for 6.8 ounces)* contains alcohol, water, fragrance, and resorcinol. This is almost pure alcohol, and very irritating to the skin; plus, resorcinol is a serious skin irritant, and one the FDA disallowed for claims in acne products in 1992.

☹ **Heavy Controlling Lotion PM Oil Control for Slightly Oily to Extremely Oily Skin** *($28 for 6.8 ounces)* contains mostly alcohol, water, talc, glycerin, thickener, and coloring agents. This won't control anything, and the alcohol makes it too drying and irritating for all skin types.

☺ **$$$ HydrapHel Skin Supplement Freshener for Extremely Dry and Dry Skin** *($30 for 6.8 ounces)* contains mostly water, slip agents, water-binding agent, anti-irritant, film former, fragrance, and preservatives. At least this one doesn't contain any alcohol; it's about time. This would be a good nonirritating toner for most skin types.

☹ **Light Controlling Lotion Toner for Slightly Dry to Oily Skin** *($26 for 6.8 ounces)* contains mostly water, alcohol, slip agents, and fragrance. The alcohol is too irritating for all skin types.

☹ **Regular Controlling Lotion PM Oil Control for Slightly Dry and Normal**

Skin *($28 for 6.8 ounces)* is an alcohol-based toner that also contains some talc and baking soda. The alcohol is too irritating and drying for all skin types but is particularly inexcusable on dry skin.

☹ $$$ **AHA Revitalizing Complex** *($95 for 1.5 ounces)* contains mostly water, silicone, thickeners, slip agent, AHAs, BHAs, water-binding agents, and preservatives. This product contains about 3% to 4% AHAs and BHAs combined, but the pH is too high for it to be an effective exfoliant, not to mention that there are far more effective and less expensive AHA or BHA versions available and I am also not one to recommend both together; use AHA for sun-damaged skin and BHA for blemish-prone skin.

☺ $$$ **Active pHelityl Cream PM Moisturizer for Slightly Dry Skin** *($32 for 2 ounces)* contains mostly petrolatum, safflower oil, thickeners, fragrance, more thickeners, and preservatives. This is a standard, emollient, petrolatum-based moisturizer. You're paying a lot of money for Vaseline.

☹ **Antioxidant Complex for Eyes, Lightening, Firming, Protective Eye Treatment for All Skin Types** *($65 for 1 ounce)* doesn't contain any skin-lightening ingredients, though it does contain some plant extracts that can irritate and swell the skin around the eye, including lemon, grapefruit, and witch hazel. The skin won't be firming, just swollen.

☺ $$$ **Antioxidant Concentrate for Eyes, Intensive Therapy for the Eye Area** *($48 for 0.5 ounce)* is a very good emollient moisturizer that contains mostly water, plant oils, thickeners, silicones, water-binding agents, anti-irritant, vitamins, and preservatives. It does contain a tiny amount of witch hazel but not enough to have an effect on the skin.

☹ **Antioxidant Moisture Complex SPF 15 Oil-Free Moisturizer for All Skin Types** *($55 for 2 ounces)* doesn't contain avobenzone, zinc oxide, or titanium dioxide, and is not recommended.

☺ $$$ **Antioxidant Moisture Complex Cream for Extremely Dry to Normal Skin** *($65 for 2 ounces)* contains mostly water, thickeners, plant oils, glycerin, slip agents, silicones, vitamins, water-binding agents, and preservatives. This is a good emollient moisturizer for someone with dry skin.

☹ **Daily Moisture Protection Lotion SPF 15 AM Moisturizer with Sunscreen for All Skin Types** *($45 for 2.5 ounces)* doesn't contain avobenzone, zinc oxide, or titanium dioxide, and is not recommended.

☺ $$$ **HydrapHel Complex PM Moisturizer for Extremely Dry and Dry Skin** *($55 for 2 ounces)* contains mostly water, mineral oil, thickeners, plant oils, vitamins, and preservatives. This is a good standard emollient moisturizer for dry skin.

☺ $$$ **HydrapHel Emulsion AM Moisturizer for Extremely Dry and Dry Skin** *($45 for 2 ounces)* contains mostly water, a tiny amount of sunscreen (not enough to protect adequately from the sun), thickeners, plant oils, glycerin, water-binding agents, anti-irritants, vitamins, silicone, mineral oil, preservatives, and fragrance Other than that, this is a good emollient moisturizer that still requires a good sunscreen if you are going to be wearing it during the day.

☺ **$$$ Moisture-Firming Throat Cream for All Skin Types** *($23 for 2 ounces)* is a good emollient moisturizer for dry skin, but there is nothing about this product that makes it special for the throat.

☺ **$$$ pHelitone Replenishing Eye Cream for All Skin Types** *($42 for 0.5 ounce)* contains mostly water, thickener, slip agent, petrolatum, plant oils, more thickeners, vitamin E, anti-irritants, more thickener, mineral oil, more thickeners, and preservatives. Pricey for a jar of petrolatum-based moisturizer, don't you think?

☺ **$$$ pHelityl Cream PM Moisturizer for Normal Skin** *($55 for 2 ounces)* contains mostly water, thickeners, silicone, more thickeners, mineral oil, more thickeners, petrolatum, and preservatives. This is a fairly standard emollient moisturizer for normal to dry skin. Can you believe they're charging that much for mineral oil and petrolatum?

☺ **$$$ pHelityl Lotion AM Moisturizer for Slightly Dry to Slightly Oily Skin** *($45 for 3 ounces)* contains mostly water, thickeners, mineral oil, vegetable oil, more thickeners, and preservatives. It's good, lightweight, and emollient for someone with dry skin, but overpriced for a very ordinary mineral oil–based moisturizer. Plus, no one with even slightly oily skin is going to be happy with this much oil in a product of any kind, and without sunscreen it is useless for daytime.

☺ **$$$ Total Skin Revitalizer Facial Hydration Enhancer for All Skin Types** *($54 for 1 ounce)* is a lightweight emollient moisturizer that contains water, slip agent, silicone, plant oil, glycerin, water-binding ingredients, soothing agent, thickeners, fragrance, and preservatives. It won't revitalize the skin, but it will keep normal to dry skin moist, just like any other moisturizer.

☺ **$$$ Total Skin Revitalizer for Eyes Hydration Enhancer for the Eye Area** *($45 for 0.5 ounce)* contains mostly water, thickeners, film former, water-binding agents, plant oil, anti-irritant, glycerin, vitamins, and preservatives. This is a good emollient moisturizer for the eyes (although there is a tiny amount of witch hazel in here it's probably not enough to be much of an irritant).

☹ **Oil-Free Sunblock SPF 25 for All Skin Types** *($22 for 4.3 ounces)* doesn't contain avobenzone, zinc oxide, or titanium dioxide, and is not recommended.

☺ **$$$ Self-Tanning Lotion SPF 8** *($22 for 4.2 ounces)* doesn't contain avobenzone, zinc oxide, or titanium dioxide, and is not recommended as a sunscreen, but it works fine as a self-tanner.

☹ **Sun Control Mist SPF 15** *($22 for 3.5 ounces)* doesn't contain avobenzone, zinc oxide, or titanium dioxide, and is not recommended.

☹ **Beta Complex Acne Treatment** *($65 for 2 ounces)* is a good, irritant-free BHA exfoliant, but the price is almost mind-boggling, plus the pH is too high for this to be an effective exfoliant. There are far less expensive versions with the appropriate pH that work. This one is a waste of time for the skin.

☹ **Beta Target Blemish Treatment** *($18 for 0.5 ounce)* contains too much alcohol, eucalyptus, peppermint, menthol, and camphor for any skin type; this is an irritation waiting to happen.

☺ **$$$ Hydra-Therapy Skin Vitality Treatment, Two Phase Moisture Mask for All Skin Types** *($36 for four applications of each phase)* is a two-part system that is so amazingly overpriced it is almost embarrassing. You mix an ordinary liquid with a simple powder that is mostly salt, apply it to your face, let it set, and then rinse. The liquid contains water, film former, anti-irritant, slip agent, and preservatives. The powder is made of magnesium carbonate (like milk of magnesia in powder form), sea salt, silica (sand), mineral salt, and calcium (powder). Ordinary ingredients, but an absurdly expensive product.

☺ **$$$ pHelitone Firming Eye Gel Mask for All Skin Types** *($30 for 0.5 ounce)* is an absurdly standard, lightweight gel for minimally dry skin. It contains mostly water, slip agents, anti-irritant, plant extracts, thickeners, and preservatives. It does contain a small amount of witch hazel but probably not enough to be a problem.

☹ **Sea Mud Mask** *($32 for 4 ounces)* is basically a standard clay mask, but it also contains alcohol and peppermint, which makes it too irritating for all skin types.

Erno Laszlo Makeup

☹ FOUNDATION: **Regular Normalizer Shake-It** *($30)* is mostly water, silicone, and talc. This is a drying foundation that goes on choppy and thin. **These colors are very good:** Honey, Neutral, Light Beige, and Suntan. **These colors are too peach or pink:** Beige, Porcelain, and Soft Beige.

☹ **Heavy Normalizer Shake-It** *($29)* contains mostly water, alcohol, talc, more alcohol, glycerin, and coloring agents. The alcohol makes this product too irritating for most skin types.

☺ **$$$ Multi-pHase Light Diffusing Foundation SPF 15** *($28)* is a liquid foundation that has a beautiful smooth consistency with a soft, sheer, matte finish. Most all of the shades are truly excellent. The only one to be careful of is Rose Beige, which can be slightly pink for most skin tones. By the way, this doesn't diffuse light or change the appearance of a wrinkle, it is just a very good foundation with a great partly titanium dioxide–based sunscreen.

☺ **$$$ Multi-pHase Oil-Free Foundation SPF 15** *($28)* is quite similar to the Light Diffusing Foundation above and actually the same comments apply to this one too, except the only shades to watch out for are Bisque and Linen, which can be slightly too pink for most skin tones.

☺ **Multi-pHase Perfecting Foundation SPF 8** *($32)* is a stick foundation that goes on fairly creamy but blends to a smooth, soft finish. Still, it can't hold a candle to the two Light Diffusing foundations above. The SPF for this one is poor, it has no UVA protection, and the colors are just the worst; all of the 12 shades are either too peach, pink, peach, or ash for all skin tones.

☺ **$$$ <u>CONCEALER:</u> Anti Cerne Concealer** *($25)* has a great smooth texture and application for a pot container–type consistency, and would be wonderful to recommend, but of the four shades only Shade 0 is a good neutral light shade; the other three are too pink, peach, or rose for all skin types.

☺ **$$$ <u>POWDER:</u> Controlling Pressed Powder** *($32)* and **Duo pHase Pressed Powder** *($32)* are fairly standard talc-based powders with silky-soft textures in great shades.

☹ **Multi-pHase Finishing Powder** *($25)* is a prism of shades in one pressed-powder compact that end up combining to create one shiny shade. It looks prettier in the compact than the effect it creates for the skin. There are four shades; only one is matte, and it looks pink on the skin; the others are pink shiny, bronze shiny, and white shiny.

☹ **<u>EYESHADOW:</u> Eyeshadow** *($22)* are pots of cream eyeshadow that are mostly shine (only two are matte). Cream eyeshadow is not the best, but some women find this a great way to apply eyeshadow. Even the salesperson discouraged me from buying any of these.

☺ **$$$ <u>LIPSTICK AND LIP PENCIL:</u> Multi-pHase Lipstick Creme and Sheer SPF 15** *($16)* are both fairly glossy-finish lipsticks. The SPF 15 doesn't include UVA protection. **Lasting Color Lipstick** *($16)* is a very good cream lipstick with a slight amount of tint so it helps the color last slightly longer than normal.

☹ **Multi-pHase Lip Liner** *($13)* is just a very standard lip pencil with a very soft, almost smushy finish, which means this pencil gets used up pretty fast.

☺ **$$$ <u>MASCARA:</u> MultipHase Mascara** *($19)* is a good mascara, but not great. It builds decent length and thickness, but nothing special or worth this price.

Estee Lauder

What sets the venerable Estee Lauder company apart from its competition is that it owns most of the cosmetics lines it competes with, and in all price ranges and attitudes. Lauder's formidable reach includes Clinique, Origins, Prescriptives, M.A.C., Bobbi Brown, and Aveda. A more recent acquisition is the drugstore line Jane, which for the first time puts Lauder in the drugstore makeup game. Of course, Estee Lauder is still the grande dame of makeup lines, with a loyal following and impressive public relations. Ask any of the salespeople who work for this seasoned cosmetics company, and they will tell you the products sell themselves. A few years ago, Night Repair and Eyezone were jumping off the shelves; then Lauder's AHA product, Fruition (discontinued in favor of the far better formulation Fruition Extra), caught fire; and now the hot seller is Day Wear, the line's antioxidant. This is a company with dedication to selling and to training its sales staff. The counter displays are not accessible without the help of a salesperson, so the sales pressure is fairly intense. Even more intense is the almost overwhelming number of age-control, antiwrinkle, micro-targeted, night-repair, quick-life, nourishing, and free radical–fighting products. It seems as if every wrinkle on your face has a product dedicated to it. Now, here's the question: If just one or two of their products could live up to their claims to get rid of wrinkles, why would you need an additional 50 products that claim to do the same thing? The Lauder lineup boasts some wonderful moisturizers, but also absurd prices for pretty standard products that can't live up to their more glorious claims.

Lauder has some great foundations and some disappointing ones as well. The best in the group are Double Wear SPF 10 (it is truly ultra-matte) and Enlighten SPF 10 (excellent for dry skin), and Impeccable SPF 20 (somewhat greasy but good for dry skin), and are all nonchemical SPFs. You have to be careful when choosing colors; some of the foundations in this collection are pink and orange. Most of the blushes are lovely, and they go on extremely soft and sheer. For more information about Estee Lauder call (800) 572-4800.

Estee Lauder Skin Care

☹ **Facewash Self-Foaming System** *($17.50 for 6 ounces)* is a fairly drying water-soluble cleanser. TEA-lauryl sulfate, the second item on the ingredient list, can be a skin irritant.

☺ **$$$ Instant Action Rinse-Off Cleanser** *($17.50 for 6 ounces)* is a plant oil–based cleanser and does not rinse off easily without the use of a washcloth. Its cleansing agent is quite mild, so this can be good for dry skin.

☹ **Micro-Moisture Cleansing Bar Normal to Dry** *($17.50 for 5 ounces)* is a standard bar cleanser made of tallow and sodium cocoate. It does contain some plant oils, which can help counteract some of the drying effect of this product, but why dry out the skin in the first place? Also, tallow can cause breakouts.

☹ **Micro-Refining Bar Cleanser Normal to Oily** *($17.50 for 5 ounces)* is practically identical to the bar above, but with a different color and a few different oils, and the same review applies.

☺ **$$$ Re-nutriv Extremely Delicate Skin Cleanser** *($32.50 for 7.5 ounces)* contains mostly mineral oil, water, beeswax, petrolatum, plant oil, thickeners, lanolin, and preservatives. Why use this very greasy product when Pond's Cold Cream is essentially the same thing for a fraction of the price?

☺ $$$ **Re-nutriv Moisture-Rich Creme Cleanser** *($27.50 for 3.4 ounces)* is similar to the one above only less greasy. The same basic review applies.

☹ **Rich Results Hydrating Cleanser** *($18.50 for 4.2 ounces)* contains a small amount of a gentle cleansing agent, but it also contains wax and other thickeners that make it hard to rinse off without the aid of a washcloth, and for some reason this one contains menthol, which can irritate the eyes.

☹ **Solid Milk Cleansing Grains** *($18.50 for 3.7 ounces)* contains mostly corn flour, film former (PVP, a possible irritant), thickeners, chalk, nonfat dry milk, fragrance, detergent cleanser, anti-irritant, and preservatives. This thick scrub uses sodium lauryl sulfate as the cleansing agent, and that is very drying for the skin; also, PVP in this amount is a skin irritant. One more warning: corn flour and milk can cause breakouts.

☹ **Splash Away Foaming Cleanser** *($18.50 for 3.4 ounces)* is a fairly drying detergent-based, water-soluble cleanser. Keep it away from your eyes, because it can sting if you get even a little in them.

☺ $$$ **Tender Creme Cleanser** *($26 for 8 ounces)* is a cleanser that needs to be wiped off with a tissue or a washcloth. It tends to leave a slightly greasy film and does not take off makeup all that well.

☺ $$$ **Verite Light Lotion Cleanser** *($22.50 for 6.7 ounces)* contains mostly water, thickener, water-binding agents, plant oils, silicone, more water-binding agents, plant extracts, more water-binding agent, and preservatives. This is an OK wipe-off cleanser that can leave a slightly greasy film.

☺ $$$ **Verite Soft Foam Cleanser** *($22.50 for 4.2 ounces)* contains mostly glycerin, petrolatum (Vaseline), detergent cleansing agents (including sodium C14-16 olefin sulfate, which is considered quite drying), water, plant extracts, and water-binding agents. This is the only product in the entire Verite grouping with a fairly irritating ingredient that is totally inappropriate for someone with sensitive skin; and the hallmark of the Verite line is sensitive skin. Also, the petrolatum can leave a greasy film on the skin.

☺ $$$ **Gentle Eye Makeup Remover** *($13.50 for 3.4 ounces)* is a standard gentle eye-makeup remover. Any gentle water-soluble cleanser should do the same thing without making you wipe and pull at your eyes with an extra product.

☹ **Deep Sweep Skin Refiner** *($18.50 for 3.4 ounces)* costs a lot of money for what is basically alcohol, synthetic scrub, and slip agents. It can dry and irritate the skin.

☺ $$$ **Gentle Action Skin Polisher** *($18.50 for 3.4 ounces)* is supposed to be a water-soluble scrub, but it doesn't rinse off well. It contains mostly water, mineral oil, thickeners, detergent cleanser, and preservatives. Although the scrubbing effect is fairly mild, the other ingredients are emollient and rather standard thickeners that can clog pores. This could be good for someone with dry skin.

☹ **Clear Finish Purifying Toner N/D** *($25 for 13.5 ounces)* contains mostly water, slip agents, plant extracts, water-binding agents, and preservatives. It does contain menthol which can be a skin irritant for most skin types.

☹ **Clean Finish Purifying Toner N/O** *($25 for 13.5 ounces)* is similar to the one above only this one adds grapefruit and papaya to the irritation quotient.

☺ **$$$ Re-Nutriv Gentle Skin Toner** *($30 for 6.7 ounces)* is an alcohol-free toner whose second ingredient is cetrimonium chloride, a cleansing agent and disinfectant. It isn't bad for the skin, it just isn't all that gentle. There probably isn't much in this product, though, which means there is even less of everything else that follows it on the ingredient list.

☺ **$$$ Verite Soothing Spray Toner** *($22.50 for 6.7 ounces)* contains mostly water, water-binding agents, plant extracts (including green tea, an anti-irritant), and preservatives. This is a very good nonirritating toner for all skin types.

☺ **$$$ Advanced Night Repair Protective Recovery Complex** *($70 for 1.7 ounces)* is a good moisturizer that contains mostly water, water-binding agents, thickeners, anti-irritants, silicone, plant oil, more water-binding agents, vitamin A, and preservatives. It also contains a small amount of sunscreen, which doesn't make sense in a product that's meant to be used at night, and can be a skin irritant. This product won't repair anything, but it is a good lightweight moisturizer for dry skin.

☺ **$$$ Age Controlling Creme** *($60 for 1.7 ounces)* contains mostly water, lanolin, slip agents, plant oils, mineral oil, several thickeners, petrolatum, water-binding agents, anti-irritant, vitamins, silicone, and preservatives. It is a very good moisturizer for someone with very dry skin, but why this product is for "age control" is anyone's guess.

☺ **$$$ Clear Difference Oil-Control Hydrator for Oily Normal/Oily and Blemish-Prone Skin** *($27 for 1.7 ounces)* is a good lightweight moisturizer for dry areas of skin but this won't control oil. It contains mostly water, silicones, thickeners, film former, anti-irritant, BHA, water-binding agents, thickeners, and preservatives. The pH of this product is about 4, but a pH of 3 would make it a more effective exfoliant. This still can be an option for blemish-prone skin.

☹ **Equalizer Oil-Free HydroGel** *($27.50 for 1.7 ounces)* is basically alcohol and silicone. The alcohol can be drying and irritating.

☺ **$$$ Estoderme Creme** *($25 for 4 ounces)* contains mostly mineral oil, water, lanolin, thickeners, slip agent, water-binding agents, plant oil, preservatives, and fragrance. This is a very emollient, rich, almost greasy moisturizer for someone with very dry skin.

☺ **$$$ Estoderme Emulsion** *($25 for 4 ounces)* is similar to the moisturizer above, and the same review applies.

☺ **$$$ Eyezone Repair Gel** *($35 for 0.5 ounce)* contains mostly water, film former, plant extract, water-binding agents, thickeners, and preservatives. I was told it would last six months because you use so little, but you would have to use none for a half-ounce to last that long. This gel won't repair the skin, but it is an OK light-weight moisturizer for slightly dry skin.

☺ **$$$ Fruition Extra Multi-Action Complex** *($70 for 1.7 ounces)*. The original Fruition has been discontinued, and the Extra is now the only version available. The original was supposed to be an exfoliating AHA product, but it didn't contain enough of the stuff to have any effect; all it was, was a good lightweight moisturizer. Fruition Extra adds salicylic acid to the mix and a higher percentage of AHA, which means more exfoliation. Finally, that makes this one a decent, though overpriced, exfoliant. I also don't recommend BHA for all skin types, but rather for someone with breakouts, and AHAs for sun damaged skin.

☺ **$$$ Future Perfect Micro-Targeted Skin Gel** *($45 for 1.75 ounces)* contains mostly water, film former, slip agent, silicone, water-binding agents, vitamins, plant extracts, more thickeners, fragrance, and preservatives. This is a good lightweight emollient moisturizer for normal to dry skin. The name of this gel is better than what you get; it sounds as if you can place it over a wrinkle, zero in, and, poof, get rid of it. Not possible.

☺ **$$$ Re-nutriv Creme** *($75 for 1.75 ounce)* contains mostly water, lanolin, mineral oil, a long list of thickeners, vitamins, silicone, water-binding agents, fragrance, and preservatives. This is a very emollient, though ordinary, moisturizer for extremely dry skin.

☺ **$$$ Re-nutriv Firming Eye Creme** *($47.50 for 0.5 ounce)* contains mostly water, water-binding agents, slip agent, several thickeners, lanolin oil, plant extract, more water-binding agents, vitamins A and E, mineral oil, more thickeners, and preservatives. This won't firm the eye area, and the fancy water-binding agents (amino acids and collagen) cannot get rid of wrinkles, but it is a very good emollient moisturizer for dry skin.

☺ **$$$ Re-nutriv Firming Throat Creme** *($53 for 1.7 ounces)* is similar to the one above, but there is nothing about this formulation that makes it better for the throat versus the face.

☺ **$$$ Re-nutriv Intensive Firming Plus** *($95 for 1.7 ounces)* contains a small amount of AHAs but not enough to be considered an exfoliant. This is just a good, very overpriced moisturizer for dry skin.

☺ **$$$ Re-nutriv Intensive Lifting Creme** *($150 for 1.7 ounces)* contains mostly water, silicone, thickeners, Vaseline, water binding agents, plant extracts, fragrance, anti-irritant, vitamins, more fragrance, and preservatives. While this is a good moisturizer, there is nothing in here that will lift skin anywhere, and the price is nothing less than obscene given the ingredient list. Lauder charges a lot less for other moisturizers they sell with a similar ingredient listing.

☺ **$$$ Re-nutriv Replenishing Creme** *($78 for 1.7 ounces)* is similar to the moisturizer above, only not as greasy, and the same review applies.

☹ **$$$ Re-nutriv Lightweight Creme** *($75 for 1.75 ounces)* is almost identical to the creme above, but slightly lighter weight. The company suggests using this for normal to oily skin, but ingredients like plant oils, lanolin oil, and thick waxes make that recommendation absurd and the price painful.

☹ **$$$ Resilience Elastin Refirming Creme** *($60 for 1.7 ounces)* contains mostly water, plant oil, slip agent, thickeners, glycerin, water-binding agents, vitamin E, plant extracts, silicone, fragrance, and preservatives. This is a good, but extremely ordinary, moisturizer for someone with normal to dry skin. Fish elastin won't help firm a fish's skin any more than it will yours.

☹ **$$$ Resilience Elastin Refirming Lotion** *($60 for 1.7 ounce)* is similar to the product above, only in lotion form, and the same review applies.

☺ **$$$ Resilience Eye Creme** *($42.50 for 0.5 ounce)* contains thickeners, emollient, silicone, film former, water-binding agents, plant extracts, vitamin E, more water-binding agents, more thickeners, and preservatives. This is a good emollient moisturizer for dry skin.

☹ **$$$ Skin Defender Sensitive Skin Protector** *($45 for 0.9 ounce)* contains mostly water, water-binding agents, silicone, slip agents, thickeners, vitamin A, more water-binding agents, anti-irritant, more thickeners, and preservatives. This is a very good moisturizer for someone with very dry skin. However, although a sunscreen is listed on the ingredient listing, there is no SPF rating on the label, so there is no way to know how much protection it provides. Therefore you must not count on this one for use during the day.

☺ **$$$ Skin Perfecting Creme Firming Nourisher** *($35 for 1.75 ounces)* is a lightweight moisturizer with one of the longest ingredient lists I've ever seen. If you are looking for every state-of-the-art moisturizing ingredient, look here: collagen, vitamins, marine extracts, plant oils, proteins, antioxidants, anti-irritant, and amino acids, all fairly high on the ingredient list. This would take care of dry skin, as well as any concerns that you might be missing out on the latest skin-care ingredients (except for AHAs), and it's cheaper than a lot of the nonsense in this line.

☹ **$$$ Skin Perfecting Lotion Lightweight Moisturizer** *($27.50 for 1.7 ounces)* contains mostly water, silicone, several thickeners, vitamins E and A, anti-irritants, plant extracts, water-binding agents, and preservatives. It is lightweight but boring. There is no SPF rating on the label although a sunscreen agent is listed, and that means there is no way to know how much protection this product provides. Do not count on it for use during the day.

☺ **$$$ Swiss Performing Extract Moisturizer** *($37.50 for 3.2 ounces)* contains mostly water, plant oils, water-binding agents, slip agents, lanolin, mineral oil, thickeners, silicone, fragrance, and preservatives. This is a very emollient, very good moisturizer for someone with dry skin.

☺ **$$$ Time Zone Eyes Ultra-Hydrating Complex** *($40 for 0.5 ounce)* contains mostly water, film former, glycerin, slip agent, aloe, thickeners, water-binding agents, plant extracts, vitamins, and preservatives. This is a lightweight moisturizer for normal to dry skin. Seaweed and fish collagen won't hydrate the skin, but the water-binding agents are nice. Some of the film formers in here can be irritating for some skin types.

☺ **$$$ Time Zone Moisture Recharging Complex** *($55 for 1.7 ounces)* is similar to the one above, only with more emollients. It would be good for dry skin.

☹ **$$$ Uncircle** *($37.50 for 0.5 ounce)* contains mostly water, film former, Vaseline, slip agents, fish cartilage, water-binding agents, more hairstyling-type ingredients, thickening agents, and preservatives. There is nothing in here that will have any more effect on circles than would any other moisturizer in this line. Petrolatum and film former is not what I or anyone else would call an exotic or excitingly new formulation, and fish cartilage can't affect anything around the eye, but you already knew that.

☺ **$$$ Verite Moisture Relief Creme** *($50 for 1.75 ounces)* contains mostly water, silicone, water-binding agents, thickeners, more water-binding agents, plant extracts (including oat extract, which is considered an anti-irritant), and preservatives. This is a very good moisturizer for someone with dry skin.

☺ **$$$ Verite Calming Fluid** *($60 for 1.7 ounces)* contains mostly water, silicones, glycerin, water-binding agents, plant extracts, vitamin E, thickeners, and preservatives. It probably won't calm anything, but it is a very good moisturizer for someone with normal to dry skin.

☹ **$$$ Creme de la Mer** *($155 for 2 ounces)* is a very costly little cream accompanied by quite a dramatic story! Max Huber, a NASA aerospace physicist, created this product, supposedly to take care of burns he received in an accident. As enticing as this dramatic story is, the reality is that this very basic cream doesn't contain anything particularly extraordinary or unique, unless you want to believe that seaweed extract (sort of like seaweed tea) can in some way heal burns and scars. Even if it could, burns and scars don't have much to do with wrinkling, and that's what this product is now being sold as: a wrinkle cream. According to Susan Brawley, professor of plant biology at the University of Maine, "Seaweed extract isn't a rare, exotic, or expensive ingredient. Seaweed extract is readily available and used in everything from cosmetics to food products and medical applications." Creme de la Mer contains mostly seaweed extract, mineral oil, petrolatum, glycerin, waxlike thickening agents, plant oils, plant seeds, minerals, vitamins, more thickeners, and preservatives. This rather standard moisturizer contains some good antioxidants, which can help heal skin by keeping air off it, but these ingredients are also found in many other moisturizers that cost a *lot* less. According to the cosmetic chemists I've interviewed, it costs pennies, not hundreds of dollars, to stick some seaweed and vitamins in a cosmetic.

☺ $$$ **Nutritious Bio Protein** *($45 for 1.7 ounces)* is Lauder's latest endeavor to convince us that you can feed the face from the outside. You can't, but it will be hard for the average trusting cosmetics consumer to not be impressed with all the milk by-products and healthy minerals like calcium and magnesium, not to mention amino acids and vitamins, in here. Of course, none of those ingredients has any impact beyond keeping water in the skin, but the emphasis on nutrition, no matter how physiologically impossible from the outside in, is a hot ticket in the cosmetics world these days. What else does this product contain? A long list of water-binding agents. These are ingredients that form a barrier on the outside of the skin, preventing water from being absorbed by the air. Is the long list necessary? In essence, one or two water-binding agents provide the same benefit as a dozen. Skin can only hold so much water. For your information, this product contains mostly water, plant oils, glycerin, silicone oil, thickeners, water-binding agents, minerals, more water-binding agents, plant extracts, more water-binding agents, vitamins, more water-binding agents, and preservatives.

☺ $$$ **Diminish Retinol Treatment** *($47.50 for 1 ounce)* came on the scene with a fanfare of claims about getting rid of lines, evening skin tone, improving skin texture, and on and on, much like the claims around several of their other products. It definitely contains retinol, but only about 1% or 2%. Other than that, the rest of the ingredients are standard, lightweight moisturizing ingredients. Would I use this product over Retin-A? No, especially not if I had sun-damaged skin, but I do think it is a very impressive lightweight moisturizer for nighttime (the lack of sunscreen makes it an evening product), and anything that gets women to switch to a lightweight moisturizer is going to be beneficial in the long run. If you are interested in Diminish purely for the retinol (and there really is no other reason), let me point you in the direction of Avon Anew Retinol Recovery Complex P.M. Treatment *($17.50 for 1 ounce)*. It has about the same amount of retinol as the Lauder product and is also lightweight, but far less expensive.

☺ $$$ **100% Time Release Moisturizer** *($32.50 for 2 ounces)* contains mostly fossilized water, silicones, slip agents, several thickeners, water-binding agents, vitamin E, and preservatives. Are you wondering what the fossilized water is all about? So was I. The package states it contains 70 minerals. Is that helpful for the skin? Hardly. Most water contains minerals, but when used in cosmetics the minerals are usually taken out to leave the skin feeling softer and make product formulation easier.

This is a good moisturizer for someone with normal to dry skin, but it is one of the more ordinary offerings in the Lauder lineup.

☺ **$$$ Enriched Under-Makeup Creme** *($25 for 4 ounces)* is definitely rich. It contains mostly water, mineral oil, lanolin, several thickeners, slip agent, water-binding agents, silicone, vitamin E, and preservatives. This is a very emollient moisturizer for someone with very dry skin.

☺ **$$$ Advanced Suncare Baby Block Lotion for Children SPF 25** *($19.50 for 4.25 ounces)* is an excellent nonchemical (meaning titanium dioxide-based) sunscreen for normal to slightly dry skin. There is nothing about this product special for children; it is a sunscreen anyone can wear.

☺ **$$$ Advanced Suncare Sun Block for Face SPF 25** *($19.50 for 1.7 ounces)* is similar to the one above and the same review applies.

☺ **$$$ Advanced Suncare Sun Block for Face SPF 15** *($19.50 for 1.7 ounces)* is similar to the one above only with an SPF 15, and the same review applies.

☺ **$$$ Advanced Suncare Sun Block Lotion Spray No Chemical Sunscreen SPF 15** *($18.50 for 4.25 ounces)* is a very good titanium dioxide–based sunscreen in a silicone base. This will leave a fairly nongreasy finish, but it can appear somewhat white on the skin.

☺ **$$$ Day Wear Super Anti-Oxidant Complex SPF 15** *($37.50 for 1.7 ounces)* contains mostly water, silicones, a very long list of thickeners, vitamins, plant extracts, water-binding agents, fragrance, and preservatives. The antioxidants are not exactly at the top of the ingredient list, nor are they any more special than in hundreds of other products, so none of that is all that super. What is good about this day cream is that it contains an SPF 15 sunscreen that is part titanium dioxide, which is one of the better ways to protect against sun damage. In that regard, this product is right on, as are most of Lauder's sunscreens.

☺ **$$$ Self-Action SuperTan for Face, Medium/Dark** *($18.50 for 1.5 ounces)*; **Self-Action Spray, Medium/Dark** *($25 for 4.2 ounces)*; **Self-Action Tanning Creme, Dark** *($17.50 for 4.2 ounces)*; **Self-Action Tanning Creme, Medium** *($17.50 for 4.2 ounces)*; and **Self-Action Tanning Creme, Very Dark** *($17.50 for 4.2 ounces)* are like all other self-tanners, they all use the active ingredient dihydroxyacetone to turn the skin brown. These work as well as any.

☺ **$$$ Almond Clay Mask** *($18.50 for 3.4 ounces)* contains mostly water, thickeners, clay, almond meal, a small amount of salicylic acid, and preservatives. This is a fairly standard clay mask with the addition of a gritty substance (almonds). The BHA is almost nonexistent and won't have much effect as an exfoliant. This is a just a standard clay mask.

☹ **Counter-Blemish Lotion** *($12 for 0.45 ounce)* contains alcohol as the first ingredient and is not recommended for any skin type.

☺ **$$$ Quick Lift 4-Minute Mask N/D** *($18.50 for 3.4 ounces)* is a standard clay mask with emollient. This can be a good mask for someone with normal to dry skin.

☺ **$$$ Quick Lift 4-Minute Mask N/O** *($18.50 for 3.4 ounces)* is similar to the mask above, and the same review applies.

☺ **Soothing Creme Facial** *($18.50 for 3.4 ounces)* is supposed to be a deep-cleansing mask. It isn't all that deep-cleansing, but it is a fairly emollient clay mask that can be good for someone with normal to dry skin. It contains mostly water, slip agent, thickeners, water-binding agents, clay, plant oil, more thickeners, anti-irritant, cleansing agents, and preservatives.

☹ **$$$ Stress Relief Eye Mask** *($27.50 for ten 0.4-ounce packets)* contains mostly water, glycerin, slip agents, water-binding agents, plant extracts, and preservatives. This is a very sticky mask that doesn't feel great on the skin. This won't affect stress in the least, and it's not great for skin either.

☺ **$$$ Triple Creme Hydrating Mask** *($27.50 for 2.5 ounces)* contains mostly water, thickeners, plant oil, slip agents, water-binding agents, fragrance and preservatives. These are good moisturizing ingredients, so they would feel good if left on the face for a while.

Estee Lauder Makeup

☹ **FOUNDATION: Impeccable SPF 20** *($27.50)* has a great name; what a pity it can't live up to such perfect coverage. This greasy, cream-to-powder foundation in a compact form blends evenly, with medium coverage. Unfortunately, it can slip into lines on the face, and the third ingredient is aluminum starch, which can cause breakouts. The color selection isn't the best, but the SPF 20 (nonchemical) rating is impressive. For someone with dry skin, this may be an option, but I would definitely give it a trial run before investing. **These colors are wonderful:** Soft Cream and Sunkissed. **These colors are either too peach, orange, or ash:** Fresh Ivory, Linen, Nude Beige, True Beige, Golden Honey, and Rich Cocoa.

☺ **Minute Makeup SPF 15** *($27.50)* is a stick makeup that takes as long to apply as any other makeup. While the name is ambiguous, the foundation is quite good and the color selection superior. It goes on smooth and even, and provides great sun protection and medium to heavy coverage. Consider this one if you have normal to dry skin. One word of warning: Lauder claims it is non-acnegenic. I disagree. Several ingredients in here could trigger breakouts, not the least of which is the active sunscreen ingredient, titanium dioxide.

☺ **Maximum Coverage with Non-Chemical SPF 12** *($25)* goes on creamy and smooth and then seems to stick to the skin, which can feel uncomfortable. It doesn't provide as much coverage as the name implies (this isn't Dermablend), although it does cover well. There is a limited assortment of colors to choose from, but most of the available colors are great. There are two color-correcting shades of green and yellow, but just ignore those.

☺ **Lucidity Light Diffusing Makeup SPF 8** *($27.50)* can't diffuse light, although it is a good liquid foundation for someone with normal to dry skin. Unfortunately this one has no UVA protection. **These colors are very good:** Gold Alabaster (excellent pale shade), Ivory Beige (slightly peach), Rich Ginger (may turn peach), Sun Bronze (may turn rose), Gold Caramel, Gold Sand, Bronze Mocha, Medium Beige (slightly rose), Sun Beige, Coffee, and Sable. **These colors are too peach or pink for most skin tones:** Neutral Beige, Gold Ivory, Cool Beige, Outdoor Beige, and Vanilla Beige.

☺ **Enlighten Skin-Enhancing Makeup with SPF 10** *($27.50)* is a superior foundation with a nonchemical sunscreen. What a shame it's rated only SPF 10; that isn't bad, but SPF 15 would be better. The application is smooth and sheer, leaving a beautiful slightly matte finish. It is best for someone with normal to combination or slightly dry skin. The color selection isn't the best, with some strange shades of pink, peach, and yellow. **These colors are too be avoided:** Vanilla Beige, Day Break, Neutral Ivory, Neutral Beige, Outdoor Beige, and Rich Ginger.

☹ **Futurist Age-Resisting Makeup SPF 15** *($32.50)* would be a great foundation to recommend because of its great color selection and texture. Regrettably, the SPF 15 doesn't include any of the UVA protecting ingredients avobenzone, zinc oxide, or titanium dioxide, and therefore it is not recommended.

☺ **$$$ Compact Finish Double Performance Makeup** *($27.50)* is a standard powder foundation with a superior soft, silky finish; it works well alone or with foundation. You are supposed to be able to use it wet or dry, but the wet never works well with these kinds of powders. All the salespeople I spoke to warned about streaking, which is what can easily happen no matter how deftly you are blending. Still, there are a number of impressive shades to choose from, and all are just beautiful. The only colors to consider carefully are Ivory Beige (may be too pink) and Ivory (can be too peach).

☺ **$$$ Double Wear Makeup SPF 10** *($27.50)* is great! It has a terrific matte texture and it truly doesn't move. Someone with normal to oily skin will be impressed with the application and the way it holds up over a long day. Great colors, too. The only negative is that it can provide too much coverage. This is not a sheer foundation.

☹ **Double Matte Oil-Control Makeup SPF 15** *($27.50)* is an excellent foundation, providing more sheer, less opaque coverage than the Double Wear above, although both are exceedingly matte; however, the SPF for this one doesn't contain any UVA protection! Why couldn't Lauder make the Double Matte a nonchemical SPF 15 like Double Wear? How disappointing!

☺ <u>CONCEALER:</u> **Smoothing Creme Concealer with SPF 8** *($16)* would be better as an SPF 15 but it is nonchemical, so that's better than nothing. It has a great creamy consistency, but it can crease, so be sure to test this one before you consider buying it.

☺ **Uncircle Concealer SPF 20** *($15)* is a standard creamy concealer in a small pot. It happens to have a great SPF with a nonchemical sunscreen base (something most concealers don't have) and a small but good range of colors. I would love to recommend it, but it can easily crease on and off for most of the day. If you have any lines under your eyes, this is not a viable option, or at least test this one before you consider it an option.

☹ **Automatic Concealer** *($13.50)* comes in three fairly pink shades. The consistency is on the dry side, but it stays on well. What a shame the colors are so poor.

☺ $$$ <u>POWDER:</u> **Double-Matte Oil-Free Loose Powder** *($18.50)* and **Double-Matte Oil-Free Pressed Powder** *($20)*, for oily skin, are both standard talc-based powders. Both have a great texture, with a dry, slightly chalky finish. Light and Light Medium can both be too peach for some skin tones. **Lucidity Translucent Loose Powder** *($26)* and **Lucidity Translucent Pressed Powder** *($20)*, for all skin types, are also standard talc-based powders. Both of these have great color selections. Lucidity is supposed to change the way light focuses on your face. It feels nice and silky smooth, but it doesn't look any different than dozens of other powders I've tested. **Enlighten Powder** *($20)* isn't enlightened in the least, though it does come packaged with a petite but useful brush for touch-ups. This is a decent, standard talc-based powder with a soft, silky feel and an extremely sheer finish.

☺ <u>BLUSH:</u> **Blush All Day** *($20)* has a smooth, dry, sheer finish and a nice array of colors to choose from. One shade in the group is a white shimmering frost. It has a remarkable amount of shine and is a good option for evening. **Blushing Natural Cheek Creme** *($20)* is a standard cream-to-powder blush in a small array of rather pretty colors that are somewhat shiny. I dislike cream blush because it can be tricky to blend and only works for flawless skin, plus shiny and creamy are not something I can recommend. However, the application for this product is just fine if this is the kind of blush you are looking for. **Just Blush! Eye and Cheek Powder** *($25)* has been narrowed down to two colors, which are soft and meant to work on both the cheek and the eye. It comes with a retractable brush that's a nice size.

☺ <u>EYESHADOW:</u> **Two-In-One Eyeshadow** *($12)* comes in a soft, attractive range of single colors that all have some amount of shine, but some definitely more than others. They have a smooth, soft application (don't count on intensity from these colors), but focus your concentration on the matte shades only. One interesting feature of these colors is that they can be applied wet and they do so nicely. That provides for a slightly more opaque coverage but also adds a smoothness you should check out. **Consider checking out:** Fawn, Camel, Sand Dollar, Eggshell, and Tearose.

☺ **$$$ EYE AND BROW SHAPER: Automatic Pencil for Eyes** *($22.50; $8 for a refill)* is a standard twist-up pencil in an elegant container. It is among the most expensive pencils on the market, but the refills are a bargain and then you have the sexy container, if you're into that kind of thing. Some of the colors are too shiny and fairly greasy, so be careful; this can smear under the eye. **Eye Defining Pencil** *($22.50)* is a standard pencil with a smooth finish in a nice array of colors. **Two-in-One Eye Pencil** *($16)* is a standard eye pencil. Each pencil has two different colors, one at each tip. **Two-in-One Eyeliner/Brow Color** *($25)* goes on wet or dry. It comes in one compact with two colors: Brown and Black. While it does work to fill in brows or line the eye, the color selection is rather limited and most any matte eyeshadow can perform the identical function. **Automatic Pencil for Brows** *($22.50; $8 for a refill)* is similar to the Automatic Pencil Liner for Eyes, only this one has a slightly drier finish. It comes in a pretty container, but penciling is not the best option for a natural-looking brow. **Brow Gel** *($13.50)* is a clear, hair spray–like product that holds the brow in place. It works fairly well, but no better than hair spray on a toothbrush.

☺ **$$$ Liquid Liner** *($13.50)* has a hidden amount of shine and can easily chip and rub off. **Waterproof Liquid Liner** *($14)* isn't all that waterproof, and has a hard-to-control brush.

☹ **Natural Brow Filler** *($13)* is a one-color fat eyebrow pencil that isn't by any means a one-size-fits-all product. The fat tip makes it hard to control the color through the brow, and the color isn't in the least natural, so it isn't for everyone.

☺ **LIPSTICK AND LIP PENCIL: Perfect Lipstick** *($15)*, **All Day Lipstick** *($12.50)*, and **Polish Performance** are wonderful: very creamy and rich. **True Lipstick Satin** or **Matte** *($16)* is supposed to have great staying power without bleeding or changing color. Well, it doesn't stay any better, nor is it more "true," than a hundred other lipsticks at the drugstore and cosmetics counters. This one bleeds right into the lines around the mouth—rather quickly, too, I might add. But for a creamy, slightly glossy texture lipstick, it is just fine. **Indelible Lipstick** *($16)* is another rendition of Maybelline's Budgeproof Lip Color and Revlon's ColorStay. Is there a reason to use Lauder's over the other two? Absolutely not; they all work just about identically. Whether it's Lauder's Indelible or Cover Girl's Marathon, they all go on moist and wet, and dry within a few seconds to form a dry, matte layer over the lips with no movement or creaminess. This texture of lipstick is not for everyone, and particularly not for those with chapped lips, but it is an option for a contemporary matte finish. **Lip Blush** *($15)* is just lip gloss in a tube, very standard, and very ordinary.

☺ **High Shine Gloss SPF 15** *($13)* doesn't have any UVA protection and is not recommended for sun protection. It is just a standard, shiny gloss.

☺ **Pink Slip for Lips** *($15)* is a fat, short pencil that is supposed to double as a lipstick and lip liner. The primary problem is that you have to sharpen it frequently, and that can be a pain. It looks more convenient than it ends up being in real life. If you are interested in giving this type of product a shot, Maybelline Lip Express and L'Oreal Crayon Grande are identical at one-third the price. **Lip Shaper Primer ($16)** is a beige-tone foundation-type product that is supposed to set lipstick and keep it from slipping into the lines around the mouth. It works no better than a matte foundation to keep lipstick on, and it would be far better to just have a lipstick that stayed in place and didn't shift as you wore it.

☺ **Lip Defining Pencil ($13)** is a standard lip pencil that comes in a great assembly of colors. **Automatic Pencil Liner for Lips ($22.50; $8 for refills)** is a very standard twist-up pencil in a very elegant container; the refills are great and inexpensive, so in the long run it probably balances out the convenience and price!

☺ **MASCARA: More Than Mascara ($15)** isn't more than mascara, it's just mascara. Nevertheless, it goes on easily while building decent length and some amount of thickness. But for the money and nice thick lashes, I'm not giving up my Maybelline Illegal Lengths!

☹ **$$$ Pure Velvet Dramatic Volume Mascara ($16)** is one of those products that belong in a "why bother" bin. There is nothing dramatic, volumizing, or velvety about it. If you don't expect much from a $16 mascara, this one will do. It doesn't clump or smear, but it also doesn't lengthen much and it definitely doesn't thicken. It's a lot like the two Prescriptives mascaras reviewed below. I think the Lauder company (which owns Prescriptives) needs to talk to the chemists who formulate their mascaras. **Individualist Lash Building Mascara ($16.50)** is a decent enough mascara, but it doesn't build very long lashes and can take quite a while to create any thickness worth mentioning. It didn't smudge, smear, or clump, so it would be a good choice if you're looking for reliability without much length or bulk. **Lash Primer ($15)** is supposed to help make lashes even longer if you apply it before the mascara. It is little more than a white mascara, which is the same as laying down a layer of regular mascara, waiting a moment and then adding more. Besides, if Lauder's mascara worked well to build length, why would you need this extra step? **Raincoat Waterproofing TopCoat for Mascara ($15)** works all right, though it can be tricky to get on over your already applied mascara. It is little more than hair spray for the lashes. My question is, why buy this product when you can get a really good waterproof mascara and apply it in one step instead of two?

☹ **$$$ BRUSHES:** Lauder has a small array of brushes. They are not the best I've ever seen, given the quality, shape, and range at the M.A.C., Trish McEvoy, Bobbi Brown, Shu Uemura, Lancome, and Prescriptives counters, or in The Body Shop, Joan Simmons, and Rialto (Canada only) brush collections. The sizes aren't the most workable, at least not for everyone, and the bristles, though soft, tend to be too full, making placement and control tricky. **Blush** *($18.50)* is a nice soft brush that would work well for blush. **Square Shading for Eye** *($12.50)* is a good all-over eyeshadow brush but can be too big for some eye shapes. **Angled Eyeshadow and Brow** *($12.50)* is a standard, soft, angled brush that can work for some eyeshadow blending and filling in a brow. **Eyeshadow Shading and Contouring** *($12.50)* is a good basic eyeshadow brush. **Face** *($18.50)* has a flat top, which makes it difficult to create a soft edge or blend easily over the face. **Eye Liner** *($12.50)* is a stiff, square brush that is too firm for eyeshadow and too large to control a line along the lashes; this one hurts. **Concealing** *($12.50)* works fine, but your finger works just as well if not better. **Tapered Blending for Eye** *($12.50)* is too long and floppy to provide much control for placement of eyeshadows.

Eucerin (Skin Care Only)

For more information about Eucerin call Beirsdorf Inc. at (800) 227-4703.

☹ **Cleansing Bar Dry Skin Therapy** *($3.88 for 3 ounces)* is a detergent-based bar cleanser. While it is still milder than others, there are far better water-soluble cleansers available. Plus, the ingredients that keep the bar in its bar form can clog pores.

☺ **Facial Moisturizing Lotion, SPF 25** *($8 for 4 ounces)* is a very good in-part titanium dioxide– and zinc oxide–based sunscreen for someone with normal to dry skin.

☺ **Eucerin Light Moisture Restorative Creme** *($6.99 for 4 ounces)* and **Light Moisture Restorative Lotion** *($6.99 for 8 ounces)* aren't all that light, but compared with the original Eucerin cream and lotion, they are amazingly light. Neither will restore anything, but they are very rich and easily absorbed, leaving a silky-smooth feel on the skin. If you want to start winterizing your skin with generous amounts of moisturizer, these are a great option. The cream contains mostly water, plant oil, glycerin, thickeners, vitamin E, more thickeners, water-binding agents, and preservatives. The lotion contains mostly water, plant oil, petrolatum, glycerin, thickeners, vitamin E, more thickeners, and preservatives. If you tend to break out, these products aren't for you. Also, they don't contain sunscreen, so daytime use on exposed parts of the body is not recommended.

☺ **Original Moisturizing Creme** *($4.19 for 2 ounces)* is an extremely heavy moisturizer that contains mostly water, petrolatum, mineral oil, thickeners, and preservatives. It would be best for someone with extremely dry, parched skin, but there are more elegant formulas than this one available.

☺ **Original Moisturizing Lotion** *($10 for 8 ounces)* contains mostly water, mineral oil, isopropyl myristate (which can cause blackheads), several thickeners, and preservatives. This product is basically just thickeners and mineral oil, which makes it a mediocre but OK moisturizer for very dry skin.

☹ **Plus Alpha Hydroxy Moisturizing Lotion** *($7.49 for 6 ounces)* contains minimal amounts of AHA in a pH that is too high for them to work as exfoliants.

☹ **Plus Alpha Hydroxy Moisturizing Creme** *($7.49 for 6 ounces)* is similar to the lotion above, and the same review applies.

☹ **Plus for the Face Alpha Hydroxy Moisturizing Treatment SPF 15** *($7.99 for 4 ounces)* is meant to be a combination sunscreen and AHA product. It falls short on both counts. It does not contain titanium dioxide, zinc oxide, or avobenzone, so it is absolutely not recommended, and the amount of AHA is too tiny for it to be effective as an exfoliant.

Exact (Skin Care Only)

For more information about Exact, call Advance Polymer Systems at (415) 366-2626.

☺ **Exact Face Wash, Medicated Antibacterial Cleanser (Triclosan)** *($4.61 for 6 ounces)* is a detergent-based water-soluble cleanser with a tiny amount of disinfectant. The disinfectant won't help much, first because there isn't much in here, and second because it would just be washed down the drain. Still, this can be a good cleanser for someone with normal to oily skin.

☹ **Exact Acne Medication Tinted Cream** *($3.54 for 0.65 ounce)* is a 5% benzoyl peroxide product but it is unlikely to be helpful because few people have skin the color of this tint. You can find similar products that don't have tints and that won't look strange on your skin.

☺ **Exact Acne Medication Vanishing Cream** *($3.54 for 1 ounce)* won't cause anything to vanish. This 5% benzoyl peroxide product can be effective for some skin types, but it contains thickening agents that may clog pores.

Exuviance by Neostrata (Skin Care Only)

The politics that take place in the cosmetics industry are sometimes mind-boggling. From an outsider's point of view, it may seem a bit boring, but from the inside, where I spend some amount of time, it is a fascinating saga of egos, money, and skin-care hopes and dreams. Exuviance has some of that drama in its history. Exuviance was created Dr. Eugene Van Scott and Dr. Ruey Yu. These two researchers owned the original use patent for glycolic acid (AHA) in relation to its use for diminishing wrinkles. As far as Scott, Yu, and their attorneys were concerned, that meant anyone who used glycolic acid in their products for wrinkles should be paying the two doctors a licensing fee. The ensuing court case never got very far, which must have been quite frustrating, because from Yu's and Scott's perspective, their research and patent was gaining profits for everyone but them. (I should point out that Avon and a handful of other companies did pay licensing fees for their use of glycolic acid.) To add fuel to the fire, Yu and Scott's own line of AHA products, Neostrata, never found much of an audience in the world of dermatology where they were exclusively marketed. The more popular lines of M.D. Formulations, Dr. Obagi, Murad, and Dermalogica, among others, showed up far more often in doctor's offices than Neostrata ever did.

Either in frustration or to better compete, Scott and Yu have repackaged themselves in Exuviance, a line of AHA products with supposedly more hypoallergenic, sensitive skin formulations. Separate from the drama and politics, how do these products rate? Well, I would hardly call these formulations "hypoallergenic." Two of the products have alcohol as the second ingredient, and all of the products have effective AHA formulations that can easily be considered AHA overkill. While all that is problematic, all of these AHA products are definitely better than the average AHA formulations that contain Scott's and Yu's new mixture utilizing gluconolactone and glycolic acid. These products have a concentration of AHAs between 6% to 8%, and a very effective pH of 4. Scott and Yu feel strongly that their new blend of AHAs works better than just plain glycolic acid but I'm skeptical about that. The research doesn't support the claim and, to some extent, AHA exfoliation is just exfoliation.

There is reason to consider these products, and especially for those of you in search of an effective AHA and sunscreen formulation, this line excels. But do be careful; I think Scott and Yu got carried away with their own creation and couldn't imagine a product of theirs without their AHA in it. For more information about Exuviance call (800) 225-9411.

☺ **$$$ Gentle Cleansing Creme, Sensitive Formula** (*$18 for 8 ounces*) contains a tiny amount of AHA, thankfully not enough to affect the eyes, but this isn't a very effective cleanser unless you use it with a washcloth.

☺ **$$$ Purifying Cleansing Gel** (*$18 for 8 ounces*) is a standard detergent-based, water-soluble cleanser with scrub particles. This is a lot to rub over the face every day, especially the eye area. Be careful with this one.

☹ **Moisture Balance Toner** (*$17.50 for 8 ounces*) contains alcohol as the second ingredient, and that makes it unacceptable for any aspect of skin care!

☹ **Soothing Toning Lotion Sensitive Formula** (*$17.50 for 8 ounces*) is a disappointing formulation that is mostly water and preservatives. How odd that all the other ingredients come after the preservatives. And the amount of AHA in this product isn't even 2% so it has no exfoliating properties.

☺ **$$$ Essential Multi-Defense Day Creme SPF 15** (*$25 for 1.75 ounces*) is a definite, though very expensive, option if you are looking for an effective 8% AHA product with a decent sunscreen. It is a good in-part titanium dioxide–based sunscreen. The moisturizing base is just a list of thickeners with some silicone, nothing very interesting, but good for someone with normal to slightly dry skin.

☺ $$$ **Essential Multi-Defense Day Fluid SPF 15** *($22.50 for 2 ounces)* is almost identical to the one above, only in lotion form.

☺ $$$ **Fundamental Multi-Protective Day Creme SPF 15 Sensitive Formula** *($25 for 1.75 ounces)*, other than containing slightly less AHA than the others, is still similar to the ones above, and the same review applies.

☺ $$$ **Fundamental Multi-Protective Day Fluid SPF 15 Sensitive Formula** *($22.50 for 2 ounces)* is similar to the one above, and the same review applies.

☺ $$$ **Evening Restorative Complex** *($27.50 for 1.75 ounces)* contains mostly water, silicone, AHA, thickeners, slip agents, lots more thickeners, plant oil, water-binding agents, preservatives, and vitamins. This is a very average moisturizer with about a 6% concentration of AHA.

☺ $$$ **Hydrating Lift Eye Complex** *($22.50 for 0.5 ounce)* isn't very different from the Evening Restorative above; for all intents and purposes they both work well for normal to dry skin and are decent AHA concentrations.

☹ **Blemish Treatment Gel** *($13.50 for 0.5 ounce)* lists alcohol as the first ingredient, which makes this product too irritating for all skin types.

☹ **Skin Lightener Gel** *(16.50 for 1.6 ounces)* would be a good 2% hydroquinone and AHA skin-lightening product if it wasn't for the alcohol it contains, which is unnecessarily irritating.

☹ **Essential Multi-Protective Lip Balm, SPF 15** *($8.50 for 0.14 ounce)* doesn't contain avobenzone, zinc oxide, or titanium dioxide, and is not recommended.

Face Stockholm

This boutique line of makeup has personality and style. The two Swedish owners, mother and daughter Gum Nowak and Martina Arfwidson, have a passion for what they do and have created an interesting niche in the cosmetics world for women who want makeup to be fun and casual. With little attitude and a large number of color choices, there are indeed some interesting products to choose from although, in the long run, there's nothing really exceptional. It's hard to tell the difference between this line and M.A.C. or Bobbi Brown or Stila, to name a few.

The skin care here is lackluster, with major problems to be found, especially with the sunscreens and with the presence of irritating ingredients. The prices are another factor: they are unreasonable for what you get. For more information about Face Stockholm call (888) 334-FACE.

The Reviews F

Face Stockholm Skin Care

☹ **Aloe Vera Cleansing Cream** *($18 for 4 ounces)* is an emollient, wipe-off, cold cream–style makeup remover that can leave a greasy film on the skin. Wiping off makeup can tug at the skin and encourage wrinkles.

☹ **Aloe Vera Cleansing Lotion Normal to Dry, Sensitive Skin** *($12 for 4 ounces)* is similar to the one above, and the same comments apply.

☺ **Foaming Facial Cleanser Normal to Oily Skin** *($12 for 4 ounces)* is a standard detergent-based cleanser that works quite well both in removing makeup and not drying out the skin.

☺ **$$$ Apricot Gel Scrub Normal to Oily** *($16 for 2 ounces)* is an exceptionally overpriced scrub of gel, thickening agents and ground-up apricot seeds. Baking soda mixed with Cetaphil Gentle Skin Cleanser would work far better and be vastly less expensive.

☹ **Eye Makeup Remover** *($8 for 2 ounces)* is a standard detergent-based makeup remover, but this one uses sodium lauryl sulfate, an exceptionally irritating one.

☹ **Aloe Vera Toner All Skin Types** *($12 for 4 ounces)* contains witch hazel, and that is a completely unnecessary irritant for the skin.

☹ **Blue Astringent Oily and Problem Skin** *($12 for 4 ounces)* contains alcohol and camphor, and that can cause lots of problems for any skin type.

☹ **Botanical Toner Normal to Oily Skin** *($12 for 4 ounces)* contains witch hazel and eucalyptus, which are both irritants that can cause problems for the skin.

☹ **Vegetable Toner All Skin Types** *($12 for 4 ounces)* contains water and plant extracts. That wouldn't necessarily be a problem, though it also wouldn't be helpful, except this toner also contains lemon oil, which is a skin irritant and not recommended.

☺ **$$$ Aloe Vera Moisture Cream All Skin Types** *($24 for 2 ounces)* is a very good emollient moisturizer for dry skin. It wouldn't work for all skin types; this one contains lots of ingredients that would be a problem for oily, combination, or blemish-prone skin types, including plant oil and lanolin.

☺ **$$$ Aloe Vera Facial Lotion All Skin Types** *($14 for 4 ounces)* is an extremely emollient moisturizer that contains mostly water, plant oils, lanolin, thickeners, vitamin E, and preservatives. It would be very good for someone with dry skin. Much like the product above, this one is not suited for all skin types.

☺ **$$$ Orchid Oil Moisturizer All Skin Types** *($24 for 2 ounces)* is similar to the one above, and the same comments apply.

☺ **$$$ Vitamin Cream All Skin** *($24 for 2 ounces)* is similar to the one above, and the same comments apply. It does contain vitamins but not enough to matter.

☹ **SPF 15 Moisture Cream All Skin Types** *($24 for 2 ounces)* doesn't contain avobenzone, zinc oxide, or titanium dioxide, and is not recommended.

☺ **$$$ Aloe Vera Gel All Skin** *($12 for 4 ounces)* is just fine except for a few plant extracts thrown in that could be skin sensitizers, although for aloe vera you would be better going to the health food store and getting the pure stuff.

☹ **AHA Cream Dry to Mature Skin** *($26 for 2 ounces)* contains both lemon and grapefruit as the second and third ingredients. Neither of these are AHAs; all they do is irritate the skin, and that's not good for any skin type.

☹ **AHA Face Lotion Normal to Oily** *($14 for 4 ounces)* is similar to the one above, and the same review applies.

☺ **$$$ AHA Eye Cream All Skin Types** *($24 for 1 ounce)* is a good moisturizer for normal to dry skin but that's about it. At least with this one there's no lemon and grapefruit. There is about a 2% concentration of lactic acid, but that isn't enough for it to work as an exfoliant.

☺ **$$$ Sage and Aloe Mask All Skin Types** *($18 for 2 ounces)* is just a bunch of thickeners and emollients; it would be good for dry skin (not for all skin types as the name implies). Someone with oily or blemish-prone skin would not appreciate the lanolin oil and plant oils this mask contains.

Face Stockholm Makeup

☺ **$$$ FOUNDATION: Liquid Foundation** *($21)* is a good but rather ordinary foundation with an even, light-to-medium application and a handful of great colors. **The only ones to avoid** are Sno, which can be too pink, and Sommar, which can be too peach.

☺ **$$$ Matte Foundation** *($21)* has a soft matte finish, but it has a heavy silicone base and so the matte finish doesn't hold up long. It may look almost identical to the Liquid Foundation in an hour or two. Both foundations end up being good for normal to dry skin. **The colors to avoid are** Sno, which is slightly pink, as well as Yellow, Mint, and Lilac. The last three are color correctors and they just add a layer of makeup that doesn't correct anything.

☺ **$$$ Powder Foundation** *($24)* has excellent shades and a wonderfully soft, dry finish. These are better used as powders than foundation and are definitely preferred over the regular Pressed Powders that are all shiny. **The only shades to avoid** are July and November, which are both fairly peach.

☹ **$$$ CONCEALER: Corrective Concealer** *($16)* doesn't correct, it just places strange shades of yellow, pink, and blue on the face. **Concealer Wand** *($12)* is a tube applicator concealer that has an extremely poor range of colors; all of them are either too pink, peach, ash, or green to recommend. **Concealer Stick** *($12)* is a standard lipstick-style concealer; most of the colors are poor, only Light Amber, Amber, and Dark Amber look like skin tone, plus this one tends to crease.

☺ $$$ <u>POWDER:</u> **Pressed Powder** *($18)* has some great colors and a dry, smooth texture but all of the shades are shiny. Doesn't that negate the reason for using a pressed powder?

☺ $$$ **Loose Powder** *($18)* has some great neutral shades with a very dry, soft finish. There are some shiny shades and strange colors for preference and fun, but they're not to be taken seriously.

☺ $$$ <u>BLUSH:</u> **Blush** *($13)* are standard single-tin blushes that have a great soft texture. The large color selection has some excellent options, although these are strongly reminiscent of many other lines and nothing unique or special.

☺ $$$ <u>EYESHADOW:</u> **Pearl Shadow** and **Matte Shadow** *($13)* are nicely identified; the matte shades are excellent and there are a lot of them.

☹ $$$ **Eye Dust** *($16)* are tins of extremely shiny powder. They are messy to use and hard to control but they do create shine all over and work as well as any. **Face Highlighters** *($16)* are greasy, iridescent tins of color that can be used any place you want to add shine. They work best for evening only.

☺ $$$ <u>EYE AND BROW SHAPER:</u> **Eye, Brow, and Lip Pencils** *($10)* are all grouped together and they are extremely standard soft-finish pencils in a wide range of colors. **Cake Eyeliner** *($11)* is a standard cake eyeliner to be used wet that creates a dramatic line along the lashes. **Brow Fix** *($12)* comes in two shades, clear and a medium brown. They work well to make brows look fuller and keep them in place, but the color choice is dismal. **Brow Shadow** *($16)* is a group of matte eyeshadows that match brow color rather nicely. This is a great way to apply brow color.

☺ $$$ <u>LIPSTICK AND LIP PENCIL:</u> **Lipstick** *($15)* has a vast range of colors that are nicely creamy and opaque. **Matte Lipstick** *($15)* has a great, soft, matte finish and a smaller color selection than the regular lipstick, but it's still a large assortment with great neutral shades. **Lipstick Veil** *($15)* is just a sheer, glossy lipstick. **Lipgloss** *($12)* is just a tube lip gloss with a great range of colors. **Pot Lipgloss** *($12)* is a slightly sticky but very glossy pot of gloss with an exceptionally vivid application of color.

☹ $$$ <u>MASCARA:</u> **Mascara Regular** *($12)* is a decent mascara that builds some amount of length and thickness, but it takes awhile. The more interesting aspect for the mascara is the color selection; lavender, silver, and eggplant are, to say the least, unique and a kick for a noticeably strange look.

☺ $$$ <u>BRUSHES:</u> The large range of brushes offered in the Face Stockholm line come in a good price range *($10 to $30)*. The eyeshadow brush selection is excellent and there are many reasons to check these out, especially for size options. However the larger face brushes tend to be stiff and coarse and are not as dense as I would prefer for easy application.

Fashion Fair

There are a handful of cosmetics lines aimed at women of color: Fashion Fair, Flori Roberts, Iman, Black Opal, and Posner. Of these, Black Opal, Iman, and Posner are the strongest for color selection, with an impressive range of matte eyeshadows, blushes, and excellent lip colors. Fashion Fair comes in a distant fourth and Flori Roberts just can't compete with the selection of colors and product types the other two companies offer. Fashion Fair has an extensive lineup, with one major drawback: almost all of the eyeshadows are intensely shiny and the lipsticks fairly greasy. I don't recommend shiny eyeshadow for women of color any more than I do for women with lighter skin tones. Shiny eyeshadows make eyelids look wrinkly, and they are always inappropriate in daytime. However, Fashion Fair has a line of fragrance-free products that is worth looking at, as well as oil-free foundations, blushes, concealer creams, and lipsticks with good textures and color choices. The display units are not user-friendly: it is necessary to have a salesperson get testers for you; also, the products are poorly organized (there are no color groupings to help you make selections).

One area of utter disappointment is the skin-care products. They are mostly greasy cold cream–like cleansers, water-soluble cleansers with strongly irritating cleansing agents, alcohol-based toners, and greasy moisturizers. Layering greasy moisturizers on darker skin tones can cause a buildup of dead skin cells, making skin look dull and uneven. Almost all of the toners are exceedingly drying and irritating, which is another cause of dull, uneven skin tones and breakouts. An even more glaring defect is the lack of sunscreens or AHA products. Surely by now Fashion Fair knows that darker skin tones still run the risk of sun damage. A major cause of ashen discolorations on dark skin tones is damage caused by the sun. For more information about Fashion Fair call (312) 322-9444.

Fashion Fair Skin Care

☺ **Botanical Cleansing Gel** *($12 for 6.7 ounces)* is a good but standard detergent-based water-soluble cleanser for someone with normal to oily skin.

☺ **Cleansing Creme with Aloe Vera** *($13.25 for 4 ounces)* is a standard mineral oil–based wipe-off cleanser that can leave a greasy film.

☹ **Deep Cleansing Lotion Balanced for All Skin Types** *($15 for 8 ounces)* is a fairly greasy cleanser that needs to be wiped off. It contains several ingredients that could cause breakouts, including lanolin and isopropyl palmitate. Calling this suitable for all skin types is absurd.

☹ **Facial Shampoo Original Formula for Normal or Oily Skin** *($10 for 2.1 ounces)* is a standard detergent-based water-soluble cleanser that uses sodium lauryl sulfate as the main cleansing agent. It can be very drying and irritating for most skin types, and I do not recommend it.

   ☺ **Gentle Facial Shampoo Mild for Dry Sensitive Skin** *($10 for 2.1 ounces)* is definitely gentler than the shampoo above and could be very good for someone with normal to oily skin.

   ☺ **Eye Makeup Remover** *($8.50 for 2 ounces)* is a standard detergent-based eye-makeup remover with silicone. It works, but wiping off makeup is not the best method anywhere on the face.

   ☹ **Gentle Facial Polisher for All Skin Types** *($13.25 for 3 ounces)* is a detergent cleanser that also contains synthetic scrub particles. It does contain menthol which can be irritating for many skin types.

   ☺ **Botanical Skin Purifier I for Normal to Oily Skin** *($11.50 for 6.7 ounces)* is just water, glycerin, plant extract, aloe, fragrance, and preservatives. This won't purify anything; it is just about as ordinary a toner as you can get.

   ☺ **Botanical Skin Purifier II for Normal to Dry Skin** *($11.50 for 6.7 ounces)* is just water, slip agents, plant extracts, fragrance, and preservatives. This can't balance skin, but it is an OK toner for the skin type indicated.

   ☹ **Deep Pore Astringent Regular for Normal to Oily Skin** *($13.25 for 8 ounces)* is primarily alcohol and fragrance, and that is too drying and irritating for all skin types.

   ☹ **Skin Freshener I Normal to Oily Skin** *($11.50 for 6 ounces)* contains mostly alcohol, which is very drying, not to mention irritating.

   ☹ **Skin Freshener II Dry or Sensitive Skin** *($11.50 for 6 ounces)* has basically the same ingredients as Skin Freshener I and can be just as drying. Alcohol isn't appropriate for any skin type, but even more so for someone with dry or sensitive skin.

   ☹ **Toning Lotion Mild for Dry Sensitive Skin** *($13.25 for 8 ounces)* is an alcohol-based toner; alcohol isn't good for even the hardiest skin type, much less dry, sensitive skin.

   ☺ **$$$ Dry Skin Emollient for Excessively Dry Skin** *($21 for 2 ounces)* contains mostly mineral oil, water, thickeners, petrolatum, vitamins, and preservatives. This is a good but extremely standard and rather greasy moisturizer for someone with very dry skin.

   ☺ **$$$ Eye Cream** *($20 for 0.5 ounce)* is a somewhat thick but very basic moisturizer that contains water, thickeners, mineral oil, plant oils, and preservatives. This is a good emollient moisturizer for dry skin.

   ☹ **Hidden Beauty Skin Enhancing Creme** *($24.50 for 1.9 ounces)* is supposed to be a blend of antioxidant vitamins and beta hydroxy acids. The amount of vitamins is minimal and I found no discernible BHA (willow bark is not the same as salicylic acid) on the ingredient list. There are vastly better BHA or AHA products on the market.

☺ **Moisturizing Creme with Aloe Vera for Dry Skin** *($18.50 for 4 ounces)* is a very emollient moisturizer that would work well on very dry skin, but not because of the aloe. It contains mostly water, thickeners, mineral oil, plant oils, slip agent, preservatives, water-binding agents, and vitamins.

☺ **Moisture Lotion for All Day Beauty** *($14.75 for 4 ounces)* contains mostly water, mineral oil, slip agent, thickeners, silicone, and preservatives. It's a standard emollient moisturizer for someone with dry skin, but rather unimpressive, and without sunscreen it is not good for all-day protection.

☹ **Moisturizing Lotion for Normal to Oily Skin** *($18.50 for 4 ounces)* is a very standard moisturizer containing mostly water, slip agent, petrolatum, several thickeners, and preservatives. What are petrolatum and lanolin doing in a product for oily skin!

☹ **Oil-Free Moisturizer** *($19.50 for 4 ounces)* is indeed an oil-free moisturizer, but it also contains isopropyl myristate and isopropyl palmitate high up on the ingredient list, and both of those thickening agents are well known for causing blackheads and breakouts.

☺ **Special Beauty Creme with Collagen** *($19.50 for 2 ounces)* contains mostly water, mineral oil, collagen, thickeners, lanolin, preservatives, and vitamins. This is a good ordinary moisturizer for someone with very dry skin. Collagen is a good water-binding agent, but it doesn't affect the collagen in your skin one little bit.

☹ **Deep Pore Cleansing Masque for Normal to Oily Skin** *($15.25 for 2 ounces)* contains mostly water, synthetic scrub particles, glycerin, aluminum chlorohydrate (also found in deodorant; it can be a skin irritant), thickeners, and preservatives. There are far better mask formulations available than this one.

☹ **Oil-Control Lotion** *($15 for 3 ounces)* contains mostly alcohol and some minerals that have some ability to absorb oil. The alcohol causes more problems than the minerals can help.

☺ **Vantex Skin Bleaching Creme with Sunscreens** *($14 for 2 ounces)* doesn't contain enough sunscreen to protect skin from any amount of sun damage, but it is a good 2% hydroquinone product in a slightly moisturizing base. You would still need a reliable sunscreen in order for this product to be effective.

Fashion Fair Makeup

☺ <u>FOUNDATION:</u> **Oil-Free Perfect Finish Souffle** *($21)* goes on thick and creamy but dries to a matte sheer finish. It can be tricky to blend, but the color selection and coverage are excellent (although it may look somewhat pasty on normal to dry skin). **These colors are superior:** Amber Glo, Honey Glo, Tawny Glo, Tender Glo, Topaz Glo, Mocha Glo, Cocoa Glo, Pure Brown Glo, Ebony Brown

Glo. **These colors are too peach for most skin tones:** Copper Glo, Brown BlazeGlo, and Bronze Glo.

☺ **Oil-Free Liquid** *($17.50)* is an excellent foundation for someone with oily skin. It goes on creamy but dries very matte, and has a good color selection. **These colors are very good:** Toffee Tone, Tender Brown, Rich Topaz, Warm Caramel, Bare Bronze, and Sheer Espresso. **These colors are poor:** Honey Amber, Tawny, Copper Tan, and Copper Blaze.

☺ **Liquid Sheer Foundation** *($12.50)* works best on dry skin, and comes in a superior array of colors. **These colors are beautiful:** Vanilla, Toffee Tone, Rich Topaz, Tender Brown, Warm Caramel, Bare Bronze, Sheer Espresso, and Ebony Brown. **These colors are not recommended:** Honey Amber, Tawny, Copper Blaze, and Copper Tan.

☹ **Perfect Finish Creme Makeup** *($15)* is a fairly greasy compact foundation, but it does blend sheer. The amount of oil in this can cause the color to turn orange. Foundations for women of color, and women with darker skin tones in particular, contain more pigment, and the oil intensifies the pigment, so wear this one for a while to see how the color will end up looking all day on your skin. **These are colors to consider:** Pure Pearl, Honey Glo, Topaz Glo, Mocha Glo, Beige Glo, Tender Glo, Cocoa Glo, Pure Brown Glo, and Ebony Brown Glo. **These colors are not recommended:** Tawny Glo, Bronze Glo, Amber Glo, Copper Glo, and Brown Blaze.

☺ **Oil-Free Perfect Finish Creme to Powder Makeup** *($20)* has a somewhat greasy finish though the colors are quite good. This can be too creamy for someone with oily skin and too powdery for someone with dry skin.

☺ <u>CONCEALER:</u> **Cover Tone Concealing Creme Fragrance-Free** *($15)* is for use under the eyes or over blemishes and scars. It has a very dry, thick consistency and provides fairly heavy coverage with a slightly sticky finish. If you need a lot of coverage this is an option; if not, this product is not in the least bit natural looking. **All of the colors are very good.**

☹ **Fragrance-Free Coverstick** *($10)* has a drier consistency for oily skin. It can be difficult to blend, and the two colors, Medium and Dark, are too peach or orange for most skin tones. The regular **Coverstick** *($10)* has fragrance and a much creamier formula. It does blend sheer, but can slip into lines around the eye. Most of the colors are either too peach or orange. The only neutral color is Very Light.

☹ <u>POWDER:</u> **Loose Powder** *($15.50)* and **TransGlo Pressed Powder** and **Loose Powder** *($12)* both contain talc and mineral oil, while **Oil-Control Loose Powder** *($17)* and **Oil-Control Pressed Powder** *($13)* are oil-free. **Fragrance-Free Pressed Powder** *($13)* is a standard talc powder. All of these powders have good textures and are available in an excellent range of colors, but they all have shine. The salesperson insisted they didn't, but the sparkle was clearly evident. Perhaps these would be OK for evening wear, but they certainly won't reduce the shine of a foundation.

☺ **BLUSH: Beauty Blush Fragrance and Fragrance-Free** *($13)* comes in a wonderful variety of colors, both fragranced and fragrance-free. They go on dry but smooth and include both vivid and subtle shades, but be careful: many of the colors are also quite shiny.

☹ **EYESHADOW: Ultimate Eyes** *($15)*, **Eye Shadow Collection Quads** *($14.50)*, **Trios** *($13.50)*, and **Touches of Color** *($13.50)* are all extremely shiny. They are a poor option for women of any color. The two shades of brown that aren't shiny each come packaged in a set of four colors, and the other three shades are shiny. I do not recommend any of the Fashion Fair eyeshadows except possibly for evening wear.

☺ **EYE AND BROW SHAPER: Slim Line Eye Liner Pencils** *($10)* are standard eye pencils with a smudge tip on one end. **Brow Pencil** *($7)* is similar to the eye pencil except one end has a brush.

☹ **Brush On Brow** *($11)* comes in two shades of powder, but both are shiny, and the one place where there is never an excuse to have shine is when trying to create a natural looking eyebrow.

☺ **LIPSTICK AND LIP PENCIL: Lipstick Cremes, Frosts,** and **Forever Matte** *($12.50)* come in a good range of colors. The Cremes are more glossy than creamy but do have opaque coverage. The frosts are all intensely shiny. Forever Matte does have a nice selection of matte shades. **Automatic Lip Colors** *($10.50)* is just a small group of standard lip glosses; one shade is clear and the other two are extremely shiny.

☺ **Lip Liner Pencils** *($8.50)* come in a small but attractive array of colors and go on smoothly.

☹ **MASCARA: Mascara** *($11)* never builds any length or thickness, and it smears faster than any other mascara I've tested.

Flori Roberts

Flori Roberts is by far the weakest of the four major cosmetics lines designed specifically for women of color, with an abundance of shiny eyeshadows, poor foundation textures and shades, and dry, grainy blushes. Women of color require stronger colors (which tend to cause grainy texture), but that doesn't mean the blushes can't be silky smooth and have stronger pigment at the same time. (Many other lines have accomplished this feat.) And darker skin tones do not require shiny eyeshadows. If the blushes can be matte, surely the eyeshadows can too. If Prescriptives, Maybelline, M.A.C., Iman, and Black Opal can create workable matte shades for women of color, so can Flori Roberts.

This line leaves much to be desired in the skin-care arena. It has more than its share of greasy moisturizers and drying toners (containing lots of irritating ingredients), which can create problems for darker skin tones that weren't there before. Irritation on darker skin tones can look flaky and ashen. None of that is good. This line needs an overhaul, but it doesn't look like it's coming anytime soon. For more information about Flori Roberts call (800) 621-6043.

Flori Roberts Skin Care

☹ **My Everything Double O Soap Gold, for Normal to Oily Skin** *($13 for 4 ounces)* is a standard bar soap with many ingredients, such as peppermint oil, eucalyptus oil, and camphor, that are very irritating and drying.

☹ **My Everything Treatment Foaming Cleanser** *($15 for 6 ounces)* is a standard detergent-based, water-soluble cleanser that can be a bit confusing for some skin types. The cleansing ingredients are on the drying side, but then there are plant oils that can compensate but also be a problem for oily skin. This one also contains spearmint oil, an unnecessary irritant.

☺ **My Everything Treatment Foaming Gel Cleanser** *($10 for 6 ounces)* is a gentle detergent-based water-soluble cleanser that contains a small percentage of lactic acid (an AHA). In a cleanser, this small amount of AHA isn't a problem; the lactic acid is more a moisturizing agent than an exfoliant.

☺ **Optima Gel Cleanser Gold Oil-Free** *($15 for 6 ounces)* is a fairly good water-soluble cleanser that should work well for someone with oily skin. It can be drying for some skin types.

☺ **My Everything Treatment Exfoliating Facial Scrub and Primer** *($12.50 for 4 ounces)* contains mostly thickener, peanut meal, water, slip agent, synthetic scrub agent, more thickeners, and preservatives. This would be an OK and gentle exfoliant, but it can be tricky to rinse off.

☹ **Double O Complex Gold for Normal to Oily Skin** *($14.50 for 8 ounces)* contains alcohol and a host of irritating ingredients, such as peppermint oil, eucalyptus oil, clove oil, and camphor. This toner does nothing for the skin other than irritate and dry it, a problem for all skin types and all skin colors.

☹ **My Everything Treatment Skin Balancing Astringent/Toner** *($12 for 6 ounces)* contains mostly water, witch hazel, slip agent, lactic acid, anti-irritant, and preservatives. This is about a 5% AHA product. The witch hazel and orange oil in here make it more irritating than necessary, and this toner is not suitable for most skin types.

☹ **Optima Refining Lotion Gold Oil-Free** *($14.50 for 6 ounces)* contains mostly water, slip agent, witch hazel, cleansing agent, and preservatives. Water and witch hazel provide no real benefit for the skin. The lotion does contain a tiny amount of protein, but it is nothing more than a water-binding agent, and there's not enough of it to help the skin.

☺ **Hydrophilic Moisture Complex Gold** *($20 for 2 ounces)* contains mostly water, glycerin, mineral oil, thickeners, collagen, preservatives, a tiny amount of AHAs, and more preservatives. This is an OK lightweight moisturizer for normal to dry skin, but as an exfoliant it doesn't even rate.

☺ **$$$ My Everything Creme** *($25 for 3.25 ounces)* contains mostly water, thickeners, glycerin, isopropyl myristate (can cause blackheads), plant oils, thickeners, vitamin A, anti-irritants, and preservatives. This would be a good emollient moisturizer for someone with dry skin who isn't prone to breakouts.

☹ **My Everything Treatment Advanced Formula Creme, Alpha-Melanix with Sunscreen** *($28.50 for 3.25 ounces)* doesn't contain enough sunscreen to protect skin from sun damage, nor does it contain any UVA protection, and it is not recommended.

☹ **My Everything Treatment Revitalized Protection Moisturizer, Alpha-Melanix with Sunscreen** *($16.50 for 4 ounces)* doesn't contain enough sunscreen to protect skin from sun damage, nor does it contain any UVA protection, and it is not recommended.

☹ **My Everything Treatment Eye Treatment Complex** *($18.50 for 1 ounce)* is just a bunch of thickeners; what a terribly formulated, overpriced, do-nothing moisturizer.

☺ **My Everything Treatment Oil Control Serum Normal to Oily Skin** *($14 for 1 ounce)* is a good lightweight gel moisturizer for normal to slightly dry skin. It contains mostly water, aloe, slip agents, water-binding agents, and preservatives.

☺ **My Everything Treatment Advanced Chromatone Plus with Alpha-Melanix Fade Cream with Sunscreen** *($14.50 for 1.7 ounces)* is a standard 2% hydroquinone fade cream in an emollient base. Hydroquinone has some ability to lighten the skin. This product contains a tiny amount of lactic acid, but not enough to exfoliate the skin or help the hydroquinone perform more effectively by improving cell turnover, and the sunscreen in here is useless for any kind of reliable protection.

Flori Roberts Makeup

☹ <u>**FOUNDATION:**</u> **Touche Satin Finish** *($15)* is a cream-to-powder makeup that stays more creamy than powdery on the skin. It provides good, even coverage, but the color choice leaves much to be desired. **These just aren't realistic skin tones for women of color;** they are all either too red, peach, or orange for most skin tones.

☺ **Maximum Matte Souffle Oil-Free Makeup** *($20)* has a gorgeous smooth texture and blends on easily and evenly. The finish is truly matte and light, and all the colors are beautiful. This foundation is absolutely worth checking out if you have normal to oily skin.

☺ **Hydrophillic Oil-Free Foundation** *($21)* has a somewhat matte finish. There are only six colors, and most are not best for darker skin tones. **These colors are good:** Chroma A and Chroma B. **These colors are too orange or copper:** Chroma C, Chroma D, Chroma E, and Chroma F.

☹ **Hydrophillic Demi Compact** *($18.50)* is creamy foundation with just a disappointing group of colors for darker skin tones. Every one is either too peach, orange, or red.

☺ **POWDER: Chromatic Loose Powder** *($17.50)* has a soft, dry finish. It comes in three shades, but Light and Medium are too peach for most skin tones. The only possible shade is Deep. **Pressed Powder** *($13)* has a dry sheer finish, but most of the colors are either too peach or too red for most skin tones.

☹ **Compact Face Powder with Oil-Control** *($15)* has a great dry texture, but blends on evenly. All four colors are a problem for darker skin tones.

☺ **BLUSH: Radiance Blush** *($13)* has some great colors for darker skin tones, but they tend to have a grainy, dry texture that can look heavy and thick. For the most part these colors would be good only for women with darker skin tones. **More Than Blush** *($14.50)* is intensely shiny and comes in only one shade.

☹ **EYESHADOW: Signature Eyeshadow Trios** *($14.50)* are all very shiny, or the color combinations strange and contrived. The only mattes of the group are #9 and #11, which are OK, just limited.

☺ **EYE AND BROW SHAPER: Eye Contour Pencils** *($8.50)* are fairly standard, but a bit drier than most on the market. This makes them a little harder to apply, but they also don't smear as fast. **Matte Brows** *(10.50)* is a powder shadow meant for use on the brows. It comes in two colors, Brown and Black, and is a great option for shaping eyebrows.

☺ **LIPSTICK AND LIP PENCIL:** Flori Roberts excels in this arena. **Lipstick** *($10)* has a wide selection of colors and a good creamy texture slightly bordering on greasy. **Matte Lipstick** *($10.50)* isn't really all that matte; it's actually creamy and slightly on the greasy side. There is also a small but nice selection of standard tube glosses called **Liquid Lip Gloss** *($10.50)* that are OK if you want a more opaque gloss, but they have a slightly sticky feel. **Lip Contour Pencil** *($8.50)* is a standard pencil that has a slightly drier texture than most.

☺ **MASCARA: Lash Set 2000 Mascara** *($12)* goes on well and builds fast, thick, long lashes; its only drawback is a slight tendency to clump, but that's sometimes the exchange for getting thick lashes fast.

Forever Spring (Skin Care Only)

Actress Connie Stevens promotes this line as the reason she looks so wonderful. Well, Connie, you do look wonderful (at least in the pictures), but I'm fairly certain it has nothing to do with these products. These are just skin-care products with ingredients similar to a hundred others on the market. I also have a rough time with the name of the company. Any cosmetics-company name that implies that you will stay forever youthful from buying a set of skin-care products, whether it's Sudden Youth, Instant Youth, Instant Lift, or Forever Spring, is selling a marketing gimmick and not a reality in any way, shape, or form.

Despite my feelings about the name for this line, there are some good products here for dry skin. The big problem in this line is the ☹ **Time Machine** *($120).* This is by far one of the bigger wastes of money I've seen in the world of cosmetics. It is supposed to exercise facial muscles through topical stimulation. Facial muscles, just like body muscles, cannot be built up through artificial exercise; if they could, why would a bodybuilder ever bother to lift weights? Even if this machine did work, the muscles would simply bulge, not lift skin (you'd look like many an older bodybuilder, with muscles *and* sagging skin). In addition, this machine can create damage by breaking delicate surface capillaries. It is supposed to increase circulation, but there are better ways to increase circulation than with voltage. Running up and down your stairs for 20 minutes will not only increase your circulation but also help your heart and build energy. For more information about Forever Spring call (800) 523-4334.

☺ **Glycerin Soap** *($4.75 for 3 ounces)* is a standard detergent-based bar soap that contains tallow, which can cause breakouts. This soap would be OK from the neck down, but not from the neck up.

☺ **Collagen Facial Cleanser** *($14.25 for 4 ounces)* is a fairly standard, greasy wipe-off cleanser that is not water-soluble. It contains mineral oil, thickeners, lanolin oil, collagen, and safflower oil. The directions say to wipe up, never down, but regardless of whether you pull the skin up or down, you're still causing it to stretch, and that causes sagging.

☹ **Honey Almond Apricot Scuffer** *($13.25 for 4 ounces)* is a detergent-based, water-soluble cleanser that uses sodium lauryl sulfate as the cleansing agent. It would be very drying and irritating for most skin types.

☺ **Ambrosia Skin Refresher** *($14.50 for 4 ounces)* is a very good irritant-free toner that contains good water-binding agents and anti-irritants.

☹ **Purely C Vitamin C Cleansing Therapy Gel with Vitamins A & E** *($15.50 for 6 ounces)* contains several ingredients that can irritate the eyes and skin, including grapefruit and tangerine. Those serve no purpose for skin other than to cause irritation.

☹ **Purely C Vitamin C Balancing & Toning Therapy Lotion, with Vitamins A & E** *($10.50 for 6 ounces)* has the same problems as the cleanser above.

☹ **Purely C Triple C AHA Vitamin Therapy Serum** *($34 for 0.5 ounce)* is a mixture of about 2% AHA and 0.5% BHA. Either way, the pH isn't low enough for this product to work as an exfoliant. What is a problem is the first ingredient: it's aluminum starch octenylsuccinate, a fairly irritating thickening agent.

☺ **$$$ Retrieve Alpha & Beta Hydroxy Combination for the Face** *($26.95 for 1 ounce)* doesn't have a pH that's low enough for it to be an effective exfoliant, but it can be a good moisturizer for someone with dry skin.

☺ **$$$ Bio Eye and Throat Intensive Lubrication Complex** *($15 for 1 ounce)* contains mostly water, several thickeners, plant oil, soothing agent, water-binding agent, vitamins, preservatives, and fragrance. This would be a good emollient moisturizer for someone with dry skin, but it isn't as interesting as some of the others in the Forever Spring collection.

☺ **$$$ Collagen Skin Quencher** *($22.75 for 4 ounces)* contains mostly water, slip agent, water-binding agents (collagen and elastin), aloe, glycerin, and preservatives. This is a good moisturizer for someone with dry skin, but the collagen and elastin can't do anything for the collagen in your skin. This moisturizer is supposed to be used with the Time Machine, and you already know what I think of that.

☹ **Collagen Spray** *($4.95 for 2 ounces)* is more like spraying water on the face than anything else. The amount of collagen water in here is negligible.

☺ **$$$ Fibro Eye Soother** *($14 for 0.5 ounce)* contains mostly water, silicone, glycerin, plant extract, water-binding agents, vitamins, preservatives, and fragrance. This product is almost all water and silicone. They can feel good, but it isn't worth the price tag for this tiny amount.

☺ **$$$ Ginseng and Vitamin C Intensive Complex with Vitamins E, A, C, and Lipolic Acid** *($31.50 for 2 ounces)* contains mostly water, plant oil, thickeners, slip agents, vitamins, fragrance, and preservatives. This is a good emollient moisturizer for dry skin and all the vitamins you could want.

☺ **Ginseng Facial Feed** *($21.25 for 4 ounces)* is a very good emollient moisturizer for dry skin, but nothing more. It contains mostly water, slip agent, plant oils, mineral oil, thickeners, ginseng, water-binding agents, silicone, vitamins, and preservatives.

☹ **$$$ Lift and Taut Spring Skin Serum** *($26.95 for 1 ounce)* contains mostly arnica extract (potential skin irritant), thickeners, slip agent, water-binding agents, plant extracts, vitamins, anti-irritant, silicone, fragrance, and preservatives. I suspect the arnica swells the skin and makes it look temporarily smoother. But irritation of any kind can be a problem for skin. Other than that, this would be a good moisturizer for someone with dry skin.

☺ **$$$ Mandarin Liposome Oxygen Booster** *($24.95 for 0.5 ounce)* contains mostly water, slip agent, thickeners, plant extracts, glycerin, plant oil, water-binding agents, and preservatives. This product lists liposomes as an ingredient, which is strange, because liposomes are a delivery system (a way of formulating a product), not an ingredient. In any case, this product can't deliver oxygen into the skin, although it would be a good moisturizer for someone with normal to dry skin. Be careful though, mandarin is a citrus and that can irritate the skin.

☺ **$$$ Petal Soft Eye Cream** *($14 for 0.5 ounce)* contains mostly water, mineral oil, thickeners, slip agent, petrolatum, water-binding agents, and preservatives. This would be a very good emollient but very standard (and therefore overpriced) moisturizer for someone with dry skin.

☺ **$$$ Super Rich Emollience** *($24.50 for 4 ounces)* contains mostly water, slip agents, plant oils, several thickeners, water-binding agents, vitamins, silicone, mineral oil, preservatives, and fragrance. This would be a very good emollient moisturizer for someone with very dry skin.

☹ **Super Rich Emollience Outdoor Protection SPF 15** *($24.95 for 4 ounces)* doesn't contain avobenzone, titanium dioxide, or zinc oxide, and is not recommended.

☺ **$$$ Forever Summer Self Tanning Lotion, Super Rich Emollience** *($23.50 for 4 ounces)*, like all self-tanners, uses dihydroxyacetone to turn the skin brown. This one works as well as any.

☹ **Acne Blemish Relief Alpha/Beta Hydroxy Acids Acne Treatment Lotion with Tea Tree Oil, French Clay, Volcanic Mud, and Aromatherapy** *($17.50 for 1 ounce)* is a mishmash of ingredients that can add up to problems, not help. The clay and BHA aren't bad, but several of the plant extracts are irritants, including arnica, lemon, orange, kiwi, clove, and cypress. It also contains sulfur, another potent irritant. This is redness and flaking just waiting to happen.

☺ **$$$ Baby Soft Facial Clay** *($15 for 4 ounces)* is a standard clay mask that contains mostly water, clays, glycerin, water-binding agent, thickener, plant extract, and preservatives. If you want a clay mask, this would be fine, and it can make the skin feel soft, but "baby soft" is stretching things a bit.

☹ **Ginseng Firming Peel-Off Facial Masque with Multi-Fruit AHAs** *($18 for 4 ounces)* is mostly plastic and alcohol with a tiny amount of AHAs. There is no reason to put this combination of ingredients on your skin.

Freeman Beautiful Skin (Skin Care Only)

For more information about Freeman products call (800) FREEMAN.

☺ **Blueberry & Lavender Facial Gel Cleanser** *($2.85 for 6 ounces)* is a standard detergent-based, water-soluble cleanser that contains its share of plant extracts. The blueberry and lavender sound nice, but lavender oil can be a skin irritant, and I suspect that if you are allergic to berries, blueberry won't be so beautiful. This could be a good cleanser for someone with oily skin, however. It can be quite drying for some skin types.

☺ **Pineapple & Papaya Foaming Enzyme Facial Wash with Alpha-Hydroxy Acids** *($2.85 for 8 ounces)* is a standard detergent-based, water-soluble cleanser that contains a tiny amount of fruit extracts, which aren't the same as AHAs, as well as papain (papaya enzyme) and bromelain (pineapple enzyme). Papain and bromelain are very unstable as exfoliants, and are more irritants than anything else. Besides, even if they were effective, in a cleanser all these ingredients would just be washed down the drain.

☹ **Skin Control Acne Formula Facial Gel Cleanser** *($2.85 for 4 ounces)* uses sodium C14-16 olefin sulfate as the cleansing agent, which is too irritating and drying for all skin types. It also contains grapefruit and menthol that can add to the irritation.

☹ **Skin + Vitamin C Complex Cleanser and Toner** *($5.99 for 8 ounces)* is a witch hazel–based toner with fairly drying detergent cleansing agents that shouldn't be left on the skin. I suspect this will be fairly irritating to many skin types.

☺ **Apricot & Sea Kelp Facial Scrub** *($3.50 for 6 ounces)* is a walnut shell–based scrub that also contains plant oil, thickeners, soothing agents, and preservatives. The plant oil makes this product good only for someone with dry skin. It can leave a greasy film.

☺ **Raspberry & Almond Face & Body Scrub** *($3.50 for 6 ounces)* uses synthetic scrub particles in a detergent cleanser base. It will exfoliate the skin, but it may be a bit on the drying side for some skin types.

☺ **Sugar Cane and Meadowsweet Alpha-Hydroxy Facial Scrub** *($3.50 for 5.3 ounces)* is similar to the product above only with no AHA to speak of, so the same basic review applies.

☹ **Skin Control Facial Gel Exfoliator** *($2.85 for 4 ounces)* contains several irritating ingredients that serve no purpose but to dry and irritate the skin, including grapefruit and mint, which, along with the synthetic scrub particles in here, would be like rubbing salt into a wound.

☹ **Skin Control Facial Gel Toner** *($2.85 for 4 ounces)* is an alcohol-based toner that includes menthol and grapefruit. Ouch!

☹ **Skin Control Pure Pore Astringent** *($2.85 for 8 ounces)* is similar to the one above and the same review applies.

☹ **Raspberry & Sugar Cane Alpha Hydroxy Lotion** *($2.88 for 18 ounces)* contains no real AHA ingredients and is not recommended.

☹ **Sugar Cane & Green Tea Alpha-Hydroxy Nighttime Facial Moisturizer**

Natural Renewal Complex *($3.50 for 3.5 ounces)* is similar to the lotion above, and the same review applies.

☻ **Alpha Hydroxy Nighttime Facial Moisturizer** *($2.85 for 3.5 ounces)* has a passable pH of 4, but no alpha hydroxy acids (the sugar cane extract it contains is as unrelated to an actual AHA as moldy bread is to penicillin).

☺ **Apricot & Vitamin E Ultra Nourishing Lotion** *($2.88 for 18 ounces)* is a good emollient moisturizer for dry skin, and includes plant oils, thickeners, and vitamins. Now that's beautiful.

☺ **Skin Control Facial Gel Moisturizer** *($2.85 for 4 ounces)* is a good but extremely lightweight moisturizer for slightly dry skin. It contains mostly water, silicone, glycerin, and preservatives. That's about as simple as it gets.

☹ **Anti-Oxidant Daytime SPF 8 Facial Moisturizer Provitamin B5 & Vitamin C** *($2.88 for 3.5 ounces)* doesn't contain avobenzone, zinc oxide, or titanium dioxide, and is not recommended.

☹ **Sunflower & Aloe Perfect Moisturizer SPF 6** *($2.85 for 4.6 ounces)* is hardly "perfect." Its SPF rating is only 6, which is not adequate to protect against sun damage, and it doesn't contain avobenzone, zinc oxide, or titanium dioxide.

☹ **Skin + Vitamin C Complex Moisturizer SPF 15** *($6.99 for 2.5 ounces)* doesn't contain avobenzone, zinc oxide, or titanium dioxide, and is not recommended.

☺ **Skin + Vitamin C Complex Eye Cream** *($7.99 for 0.5 ounce)* is a good emollient moisturizer for dry skin. It contains mostly water, plant oil, thickeners, water-binding agents, vitamins, soothing agent, silicone, preservatives, and fragrance.

☺ **Skin + Vitamin C Complex Night Repair** *($7.99 for 2 ounces)* won't repair anything, but it is a good moisturizer for dry skin.

☺ **Avocado & Oatmeal Mineral Mud Mask** *($2.85 for 6 ounces)* is a standard clay mask with a small amount of oil, which can prevent it from being too drying. If you want to use a clay mask, this is a good one for an exceptionally reasonable price.

☻ **Blackberry & Tangerine Mud Mask** *($2.85 for 6 ounces)* is a standard clay mask that also contains a small amount of plant oil, slip agents, plant extracts, minerals, preservatives, and fragrance. Some of the plant oils, such as peppermint and tangerine, can be skin irritants.

☹ **Cucumber & Ginseng Peel-Off Masque** *($2.85 for 6 ounces)* is mainly alcohol and plastic, and there is never a reason to put these kinds of ingredients on your skin. I know it's fun to peel masks of this kind off the skin, but this just isn't good for the skin.

☹ **Sugar Cane & Guava Alpha-Hydroxy Peel-Off Masque** *($2.85 for 6 ounces)* is identical to the mask above except that it contains fruit extracts. That doesn't make this an AHA product, because there is no way to tell exactly what these fruit extracts are.

☹ **Skin + Vitamin C Complex Pore Masque and Clarifier** *($5.99 for 2.5 ounces)* is mainly alcohol and plastic, and there is never a reason to put these kinds of ingredients on your skin. I know it's fun to peel masks of this kind off the skin but this just isn't good for the skin.

Galderma (See Cetaphil)

Gale Hayman of Beverly Hills

I found Gale Hayman's brochure for her skin-care products a bit implausible. It states "the impression you get in Beverly Hills is obvious. From the very glamorous to the trend-setting elite, the women of Beverly Hills boast a quality found nowhere else in the world. It's an ageless appearance, a beauty that transcends time." Clearly, with a title attached to a highbrow town, the impression you're supposed to get is that Hayman's products have in some way contributed to this lean and "ageless" look. That's almost funny. What isn't so funny is that in all of the hyperbole about these products there's not one sunscreen in the group. So much for ageless beauty. You're supposed to believe that the elastin, amniotic fluid, DNA, and DHEA in these products can help restore skin. If it were only that easy! In regard to the ladies of Beverly Hills, first, having spent a great deal of time in Beverly Hills, I can assure you that the glamorous and not so glamorous have all seen a plastic surgeon and most every inch of their anatomy from head to toe has either been lifted, suctioned, cut and pasted, or resurfaced more times than you can count. Their beauty has nothing to do with this line of products or any other line. Second, even if this line had some secret miracle, the ladies of Beverly Hills aren't shopping at Sears, where this line is often sold.

Speaking of Beverly Hills, Hayman's real claim to fame is that she was married to Fred Hayman, the founder of Giorgio perfume and retail stores. She started her skin-care line after their divorce. If you want more information about Hayman's products you can call (800) FOR-GALE or (800) 755-5009.

Gale Hayman Skin Care

☺ **$$$ Total Eye Make-up & Facial Cleanser** *($18.50 for 6.76 ounces)* is a good detergent-based cleanser that would work well for most skin types. This cleanser contains amniotic fluid, and for some reason that is supposed to sound helpful for skin; it isn't, and for me it is just offensive.

☺ **$$$ Total Skin Toner Freshener & Firmer** *($18 for 6.76 ounces)* is virtually identical to the cleanser above and the same review applies.

☺ **$$$ Eyelift Gel** *($25 for 0.5 ounce)* is just water, film former, water-binding agents, plant extracts, and thickeners. This is an OK lightweight moisturizer, but the film former simply places a layer over skin that can make it look smoother, it isn't a lift and doesn't change skin.

☺ **$$$ Line Lift** *($27.50 for 0.07 ounce)* contains water, DNA, elastin, plant oils, and preservatives. DNA and elastin can't change skin, period. This can be a good lightweight moisturizer but that's it.

☺ **$$$ Youth Lift** *($45 for 1 ounce)* is almost identical to the one above; the same comments apply.

☺ **$$$ Youth Lift Firming Night Treatment** *($55 for 1 ounce)* contains mostly water, plant oil, egg yolk, thickeners, water-binding agents, and preservatives. This is a good emollient moisturizer for dry skin with a Beverly Hills price tag.

☺ **$$$ Youth Lift Total Moisturizer** *($35 for 2 ounces)* is similar to the one above and the same review applies.

☺ **$$$ 5-Minute Pore Cleanser Exfoliating Mask** *($22 for 2 ounces)* is a clay mask with almond pieces and synthetic scrub particles. Leaving scrub particles sitting on the skin isn't the best way to exfoliate skin, but it won't necessarily hurt the skin either.

☺ **$$$ Lip-Lift** *($16 for 0.04 ounce)* is just a good mineral oil–based lip balm.

Gale Hayman Makeup

☺ **Light Coverage Treatment Makeup** *($15)*. Most of the colors for this light, sheer foundation are quite good. It is best for someone with normal to dry skin who isn't looking for much coverage. **The only colors to stay away from are** Porcelain, Beige, and Medium Beige.

☹ **Treatment Concealer Cream** *($12.50)* isn't much of a treatment, and the colors are all too peach or pink to recommend for any skin tone.

☺ **Semi Translucent Face Powder** *($17)* has a soft, smooth, dry texture. Sun Bronze is part of this group but it is just a shiny brown powder. Since when does a tan have to look iridescent?

☹ **MonoChrome Shadow Liner** *($16)* colors are all extremely shiny (even the matte shades) and have an uneven, choppy application.

☺ **$$$ Color Control Blusher** *($17)* has a grainy finish with some amount of shine. These are fairly vivid colors that grab easily and need to be blended out well.

☺ **Automatic Eye Pencil** *($7.50)* and **Automatic Brow Definer** *($16)* come in only two shades, so there isn't much to choose from, but this is a good, albeit standard, dry finish pencil.

☺ **Treatment Lip Glaze** *($13)* is supposed to be a lip gloss that doesn't bleed into the lines around the mouth. Don't believe it for a second; one application and it will be up into the lines around your mouth before you know it, but it is still a good lip gloss. **Treatment Lip Color** *($10)* is a good creamy lipstick with a slightly glossy finish. **Automatic Lip Definer** *($13)* has a drier finish than most, but is still just a very standard lip pencil that comes in only four shades.

☹ **$$$ Dramatic Lash Mascara** *($13)* is just an OK mascara; it does build some length and thickness, but I wouldn't call it dramatic or worth the extra price.

Garden Botanika

Garden Botanika has been opening stores at an incredibly fast pace. They opened over 200 stores between 1996 and 1997 (according to an article in *The Seattle Times*). As of now they have almost 500 stores in 48 states. Garden Botanika is like The Body Shop but with a Northwest flair (it is, after all, a Seattle-area company). The prices are extremely reasonable, and the packaging a little more upbeat than its competition. Between the prices and the consumer demand for "natural" products" (regardless of how senseless that demand is) you're likely to find enough plants and aromatherapy here to satisfy.

In the long run, Garden Botanika is just one of several cosmetics companies that have done their own versions (read "knock-offs") of The Body Shop—a boutique skin-care/makeup shop where beauty and environmentalism merge in a mélange of exotic-sounding and -smelling concoctions. Actually, The Body Shop itself was not an original idea, but was somewhat of a knock-off of Caswell Massey. What all these stores offer is an intimate shopping atmosphere, low-key salespeople, reasonable prices, and all the vegetable, botanical, herb, fruit, and random plant extracts you could ask for.

As far as products go, Garden Botanika has made some impressive headway in the makeup field, usually not the strong suit of natural cosmetics lines of this type (though The Body Shop has leapt ahead in that area too). There are some great colors here, but most of them are best for Caucasian and Asian women, and not for women of darker skin colors. The color groupings are impressively arranged on a standup wood podium. Regrettably, the display is inconvenient to use, with no shelf space for purses, hands, arms, or note taking. The colors are divided in two sectors: one half of the dais holds pink and rose tones and the other half yellow and peach tones. Very functional for those who want to be careful about choosing the right colors.

In terms of skin care, let me preface my review here by saying I have been thoroughly impressed with much of the research concerning salicylic acid (BHA) as an effective, pore-penetrating exfoliant that can reduce blackheads and blemishes by removing skin cells that line the pore. Salicylic acid is a specific ingredient, just like glycolic acid and lactic acid, but glycolic acid comes in a handful of other forms with long technical names. Not salicylic acid. This is one ingredient that is always easy to identify, because it has only one form. Of course, the pH of a BHA product can be hard to discern (it needs to have a pH of 3 to be effective), but if salicylic acid is in the ingredient list, you can be assured it's the real deal. That clarification is my way of explaining why you should ignore some of Garden Botanika's new Skin Correcting line of skin-care products and pay attention to only a couple of them. This line of blemish products is supposed to contain salicylic acid, yet, except for two of them, it does not, and of the two that do, only one has a pH in an effective range. What most of these products do contain is willow bark extract. Why? Salicylic acid is derived from willow bark. But even though the two may have some rudimentary connection, that's where it starts and stops. Willow bark sounds more friendly and natural than salicylic acid, but implying that they are the same cheats the consumer. The ingredient to look for is salicylic acid, not willow bark, if you want to choose a product that can better effect exfoliation inside the pore. Inconveniently, there is no easy way to check for pH. For more information about Garden Botanika call (800) 968-7842.

Garden Botanika Skin Care

☹ **Skin Correcting Cleansing Bar** (*$4 for 4.2 ounces*) is a standard bar cleanser that contains ingredients that can be quite drying and may clog pores. It does contain a disinfectant, but disinfectants work only when left on the skin, and you would not want to keep this cleanser on your face for even a second.

☺ **Skin Correcting Deep Cleansing Face Wash** (*$10 for 8 ounces*) is a standard detergent-based, water-soluble cleanser. The detergent cleansing agents used can make it drying for some skin types. It does have a host of plant extracts, but none of these are helpful for blemishes or beneficial for any skin type.

☺ **Skin Correcting Purifying Toning Lotion** (*$10 for 8 ounces*) does contain the real thing, salicylic acid, and it is listed as the active ingredient with a pH of 3! It comes in a simple slip-agent base with a host of plant extracts. What counts is the BHA, and this is a very good lightweight one to consider. If you aren't allergic to the plants in this product, it is a definite consideration.

☺ **Skin Correcting Essential Moisture Lotion** (*$10.50 for 1.75 ounces*) is a standard, rather ordinary moisturizer that contains mostly water, thickeners, plant extracts, water-binding agents, silicone, soothing agents, and preservatives. Unless you have dry skin, this is a truly unnecessary step. If you do have dry skin and want to try it, it is an option, but only over dry areas. The host of plant extracts in this lotion can be a problem for some skin types.

☹ **Skin Correcting Intensive Blemish Treatment** (*$7.50 for 0.5 ounce*) is another real BHA product but the pH is too high to make it an effective exfoliant.

☹ **Skin Renewing Gentle Foaming Cleanser, with Alpha Hydroxy Acid** (*$10 for 8 ounces*) is a standard detergent-based cleanser. The cleansing agent is TEA-sodium lauryl sulfate, which can be very drying and potentially irritating for most skin types.

☹ **Skin Renewing Cleansing Bar** *($4 for 4.2 ounces)* is a standard bar cleanser that can be drying for all skin types, and the ingredients that keep the bar in its bar form can clog pores.

☺ **Skin Renewing Clarifying Toning Lotion** *($9 for 8 ounces)* is basically just water and glycerin with a bunch of plant and fruit extracts thrown in. It should be fine for most skin types, if you are not allergic or sensitive to the plants.

☹ **Skin Renewing Moisture Replenisher SPF 8** *($12.50 for 1.75 ounces)* has only minimal sun protection; with all the SPF 15 around, why bother?

☺ **Skin Renewing Clarifying Facial Mask** *($8.50 for 2 ounces)* is a standard clay mask that can be good for someone with normal to slightly dry skin. It won't renew the skin, and even though it does contain tiny amounts of plant extracts, none of them can exfoliate skin.

☺ **Chamomile Cleansing Milk** *($8.50 for 8 ounces)* is a plant oil–based standard wipe-off cleanser. It will take off makeup, but wiping and pulling at the skin is not good.

☺ **English Violet Cleansing Milk** *($8.50 for 8 ounces)* is similar to the one above and the same comments apply.

☺ **Linden Flower Cleansing Milk** *($9.50 for 8 ounces)* is similar to the one above and the same comments apply.

☹ **Citrus Cleansing Gel** *($9 for 4 ounces)* is a standard detergent-based water-soluble cleanser. It also contains a small amount of orange oil, which may smell nice, but can also irritate the eyes.

☺ **Cucumber Cleansing Gel** *($10 for 8 ounces)* is a standard detergent-based water-soluble cleanser that can be good for someone with normal to slightly dry or oily skin.

☹ **Oatmeal & Glycerine Cleansing Bar** *($4 for 4 ounces)* is fairly alkaline, which is drying for all skin types, and the ingredients that keep the bar in its bar form can clog pores.

☺ **Gentle Eye Makeup Remover** *($6 for 4 ounces)* is a very standard detergent cleanser makeup remover. It will do the job, but I never recommend wiping off makeup.

☺ **Jojoba Scrub** *($7.50 for 2 ounces)* is a gentle scrub that could work well for someone with normal to dry skin, but some of these ingredients could clog pores. I still wouldn't use this one over Cetaphil Gentle Skin Cleanser mixed with baking soda.

☺ **Elder Flower Toning Lotion** *($9.50 for 8 ounces)* is just glycerin and fragrance; it's OK for someone with normal to dry skin, but it's mostly a do-nothing formulation.

☺ **Honey and Rosewater Toning Lotion** *($9.50 for 8 ounces)* is similar to the one above and the same comments apply.

☹ **Witch Hazel & Thyme Toning Lotion** *($9.50 for 8 ounces)* contains witch hazel, which is irritating enough, but this one also contains camphor and is not recommended.

☹ **AHA Skin Renewing Balancing Creme, SPF 8** *($12.50 for 1.75 ounces)* has only minimal sun protection; with all the SPF 15 around, why bother?

☺ **AHA Skin Renewing Treatment for the Face** *($12.50 for 1 ounce)* is mostly a good emollient moisturizer for dry skin, similar to the Moisture Replenisher above, but minus the sunscreen. The second ingredient is mixed fruit extracts, so it's impossible to know whether or not this is a good 8% AHA product. Garden Botanika says it is, but I would prefer to know if it contains glycolic acid or lactic acid instead of some mysterious mixed fruit stuff.

☹ **Angelica Moisture Creme** *($9 for 2 ounces)* is one of the more dull and uninteresting moisturizers for dry skin I've seen; it contains mostly water, plant extracts, thickeners, and preservatives. This is not a product I would recommend.

☹ **Botanical Moisture Mist** *($8.50 for 8 ounces)* just lets you spray some aloe and witch hazel on your skin with some plant extracts. I wouldn't recommend it. If you want aloe, there are better forms than this one.

☺ **Calendula Moisture Cream for Dry Skin** *($10 for 2 ounces)* is a good moisturizer for dry skin that contains mostly water, plant oils, thickeners, water-binding agents, vitamin, preservatives, and fragrance.

☺ **Hydrating Cream with Aloe** *($10 for 2 ounces)* is a good, basic moisturizer for dry skin. It contains mostly aloe, water, plant oil, thickeners, vitamin, water-binding agents, fragrance and preservatives.

☺ **Nutrient Night Creme** *($10 for 2 ounces)* is similar to the one above and the same basic review applies.

☺ **Ivy and Yarrow Moisture Creme** *($9.50 for 2 ounces)* is a good, though basic, moisturizer for dry skin; it contains mostly water, thickeners, water-binding agents, preservatives, and fragrance. Ivy and Yarrow can be irritants but there aren't enough of them in here to have an effect.

☺ **Meadow Sweet Night Cream** *($10 for 2 ounces)* is similar to the two above and the same review applies.

☺ **Nourishing Eye Creme** *($9.50 for 1 ounce)* is similar to the ones above and the same review applies.

☹ **Night Normalizing Gel** *($10 for 2 ounces)* contains too many potentially irritating ingredients, including lemon, to be recommended.

☹ **Oil-Absorbing Moisture Gel** *($9.50 for 2 ounces)* is similar to the gel above and the same comments apply.

☺ **Skin Balancing Moisture Cream** *($9.50 for 2 ounces)* contains mostly water, aloe, thickeners, vitamin, plant extracts, fragrance, and coloring agents. None of this can balance skin, it is merely an ordinary moisturizer for slightly dry skin.

☺ **Soothing Herbal Eye Gel** *($8.50 for 1 ounce)* is similar to the one above, only in gel form.

☺ **Vitalizing Night Creme** *($11 for 2 ounces)* contains mostly water, thickeners, vitamins, plant oil, and preservatives. This is a good moisturizer for someone with dry skin.

☺ **Chamomile Moisture Mask** *($8.50 for 2 ounces)* is just waxes and plant oils. It is moisturizing, but I think it's more of a why bother?

☺ **Desert Mud Mask,** *($7.50 for 2 ounces)* is a standard clay mask that can be good for someone with oily skin.

☺ **Skin Correcting Activated Charcoal Mask** *($10 for 3.4 ounces)* is a standard clay mask that also contains some charcoal. Everything I've ever seen about charcoal indicates it's not a great substance for skin, but I haven't seen information that suggests it's damaging either.

☺ **Soothing Botanical Gel Mask** *($8.50 for 2 ounces)* is a very standard mix of thickening agents and plant extracts. It may feel refreshing but it won't do much for skin.

Garden Botanika Makeup

☺ <u>FOUNDATION:</u> **Moisturizing Foundation SPF 8** *($10)* is a liquid foundation with a very nice, soft application. Most of the colors are fine, particularly Linen, Vanilla, and Honey, but Alabaster is too pink, Willow is too peach, and Sand and Flax can turn peach. The SPF 8 isn't the best (it should be at least SPF 10, but 15 is better), although it does contain titanium dioxide. **Oil-Free Foundation SPF 8** *($11)* isn't all that different from the Moisturizing Foundation above; they have a similar texture and finish. This isn't the best for someone with oily or combination skin but it can be suitable for someone with normal to dry skin. However, the same concerns about SPF and color choice apply here.

☺ **Natural Color Powder Plus** *($12.50)* is a pressed powder–style foundation that has a rich, soft texture in a small but good selection of colors. It can be used alone or over foundation. It does have a small amount of oil, so it may not be preferable for someone with normal to oily skin. The only two colors to watch out for are Sand Dollar and Sesame, which may be slightly too pink for some skin tones.

☹ <u>CONCEALER:</u> **Color Corrector Stick** *($7.50)* and **Color Corrector Creme** *($7.50)* are shades of pink, yellow, and green that are an unnecessary extra layer of makeup. Too many layers of makeup can feel thick and heavy on the skin. If the foundation color is right (meaning neutral with no overtones of peach, pink, rose, or ash), and the consistency is smooth and even, there is no need for this step. **Concealer** *($8.50)* comes in a wand applicator, but the colors are fairly peach and not the best to consider for any skin tone.

☺ <u>POWDER:</u> **Pressed Powder** *($8.50)* comes in three good shades with a dry, soft finish.

☹ **Translucent Loose Powder** *($9)* has a very dry, choppy finish, and all the shades are shiny, which negates the effect of dusting down shine with a powder.

☺ <u>BLUSH:</u> **Natural Color Blush** *($8.50)* comes in some great, neutral, earth-toned, matte shades. There are only a handful of shiny colors to steer clear of. **Face Shimmer** *($8.50)* is very iridescent eyeshadow. The shine is overkill, but then everyone seems to need shine these days so why not this line.

☺ <u>EYESHADOW:</u> **Natural Color Eyeshadow** *($7.50)* has a small but workable group of matte eyeshadows. It also has its share of shiny shades but they are easily avoidable. Check out Birch, Papyrus, Dogwood, Logan Berry, and Smoky Quartz. **Shadow Primer** *($8.50)* has a cream-to-powder finish that can be helpful to keep eyeshadows on if you are using a moisturizing foundation; if you are using a more matte-finish foundation this isn't necessary.

☺ **Eye Shadow Stacker** *($10 for a set of six)* is an assortment of six stackable, cream eye-shadows that have a slight, and I mean slight, powdery finish. The colors are quite neutral, with two being somewhat shiny and the rest fairly matte. This is a tricky way to blend on eyeshadow, but if you want to experiment with cream eyeshadows this is the least expensive way to go about it, and these are as good as any. Be careful, these easily crease and they easily slip off while you're applying them.

☺ <u>EYE AND BROW SHAPER:</u> **Brow Gel** *($7.50)* comes in one shade, Clear. It works fine but is clearly limited. **Natural Color Eye Pencil** *($6)* is just a standard, slightly dry finish pencil in a small but good range of colors.

☺ **$$$** <u>LIPSTICK AND LIP PENCIL:</u> **Sheer Lip Crayon** and **Matte Lip Crayon** *($7.50)* are just a sheer gloss and a matte lipstick in the shape of fat pencils. These require sharpening, which makes them inconvenient to use. **Lip Shimmers** and **Lip Shines** *($10 for a set of six colors)* are a stack of six pots of shiny glosses (that's the Shimmers) or nonshiny glosses (the Shines). They are fun to use if you are into gloss, and the price is almost too lip-smacking to pass up. **Lip Polish** *($6.50)* is just a standard gloss in a tube, but a rather good one considering the consistency and price. **Natural Color Lipstick** *($7.50)* is an excellent group of creamy lipsticks with good opaque coverage. **Natural Color Lip Pencil** *($6)* is just a standard, slightly dry finish pencil in a small but good range of colors.

☺ **Lip Primer** *($7.50)* is an option only if lipstick tends to turn color on you. It lays down a neutral beige tone that you then apply lipstick over. It doesn't stop lipstick from feathering.

☺ <u>MASCARA:</u> **Mascara** *($7)* is just an OK mascara. It doesn't build much length and definitely no thickness, and the tube can get pretty gloppy and messy.

☹ **Lash Primer** *($7.50)* is an extra step that shouldn't be necessary. If a company makes a good mascara, that should be all it takes to make beautiful long, thick lashes.

☺ <u>BRUSHES:</u> This isn't the best assortment of brushes, but there are some that are definitely worth a consideration. The **Dome Brush** *($15)*, **Shadow Brush** *($6)*, **Fluff Brush** *($5)*, **Lip Brush** *($5)*, and the **Angle Brush** *($5)* are all excellent, with great shapes, soft bristles, and nicely packed to hold powder well.

☹ However, the **Blush Brush** *($7)* is too small, the **Shadow Contour** *($6)* too floppy to control, and **Blender** *($8)* is too big for the eyes yet too small for the face.

Givenchy

The name Givenchy rolls off the tongue like an infusion of French wine and haute couture fashion. Yet, as eloquent and refined as it sounds, when it comes to cosmetics style doesn't equal substance and it turns out the Givenchy products have more accent than quality. Skin care is the most disappointing aspect of this line, although the packaging is some of the most elegant in the industry. What a shame packaging won't help your skin. Ordinary formulations abound, and despite the presence of some exotic sounding ingredients these are mostly waxy bases with little to no current formulations. As fascinating as it may sound to have some ginseng, coltsfoot, or hawthorn extract, or placental enzymes and thymus peptides, which show up repeatedly in scant amounts, your skin would be far happier with more interesting water-binding agents and anti-irritants than the standard concoctions this line is filled with. And not one of the sunscreens has any UVA protecting ingredients. Placenta and thymus—is anyone intrigued by these types of ingredients anymore? I imagine cosmetics manufacturers these days throwing plants into just about anything. But these prices are embarrassing for what you get.

The makeup also leaves much to be desired, with narrow color options, minimal colors for darker skin tones, pink and peach toned foundations, shiny eyeshadows, and just average pressed powders. For more information about Givenchy products call (212) 759-7566.

Givenchy Skin Care

☹ **Gentle Cleansing Gel** *($28 for 4.2 ounces)* may be gentle by some standards, but not any I've heard of. This very standard detergent-based cleanser includes a form of tallow which can irritate and clog pores. There are far more elegant cleanser formulations out there for a fraction of this price.

☹ **Gentle Cleansing Milk** *($28 for 6.7 ounces)* is an extremely confused cleanser and isn't gentle. It contains mineral oil, which can leave a greasy film on the skin, and it uses sodium lauryl sulfate as the cleansing agent. Sodium lauryl sulfate is notorious for being one of the more irritating cosmetic ingredients.

☹ **Regulating Cleansing Gel, Purifying Care for Radiant Skin Combination and Oily Skins** *($20 for 4.5 ounces)* is a standard detergent-based cleanser that can be drying for most skin types. Don't count on this to purify or regulate any aspect of skin.

☺ **$$$ Gentle Eye and Lip Makeup Remover Gel** *($15 for 1.3 ounces)* is a standard detergent-based makeup remover with a handful of plant extracts thrown in for effect.

☺ **$$$ Gentle Exfoliating Massage** *($27 for 1.7 ounces)* is a standard synthetic-based scrub mixed in with a bunch of waxy thickening agents and mineral oil. It can exfoliate but for this price and this less than impressive formulation you would be better off with Cetaphil Gentle Skin Cleanser and baking soda!

☺ **$$$ Balancing Mist** *($30 for 5 ounces)* is just silicone with some plant extracts and standard water-binding agents. It is a good irritant-free toner for someone with dry skin.

☺ **$$$ Gentle Toning Lotion** *($28 for 6.7 ounces)* is a standard, irritant-free glycerin-based toner, with some silicone and a few water-binding agents. It would be good for someone with dry skin.

☹ **Regulating Mist** *($30 for 5 ounces)* is similar to the one above except that this one contains witch hazel and that won't regulate anything, though it can be a skin irritant.

☺ **$$$ Double Sequence Eye Contour Firming Balm** *($75 for 60 doses)* is a two-step process that comes in medical-looking doses. As therapeutic as this appears to be, the ingredients are less than remarkable. This is a combination that may make for a good moisturizer but it won't firm anything. Dose 1 contains several thickening agents, water-binding agents, emollients, preservatives, and plant extracts. Dose 2 is almost identical. There are minuscule amounts of vitamins and anti-irritant but not anything unusual or special for skin.

☺ **$$$ Lifting Double Sequence** *($100 for 0.5 ounce total, 30 treatments)* is a lighter-weight version of the Eye Balm above. These two Doses are good moisturizing formulations with some interesting water-binding agents, but this is by far more image than substance. You are actually spending $3,200 for a pound of this stuff, and all you'll be getting is a moisturizer for normal to slightly dry skin. For this kind of money you would have enough for a face-lift in less than a year or two.

☺ **$$$ Fundamental Care** *($69 for 1.7 ounces)* is a very standard, almost boring lightweight moisturizer. This is a nice formulation for someone with normal to slightly dry skin. It contains mostly thickening agents, glycerin, silicone, and good water-binding agents. It does contain a tiny amount of lactic acid, but nowhere near enough to be considered an exfoliant.

☹ **Hydra Tricellia Creme SPF 15** *($45 for 1.7 ounces)* does not contain avobenzone, zinc oxide, or titanium dioxide, and is not recommended.

☹ **Hydra-Tricellia SPF 15 Tri-Activating Hydration Lotion, Oil-Free** *($58 for 2.5 ounces)* does not contain avobenzone, zinc oxide, or titanium dioxide, and is not recommended.

☹ **Matte Regulating Day Care** *($38 for 1.7 ounces)* is indeed matte: the second ingredient is aluminum starch octenylsuccinate, a thickening agent that has some absorbing properties (like alum), but it is more likely to absorb the moisture in this product than the oil on your skin, plus it can be an irritant. It also contains witch hazel, silicone, and thickening agents.

☺ **$$$ Nutritive Care** *($54 for 1.7 ounces)* is a standard mineral oil–based moisturizer that contains thickening agents, and a tiny amount of water-binding agents. It's fine for dry skin, but absurdly overpriced for what you get.

☺ **$$$ Protective Day Care** *($43 for 1.7 ounces)* does not include sunscreen, so this only counts for evening care. It is a standard petrolatum-based moisturizer with thickening agents and a tiny amount of water-binding agents. This is so standard as to be almost embarrassing.

☹ **Relaxing Complex** *($44 for 1.7 ounces)* contains nothing relaxing, although it does contain alcohol, which can dry and irritate skin.

☺ **$$$ Hydra-Tricellia Mask** *($40 for 2.8 ounces)* contains mostly emollients, minuscule amounts of some good water-binding agents, and clay. It does contain a tiny amount of alcohol but probably not enough to be a problem. This could be a good mask for someone with normal to slightly dry skin, but this is mostly a why bother.

☺ **$$$ Hydrating Cream Mask** *($40 for 1.7 ounces)* is a mineral oil–based mask with thickening agents and plant oils. It does contain a tiny amount of lactic acid, but not enough to make it an exfoliant.

☹ **Regulating Purifying Mask** *($38 for 2.8 ounces)* is mostly alcohol, witch hazel, and clay, which makes it too irritating and drying for any skin type.

☺ **$$$ Whitening Concentrate** *($48 for 1 ounce)* is a hydroquinone-based skin-lightening product. When used with sunscreen this can be an effective way to improve the appearance of sun-damaged skin discolorations.

☹ **Roll-on Exact Eye and Lip Contour** *($43 for 0.5 ounce)* is supposed to help diminish wrinkles, but the only thing it will diminish is your pocketbook. It is a good moisturizer for dry skin but that's about it.

Givenchy Makeup

☹ <u>FOUNDATION:</u> **Perfect Moisturizing Foundation** *($42)* isn't what I would call perfect. While it does have a very creamy, smooth finish, it comes in a limited group of colors. Of the eight shades only six are the color of skin; Beige and Beige Cannelle are either too pink or peach for most skin tones. **Concealing Matte Finish Foundation** *($42)* lives up to its name. It does have a surprisingly soft matte finish, but it can show shine sooner than other matte foundations. The color selection is very small and you should stay away from Vanille and Epice, which are both too orange for most skin tones.

☹ <u>CONCEALER:</u> The **Concealer** *($28)* has a poor color selection and tends to crease.

☺ $$$ <u>POWDER:</u> **Pressed Powder** *($35)* comes in only one shade, and while it does have a very dry, sheer finish, one color will not fit everyone. **Compact Face Powder Prism** *($40)* has a dry, smooth finish, but the sets of colors are strange and difficult to use, and all but one are exceptionally shiny, which seems to defeat the purpose of a powder: reducing shine on the face.

☺ $$$ <u>BLUSH:</u> **Blush Prism** *($42)* is a selection of six very shiny blush colors. It does have a satiny, soft texture, but the shine is, well, just too shiny.

☹ <u>EYESHADOW:</u> **Duo Couture Eyeshadow Prism** *($30)* is a compact eyeshadow with an interesting twist. Each shade has two versions in the one compact; one side is shiny and the other matte. It ends up being too shiny either way you look at it. **Eyeshadow Prism** *($38)* is a five-color eyeshadow compact. Each of the colors is so tiny that you can easily miss the separation. The center color is intensely shiny and the other colors don't necessarily work together. Divided or not, this is a compact that is prettier to look at it than it is to use.

☺ $$$ <u>EYE AND BROW SHAPER:</u> **Eye Brow Pencil** *($18)* is just a standard pencil with a dry finish, which is nice for a brow pencil. One end of the pencil is a comb to help smooth out the line the pencil creates. **Eye Liner Pencil** *($19)* has a dry, hard finish, which isn't great for eye lining. One end of the pencil is a sponge tip, convenient for softening up the hard line this pencil is likely to create. **Eye Liner Extreme Perfect** *($24)* is a liquid liner that goes on quite nicely, not too hard or heavy, but soft and even. The three shades are black, brown, and white. I understand the black and brown, but the white is definitely not for everyone when it comes to your average daytime look.

☺ $$$ <u>LIPSTICK AND LIP PENCIL:</u> **Long Lasting Lipstick** *($21)* is a very good creamy lipstick with a slight matte finish. It doesn't last any longer than most lipsticks in any price range. **Long Lasting Gloss** *($21)* is a standard, exceedingly overpriced lip gloss. **Rouge A Levres** *($19)* is a fairly creamy moist lipstick. **Lip Liner Pencil** *($18)* is a standard pencil with a dry, soft finish. One end is a lip brush, which is a nice convenience, but lots of much less expensive pencils have the same advantage, and I mean lots less expensive.

☺ $$$ <u>MASCARA:</u> The **Mascara** *($19)* is quite good. It builds fairly long, thick lashes with little effort. It also doesn't clump or smear. However, there are lots of mascaras for one-fourth the price that match or surpass this mascara's performance.

Guerlain

If any cosmetics line can be considered sensual, luxurious, and elitist, Guerlain is it. Without even taking quality into consideration, it is hard to ignore the lavish gold packaging, intricate design, and awesome price tag that accompany everything from eyeliner to powder. A refillable powder compact sells for over $140 and a lipstick compact sells for $80! They are exquisite containers bedecked with gold and faux jewels. If it were chic to powder your nose and put lipstick on in public, you would be the talk of the party. But that's the problem with overkill packaging: it is essentially a waste, because no one but you and your makeup bag see it. All that counts when it comes to makeup is how it looks on your face. Beautiful containers are nice, but if the product is only a blush and the lipstick only a lipstick, there is no real reason to lust after a container.

Guerlain's skin-care products contain standard cosmetic ingredients that you've seen before for a fraction of the cost in hundreds of other products. What is most shocking is the line's blatant lack of sunscreen options. There are dozens and dozens of moisturizers in this line, and no sunscreens as part of the daily routine. That is unconscionable from a skin-care point of view. Repetitive formulations are the hallmark of the Guerlain line, despite specialty claims for each product grouping. In terms of the color line, the strong points are the blushes and foundations, while the weaknesses are the shiny eyeshadows and pressed powder. To be fair, I should add that Guerlain is not the most expensive product line at the cosmetics counters, although it's definitely up there, with several products costing over $100.

I've been asked repeatedly why I bother to review extravagant, expensive lines like Guerlain, La Prairie, and Orlane. Why would someone who's looking to save money and find the best buys want to know whether or not Guerlain has good products? The women who can afford Guerlain, or who hope that spending that kind of money on skin care can save their youth, probably aren't reading this book. They do not want to hear that they are wasting their money on a poor product or spending ten times more than they need to for a good one.

My position is that, regardless of expense, women who can afford to spend (waste) a lot of money deserve consumer information, and that, no matter what the price, it is never OK for women to be misled or be misinformed. For me personally, it is essential to stay informed about what is currently available in the world of cosmetics, because I never know where I might find the best products, those that would set the standard for my reviews. So don't worry if you can't afford this line; you won't be left out to wrinkle alone in the cold. For more information about Guerlain call (800) 882-8820.

Guerlain Skin Care

☺ **$$$ Evolution Complete Cleanser** *($34 for 8.2 ounces)* is a standard mineral oil–based cleanser that doesn't rinse off well without the help of a washcloth, and it can leave a greasy film on the skin. This is a lot of money for a product that's basically cold cream.

☺ **$$$ Evolution Purifying Foaming Gel** *($32 for 5.4 ounces)* is a standard detergent-based cleanser that would be good for someone with normal to oily skin. It can be drying for some skin types.

☺ **$$$ Evolution Exfoliating Creme for the Face** *($29 for 1.7 ounces)* is a standard scrub that uses synthetic particles as the exfoliant. Other than that, it contains a long list of thickeners and detergent cleansing agents. It can be good for someone with normal to dry skin.

☹ **Evolution Clarifying Toner** *($33 for 8.5 ounces)* is a standard alcohol-based toner that is too irritating for most skin types. This won't clarify anything, but it can be quite irritating and drying.

☹ **Evolution Refreshing Tonic Vitale** *($33 for 8.5 ounces)* is a standard alcohol-based toner that is too irritating for most skin types. There is nothing refreshing about this toner, but it can be quite drying and sensitizing.

☺ **$$$ Evolution Sublicreme No. 1 Light Day and Night Care** *($52 for 1.7 ounces)* contains mostly water, a long list of thickeners, water-binding agents, fragrance, more thickeners, and preservatives. There are several good water-binding agents, which makes this a good lightweight moisturizer for normal to dry skin. It does contain a minuscule amount of DNA—but we all know DNA can't help repair skin cells, right? And without any measurable sunscreen, this product is not appropriate for day wear, and if warn during the day, the lack of sun protection will actually destroy DNA.

☺ **$$$ Evolution Sublicreme No. 2 Rich Day and Night Care** *($52 for 1.7 ounces)* is almost identical to the moisturizer above except that it is slightly more emollient, and the same review applies.

☺ **$$$ Evolution Sublifluide Day and Night Care** *($50 for 1.7 ounces)* contains mostly water, several thickeners, slip agents, more thickeners, water-binding agents, fragrance, a tiny amount of sunscreen, vitamins A and E, and preservatives. This is a good lightweight moisturizer for someone with normal to slightly dry skin, but that's about it.

☺ **$$$ Evolution Divinaura Beauty Enhancer** *($59 for 1 ounce)* contains incredibly standard ingredients—water, slip agents, thickeners, preservatives, fragrances, and—are you ready for this?—gold. How much gold? Six milligrams, which is about 0.000353 ounce. What is this microscopic amount of gold supposed to be for? Stimulating and energizing the skin, according to the label. Skin can't absorb gold, though, so I imagine that rubbing a gold necklace over my face should do the same thing, and save me a lot of money in the bargain.

☺ **$$$ Evolution Sublilift A.R.T. Recontouring Serum for the Face** *($59 for 1 ounce)* contains mostly water, a long list of thickeners, vitamin E, fragrance, and preservatives. As in many Guerlain products, most of the interesting water-binding agents are found at the end of the ingredient list, meaning they're in such small amounts they are barely worth mentioning. This is a good, but extremely ordinary, moisturizer for someone with normal to dry skin; it won't recontour or reshape anything.

☺ **$$$ Evolution Specific Eye Contour Care Emulsion** *($37 for 0.5 ounce)* contains mostly water, thickeners, silicone, lanolin, standard water-binding agents, more thickeners, more water-binding agents, vitamin E, and preservatives. It's a good emollient moisturizer for dry skin but that's about it.

☺ **$$$ Evolution Fresh Complexion Mask** *($37 for 1.7 ounces)* contains mostly water, slip agents, glycerin, thickeners, and preservatives. It's a very ordinary but good lightweight mask for someone with normal to slightly dry skin.

☺ **$$$ Evolution Treatment Mask with Revitenol** *($37 for 1.8 ounces)* is an extremely standard clay mask that also contains thickening agents, film former, more thickeners, vitamin E, fragrance, and preservatives. It does contain a minuscule amount of DNA, but that has no effect on the skin. There is no such ingredient as "revitenol" that can change skin.

☺ **$$$ Issima Creme Cleanser** *($49 for 6.8 ounces)* is a standard mineral oil–based cleanser with ordinary thickeners and slip agents. It doesn't rinse off well without the aid of a washcloth, and it can leave a film.

☺ **$$$ Issima Moisturizing Lotion** *($42 for 6.8 ounces)* contains mostly water, slip agent, thickener, fragrance, and preservatives. This product is almost embarrassingly ordinary. It is an irritant-free toner, but it contains nothing to comment about one way or the other.

☺ **$$$ Issima Aquaserum Long Term Rehydrating Formula** *($125 for 1.7 ounces)* contains mostly water, thickener, mineral oil, more thickeners, vitamin E, water-binding agent, a tiny amount of sunscreen, plant oil, more thickeners, AHAs, fragrance, and preservatives. This is a good mineral oil–based moisturizer for someone with normal to dry skin, but the price is so absurd and the product so ordinary that buying it would be like spending $125 on a box of Duncan Hines chocolate cake mix. The amount of AHAs in this product is about 1%; that makes it an OK water-binding agent, but that's about it.

☺ $$$ **Issima Intensive Protective Emulsion** *($89 for 1.7 ounces)* contains mostly water, thickeners, plant oil, a very long list of other thickeners, silicone, vitamin E, AHAs (too small an amount to be considered an exfoliant), fragrance, and preservatives. This is a good moisturizer for someone with dry skin, but the price could make you feel worse than any amount of flaky skin ever could.

☺ $$$ **Issima Intensive Revitalizing Creme** *($125 for 1.7 ounces)* is similar to the product above, and the same review applies.

☺ $$$ **Issima Midnight Secret Late Night Special Treatment** *($89 for 1 ounce)* contains mostly water, thickeners, mineral oil, silicone, vitamin E, fragrance, a tiny amount of AHAs, and preservatives. This is a good, extremely ordinary moisturizer for normal to dry skin, but nothing more. The secret must be that there's nothing interesting inside the bottle.

☹ $$$ **Issima Serenissime Restructuring Treatment with Active Genesium** *($175 for 1 ounce)* ends up costing $2,800 a pound for extremely standard ingredients and something called "genesium," which supposedly can tackle all the things that cause the skin to age. Not on your life! Serenissime does not contain a sunscreen. Without a sunscreen it can't handle the number-one cause of aged-looking skin, and that's sun damage. It does have some good water-binding ingredients and some antioxidants, but they are overwhelmed by the waxy thickening agents and mineral oil, which you can find in a hundred other products. Even the interesting ingredients come after the fragrance and preservatives, meaning they are barely present.

☺ $$$ **Issima Eye Contour Treatment, Anti-Wrinkle Eye Contour Fluid** *($68 for 0.5 ounce)* contains water, slip agent, plant extract, thickeners, vitamin E, water-binding agents, more thickeners, more plant extracts, vitamin A, and preservatives. This is a good lightweight emollient, but the price tag is way out of line for these average ingredients.

☺ $$$ **Issima Intenserum Beauty Treatment** *($175 for ten 0.08-ounce ampoules)* is, to say the least, inanely overpriced. For $3,300 per pound, you get mostly water, slip agents, thickeners, silicone, vitamin E, fragrance, water-binding agents, and preservatives. It isn't worth it. To be fair, it is a good lightweight moisturizer for someone with normal to dry skin, but these ingredients do not warrant a price tag that's even one-tenth of that amount.

☹ $$$ **Issima Neck Firming Creme** *($89 for 1.7 ounces)* contains mostly water, thickeners, preservatives, water-binding agents, and vitamins. The preservative is way too high on this ingredient listing, indicating this stuff is 99% wax! And for $89. Why this is for the neck as opposed to any other part of the body makes no sense.

☹ $$$ **Issima Super Aquaserum Optimum Hydrating Revitalizer** *($125 for*

1.7 ounces) contains mostly water, plant oil, glycerin, slip agent, a long list of thickening agents, AHAs, water-binding agents, vitamin E, more thickeners, fragrance, and preservatives. This is about a 2% to 3% AHA product, which means it doesn't contain enough AHAs to exfoliate, although the AHAs are good water-binding agents. I can't even comment about the prices anymore—they are too preposterous to believe and completely unwarranted.

☺ **$$$ Issima Revitalizing Moisturizing Mask** *($65 for 2.5 ounces)* is moisturizing but hardly revitalizing. This product contains a host of thickening ingredients, minimal vitamins, and water-binding agents. That's not bad, just not worth $65. This would be a good mask for someone with dry skin.

☹ **Odelys Gentle Foaming Cleanser** *($29 for 5 ounces)* is a standard detergent cleanser that also contains tallow and lanolin. Both tallow and lanolin can cause breakouts and allergic reactions. The Odelys product line is supposed to be for sensitive skin, but I think Guerlain must have overlooked their own problematic ingredient listing.

☺ **$$$ Odelys Instant Relaxing Cleanser** *($32 for 7 ounces)* is a standard mineral oil–based wipe-off cleanser with a small amount of detergent cleansing agent. This can leave a greasy film on the skin and is more like a cold cream than anything else.

☺ **$$$ Odelys Delicate Eye Makeup Remover** *($19 for 2.5 ounces)* contains mostly water, slip agent, detergent cleanser, and preservatives. It will take off eye makeup.

☺ **$$$ Odelys Soothing Toner** *($29 for 6.8 ounces)* is a good irritant-free toner that contains mostly water, slip agents, vitamin E, and preservatives.

☺ **$$$ Odelys Perfect Care #1 Day and Night (Light)** *($52 for 1.7 ounces)* contains mostly water, thickeners, slip agents, more thickeners, plant oil, vitamin E, more thickeners, and preservatives. This is a good, but extremely ordinary, moisturizer for someone with normal to dry skin, but because it doesn't contain sunscreen you would be ill-advised to use it during the day.

☺ **$$$ Odelys Perfect Care #2 Day and Night (Rich)** *($52 for 1.7 ounces)* is similar to the moisturizer above, only more emollient, and the same review applies.

☺ **$$$ Odelys Perfect Care No. 3 Super Rich, Day and Night** *($52 for 1.7 ounce)* is similar to the moisturizer above, and the same review applies.

☺ **$$$ Odelys Stabilizing Serum** *($56 for 1 ounce)* is more of a lotion than the other products above. This one is supposed to act as a protective barrier between skin-care products and the skin. It doesn't, though it is a good lightweight moisturizer for someone with normal to slightly dry skin. The standard ingredient listing doesn't in any way justify the price.

☺ **$$$ Odelys Perfect Eye Contour Care** *($35 for 0.7 ounce)* contains mostly water, thickeners, film former, slip agents, more thickeners, and preservatives. This is a good ordinary moisturizer for someone with dry skin.

☺ $$$ **Odelys Moisturizing Creme Mask** *($33 for 2.6 ounces)* contains mostly water, thickeners, plant oil, slip agents, more thickeners, clay, mineral oil, vitamins, more slip agents, fragrance, and preservatives. This is a good emollient clay mask for someone with normal to dry skin.

☹ **Odelys Soothing Gel Mask** *($37 for 2.5 ounces)* contains mostly water, slip agents, thickeners, preservatives, anti-irritants, and plant extracts. Though the anti-irritants are nice, this product also contains plant extracts that could be irritating to the skin, including arnica, ivy, and witch hazel, and that doesn't make any sense.

☹ **Guerlain's Age Defense 12 M Time Response SPF 8** *($49 for 1 ounce)* is not only an ordinary moisturizing formulation, it is a poor sunscreen that won't defend against anyone's age, especially not at SPF 8. It contains neither avobenzone, titanium dioxide, nor zinc oxide, so it can't adequately protect from UVA damage, which causes skin cancer and wrinkles.

☹ **Les Gestes Purete Complete Cleanser and Toner, Gentle for the Eyes and Face** *($29 for 6.8 ounces)* is not in the least complete. This cleanser doesn't clean all that well and is mostly thickeners and slip agents.

☺ $$$ **Les Gestes Purete Foaming Gel, Refreshing for the Face** *($29 for 6.8 ounces)* is a standard detergent-based cleanser. It can be good for someone with oily skin.

☹ $$$ **Les Gestes Purete Awakening Toner, Radiant for the Face** *($29 for 6.8 ounces)* is little more the glycerin, perfume, and preservatives, and a waste of money.

☹ $$$ **Alphabella Gentle Action with AHA for Dry or Weakened Skin** *($62 for 1 ounce)* is not even an average AHA product. This highly fragranced lightweight moisturizer contains about 2% to 3% AHAs. That makes it a poor exfoliant but a good water-binding agent; still, at these prices, it should do what you expect an AHA product to do.

☹ $$$ **Alphabella Intense Action with AHA for Combination or Oily Skin** *($58 for 1 ounce)* is similar to the moisturizer above, but with 3.5% AHAs. That makes it not even a competitor in the AHA arena and the emollients and thickeners in this product are a problem for combination and oily skin.

☺ $$$ **Hydrobella Creme Souple #1 Light Creme** *($50 for 1.7 ounce)* contains thickeners, slip agents, water-binding agents, preservatives, and vitamins. This would be a good moisturizer for someone with normal to dry skin.

☺ $$$ **Hydrobella Creme Onctueuse #2 Rich Creme** *($50 for 1.7 ounce)* is similar to the #1 Creme above only slightly more emollient; the same basic review applies.

☺ $$$ **Hydrobella Creme Grand Comfort #3 Ultra Rich Creme** *($50 for 1.7 ounce)* is similar to the #2 Creme above only slightly more emollient, and the same basic review applies.

Guerlain Makeup

☺ **$$$ FOUNDATION: Issima Foundation** *($53)* has a creamy, moist texture and the colors, though extremely limited, are all excellent.

☺ **$$$ Perfect Light SPF 8 Foundation** *($44)* has a sheer, soft, slightly matte finish, and a slight amount of shine, which I suspect Guerlain wants you to think diminishes the appearance of lines; it doesn't. Still, the shine is minimal and the appearance quite attractive for dry skin, and **all of the colors are excellent.**

☺ **$$$ Treatment Powder Foundation** *($47)* is a standard pressed powder with a satin-smooth finish, but this is not a treatment. The color choice is great, but watch out for 3; it can be too pink for some skin tones.

☹ **Teint Hydro-Lifting Firming Foundation** *($42)* won't lift your face, but it does blend on soft and sheer with a moist finish. What a shame the colors are so awful; only one, Vanille 2, even begins to look like skin color, **all of the other colors are way too peach or pink.**

☹ **CONCEALER: Corrective Concealer** *($25)* comes in only two shades. It blends on very smooth and creamy but dries to a matte finish and creases into lines during the day. **Protective Base for the Eyelid** *($23)* goes on creamy and then dries to a matte finish, and that wouldn't be bad, but the colors are strange; one is pink, the other shiny bronze! These serve no real purpose other than to get in the way of your eyeshadow colors.

☺ **$$$ POWDER: Pressed Powder** *($38)* is pretty standard, with a soft, dry texture. The color choice is limited but quite nice.

☹ **Loose Powder** *($40)* comes in three colors, but all of them have shine and the colors tend to be too pink for most skin tones. **Meteorites** *($42)* are small multicolored beads that mix together to make one shiny, sheer, white shade. It's a cute product but nothing to take seriously, except for maybe an evening look, though there are far less expensive ways to make the skin shine than this. **Terracotta Bronzing Powder** *($31.50)* comes in three shades that are all shiny to ultra-shiny.

☺ **$$$ BLUSH: Cream Powder Blush** *($30)* has a very heavy, grainy, dry finish and is hopefully being discontinued now that Guerlain has their Mozais blush, reviewed below in the eyeshadow section.

☺ **$$$ EYESHADOW AND BLUSH: Mozais** is a compact you can build yourself with three shades of **Eyeshadows** *($16)* and one shade of **Blush** *($19)*. There are some beautiful matte shades to check out that have a smooth dry finish, and the blushes are silky smooth with lovely shades to choose from.

☹ **Contouring Eyeshadow Powder-Creme** *($25)* comes in a tube, blends on like a thick liquid, and dries to a powder finish. **Most of the colors are shiny, except for one:** Brun Tabac.

☺ **$$$ <u>EYE AND BROW SHAPER:</u>** The small, attractive containers contain a tiny vial of ordinary but good **Liquid Eye-Liner** *($24)*. One drawback with the container is that it's too small for easy application. The colors range from basic black to shiny silver and gold. **Eye and Brow Pencils** *($18)* are, well, eye and brow pencils. The Eye Pencil goes on fairly creamy and the brow pencils go on rather dry, and both are absurdly overpriced.

☺ **$$$ <u>LIPSTICK AND LIP PENCIL:</u>** KissKiss Hydrodoux *($21)* has a beautiful creamy opaque finish. This is my kind of cream lipstick! **KissKiss Haute Tenue** *($19)* is almost identical to the Hydrodoux. **Multicolor Lip Gloss** *($19)* is an attractive-looking gloss that looks like a rainbow of colors in the tube. Of course, it goes on as one color just like any other gloss. **Lip Liner Pencil** *($18)* goes on thicker and greasier than most but comes in a nice array of colors.

☺ **$$$ <u>MASCARA:</u>** Super-Cils Mascara *($21)* takes forever to build any length, and even then it never makes much difference. The container is handsome, but that won't help your lashes look any better. This isn't a bad mascara, just a boring one. It doesn't smudge or smear.

H$_2$O Plus (Skin Care Only)

Like many boutique-oriented skin-care lines, H$_2$O Plus is having its problems. Stores are closing faster than they are opening. The boutique skin-care business has become saturated with a plethora of The Body Shop wannabe-type lines. Garden Botanika, Bath and Body Works, Victoria's Secret, Aveda, Origins, and I Natural are just some of the freestanding skin-care and makeup stores filling malls across the country. Each one tries to offer an interesting twist, from aromatherapy to exotic concoctions, yet the result is little innovation accompanied by healthy sounding claims and lots of plant extracts.

H$_2$O Plus relies on ocean water for its niche theme. Once you see the H$_2$O Plus displays, the company's marketing angle becomes crystal clear. The gurgling tubes of colored water are very attractive, and they solidly establish the company's notion of water being all important, particularly marine water.

Like most cosmetics companies in the '90s, H$_2$O Plus uses plant extracts and oils to give consumers the natural slant they've come to expect. Regardless of what the brochure says, are these products botanically based? Mostly they aren't, but there are sea plants in an array of algae extracts. Are the products good? Some are. Are they reasonably priced? For a department-store line, yes, they are. The major question to be answered is, Will these products provide skin with more moisturizing (water-retaining) benefits than other products on the market? The answer is no, but given the fear many women have of losing the moisture in their skin, the alluring name brings eager buyers flocking to the H$_2$O Plus counters and storefronts. For more information about H$_2$O Plus call (800) 242-BATH.

☺ **Marine Cleansing Gel (Oil-Free)** *($16.50 for 5.7 ounces)* is a standard detergent-based water-soluble cleanser that can be good for someone with oily skin. It has its share of plants and minerals but they don't help in the cleansing or have any effect on oily skin.

☺ **Sea Mineral Cleanser (Oil-Free)** *($14 for 12 ounces)* is similar to the one above minus the cleansing agent. That may make it more gentle but it also makes it less effective at cleansing the skin.

☹ **Water-Activated Eye Makeup Remover (Oil-Free)** *($12.50 for 4 ounces)* is a standard detergent-based liquid that can remove makeup. This one contains more detergent cleansing agents than most, as well as eucalyptus, which makes this potentially very irritating for the eye area.

☹ **Sea Mineral Scrub (Exfoliate)** *($15 for 4 ounces)* uses TEA-lauryl sulfate as the detergent cleansing agent, which is too drying and potentially irritating for most skin types.

☺ **Marine Toner (Alcohol-Free)** *($15 for 12 ounces)* contains mostly water, slip agent, sea plants, minerals, fragrance, and preservatives. There are several fragrant components in here that could be potentially irritating. This isn't a terrible toner just a confusing one.

☺ **Natural Alpha Hydroxy Acids Smoothing Face and Body Wash (AHA)** *($18 for 5.7 ounces)* does contain a small amount of AHAs, but they are useless in cleanser because their effectiveness is washed away.

☺ **$$$ Natural Alpha Hydroxy Acids Smoothing Facial Cleanser** *($18 for 6 ounces)* does contain a small amount of AHAs, but they are useless in cleanser because their effectiveness is washed away.

☺ **$$$ Natural Alpha Hydroxy Acids Smoothing Hydrocomplex (AHA)** *($22.50 for 1 ounce)* does not contain a low enough pH to make this an effective exfoliant, though it can be a good moisturizer for someone with dry skin.

☺ **Face Oasis Hydrating Treatment (Oil-Free)** *($25 for 2 ounces)* contains mostly water, film former, slip agent, water-binding agents, silicone, plant extract, thickeners, and preservatives. This would be a good lightweight moisturizer for someone with slightly dry or combination skin.

☺ **$$$ Green Tea Antioxidant Face Complex** *($30 for 2 ounces)* contains mostly thickeners, silicone, slip agents, vitamins , water-binding agents, and a teeny amount of green tea. This would be a very good moisturizer for someone with dry skin.

☺ **$$$ Hydro Essential Eye Treatment (Hydrate)** *($20 for 0.5 ounce)* is a good emollient moisturizer for someone with dry skin. It contains mostly thickeners, slip agents, water-binding agents, emollients, plant extracts, vitamins, and anti-irritants.

☺ **Marine Daily Hydrator (Oil-Free)** *($18.50 for 4 ounces)* may technically be oil free, but it contains isopropyl palmitate, and that can cause breakouts. With its requisite plant extracts, vitamins, and water-binding agents, this would be a good moisturizer for someone with normal to slightly dry skin.

☺ $$$ **Marine Daily Moisture Cream (Moisturize)** *($20 for 2 ounces)* contains mostly water, thickeners, sea plant extracts, silicone, slip agents, water-binding agents, vitamins, and preservatives. This would be a good moisturizer for someone with normal to slightly dry skin.

☹ **Marine Enzyme Serum (Anti-Oxidant)** *($22.50 for 1 ounce)* doesn't contain any more antioxidants than other products in this line. It would have been a good moisturizer for someone with normal to dry skin but it contains eucalyptus which can be a skin irritant.

☺ **Marine Moisture Mist (Hydrate)** *($11 for 6 ounces)* is a good irritant-free toner that would be good for most skin types.

☺ **After Sun Refresher Gel (Oil-Free)** *($10 for 4 ounces)* is indeed a decent, irritant-free gel of mostly water, aloe and glycerin. It would be fine as a lightweight moisturizer for someone with normal to oily skin.

☹ **Lip & Eye Stick, SPF 15** *($9.50 for 0.5 ounce)* is a sunscreen that doesn't contain titanium dioxide, zinc oxide, or avobenzone, and it is not recommended.

☹ **Oil-Free Sun Gel, SPF 4** *($10 for 6 ounces)* contains less than SPF 10 and is not recommended.

☺ **Post-Sun Hydrator** *($10.50 for 6 ounces)* is a very good standard moisturizer for dry skin. It contains water, thickening agents, slip agents, silicone, emollients, vitamins, and preservatives.

☺ **Sunless Tanning Lotion, Light** *($12.50 for 6 ounces)* and **Sunless Tanning Lotion, Dark** *($12.50 for 6 ounces)* are like all self-tanners; this one uses dihydroxyacetone. It works as well as any, though this lotion contains lemon extract, which can make it irritating for the face.

☹ **Waterproof Sunblock, SPF 30** *($10 for 4 ounces)* does not contain avobenzone, titanium dioxide, or zinc oxide, and is not recommended.

☹ **Water-Resistant Sun Shield, SPF 15** *($8.50 for 4 ounces)* does not contain avobenzone, titanium dioxide, or zinc oxide, and is not recommended.

☹ **Water-Resistant Sunscreen, SPF 8** *($9 for 4 ounces)* does not contain avobenzone, titanium dioxide, or zinc oxide, and is not recommended.

☹ **Oil Controlling Mattifying Lotion (Oil-Free)** *($15 for 2 ounces)* contains sea plants, thickener, and preservatives. Nothing in here will control oil in the least; it is just a gel with some plants. That's not bad, just not helpful in any way.

☺ **Sea Mineral Mud Mask (Purify)** *($25 for 4 ounces)* is a standard clay mask with a small amount of witch hazel, probably not enough to be an irritant. This is an OK mask for someone with oily skin but it won't purify a thing, though it can absorb oil.

H+ Beauty System (Skin Care Only)

I apologize if it gets boring, if not downright repetitive, for you to hear me continually belaboring the exaggeration and hyperbole that accompany all the makeup and skin-care infomercials I've ever seen. One after another, they portray ordinary (though overpriced) skin-care lines as being little short of miraculous. These incessant, clearly overblown claims would be laughable if so many women weren't taking them seriously. Nonetheless, the infomercial for H+ Beauty System (the H+ stands for Health Plus) really caught my attention. Not because of the standard celebrity endorsement, in this case by Cathy Lee Crosby (I know she's a celebrity, but I can't remember why) or because of the typical skin-care expert's seal of approval from Veronica Barton (whom I'm sure is a skin-care expert of some repute, although I haven't seen any of her work, so we'll just have to take her word for it). Rather, I was impressed by the creator of this line, Dr. Walter Smith. I am familiar with Dr. Smith's work as a cosmetic chemist and researcher. Most of the information I've shared with you about AHAs comes from Dr. Smith's research. Although he is definitely an industry insider, with years of employment at Estee Lauder and Procter & Gamble, and certainly subject to the industry's passion for embellishment and aggrandizement, a good deal of his research has withstood the typical distortion and what some would kindly call poetic license.

Where does that place Dr. Smith's H+ products? Right smack dab in the middle of infomercial never-never land. It's not that these products are bad, but they simply aren't anything special. I'm not sure what I was expecting or hoping for, but I was incredibly disappointed, not to mention exasperated by the claims these products make for clearing up acne. There is nothing in these products that can take on that task. Also, despite Dr. Smith's research on AHAs, and direct quotes from him about the limitations of salicylic acid in comparison with AHAs, his toner contains both alcohol and salicylic acid. There isn't a true AHA product in the bunch.

For the most part, these products would be best for someone with normal to dry skin, and there are some good choices. However, someone with normal to oily skin would find their skin layered with emollient products when none were needed. These products contain no coloring agents or fragrance, and that is exemplary. However, the pricing—at $24 to $44 for a few ounces of product—is insulting.

Whatever you decide about H+, always pick and choose what serves your skin best and avoid the tendency to believe in skin-care miracles. If you want to check out these products for yourself, you can do so by calling (800) 447-6670.

☺ $$$ **Skin Purifying Cleanser** (*$24 for 6.78 ounces*) is a good cleanser for someone with normal to dry skin. It doesn't remove makeup very well, but can be useful on a clean face.

☺ $$$ **Purifying Foaming Cleanser** (*$24 for 6.76 ounces*) is a standard detergent-based cleanser that can work well for someone with normal to oily skin.

☹ **Gentle Exfoliating Polish** (*$30 for 6.76 ounces*) isn't in the least gentle. It contains cetrimonium bromide (a skin irritant), plus plant oil that can make it too greasy. It is not as effective or as reasonably priced as mixing Cetaphil Gentle Skin Cleanser with baking soda.

☹ **New Beginnings Toner** (*$44 for 6.76 ounces*) is a standard alcohol-based toner that also contains salicylic acid. Salicylic acid is a potent exfoliant and can be useful for certain skin types. However, alcohol is always a problem for the skin, and can cause irritation and dryness.

☹ **New Beginnings Toner Extra Strength** (*$44 for 6.76 ounces*) is virtually identical to the toner above, except for a higher concentration of salicylic acid.

☺ $$$ **Nyaluronic Beauty Serum** (*$44 for 1.1 ounces*) contains mostly water, slip agents, plant extracts, water-binding agents, more slip agents, more plant extracts, anti-irritant, vitamin C, and preservatives. This is a good, lightweight gel moisturizer for someone with normal to slightly dry skin. It is really more of a toner than anything else, and the recommendation is to use it around the eyes, which is fine, especially under makeup.

☺ **Revitalizing Cream** (*$44 for 1.69 ounces*) contains mostly water, plant extracts, plant oils, silicone oil, several thickeners, slip agents, salicylic acid, more thickeners, and preservatives. Please, one exfoliating product used on a regular basis per face. Two salicylic acid products, in this and the toner, is a likely flaky mistake. Salicylic acid is also best for someone with breakouts, and this formula is too emollient for someone with that skin type.

☺ $$$ **Vitamin Enriched Day Cream** (*$44 for 1.69 ounces*) has minimal amounts of vitamins, which may be fine, but without sunscreen it makes a terrible day cream. Without sun protection you might as well say, "Wrinkles, come and get me."

☺ $$$ **Firming Eye Gel** (*$38 for 1.1 ounces*) contains mostly water, plant extracts, slip agent, film former, water-binding agent, and preservatives. This is a fine lightweight gel for slightly dry skin, though nothing special or unique. It claims to firm the skin and eliminate dark circles. Can you believe they're asking $38 for this?

☺ $$$ **Liposomal Beauty Serum** (*$44 for 1.1 ounces*) is almost identical to the Firming Eye Gel above, and the same basic review applies.

☺ **$$$ Extra Rich Night Cream** *($44 for 1.69 ounces)* contains mostly water, thickeners, silicone oil, plant oil, glycerin, plant extract, thickeners, more silicone oil, more thickeners, water-binding agents, more plant extract, more thickeners, and preservatives. It would be a good moisturizer for someone with normal to dry skin, but it isn't extra-rich or worth the cost, even if you happen to be extra-rich.

☹ **Ultra Sunup Sunscreen, SPF 20** *($24 for 4 ounces)* doesn't contain avobenzone, titanium dioxide, or zinc oxide, and is not recommended.

☹ **Waterproof Sunup Sunscreen, SPF 15** *($24 for 4 ounces)* doesn't contain avobenzone, titanium dioxide, or zinc oxide, and is not recommended.

Hard Candy (Makeup Only)

I'm not twentysomething, and haven't been for some time. That's probably why it's hard for me to relate to product lines like Urban Decay and Hard Candy, which are decidedly twentysomething or under cosmetics. The dazzling, glittered look of Hard Candy and the grunge look of Urban Decay are nothing more than image. Underneath the clever packaging, aimed at a very specific young female consumer, are basic products with fairly standard and ordinary characteristics. These lines prove my contention that targeted packaging can make a bland eye or lip pencil seem more alluring and worthy of an impulse purchase. I can imagine a younger woman thinking that Hard Candy products are cool and hip, while finding Estee Lauder products rather staid and boring.

While I can't relate to the attraction, I do know about product quality and performance, and Hard Candy offers nothing more than image. The cosmetics themselves, which range in price from $15 to $35, are overpriced, given the quality and type of products, but if you are looking for avant-garde, unconventional colors, this line is a must-see. How many other lines have shiny peacock blue lip pencils? Actually, the trend toward nonconformist colors is not all that unorthodox anymore: everyone from Revlon Street Wear to M.A.C. and Forever Paris has their share of neon, glittery makeup in very nontraditional colors. I won't comment on the color selection, since that's a matter of personal preference in this case and understandably not mine, but here are my reviews for those wondering what kind of quality is lurking underneath the packaging. For more information about Hard Candy call (800) 823-7441.

Hard Candy's ☺ **$$$ Eye Gliders** *($16)* is a standard eye-lining pencil with a good deal of sparkle. The ☺ **$$$ Lipstick** *($16)* is fairly greasy, and the ☺ **$$$ Lip Liner** *($11)* goes on very thick and comes in a convenient twist-up stick. ☹ **Eyeshadow Quartet** *($35)* is a set of colors that take shine to the extreme. The texture makes blending difficult, they don't adhere well, and the shine tends to get all over, but they absolutely do shine. The ☹ **Mascara** *($15)* is pretty standard and doesn't build much length, but when you're applying purple or gold mascara, maybe length isn't the point. The ☹ **Brow Powder Pencil** *($16)* comes in the only group of normal colors; these really are brow colors (what, no purple eyebrows?), but they have shine. Much like the lip liner in this line, the brow pencil goes on fairly thick and isn't all that powdery or soft looking. One end of the pencil is a brush, which can soften the effect, but a soft application in the first place would be better.

Hydron (Skin Care Only)

Hydron is sold on QVC, and it is simply captivating to watch the host of the show swear by it while enthusiastic callers echo the sentiment. The presentation is *very* convincing, but before you pick up your phone and order, you need more information than just what the company wants you to know.

The Best Defense Collection by Hydron supposedly can restore your skin's natural moisture balance by creating a water-insoluble film over the surface of your skin. According to the company, "Hydron is a polymer, which is an extremely high-molecular-weight compound." What Hydron really is, is polyhydroxyethylmethacrylate. That makes it basically a film former like most other acrylates that show up in skin-care products. The other aspect of Hydron is that, like any polymer, it is too large to penetrate the skin, so it sits on top and covers the surface. That water-insoluble film also has water-binding properties, which are nice and can benefit dry skin, but the film is hardly miraculous or rare or the only way to keep water in the skin.

Hydron's advertising gimmick is to compare skin to rawhide, demonstrating what happens to rawhide if you put water versus other types of ingredients on it. Skin cannot be compared to rawhide (nor to a dead leaf, contrary to a Pond's demonstration years ago on a dried-up oak leaf). First, skin is constantly being produced and shed (it is mostly a living organ of the body); rawhide, on the hand is completely dead. Further, the causes of wrinkling have nothing to do with dry skin. *Dry skin and wrinkles are not associated.* The Hydron ad demonstrates that oil does not provide water (moisture) to the skin, and although that is true, it is not exactly shocking news. However, it does take oil or other water-binding agents to *keep* water in the skin. For dry skin, the issue is getting water to the skin and keeping it there. That process can be as simple as spraying the face with water before you use a moisturizer. (You don't need to spray expensive toners on your face; water will do, and the moisturizer will trap the water underneath.)

Although Hydron claims to be a unique water-delivery system, it is by no means the only one. It uses liposomes, which were developed by Lancome/L'Oreal more than 15 years ago. One more point: All of the ingredients listed on Hydron's products are completely standard. That doesn't make them bad, but they're not the skin sensations they claim to be. For more information about Hydron call (800) 367-9444.

☺ **Best Defense Gentle Cleansing Creme** *($16.50 for 6 ounces)* is supposedly a rinseable cleanser that contains mostly thickeners and a detergent cleansing agent. It can be a good cleanser for someone with normal to dry skin, but it can leave a film on the skin.

☺ **Best Defense Gentle Eye Make Up Remover** *($17 for 4 ounces)* is just water, silicone and a detergent cleansing agent. It will take off eye makeup, but if the gentle cleanser above did its job this wouldn't be necessary.

☺ **$$$ Best Defense Micro-Exfoliating Creme** *($16.75 for 3.6 ounces)* contains mostly water, thickeners, synthetic scrub agent, more thickeners, slip agent, detergent cleansing agent, and preservatives. It can be a good standard scrub for someone with dry skin.

☺ **Best Defense Botanical Toner** *($14.50 for 6.5 ounces)* contains mostly plant water, slip agents, water-binding agents, film former, detergent cleansing agent, and preservatives. There are plenty of plant extracts in it for people who believe that's important. If you are not allergic to plants, this would be a good nonirritating toner for most skin types.

☹ **Best Defense Tri-Activating Skin Clarifier** *($37.75 for 1 ounce)* is Hydron's version of an AHA product, but the ingredient list just says it contains sugarcane extracts, and doesn't tell you *what* has been extracted from the sugarcane. It sounds natural, but if you want to be certain you're getting an effective AHA product, look for glycolic or lactic acid on the ingredient list, not fruit or sugarcane extract.

☹ **Best Defense All Over Moisturizer Oil-Free** *($15.50 for 2.25 ounces)* contains mostly water, slip agents, alcohol, thickeners, film former, lanolin, and preservatives. This may indeed be oil-free, but it contains lanolin and isopropyl palmitate, which can be a problem for someone with oily skin. This would be appropriate only for someone with normal to dry skin.

☺ **$$$ Best Defense Facial Moisturizer Oil-Free with SPF 15** *($29 for 2 ounces)* doesn't contain avobenzone, titanium dioxide, or zinc oxide, and is not recommended.

☺ **$$$ Best Defense Fragile Eye Moisturizer, Wrinkle Fighting Complex** *($26 for 0.5 ounce)* contains mostly water, slip agent, aloe, thickener, water-binding agents, more thickeners, plant oil, more water-binding agents, film former, vitamins A and E, more thickeners, and preservatives. This is a good emollient moisturizer that can be used all over the face, not just around the eyes. What a shame you get so little for so much money.

☺ **$$$ Best Defense Line Smoothing Complex** *($37.75 for 0.5 ounce)* is a good lightweight moisturizer for normal to dry skin. It contains mostly water, water-binding agents, slip agents, plant extracts, thickeners, and preservatives.

☺ **$$$ Best Defense Moisture Balance Restorative Overnight Liposome Complex** *($36 for 2 ounces)* contains mostly water, slip agent, aloe, plant oils, thickener,

water-binding agents, more thickeners, more water-binding agents, film former, vitamins A and E, and preservatives. This would be a good emollient moisturizer for
someone with dry skin.

☹ **Best Defense Self-Adjusting Tinted Moisturizer** *($24.50 for 2 ounces)* doesn't
contain avobenzone, titanium dioxide, or zinc oxide, and is not recommended.

☹ **Best Defense Sportscreen SPF 15** *($15 for two 3-ounce tubes)* doesn't con-
tain avobenzone, titanium dioxide, or zinc oxide, and is not recommended.

☹ **Best Defense Sportscreen SPF 30** *($15 for two 3-ounce tubes)* doesn't con-
tain avobenzone, titanium dioxide, or zinc oxide, and is not recommended.

☺ **Best Defense Sunless Tanning Creme** *($17.50 for 4 ounces)* works as well as
any self-tanner, using the same active ingredient to turn skin brown.

☹ **Best Defense Five-Minute Revitalizing Masque** *($24 for 2.65 ounces)* is a
standard clay mask that also contains plant extracts, glycerin, thickeners, silicone,
and preservatives. The plant extracts include eucalyptus, balm mint, pine needle,
sage, and thyme, all potential skin irritants. The mask also contains some water-
binding agents and a detergent cleansing agent. The water-binding agents are nice,
but the detergent cleansing agent is sodium lauryl sulfate, which can be a skin irritant.

☹ **Best Defense Menthol Ice** *($15 for 4 ounces)* contains both menthol and
alcohol, both drying and irritating; that may be OK for sore muscles, but keep this
one off the face or abraded skin.

☹ **Best Defense Tender Lip Care** *($15.75 for two 0.5-ounce tubes)* doesn't con-
tain avobenzone, titanium dioxide, or zinc oxide, and is not recommended.

IGIA

There probably isn't a woman in the United States right now who hasn't seen the
ads in one form or another for the IGIA Hair Removal System, IGIA Sun System
Facial Tanner, IGIA Clear Blemish Remover, or IGIA Epil-Stop. IGIA seems to have
perfected the art of selling snake oil convincingly. Because I'm afraid some of you
might actually consider using this product, I am purposely leaving out the customer
service number for these products; if you want more information you'll have to search this out for yourself, which shouldn't be hard; these products are advertised in
fashion magazines and mail order catalogues throughout the United States and Canada.
Let's start with the IGIA Sun System, because this product speaks to the ethics of this
company more than the other two, which, though useless, at least aren't harmful.

☹ **$$$ IGIA Sun System Facial Tanner** *($149)* claims to "[do] in minutes
what usually takes hours to acquire. Compact, easy to use, and safe. Comes with a
convenient 30-minute timer so there's no need to worry about burning. You control
the amount of color you receive, while its four UV lamps help you get that even tan.
Stop wasting money on unhealthy tanning salons and get better results in the privacy

of your own home with the IGIA Sun System." According to the FDA, the FCC (Federal Communications Commission), the American Academy of Dermatology, and the Skin Cancer Foundation, suntanning machines are nothing more than skin cancer machines, and should be made illegal. They radiate the most damaging effects of the sun only inches away from your body, and, worse, they are available day after day, month after month, in areas of the country where you would not normally see the sun on a daily basis, exposing body parts that are usually covered. Not only do they put users at serious risk for skin cancer, but in all likelihood they age the skin faster than normal sun exposure would because of the proximity of the radiating light source. This is a senseless machine to make readily available to an unsuspecting public that believes something is safe when the contrary is true. There is no such thing as a safe tan generated by any kind of UV exposure. This machine alone casts a great shadow over IGIA. In fact, trust is the one thing this kind of company is *not* radiating.

☹ **IGIA Epil-Stop Hair Removal Cream** *($29.95 for 4 ounces)*. The Food and Drug Administration issued a recall on September 13, 1997, for this product, manufactured by International Chemical Corporation, Amherst, New York. Previously, on September 4, 1997, the California Poison Control Office had issued a press release warning that Epil-Stop "is adulterated in that it has high pH levels which may cause skin irritation and burning." Check out the FDA home page at *http://www.FDA.gov* for more information.

IGIA Epil-Stop products were advertised on television, magazines, and over the Internet, with claims about removing hair and stopping hair growth naturally and painlessly. If only all that were true, my midweek stubble would be a thing of the past. It isn't. Epil-Stop is a horrendous example of marketing claim abuse, which isn't surprising, at least not to this cosmetic watchdog. It turns out that Epil-Stop worked like any other drugstore depilatory: by dissolving hair with a high pH ingredient base. Unlike other drugstore products, however, Epil-Stop took their pH to a higher level, eating away not only the hair but the skin as well.

☹ **$$$ IGIA's Hair Removal System** *($119)* is supposed to be a "painless home electrolysis system that helps keep hair from growing back! Unlike common [tweezing] and depilatory devices that can cause skin irritation, this system uses mild radio frequency pulses that [are] absolutely safe and [are] delivered through the tweezers to remove hair without touching the skin." Well that much is true. This overpriced machine delivers low-wattage radio waves through the hair shaft. Does that kill off a hair follicle? There is no research indicating that these machines do anything but tweeze the hair. The low voltage may make these machines ineffective, but they are also extremely low risk. In comparison to the other IGIA products this one is the safest in the bunch. Keep in mind these kinds of self-electrolysis machines have been advertised for years and years. I remember them from when I was a kid. The chances of operating these successfully yourself are at best slim. You probably would end up just tweezing instead of zapping the hair because getting the device to work right is extremely tricky and incredibly time-consuming. Given the time it takes for a hair to grow back, it could take months before you knew if it was really working. What a waste.

☹ $$$ IGIA Clear Blemish Remover ($99), while more benign than the Sun System, is a shocking waste of money. Here's the marketing language used in their brochure: "The IGIA Clear Blemish Remover uses a non-invasive process [a dull, metal-tipped, plastic wand] that produces negative ions to destroy bacteria and remove unattractive blemishes within seconds. Once the bacteria [are] destroyed the natural healing process can occur through the pores. The IGIA Clear Blemish Remover works best on small raised spots and typical skin problems such as pimples, blemishes, blackheads, ingrown hairs, and mild acne." The brochure carries on further, saying "this is the safe, painless way to remove unsightly skin spots and let your natural beauty shine through. Includes one bottle of cleanser and one moisturizer lotion, and comes in an attractive, slim, white plastic case." Where have we heard about negative ions before? In a past issue of my newsletter *Cosmetics Counter Update* I reviewed a product being sold by Sharper Image, called a Hair Wand, that claims to get rid of dandruff and repair damaged hair with negative ions. Amazing what a bunch of ions can do. The idea that ions (which are nothing more than a group of atoms, with a positive, negative, or neutral electric charge) can penetrate a pore and kill blemish-causing bacteria is preposterous. Even if ions could do that, bacteria are only part of the reason a blemish occurs. This expensive little implement doesn't address hormonal issues, the pore lining, oil production, or the use of skin-care products that can clog pores and cause breakouts. All it will remove is money from your wallet.

What about the two skin-care products packaged with the machine? The ☹ $$$ **Cleansing Lotion** contains mostly alcohol, water, witch hazel, glycerin, and menthol. If your skin isn't red and irritated before you use this product, it will be after, or worse. The ☹ $$$ **Deep Moisturizing** product contains mostly water, mineral oil, sesame oil, slip agents, thickeners, lanolin, petrolatum, preservatives, and coloring agents. Are they serious? Sesame oil and lanolin are notorious for clogging pores, and petrolatum and mineral oil leave a greasy feel on the skin. This rather dated formulation may be good for someone with seriously dry skin, but it is the worst imaginable for someone struggling with breakouts.

Il Makiage (Makeup Only)

Il Makiage is sold primarily through television presentations. This color line attempts to market itself as the makeup artist's makeup line, but it isn't my kind of cosmetics line, nor is it that of many of the other professional makeup artists I've worked with. It does offer a large range of matte blushes in a wonderful range of colors, as well as matte eyeshadows in a nice selection of neutral shades that have a great texture and blend easily. Unfortunately, the foundations are poor, the mascara doesn't build any length or thickness no matter how much you put on, the brushes are mostly just OK, and the concealers are heavy and greasy and tend to crease.

A special feature of the Il Makiage color line is an assortment of makeup kits that are quite attractive and convenient, but should nevertheless be avoided for the same reason I advise against buying sets of eyeshadow: not all of the items and colors will be appropriate for you. Apart from my feelings about the quality of the products, it is incredibly risky to buy color cosmetics from a brochure or a television show. At the very least you need to see, and preferably try on, foundations and lipsticks, and often blushes and eyeshadows too. If you are in an area where Il Makiage is sold through a hair salon or spa, you may want to consider checking it out. To find a location near you, call (800) 722-1011 or (212) 371-3992.

☺ **FOUNDATION: Liquid Foundation** *($16)*, **Creme Foundation** *($30)*, and **Dual Finish Foundation** *($25)* are products I can't recommend because of the risk involved when you can't try them on. You are taking a shot in the dark. Getting the foundation wrong is a grievous error in makeup application. If I were you, I wouldn't risk it.

☹ **Even Tones** *($11.50)* are standard color correctors that are supposed to be worn under foundation to even out skin tone. Almost without exception, foundation does a fine job of evening out skin tone (especially when the foundation matches your skin exactly). These add an unnecessary layer of makeup, and the effect isn't very convincing anyway.

☹ **CONCEALER: TV Touch Concealer** *($11)* and **TV Touch Compact Combination** *($25 for two colors)* are too heavy and greasy for everyday use. The colors are interesting, but I suspect the pink, yellow, violet, and rose shades are for corrective use, a technique that really isn't used anymore (at least not in any of the TV makeup rooms I've been in over the past several years).

☺ **POWDER: Translucent Face Powder** *($15)* is a standard talc-based powder that has a soft texture and goes on fairly translucent. There are some strange colors, such as a vivid pink and a deep lavender, but also some good neutral ones. Again, because you can't see or try it before you buy it, you could end up having to send it back.

☺ **BLUSH: Color Rouge** *($13)* comes in a large assortment of attractive matte colors that go on soft but can still build good depth for darker skin tones.

☺ **EYESHADOW: Color Shadow** *($13)* is available in some great neutral matte colors, but there are also glaring shades of blue, green, and orange, and some iridescent choices. The matte neutral shades are all worth checking out; they go on very soft and blend easily.

☹ **EYE AND BROW SHAPER:** **Cake Eye Liner** *($11)* is just what it says: a cake eyeliner that creates the perfect Marilyn Monroe look (shades of the early '60s!). The line looks quite dramatic and is surprisingly easy to apply. **Brow Set** *($13)* is little more than bottled hair spray with a brush, but it will keep brows in place. **Jumbo Pencils** *($10)* are hard to sharpen, and the color selection for these is poor.

☺ **Slim Pencils** *($11)*, for lips, eyes, and brows, are standard pencils that go on easily without being too greasy. Color selection is limited, but all of the shades (except for the vivid blue) are quite good.

☺ <u>LIPSTICK AND LIP PENCIL:</u> **Lipstick** *($13)* comes in four types: creams, iridescents, sheers, and mattes. The creams have a nice texture but can be slightly greasy; the iridescents are just that and are also on the greasy side; the sheers are more like gloss; and the mattes, though quite matte, come in only five shades, all of which are rather dark. These are all just OK and not particularly exciting. **Lip Gloss** *($10)* is very glossy and comes in a nice range of colors.

☺ <u>MASCARA:</u> **Mascara** *($12)* doesn't smear, but it also doesn't build any length or thickness.

☺ <u>SPECIALTY PRODUCTS:</u> **Summer, Fall, Winter,** and **Spring Face Kits** *($50)* offer very nice blush and eyeshadow colors, but the way the kit is arranged the lipstick and concealer are open containers placed right next to the blush and eyeshadows. That means every time you put a brush into the blush or eyeshadow, it gets all over the lipstick and concealer. Also, the likelihood that you will use all the products is slim.

☺ **Model Kit** *($85 to $125)* comes in three different color groupings: Neutral Light, Neutral Dark, and Mauve. You will probably be disappointed with what you get for this price: a tiny concealer, small brushes, a lip pencil, an eye pencil, mascara, a fairly glossy lipstick (in a tiny pot, so it is inconvenient), four matte eyeshadows, two shiny eyeshadows, two blushes, and a black cake eyeliner. The matte eyeshadows are nice, but the blushes are just OK, I never recommend shiny eyeshadows, the mascara is not the best, and the brushes are only passable.

☺ **Lip Kit** *($45)* offers a good selection of little pots of color. They are all on the greasy side, but if you like playing with a lot of different colors and don't have a problem with lipstick bleeding, this just may be an option.

Iman

Only a handful of women are known by their first name alone: they include Madonna, Cher, Ann-Margaret, and, of course, the exquisite, regal Iman. Considered a classic Ethiopian beauty, Iman broke the color line, along with model Beverly Johnson, gracing the covers of fashion magazines that had previously deemed black women unacceptable as cover models. She also became known for her social life as part of Europe's and New York's jet set (with David Bowie as her escort). Although on the surface she appears imperious and removed, in recent years she has been active in food and aid relief for her war-torn, impoverished homeland, and has fought for the rights of Ethiopian women regarding the horror of female circumcision. Iman is no ordinary woman.

Venturing into the world of makeup seems a natural for this elegant, savvy aristocrat. And in some areas Iman has achieved breakthroughs that other cosmetics lines could learn from. Regrettably, her line loses considerable ground with its skin-care products, called Liquid Assets. Whoever put these products together for her doesn't seem to have had a plan, or to have realized that different skin types exist. The cleansers are disappointing, the toners are mediocre, the AHA products are limited, and the oil-free products contain ingredients that can cause breakouts. Additionally, not one of the daytime moisturizers contains sunscreen, even though women of color are also subject to sun damage. In fact, sun damage is often responsible for darker skin tones becoming ashen, and lighter-skinned women of color run a risk of skin cancer. Like most of the skin-care lines glutting the cosmetics market right now, these products have the requisite plant extracts. But don't get too excited if you're a consumer who thinks plant extracts are what good skin care is all about; most of the green stuff comes after the preservatives, which means there isn't much.

Iman's line excels when it comes to her color collection. Most of the blush, eyeshadow, and lip colors are stunning, with a majority of matte neutral shades in a wide variety of tones that don't include blues, greens, or purples. These products are appropriate for a wide range of skin colors, from Asian to Latin and all shades of African-American skin. For more information about Iman call (212) 582-3473 or (800) 621-6043.

Iman Skin Care

☹ **Cleansing Bar with Grapefruit Normal/Oily Skin Formula** *($8.50 for 3.5 ounces)* is a standard detergent-based cleansing bar that contains tallow along with some plants and grapefruit. The grapefruit supposedly makes it good for oily skin types, although there isn't much in this bar. (If there were, it would be a skin irritant. Ever get grapefruit juice on an open cut? Ouch.) Also, tallow can cause breakouts. I don't recommend soap; however, if you have a penchant for it, there are better, gentler, tallow-free soaps on the market.

☹ **Cleansing Bar with Rose Petal** *($8.50 for 3.5 ounces)* is almost identical to the Cleansing Bar with Grapefruit (including the grapefruit), and the same review applies.

☹ **Eye Makeup Remover with Aloe Vera** *($10 for 3 ounces)* contains mostly water, slip agents, detergent cleansing agents, and preservatives. This would be a good, standard eye-makeup remover, but it also contains lemon and grapefruit, which can definitely be irritating for the eye area.

☺ **Liquid Assets Gentle Cleansing Lotion** *($13 for 3 ounces)* is a poor group of thickening agents that don't have much cleansing ability. Without a washcloth this cleanser will not help get your face clean.

☹ **Liquid Assets Skin Refresher Lotion** *($12.50 for 3 ounces)* contains mostly water, slip agents, plant extract, plant oil, menthol, soothing agent, aloe, more plant extracts, and preservatives. The orange oil and menthol are serious skin irritants.

☺ **$$$ Instant Replay AHA Perfecting Lotion** *($35 for 1 ounce)* has about a 4% concentration of AHA in a good pH. It isn't going to perfect anything and it contains grapefruit and lemon which can be skin irritants.

☺ **Eye Firming Cream with Cucumber** *($15 for 0.5 ounce)* won't firm anything, but it is a good, ordinary emollient moisturizer for someone with normal to dry skin. It contains water, thickeners, castor oil, silicone, and preservatives. There are plants (including cucumber) and vitamins in it, but not very much of them.

☹ **Night Time Complex Oil-Free Moisturizer** *($20 for 1.8 ounces)* contains several thickening agents (isopropyl myristate and shea butter) that can cause breakouts. It also contains lemon and grapefruit, which can be skin irritants.

☹ **Oil-Free Advanced Moisture Complex** *($16.50 for 3 ounces)* contains isopropyl myristate (fourth on the ingredient list) and shea butter, which are great for dry skin but are both known to cause breakouts. Neither are great for oily to combination skin despite the claim about being oil-free.

☺ **PM Renewal Cream** *($20 for 1.8 ounces)* is a very good emollient moisturizer for someone with very dry skin. It contains mostly water, thickeners, safflower oil, wax, slip agent, more thickeners, lanolin, castor oil, vitamin E, plant extracts, and preservatives. Like most of the products in this line, this one also contains grapefruit and lemon, which can be skin irritants.

☹ **Perfect Response Oil-Free Cleanser, for Acne Prone, Very Oily Skin** *($15 for 4 ounces)* includes as the primary detergent cleansing agent sodium C14-16 olefin sulfonate, plus peppermint extract and lemon extract, and all of those are exceedingly irritating. This product is not recommended for any skin type.

☹ **Perfect Response Gentle Toner, for Acne Prone, Very Oily Skin** *($15 for 6 ounces)* contains a small amount of salicylic acid, but it also contains witch hazel, a skin irritant. The pH of this product also isn't low enough to make it a good exfoliant.

☹ **Perfect Response Oil-Free Hydrating Gel, for Acne Prone, Very Oily Skin** *($18 for 1.7 ounces)* is a gel formulation containing water-binding agents, vitamins, and slip agents. It also contains several irritating ingredients, including alcohol and sulfur. The sulfur can be a disinfectant but it is also a skin irritant; the alcohol is just irritating.

☹ **Perfect Response Blemish Gel, for Acne Prone, Very Oily Skin** *($12 for 0.5 ounce)* would be a great 5% benzoyl peroxide gel to disinfect blemishes, except that it also contains peppermint and lemon, which are unnecessary irritants that can make acne-prone skin redder and tend to break out more.

☹ **Perfect Response Clay Masque, for Acne Prone, Very Oily Skin** *($12 for 4 ounces)* is an OK clay mask with 2% salicylic acid. It doesn't have a low enough pH for the BHA to be an exfoliant but the clay mask can absorb oil. It also contains a small amount of peppermint and lemon, which are unnecessary skin irritants.

☹ **Perfection Even-Tone Fade Cream** *($20 for 2.1 ounces)* is a standard 2% hydroquinone product in a good emollient base. What a shame it has to contain lemon and grapefruit to add skin irritation to an otherwise good product.

☹ **Perfect Response Even-Tone Fade Gel with AHA** *($20 for 1.7 ounces)* is similar to the one above, only this gel contains spearmint, which is a skin irritant. Though the product claims it contains AHAs, it uses sugarcane extract, which is not the exfoliating ingredient glycolic acid.

☹ **All Day Moisture Complex, SPF 15** *($16.50 for 3 ounces)* doesn't contain avobenzone, titanium dioxide, or zinc oxide, and is not recommended.

☹ **Oil-Free Hydrating Lotion, SPF 15, for Acne Prone, Very Oily Skin** *($20 for 1.7 ounces)* doesn't contain avobenzone, titanium dioxide, or zinc oxide, and is not recommended.

☹ **Sun Defense Lip & Eye Stick, SPF 15** *($15 for 0.14 ounce)* doesn't contain avobenzone, titanium dioxide, or zinc oxide, and is not recommended.

☹ **Sun Defense Lotion, SPF 25** *($20 for 4 ounces)* doesn't contain avobenzone, titanium dioxide, or zinc oxide, and is not recommended.

☹ **Time Control Peeling Masque with AHA** *($18 for 2.8 ounces)* has polyvinyl alcohol (plastic) and alcohol as the first two ingredients, while the amount of AHA is less than 2%, adding up to a useless mask.

☹ **Time Control Renewal Complex** *($29.50 for 1 ounce)* contains only about 3% AHA in a pH that's too high to make this an effective exfoliant.

☺ **Time Control Sloughing Gel** *($18 for 2.8 ounces)* is a standard synthetic scrub. If any of the AHA or BHA products in Iman's line worked, this scrub wouldn't be necessary; either way, Cetaphil Gentle Skin Cleanser and baking soda is a better option than this.

☹ **Under Cover Agent Oil-Control Lotion** *($16 for 1 ounce)* is a liquid version of Phillips' Milk of Magnesia that uses magnesium aluminum silicate instead of magnesium carbonate to absorb oil. It would do the trick, but it also contains balm mint and camphor, which are skin irritants.

Iman Makeup

☹ **FOUNDATION: Second to None Cream to Powder Foundation** *($17.50)* doesn't feel anything like a cream or a powder; it feels more like spackle. It does blend out thin, but not easily. The colors would be worth checking out if the texture weren't so exceedingly thick and heavy. What a shame!

☺ **Second to None Oil-Free Makeup with SPF 8** *($16.50)* has a very matte, dry finish, and would work well for someone with oily to combination skin, but the SPF 8 has a disappointing low number and it doesn't contain any UVA protection. For just a foundation (forgetting the sunscreen component) it is by far a better option than the Cream to Powder Foundation above. **These colors can be too peach, ash, or red for most skin tones:** Sand 4, Clay 2, Clay 3, Clay 5, Earth 1, Earth 2, and Earth 6.

☹ **CONCEALER: Corrective Concealer Camouflage** *($12)* goes on very dry and thick. If you have any lines under the eye, this concealer will make them look worse. However, it doesn't slip into the lines, so there is no creasing. If you don't have lines this could be an option.

☺ **POWDER: Luxury Pressed Powder Oil-Controlling** *($15)* is a talc-based powder that has a great range of colors and a smooth, silky, even texture.

☺ **BLUSH: Luxury Blushing Powder** *($15)* comes in a spectacular array of colors, is a pleasure to apply, and has great staying potential. However, the texture can be too dry for someone with dry skin.

☺ **EYESHADOW: Eyeshadow** *($10)* comes in an incredible array of matte neutral eyeshadow colors. **These colors are wonderful for all skin tones:** Apple, Cedar Chip, Mahogany, Vanilla, Chili, Cocoa, Brazil Nut, Almond, Walnut, Cashew, Oak, Plum, Raspberry, Grape, Iris, Orchid, Wisteria, Onyx, Pearl. **These eyeshadows are too shiny:** Nutmeg, Twigs, Violet, and Tiger Eye.

☺ **EYE AND BROW SHAPER:** The standard **Perfect Eye Pencils** *($8.50)* come in a nice range of colors and have a good dry texture that goes on easily. **Perfect Brow Pencil** *($8.50)* comes in three colors and is virtually identical to the Eye Pencils.

☺ **LIPSTICK AND LIP PENCIL:** Most of the **Luxury Moisturizing Lip Colors** *($10)* are stunning, with a wide range of matte neutral shades and a wonderful creamy but matte finish. Avoid the frosted ones, which are exceedingly greasy. **Perfect Lip Pencil** *($8.50)* comes in a nice array of colors and has a smooth, slightly creamy texture.

☹ **MASCARA: Perfect Mascara** *($12)* isn't perfect. It does go on easily and builds lashes quickly, but it tends to smear during the day.

Jafra

Regardless of what in-home line of products you choose to try out, each makeup/skin-care demonstration begins the same way. An array of products is set in front of you, and a presentation placard of information is placed next to the salesperson or, to use the preferred term, beauty consultant. You are then taken through a rather fun, hands-on demonstration of product usage after your skin type has been assessed. Of course, skin typing is almost always hit-or-miss, but I'll get to that in a minute. The skin-care routine generally involves a minimum of six products and, more often than not, "if you really want great skin," an average of seven products, although that rarely includes an adequate sunscreen. Once your face is clean and loaded up with several moisturizers, including an exfoliator, "firming" gel, protective cream, and eye lotion, the makeup application begins.

Jafra's routine is no exception, although this just as accurately describes the techniques of Mary Kay, Shaklee, Amway, and all the others. Like its peers, Jafra offers some products that are great, some that are good, some that are bad, and some that are really bad.

What is unique to Jafra is the way its salespeople determine skin type. They have a cute little machine called a Skin Programmer. It supposedly measures the moisture level of the skin by assessing its electrical conductivity. You hold a metal cylinder in one hand while the salesperson holds a plastic handle with a metal tip on your face. You don't feel a thing, but a very small electrical charge is generated. How long it takes that electrical charge to complete its circuit—from your cheek or chin to your hand—rates a number. The theory is that the less water (moisture) you have in your skin, the slower the electrical charge; the more water in your skin, the faster the electrical charge. Unfortunately, it only *sounds* good. It doesn't really tell you much about the true condition of your skin. There is so much room for error it's almost a joke. The way your skin registers an electrical current will be different depending on the time of day, what skin-care products you have on, and even the weather. My skin was rated as normal to dry. I explained that I've never had dry skin in my life. I was told that my skin may look oily, but it is only compensating for the dry skin underneath.

That would be fine if oil production worked that way, but it doesn't: oil production is regulated by hormones, not some biological homeostasis. If that weren't so, women with dry skin would automatically have oily skin too, since their oil glands would react to the state of dryness, but, as anyone with dry skin would tell you, that is clearly not the case. You would do much better to follow the skin-type suggestions in Jafra's brochures, which are standard, and ignore the output of the Skin Programmer.

Jafra's color collection has a few fairly interesting selections. It is a rather straightforward line, with all the basics and some good options for a wide range of skin tones. The color line is divided into Warm, Cool, and Neutral, which is helpful, except that some of the Neutrals tend to be warm rather than truly neutral. For more information about Jafra call (800) 551-2345.

Jafra Skin Care

☺ **Cleansing Gel** (*$12.50 for 4.2 ounces*) is a good water-soluble, detergent-based cleanser for someone with normal to oily skin. It does contain a small amount of chamomile oil, probably more for fragrance than as an oil, but it can be a problem for some skin types.

☹ **Cleansing Lotion for Dry to Normal Skin** (*$12.50 for 8.4 ounces*) is an oil-based cleanser that needs to be wiped off and can leave skin feeling greasy. I never recommend wiping off makeup for any skin type, and assuredly not for someone with normal skin.

☹ **Cleansing Lotion for Normal to Oily Skin** (*$12.50 for 8.4 ounces*) is meant to be wiped off with a washcloth, and that's essential, because it won't come off with simple splashing, as any self-respecting water-soluble cleanser should, especially one for oily skin. This cleanser leaves skin feeling greasy, which is not great for someone with oily skin.

☹ **Cleansing Cream for Dry Skin** (*$12.50 for 4.2 ounces*) is a thicker version of the lotion above; the same review applies, but even more so. While the greasy film may not be a problem for dry skin, wiping off makeup is.

☹ **Soothing Results Cleansing Lotion** (*$12.50 for 8.4 ounces*) is a wipe-off makeup remover that contains lemon peel; that isn't soothing for the skin but an irritant.

☺ **Eye Makeup Remover Gel** (*$8.50 for 0.75 ounce*) is a mineral oil–based eye-makeup remover. Using it is pretty much like using plain mineral oil, except that it's in a gel form. It's still mostly mineral oil, effective but greasy. Plain mineral oil is cheaper.

☺ **Gentle Exfoliating Scrub for All Skin Types** (*$12.50 for 2.5 ounces*) is indeed gentle, but also fairly greasy. It contains standard synthetic scrub particles, plus several plant oils and other emollient thickeners that make it very hard to rinse off. It can leave a greasy film on the skin.

☺ **Skin Freshener for Dry Skin** (*$13 for 8.4 ounces*) is a very good toner for someone with normal to dry skin. It contains mostly water, water-binding agents, plant extracts, fragrance, detergent cleansing agents, and preservatives. It does contain a tiny amount of ammonium alum, which can be an irritant, but the amount is so small it won't be a problem for most skin types.

☺ **Skin Freshener for Dry to Normal Skin** (*$13 for 8.4 ounces*) contains mostly water, water-binding agent, witch hazel, rose water, plant oils, soothing agent, and preservatives. Witch hazel and sandalwood oil (one of the plant oils) can both be skin irritants.

☹ **Skin Freshener for Normal to Oily Skin** (*$13 for 8.4 ounces*) contains a lot of alcohol, which can dry and irritate the skin (causing it to become more oily). It also contains plant oils, the last thing somebody with oily skin would want on her face.

☹ **Skin Freshener for Oily Skin** *($13 for 8.4 ounces)* contains a lot of alcohol and plant extracts that can all be potent skin irritants for all skin types. It also contains lemon extract and menthol, which only add fuel to the fire.

☺ **Soothing Results Calming Toner for Sensitive Skin** *($13 for 8.4 ounces)* is a good toner for normal to dry skin. It contains mostly water, water-binding agents, plant extracts, fragrance, and preservatives.

☹ **Rediscover Alpha Hydroxy Complex** *($31 for 1 ounce)* contains several fruit extracts, but there is no way of knowing what they are. As I've mentioned throughout this book, although alpha hydroxy acids are derived from fruit, there are innumerable fruit extracts that have nothing to do with AHAs. This product also contains lavender oil, which can make the skin sensitive to sun exposure.

☹ **Advanced Time Protector Daily Defense Cream, SPF 15** *($36 for 1.7 ounces)* doesn't contain avobenzone, zinc oxide, or titanium dioxide, and is not recommended.

☹ **Day Cream Moisturizer for Dry to Normal Skin SPF 6** *($15 for 1.7 ounces)* is inadequate for protection from sun damage.

☹ **Day Lotion for Normal to Oily Skin SPF 6** *($15 for 4.2 ounces)* is inadequate for protection from sun damage.

☹ **Day Lotion for Oily Skin SPF 6** *($15 for 4.2 ounces)* is inadequate for protection from sun damage.

☺ **Extra Care Cream** *($8 for 0.5 ounce)* contains mostly petrolatum, mineral oil, thickeners, plant oil, and preservatives. This is a very emollient moisturizer for someone with very dry skin.

☺ **Night Cream for Dry Skin** *($15 for 1.7 ounces)* is a good, though standard, moisturizer for someone with normal to dry skin. It contains mostly water, lots of thickeners, water-binding agents, fragrance, and preservatives.

☺ **Night Cream Moisturizer for Dry to Normal Skin** *($15 for 1.7 ounces)* contains mostly water, several thickeners, slip agent, silicones, more thickeners, several water-binding agents, soothing agents, and preservatives. Someone with normal skin will probably find this too emollient, but it is a good moisturizer for someone with dry skin.

☺ **Night Cream for Normal to Oily Skin** *($15 for 1.7 ounces)* contains mostly water, slip agents, film former, silicone oils, water-binding agents, soothing agent, thickeners, plant oil, vitamin E, and preservatives. Women with oily skin could find themselves with clogged pores and more oil than they started out with, but it could be a good moisturizer for normal to dry skin types.

☺ **Night Lotion** *($15 for 4.2 ounces)* contains mostly water, several thickeners, slip agent, silicones, more thickeners, several water-binding agents, soothing agents, and preservatives. This is a good moisturizer for someone with normal to dry skin.

☺ **$$$ Skin Firming Complex** *($31 for 1 ounce)* contains mostly water, several water-binding agents, thickeners, soothing agent, silicone, and preservatives. This would be a very good lightweight moisturizer for someone with normal to oily skin.

☺ $$$ **Eye Revitalizing Concentrate** *($17 for 0.75 ounce)* contains mostly water, thickeners, plant oil, more thickeners, several water-binding agents, and preservatives. This is a good emollient moisturizer for someone with normal to dry skin.

☹ $$$ **Royal Jelly Moisture Balm Lotion, Original Formula** *($60 for 1 ounce)* contains mostly water, several thickeners, royal jelly, more thickeners, water-binding agents, and preservatives. You may be wondering why this otherwise standard moisturizer sells for $60 an ounce. Jafra touts royal jelly as a miracle ingredient. The salesperson told me it could heal burns, get rid of scars, and erase wrinkles. It sure sounds like a miracle. Is it? Well, bee larvae who get fed *fresh* royal jelly turn into queen bees. But if you try to sneak *stored* royal jelly into them, they don't turn into queens. As natural and intereting as that all sounds, there is still no evidence that royal jelly has any miracle benefit to the skin.

☺ $$$ **Royal Jelly Milk Balm Moisture Lotion Dry and Normal to Dry** *($60 for 1 ounce)* is a good moisturizer for normal dry skin, but if you are expecting something special from the royal jelly, give it up. This is a gimmick that doesn't translate to good skin care. There are far more interesting water-binding agents and emollients in this product that make it worthwhile than the bee-stuff.

☺ $$$ **Royal Jelly Milk Balm Moisture Lotion Normal to Oily and Oily** *($60 for 1 ounce)* is similar to the one above and the same review applies.

☺ $$$ **Royal Jelly Milk Balm Moisture Lotion, Unscented** *($60 for 1 ounce)* is a very heavy, ordinary moisturizer that contains mostly water, mineral oil, thickeners, lanolin, wax, and preservatives. Of course there is some royal jelly, but it's unimportant. This can be an option for very dry skin, but it can clog pores and dull skin.

☺ $$$ **Time Corrector Firming Moisture Cream** *($38 for 1.7 ounces)* won't correct one minute on your face, or firm anything, but it is a good moisturizer for dry skin. It contains mostly water, thickeners, glycerin, a long list of water-binding agents, film former, and preservatives.

☹ **Ecko The Gecko Kids Sunblock** *($10.50 for 3.5 ounces)* doesn't contain avobenzone, zinc oxide, or titanium dioxide, and is not recommended.

☹ **Sunblock Cream SPF 15, Advanced UVA/UVB Protection** *($11.50 for 4.2 ounces)* doesn't contain avobenzone, zinc oxide, or titanium dioxide, and is not recommended.

☹ **Sunblock Cream SPF 30, Advanced UVA/UVB Protection** *($12 for 4.2 ounces)* doesn't contain avobenzone, zinc oxide, or titanium dioxide, and is not recommended.

☹ **Sunscreen Cream SPF 8, Advanced UVA/UVB Protection** *($10.50 for 4.2 ounces)* doesn't contain avobenzone, zinc oxide, or titanium dioxide, and is not recommended.

☹ **Clear Blemish Treatment** *($9.50 for 0.5 ounce)* has a pH of 3, which is great, but it also contains alcohol and that's a problem for healing breakouts.

☹ **Clear Pore Clarifier** *($15 for 1.7 ounces)* has a pH of close to 5, which means it isn't low enough for the BHA (salicylic acid) to have an effect. This product also contains clove oil, which can be a skin irritant.

☺ **Deep Cleansing Mask for Normal to Oily Skin** *($12.50 for 2.5 ounces)* is a fairly standard clay-based mask that also contains a small amount of plant oil, silicone, plant extracts, and lots of thickening agents. This would be an OK clay mask for someone with normal to dry skin. However, someone with oily skin would not be pleased with any amount of oil or with the emollient thickeners this mask contains.

☺ **Refreshing Moisture Mask for Dry and Dry to Normal Skin** *($12.50 for 2.5 ounces)* contains mostly water, plant oil, several thickeners, clay, more plant oils, slip agents, water-binding agents, minuscule amounts of plant extracts, vitamin E, and preservatives. Although I'm not one to recommend clay masks for dry skin, this one contains such a small amount of clay that it would be quite a good emollient mask.

☺ **Soothing Results Cooling Yogurt and Honey Mask, for Sensitive Skin** *($12.50 for 2.6 ounces)* is a clay mask with several plant oils, thickeners, and water-binding agents. Clay isn't the best thing for sensitive skin, and can be a skin irritant, but this would be a good mask for someone with dry skin.

Jafra Makeup

☺ FOUNDATION: **Supertone Moisturizing Makeup SPF 6** *($11.75)* and **Supertone Makeup Oil Controlling SPF 6** *($11.75)* have SPF 6 with no UVA protection, and that makes both of these a poor choice as far as sun protection is concerned. These two foundations are quite good at providing even, light to medium coverage, and the color selection is very good. **Avoid these colors:** Porcelain, Alabaster, Cashmere, Bisque, Honey, Ginger, Bronze, Cognac, Sable, and Pecan.

☹ **Total Foundation Cream to Powder SPF 12** *($13.50)* has a decent SPF with a titanium dioxide base. It also has a soft, sheer finish. Sadly, all of the colors are either too peach, pink, or ash to recommend.

☹ CONCEALER: **Cream Concealer** *($8.50)* comes in a stick form, with three rather mediocre colors: Fair is too pink for most skin tones, Medium is too peach, and Dark, although neutral, isn't all that dark and would be appropriate only for medium skin tones. The texture is somewhat thick and heavy, and it does tend to crease. **Total Concealer** *($9.50)* is a tube applicator concealer, and the color choice isn't much better than the Cream Concealer.

☺ **White Souffle** *($9)* is a liquid concealer that is indeed white, but it goes on very subtly, requiring just a tiny bit to lighten a shadow under the eye or along the corners of the mouth or nose. It is appropriate only for use over or under foundation.

☺ **POWDER: Pressed Powder** *($11.75)* is a standard talc-based powder with a soft but dry texture; it comes in three excellent shades. **Translucent Face Powder** *($11.75)* is not the least bit moisturizing. It has a very drying, granular texture, although the finish is indeed translucent.

☺ **BLUSH: Powder Blush** *($10.50)* has a great soft texture and blends on smoothly and evenly. All of the colors are great, though it is lacking neutral or softer shades. There is a great selection for darker skin tones (a couple have a slight amount of shine that doesn't show up much on the face), and Terra-cotta, Desert, and Copper Blaze are excellent contour colors.

☺ **EYESHADOW:** All of Jafra's eyeshadows come packaged in **Eyeshadow Trios** *($10.50)*. The line simply does not sell single eyeshadow colors, which is disappointing. Some of the combinations are best described as too weird or too shiny. However, despite the fact that I think buying sets of three is a great way to waste money (you rarely use all of the colors), there are a handful of surprisingly neutral, workable groupings. **These are the only good matte color combinations:** Bazaar, Caravan, Mirage, and Neutral Ground.

☺ **EYE AND BROW SHAPER: Eye and Brow Pencils** *($6.50)* are standard pencils with a dry finish. There is a nice array of colors, but for the Eye Pencils avoid the blue and green shades. **Liquid Eyeliner** *($8)* is a standard tube liner that goes on dramatically and tends not to chip or flake.

☺ **LIPSTICK: Long Lasting Moisturizing Lipsticks** *($7.50)* has a great creamy, opaque finish. **Always Color Stay On Lipstick** *($9)* is Jafra's version of Revlon's ColorStay. This one works quite well, with a soft, ultra-matte finish. It tends not to chip or peel like a lot of ultra-matte lipsticks do. **Lip Gloss** *($7)* is a standard lip gloss that works as well as any. Standard **Lip Pencils** *($6.50)*, identical to the eye pencils, come in a small but attractive color selection.

☹ **Time Protector Lipsticks SPF 15** *($10)* is more lip gloss than lipstick, plus the SPF doesn't include UVA protection.

☹ **MASCARA: OptiMascara** *($7)* does build beautiful long, thick lashes, but alas it smears and flakes terribly throughout the day. **Waterproof Mascara** *($7)* is neither all that waterproof nor does it build length or thickness.

☹ **BRUSHES: Deluxe Face Powder Brush** *($10.50)* has a soft feel but is really too large and floppy to control placement of powder. **Blush Brush** *($6)* is too stiff and hard, feeling scratchy and uncomfortable against the skin.

Jane (Makeup Only)

Jane is a color line of cosmetics aimed at teenagers that was purchased by Estee Lauder in 1997. The brochures accompanying the display for these products have bright young faces bemoaning the beauty problems of adolescence and extolling cute makeup and skin-care solutions. For example, one pamphlet examined the reasons for wearing makeup with these probing fill-in-the-blank questions: "Is looking cute the best way to get a guy?" or "How can I look older?" Inside were these answers. "Looking cute doesn't hurt. But if that's all it took to get and keep a boyfriend, we'd all be in deep dodo." And "Why do you want to look older? If you're trying to get into a real hip club, a little lipstick will definitely make you look like you've been there before." Not exactly your typical prosaic cosmetic rhetoric, but just obnoxious enough to attract young girls who can't relate to L'Oreal and are tired of Cover Girl.

While the brochures might be directed at teenagers and the product line's name may have been chosen to appeal to them, the simple black packaging, neutral colors, and vivid, creamy lipstick colors seem to be much more in alignment with what adults would be interested in. The prices are more than reasonable, and many of the colors are appropriate for a wide range of skin tones, but I get the feeling you won't be able to find these products much longer, because adults will discover they don't quite live up to all their needs, and they aren't what most teens are looking for either. Perhaps Lauder will move in and make some much needed improvements to the Jane selection. For more information about Jane call (800) 820-JANE.

☹ **FOUNDATION: Oil-Free Foundation** *($2.99)* is a mess of a foundation. It goes on very choppy and easily slips into pores, looking dotted and pasty. What a shame, because there are some great neutral colors in this small group.

☺ **True to You Sheer Finish Foundation** *($2.99)* has a rather good range of neutral colors and a nice, smooth texture that goes on quite sheer and smooth. There are generally no testers, and I rarely recommend foundations you can't try on before buying. Sometimes they sell small samples, and you can take advantage of that to find a great color that matches your skin exactly.

☺ **CONCEALER: No Show Concealer** *($2.29)* comes in stick form, but has a surprisingly satiny texture. It comes in three decent colors and has a slight tendency to slip into the lines around the eyes as the day goes by, although it's not as bad as most (it isn't a problem if you don't have any lines, so it just depends on how old you are). **Clueless Two Way Concealer** *($2.29)* is a decent concealer, with soft coverage and good staying power, but it does tend to slip into the lines around the eyes. The color choices are limited, but the ones that are there are all neutral and work well.

☹ **POWDER: Oil-Free Finishing Powder** *($2.29)* has a soft, silky, dry texture and goes on quite sheer and even. The colors seem to all be shades of peach now. I'm not sure what happened, but this is not good.

☺ **Staying Powder Loose Powder** *($2.99)* is a very good dry-finish, standard, talc-based powder. It is best for someone with oily skin. Of the four shades the only one to be wary of is Light, which can be too peach for most skin tones.

☺ **BLUSH: Blushing Cheeks** *($2.29)* offers a good, muted, matte color selection, and all the shades go on fairly smooth and even.

☺ **EYESHADOW: Eyeshadows** *($2.29)* are all slightly shiny, which isn't the worst, but not the best. Still the colors go on soft and blend on easily. These are as good an option for eyeshadow as any!

☺ **EYE AND BROW SHAPER:** The fairly standard **Gliding Eye Liner, One Liners Eye Liners** (twist-up container), and **High Brow Pencils** *($2.39)* all go on well without being greasy or choppy, and are an option regardless of age. Of course, brow powders are preferable, and I still recommend using darker eyeshadow colors as liners, but for pencils these are as fine as any.

☺ **LIPSTICK AND LIP PENCIL: Satin Lipstick** *($2.29)* is probably too creamy and full-colored for teens and too greasy and glossy for adults; the colors are good, but the texture can be a problem. **Shimmer Lipstick** *($2.29)* is simply the Satin Lipstick above with frost. **Sheer Lipstick** *($2.29)* is not a lipstick at all but a very emollient gloss, but it has a nice sheer finish for a teenager. **Matte Lipstick** *($2.29)* is nice and creamy but not the least bit matte; it doesn't feel any different from the Satin Lipstick and it can easily bleed into the lines around the mouth (if you have lines that is). **Gloss Over** *($2.39)* is just a very emollient pot of gloss, which makes it very good for a glossy looking mouth. **Quik Stix** *($2.69)* is a fat lipstick/lip liner pencil, and while I'm not fond of pencils you have to sharpen, this has a good soft matte finish in a small but good array of colors, and the price! At this price you can buy all of them.

☺ **One Liners Lip Liners** *($2.99)* come in twist-up containers, so they don't require sharpening, plus they have a wonderful smooth texture and a great color selection. **Shaping Sticks** *($2.29)* are standard pencils with a great texture, not too dry and not too greasy, that come in a nice assortment of colors.

☺ **One-for-All** *($2.69)* has a creamy application with a somewhat dry finish. It is supposed to be used for the eyes, lips, and cheeks. The container is really too big for some shapes of lips, but if you can pick up the knack for applying this product, it does work well in all categories.

☺ **MASCARA: Flashes Ultra Rich Mascara** *($2.29)* is surprisingly good; it goes on fast, building thick, even lashes with little to no smearing.

☺ **BRUSHES:** Jane's brushes aren't awful, they are just the wrong shape and have a poor consistency. The eyeshadow brushes are all too small or too thin, while the powder and blush brushes are soft enough but not the best size or density of bristles.

Janet Sartin

For awhile I was receiving a lot of questions about Janet Sartin's products. The number of letters has subsided, which I take to mean women are realizing there isn't much here for the skin, especially given the price. Whatever was generating the interest, it certainly wasn't the makeup products, which include a foundation almost indistinguishable from Clinique Pore Minimizer (both are just colored talc suspended in alcohol), shiny eyeshadows, and exceptionally greasy lipstick. If this line has any raison d'être, it may be the huge selection of skin-care products. With this kind of variety, women tend to think there must be something within the mélange that will work for them.

When it comes to price, I almost choked. To say the least, this is a high-end line and absurdly overpriced. Yet the products are just standard—alcohol-based astringents, standard AHA products, bar soaps, mineral oil–based cleansers, and mineral oil– and lanolin–based moisturizers—without much of anything interesting. Given the prices, you would at least want the latest water-binding agents, anti-irritants, and sunscreen formulations. Even the packaging is ordinary and clumsy. (At least when you buy Chanel or Dior, the packaging has an elegance all its own despite the contents.) In some ways this line is almost schizophrenic: the astringents and masks are all exceptionally drying and irritating, while the cleansers and moisturizers are rather greasy and emollient. I can't imagine how someone's skin wouldn't be disturbed by most combinations of these products.

One of the more provocative sections in Sartin's brochures are the lists of foods that are said to be best for specific skin types. For example, she suggests that vegetable soup, fish, cooked cereals (grains), and fruit are great, but oily nuts, fried foods, and chocolate can cause problems. This kind of blatant fiction sets skin care for those with oily and acned skin back to the Stone Age. A healthy diet low in fat and excess sugar is good for the body, but there is no evidence that fatty or sugary foods can affect even one oil gland. In fact, quite the contrary. Dermatologists and researchers searched for decades to find a dietary correlation between food and skin, and none exists. You may have food allergies that can show up on the skin, but they are more likely to be associated with shellfish, milk, wheat, and some vegetables, such as tomatoes. While I'm on the subject of food, although I advocate drinking lots of water for good overall health, no matter how much you drink it won't pass through the skin. Excess water is just eliminated; it doesn't travel to skin cells.

The Sartin product line is available at some Nordstrom stores and Bloomingdale's. But you don't have to rush out to jump on the bandwagon, because there isn't much here worth considering. For more information about Janet Sartin products call (800) 321-1779.

Janet Sartin Skin Care

☹ 1012 Soap, Specially Formulated Soap for Oily Skin *($14 for 3.25 ounces)* is basically lard and lye. Lye dries the skin and lard can clog pores. The price is excessive.

☹ **Gentle Cleansing Soap, for Normal to Combination Skin** *($14 for 3.6 ounces)* is similar to the soap above and the same review applies.

☹ **Superfatted Soap, Specially Formulated Soap for Dry Skin** *($14 for 3 ounces)* is similar to the 1012 Soap above, except with plant oil, and the same review applies.

☹ **Cleansing Oil, Nourishing Cleanser for Normal to Dry Skin** *($27 for 7 ounces)* is a joke, right? How can they charge $27 for mineral oil and peanut oil? Did they think no one would notice? This product requires wiping and pulling at the skin, which can cause sagging, and it can leave a greasy film.

☹ **Gentle Cleanser, for Normal to Oily Sensitive Skin** *($23 for 7 ounces)* is anything but gentle. It is mostly just water, alcohol, and glycerin. Alcohol is irritating, but this line seems to be in love with it, although many other cosmetics lines have let go of this offending ingredient.

☺ $$$ **Milk Cleanser, for Normal to Combination Skin** *($25 for 6.5 ounces)* is a detergent-based cleanser that uses sodium lauryl sulfate, which is fairly drying for most skin types; however, there doesn't seem to be much in here, so it shouldn't be a problem. It also contains a minuscule amount of milk, but milk has no cleansing or moisturizing effect on the face, so it doesn't matter anyway. This can be an OK cleanser for someone with normal to dry skin, but at these prices I would use Cetaphil Gentle Skin Cleanser before this stuff any day.

☺ $$$ **Sensitive Skin Cleansing Treatment** *($23 for 7 ounces)* is basically a lightweight toner that uses a standard detergent cleansing agent and glycerin to remove excess makeup. It is OK but incredibly ordinary and overpriced, and you'll need to use a lot of it to clean your face even once.

☺ $$$ **Gentle Eye Makeup Remover** *($17 for 4 ounces)* is a standard, completely ordinary eye-makeup remover. It's not bad, but wiping off makeup is always risky for the skin, in terms of sagging, especially in the eye area.

☺ $$$ **Gentle Eye Makeup Remover Pads** *($17 for 60 pads)* is similar to the remover above only it provides the wipe-off pads.

☹ **Clear Astringent, Treatment Cleanser for Normal to Oily Skin** *($23 for 7 ounces)* is a serious problem for most skin types. It contains mostly water, alcohol, and glycerin. Alcohol irritates skin causing redness, dryness, and flaking.

☹ **Controlling Astringent, Pore Refining Lotion for Excessively Oily Skin, Day and Night Treatment** *($28 for 7 ounces)* is almost identical to the product above, but this one contains talc. Talc can absorb oil, but it can also cause makeup to go on poorly when trying to blend over it. The same review as above applies.

☹ **Skin Application Clarifying Lotion, for Excessively Oily and Blemished**

Skin *($27 for 7 ounces)* is similar to the two astringents above, but with salicylic acid. Salicylic acid as an exfoliant has some good points, but in an alcohol base it can only cause problems, irritating the skin and causing more oil production.

☹ **White Astringent, Pore Refining Lotion for Normal to Oily Skin, Night Treatment** *($28 for 7 ounces)* is almost identical to the product above, and the same review applies.

☺ $$$ **Active Skin Replenishing Cream, Super Rich Nourishing Cream** *($39 for 1.85 ounces)* is incredibly emollient, and best only for someone with extremely dry skin. What this moisturizer is doing in the middle of all these drying soaps and toners is at best confusing. This product contains many ingredients that could cause breakouts, including isopropyl myristate, lanolin, sesame oil, and beeswax.

☺ $$$ **Continual Action Cream Age Protection with Kalaya Oil** *($45 for 1.7 ounces)* is a very good emollient moisturizer for dry skin but not because of the kalaya oil (emu oil), although it is a good moisturizing ingredient.

☺ $$$ **Eye Care for Sensitive Eyes, Enriched with Kalaya Oil** *($45 for 1 ounce)* is similar to the one above except more emollient, though the same basic review applies.

☺ $$$ **Eye Rest Pads** *($16 for 60 pads)* contain aloe, tea, fragrance, and preservatives. What can I say, these won't hurt the skin, unless you are allergic to the tea or rose water, but they won't do anything but your waste your time and money.

☺ $$$ **Highly Active Collagen Cream** *($44 for 1.85 ounces)* contains mostly water, lanolin, mineral oil, thickeners, petrolatum, collagen, and preservatives. This is a good emollient moisturizer for someone with super-dry skin, but there is nothing in here that will alter the aging process in the least.

☺ $$$ **Hydrating Lotion Advanced Skin Conditioning** *($38 for 1.75 ounces)* is a good moisturizer for someone with dry skin. It contain water, slip agents, silicone, thickeners, plant extracts, more thickeners, water-binding agents, and preservatives.

☺ $$$ **Nutri Performance Cream, Soothing Emollient to Help Nourish Dry Skin** *($39 for 1.85 ounces)* contains mostly water, thickeners, petrolatum, slip agents, thickeners, lanolin oil, more thickeners, and preservatives. This is an ordinary but extremely emollient moisturizer for someone with super-dry skin. It contains several ingredients that could cause problems for someone who tends to break out.

☺ $$$ **Nutri Performance Eye Care Cream** *($35 for 0.5 ounce)* contains mostly water, lanolin, thickeners, plant oils, lanolin oil, water-binding agents, vitamin A, and preservatives. This is a very emollient moisturizer for someone with super-dry skin, but it contains several ingredients that can cause breakouts. It does contain a minuscule amount of vitamin A and some trendy water-binding agent, but not enough to mention.

☺ **$$$ Revitalizing Cream with Plant Extracts** *($44 for 1.7 ounces)* is a moisturizer that contains three different AHAs, totaling about 5% AHAs in a moisturizing base of petrolatum, thickeners, and silicone. The plant extracts are so far down the ingredient list they're hard to see. In many ways this product is extremely similar to Pond's Age Defying Cream, but at four times the price.

☺ **$$$ Revitalizing Lotion with Plant Extracts** *($32 for 1 ounce)* is similar to the one above only in lotion form.

☺ **$$$ Revitalizing Lotion Advance Strength with Plant Extracts** *($35 for 1 ounce)* is similar to the one above except it contains about 8% AHA and includes glycolic acid; the same basic review applies.

☺ **$$$ Superfatted Cream, Rich Nourishing Cream for Dry Skin** *($70 for 4 ounces)* is one of the most overpriced standard formulations around. All this product contains is petrolatum, lanolin, mineral oil, and beeswax! It is great for very dry skin, but the price is just a joke.

☹ **SPF 15 Oil Free Sunspray** *($18 for 4 ounces)* doesn't contain avobenzone, titanium dioxide, or zinc oxide, and is not recommended.

☺ **$$$ SPF 15 Self-Tanning Sunblock with Plant Extracts, Medium Shade** *($19 for 4 ounces)* is a standard dihydroxyacetone self-tanner that includes sunscreen in the formula. The sunscreen does include titanium dioxide, but it can be a mistake to use this as your only sunscreen. If you're spending long days outside it needs to be reapplied, and there is only so much tan you can build with these products.

☺ **$$$ SPF 15 Sunblock Face Cream with Plant Extracts** *($39 for 1.85 ounces)* contains titanium dioxide in part, plus a host of standard thickening agents. If you use this sunscreen right it will be gone in less than a week, which makes this a very expensive way to get protection from the sun.

☺ **$$$ Sunblock SPF 15 Waterproof Lotion with Plant Extracts** *($18 for 4 ounces)* is similar to the one above only in lotion form. The same basic review applies, except that this one is far more reasonably priced. It's still on the high end, given the amount of your body that needs to be covered to protect from sun damage. There is nothing about this product that limits its use to just the face.

☺ **$$$ Sunblock SPF 25 Waterproof Lotion with Plant Extracts** *($18 for 4 ounces)* is similar to the one above, only with a higher SPF.

☹ **SPF 15 Waterproof Sunspray with Plant Extracts** *($18 for 4 ounces)* doesn't contain avobenzone, titanium dioxide, or zinc oxide, and is not recommended.

☹ **SPF 25 Sunblock Lotion** *($18 for 4 ounces)* doesn't contain avobenzone, titanium dioxide, or zinc oxide, and is not recommended.

☹ **SPF 30 Stick with Plant Extracts, for Lips and Sensitive Areas** *($12 for 0.15 ounce)* doesn't contain avobenzone, titanium dioxide, or zinc oxide, and is not recommended.

☺ **$$$ Normalizing Mask Liquid, for Excessively Oily Skin** *($15 for 4 ounces of the liquid; $15 for 3 ounces of the powder)* are a liquid and powder you mix together to create a mask that is supposed to absorb oil. It is basically just clay, water, and pH balancer. It can absorb oil, but not as well as plain old milk of magnesia (which is liquid magnesium).

☹ **Normalizing Mask, for Normal to Oily Skin** *($22 for 2.5 ounces)* is just water, clay, and alcohol. It won't normalize anyone's skin, but it can be extremely irritating.

☺ **$$$ Triple Performance Moisture Mask with Kalaya Oil** *($25 for 1.7 ounces)* is a good emollient mask for dry skin. It contains several emollient ingredients that could trigger breakouts, so this is only appropriate for very dry skin. Emu oil (kalaya) is a good emollient but there is nothing about this oil that provides miraculous properties for the skin.

☺ **$$$ Moisture Mask for Dry Skin** *($22 for 2.2 ounces)* is a good emollient mask for dry skin. It contains several emollient ingredients that could trigger breakouts, so this is only appropriate for very dry skin.

☹ **Cellulite Streamlining Complex** *($42 for 6.8 ounces)* is a lot of money for what turns out to be an AHA-based moisturizer. It does contain microscopic amounts of seaweed, algae, and kelp, but they have no effect whatsoever on cellulite. This product is quite similar to Alpha Hydrox Lotion, but five times as expensive.

☺ **$$$ Lip Sartinizer, Lip Balm for Dry and Chapped Lips** *($19 for 0.5 ounce)* is an extremely standard petrolatum- and wax-based balm for the lips. At $19 you are buying little more than Vaseline.

Janet Sartin Makeup

☹ **FOUNDATION: Dual Performance Treatment Makeup Extra Coverage** and **Regular Coverage** *($36 and $32 for 7 ounces)* come in the largest foundation containers I've ever seen, but neither formula qualifies as a "treatment." They are virtually indistinguishable from Clinique's Pore Minimizer foundation, and they have the same problems. Both contain mostly alcohol, which can cause irritation, dryness, and increased redness. There is no reason for any skin type to consider these foundations.

☹ **NutriPerformance Treatment Makeup** *($31)* has a very sheer, soft matte finish with a slight sheen, but it comes in only five shades, which is absurdly limited, and three of those colors are extremely peach or rose. Sand and Beige are the only possibilities. It won't reduce wrinkles, and the second ingredient, isopropyl myristate, is notorious for causing breakouts.

☹ **Blemish Fix** *($10)* is almost identical to the Dual Performance Makeup, and the same review applies. This one also comes in just five colors, and you only get 0.5 ounce. It won't fix any blemishes and may make matters worse.

☹ <u>CONCEALER:</u> **NutriCover Eye Cream** *($21)* comes in three shades that are unacceptable for most skin tones, and is unusually greasy, easily creasing into the lines around the eyes.

☺ $$$ <u>POWDER:</u> **Dual Performance Compact Powder** *($24)* is a good standard powder that comes in only three OK shades. Don't expect this one to control oil any better than any other pressed powder. **Face Powder Loose** *($21)* is a good soft powder, but rather messy and inconvenient to use.

☺ $$$ <u>BLUSH:</u> The standard **Refined Powder Blush** *($19)* comes in a nice array of 12 colors. It has a slightly dry finish, and while in general I prefer blush that feels silky, this one still works. The shades do have a slight bit of shine, but it ends up being barely noticeable on the skin.

☺ <u>EYESHADOW:</u> Although the Sartin concept of creating your own eyeshadow compact by selecting the shades you want *($10 per color)* and putting them in a compact you purchase *($2.50 for a duo; $3 for a trio)* is nice, most of the colors are extremely shiny and should be avoided. **The only matte colors to consider**, and they are rather attractive and go on nicely, are Toast, Dark Brown, Teakwood, Cocoa, Light Gray, Gray, Dark Gray, Sea Gray, Tan, Cashew, Cameo, Golden, and Pumpkin.

☺ $$$ <u>PENCILS:</u> There are four standard **Eyeliner Pencils** *($12)* and three standard **Lip Liner Pencils** *($12)*. It doesn't get much sparser than this. They are fine but boring. **Cake Eye Liner** *($16)* is just what the name says, but the colors are all way too obvious. Violet, Royal Blue, Midnight, and Turquoise are all too colorful. Midnight Gray is the only one to consider.

☹ <u>MASCARA:</u> **Extra Performance Mascara** *($15.50)* is one of the all-time worst mascaras I've ever tested. You can apply this one for hours and actually lose length, and it smears and smudges.

☺ $$$ <u>BRUSHES:</u> If this line has any strengths, it is in their brush selection *($12 to $19)*. These are, for the most part, very good brushes, with a silky feel and a firm but soft bristle density.

Jergens (Skin Care Only)

The Andrew Jergens Company created the Biore Strips, those strips of gauze-like paper meant to pull blackheads out of the nose and face. Jergens decided to create an identical version with an accompanying skin-care line under their own brand name. You won't find much of a difference between these, and it is unclear why Jergens would want to compete against themselves, but my comments about the Biore Strips apply to the Jergens Pore Strips as well. For more information about Jergens call (800) 742-8798.

☺ **All-Purpose Face Cream** *($2.79 for 6 ounces)* is definitely all-purpose; it's also fairly greasy and thick. It contains mostly mineral oil, water, thickeners, and fragrance. It would be OK for someone with dry skin, but only minimally so.

☺ **Gentle Foaming Face Wash** *($3.89 for 6 ounces)* is a standard but OK detergent-based water-soluble cleanser. There are tiny scrub particles in this cleanser that feel somewhat scratchy. This can be drying for some skin types, but it is still worth considering.

☹ **Naturals Soap with Aloe & Lanolin for Normal to Dry Skin** *($1.89 for 9.5 ounces)* is a standard tallow-based bar soap that also contains some lanolin. The lanolin won't undo the drying effect of the soap or prevent the breakouts tallow can cause.

☹ **Naturals Soap with Vitamin E & Chamomile for Sensitive Skin** *($1.89 for 9.5 ounces)* is almost identical to the soap above, and the same review applies. Nothing about this soap makes it appropriate for sensitive skin.

☺ **Aloe Enriched Lotion, for Very Dry Skin** *($2.99 for 6 ounces)* contains mostly water, glycerin, thickeners, lanolin, silicone, mineral oil, more thickeners, fragrance, and preservatives. This is a good basic moisturizer for very dry skin.

☹ **Daily Nourishing Cream Alpha & Beta Hydroxy Complex** *($6.59 for 2 ounces)* contains a minimal amount of AHA and a form of salicylic acid that is not effective in exfoliation, but the pH is too high to make any of this work for cell turnover.

☹ **Original Scent Lotion, for Dry Skin** *($2.99 for 6 ounces)* is a very standard moisturizer with alcohol as the second ingredient. It's probably there as an emulsifier, but my concern is that in this quantity it could be irritating for the skin.

☹ **Protective Moisture Lotion SPF 15 with Vitamin E** *($6.59 for 4 ounces)* doesn't contain avobenzone, zinc oxide, or titanium dioxide in the active ingredients, and is not recommended.

☺ **Replenishing Moisture Lotion Vitamin E Enriched** *($6.59 for 4 ounces)* is a very standard moisturizer of mostly water, glycerin, thickeners, vitamin E, silicone, fragrance, and preservative. It can be OK for slightly dry skin.

☺ **Ultra Healing Cream, for Extra Dry Skin** *($4.99 for 8 ounces)* is a good basic, petrolatum-based moisturizer for very dry skin, but the amount of AHA is too small and the pH to high for it to be an exfoliant.

☺ **Ultra Healing Lotion, for Extra Dry Skin** *($2.99 for 6 ounces)* is similar to the one above and the same basic review applies.

☺ **Ultra Healing Lotion, Fragrance Free, for Extra Dry Skin** *($3.49 for 10 ounces)* is similar to the one above and the same review applies.

☺ **Vitamin E Enriched Lotion, for Very Dry Skin** *($2.99 for 6 ounces)* is similar to the one above and the same review applies.

☹ **Pore Cleansing Strips** *($3.99 for 5 nose strips)* are the Biore strips, repackaged under the Jergens label, so please refer to that "unhappy face" review.

Joan Simmons Brushes

Imagine a tailor without a sewing machine or a needle and thread, or a stockbroker without a computer and *The Wall Street Journal*. Every task requires appropriate tools in order to perform the labor properly. Applying makeup is no different. Using professional-size brushes is the only way to apply makeup successfully, period. The little sponge-tip applicators, tiny blush brushes, and scratchy eyebrow brushes that come with cosmetics are a total waste and serve no purpose for professional makeup application. Joan Simmons Brushes *($5.50 to $27.50)* are as good an option as you will find for professional-size brushes, and they are reasonably priced. I have found these brushes at major department stores all over the country. Look for them at Nordstrom, Macy's, Saks, or any upper-end department store in your area.

☺ There are more than a dozen brushes, and most are very good, but some are positively a waste of money. **Foundation Applicator** *($7)* has a big sponge on one end of the handle. Although the idea isn't bad, a thin, round, hand-held sponge is easier to use and for a fraction of the price. **Whirly EyeLash Separator** *($3.40)* is a dry mascara brush meant to separate the lashes if they clump together. You could easily take an old mascara brush, wash it, and use it instead for free. **Blush Blender** *($10)* is a flat-edged, severely shaped brush that can't blend blush well at all. The best it can do is stripe on the color. All of the other brushes are superior and, depending on your makeup needs, worth a close look. Call (609) 655-5252 to find out if these brushes are distributed in your area.

Jurlique (Skin Care Only)

Jurlique's world is immersed in concepts like "natural," "miracles," and "belief." Jurlique is supposed to be the "purest skin care on earth, suitable for all skin types, and completely nonacnegenic. No chemicals, artificial preservatives, colors, or fragrance added." The products don't seem as important as the faith and virtue and environmental sensibility projected in the claims.

I found these claims to be completely unwarranted and contradictory. I won't get into the whole natural thing again—well, maybe a little. All of the plants in the products sound really nice, and they are mostly grown in Australia (Jurlique is an Australian company), but there is no evidence that they are beneficial for the skin or preferable to synthetic ingredients. Also, these products are supposed to be nonchemical. Even water is a chemical from a formulary point of view, but Jurlique seems to be saying that anything that doesn't sound like a plant isn't natural. Well, what kind of plant is polysorbate-20? What kind of plant is cetyl palmitate? And what about lactic acid? Lactic acid may start with milk, but I wouldn't put it on my cereal in this form. (Though even if you could eat it, that doesn't mean it would be good for your skin; you can eat a lemon, but put it on your skin or near your eyes and it burns.)

Also, despite Jurlique's claims of being nonacnegenic, many ingredients in these products can indeed clog pores or cause breakouts, including safflower oil, avocado oil, alcohol, orange oil, and jojoba oil. Furthermore, these products absolutely do contain fragrance. What do the owners of Jurlique think lavender oil (a photosensitizer) and geranium oil are? You can attribute any miracle to these ingredients you like, but they are volatile oils, they impart fragrance, and they are potentially skin irritants. So much for nonacnegenic, fragrance-free, and good for all skin types.

Whether or not Jurlique is the purest skin care on earth is inconsequential. What I found bizarre is the notion that these products are based on "alchemy." That's what their brochure says! My dictionary says alchemy is witchcraft and magic. How's that for scientific validation and research? They claim alchemy is a lost ancient science. Personally, I am not into lost ancient sciences. Back in alchemy's heyday, being sick with just about any disease meant death. Many people didn't live much past 40, women died in childbirth, infant mortality rates were sky-high, and the sun was thought to revolve around the Earth. The notion that modern science is bad compared with the magic of the past is unrealistic, naive thinking.

When you get through all of Jurlique's hype, which borders on the cultish, what is most fascinating is that these products do not utilize a reliable preservative system. Honey and alcohol seem to be the main ingredients used to preserve their products. However, alcohol and honey are not considered stable or dependable preservatives by anyone but Jurlique. Luckily, the products do come in tiny containers ($15 for a 1.4-ounce container of cleanser). You may very well use these up in one or two weeks, before they have a chance of becoming contaminated. Of course, that makes your yearly expenditure on skin care rather frighteningly high.

Now, lack of preservatives is an interesting concept, but it is also risky. Bacterial contamination is a serious concern (you wouldn't want to get a contaminated product in your eyes, for instance), especially with a product that is primarily food. How long would a cup of tea or plant oil last in your bathroom before it got moldy and started to smell bad? According to every cosmetic chemist I've ever interviewed, a good preservative system (one that prevents bacterial growth) is essential to prevent this from happening. Jurlique's boxes say the products should be stored below 30 degrees Centigrade or below 86 degrees Fahrenheit. Those temperatures won't help preserve anything. Some companies, like Fancl International, a Japanese company that doesn't utilize preservatives, honestly recommend you store their products in a refrigerator to prevent contamination.

For people who are allergic to preservatives, preservative-free formulations could be a godsend. For them, the possibility of an allergic reaction to a preservative is the lesser of the two evils if contamination is a concern. But if you aren't allergic to preservatives, nothing in these products will lower your risk of an allergic reaction. Quite the contrary: there are lots of other things in here that can cause your skin to react.

I have to admit, my reviews of the Jurlique products may sound repetitive. They are a strange blend of foods like tahini (that's sesame butter) and wax-like thickening agents, including synthetic ingredients like polysorbate, cetyl palmitate, glyceryl monostearate, and xanthan gum. I never recommend this much oil on the face for anything but very dry skin. Most of these products contain thick, fatty acid–type plant oils that can cause breakouts or clog pores. They can also form whiteheads. Furthermore, the formulas are astonishingly similar. Product after product contains the same oils and plant combinations. Finally, I really am concerned about the lack of preservatives. Other than that, if you are looking for natural, and you have a sizable budget to boot, Jurlique offers enough natural products to satisfy the natural fanatic in anyone. If you want more information about Jurlique call their Atlanta store at (800) 854-1110.

☹ **Face Wash Cream Deep Purifying Treatment** *($15.39 for 1.4 ounces)* contains mostly almonds, water, plant extracts, sesame butter, alcohol (as the preservative), water-binding agent, aloe, more plant extracts, honey, lactic acid, thickener, and fragrance. There isn't enough lactic acid in here to be a problem for the eyes, but this is primarily a wipe-off product with nuts as the scrub agent. You know what I think of wiping and scrubbing.

☹ **Cleansing Lotion Make-up Remover** *($21.55 for 3.4 ounces)* contains mostly water, tea water, plant oils, water-binding agent, alcohol (as the preservative), thickener, emollient, and fragrance. Oils will indeed let you wipe off makeup, but I never recommend wiping because daily pulling at the skin can cause sagging.

☺ **Day Care Conditioner Herbal Water** *($23.59 for 3.4 ounces)* contains mostly water, tea water, water-binding agent, alcohol, aloe, soothing agent, and fragrance. In this form the alcohol is most likely an irritant. Still, it seems to be a minimal amount, and if you aren't allergic to all the plants in here, this can be an OK toner.

☺ **$$$ Herbal Extract Recovery Mist** *($33.89 for 1 ounce)* is similar to the product above but minus the alcohol. This can be a good toner for someone with normal to dry skin.

☹ **Pure Rosewater Freshener Spray** *($21.69 for 3.4 ounces)* contains mostly rose water, quince gel (quince is fruit like apple or pear), aloe, lactic acid (not enough to be an exfoliant), and fragrance. Rose water smells nice, but I wouldn't recommend putting fragrance on anyone's face.

☺ $$$ **Chamomile-Rose Aromatic Hydrating Concentrate** *($30.75 for 1.7 ounces)* contains plant extracts, water, plant oil, fragrance, thickener, and alcohol (as the preservative). This can be a good though highly fragrant moisturizer for dry skin, but a problem for sensitive skin.

☺ $$$ **Day Care Face Cream** *($23.59 for 1.4 ounces)* contains mostly water, tea water, plant oils, water-binding agent, thickener, aloe, more plant oils, emollient, thickeners, and fragrance. This would be a good emollient moisturizer for someone with dry skin.

☺ $$$ **Day Care Face Lotion** *($24.69 for 1 ounce)* is virtually identical to the product above, but in lotion form.

☺ $$$ **Eye Gel** *($43.09 for 0.53 ounce)* contains mostly water, tea water, quince gel, aloe, plant oil, several water-binding agents, thickener, and plant extracts. This can be a good lightweight moisturizer for someone with normal to slightly dry skin who doesn't have a problem with the grapefruit extract or evening primrose oil.

☺ $$$ **Herbal Extract Recovery Gel** *($33.89 for 1 ounce)* contains mostly tea water, water-binding agent, aloe, plant oils, and fragrance. This can be a good lightweight moisturizer for someone with normal to slightly dry skin.

☺ $$$ **Herbal Recovery Gel** *($46.69 for 1 ounce)* is virtually identical to the product above except for the price. This one does contain lactic acid, but not enough and not in the right pH to be an exfoliant.

☹ **Lavender-Lavandin Aromatic Hydrating Concentrate** *($30.75 for 1.7 ounces)* is primarily lavender oil, water, thickener, and alcohol (as the preservative). Lavender oil is not only highly fragrant, it is also a photosensitizer. This product is not recommended.

☺ $$$ **Moisturizer Cream** *($19.19 for 1.4 ounces)* contains mostly water, tea water, water-binding agent, plant oil, thickener, aloe, more plant oils, lactic acid, and fragrance. This is a good emollient moisturizer for someone with dry skin. It does contain lactic acid, but not enough and not in the right pH to be an exfoliant.

☺ $$$ **Wrinkle Softener Beauty Cream for Face, Eye Area and Decollete** *($18.49 for 0.2 ounce)* contains mostly water, tea water, plant oil, water-binding agents, thickeners, emollient, aloe, lactic acid, and fragrance. This product is sold in an amount that is beyond small, but a pound of it would cost more than $1,500. For some tea water and plant oils! It is a good moisturizer for dry skin, but nothing in it is unique or special enough to rate even a fraction of the price.

☺ $$$ **Moist Face Sun Lotion, SPF 15+ Broadband UV Sunscreen** *($24.69 for 1 ounce)* is a good titanium dioxide–based sunscreen for someone with normal to dry skin, but the price and size are absurd.

☺ $$$ **Deep Penetrating Cream Mask** *($28.75 for 1.7 ounces)* contains clay, water, tea water, plant oil, water-binding agent, emollient, aloe, lactic acid, thickener, and fragrance. This would be a good mask for someone with dry skin.

☹ **Moor Purifying Mask** *($28.75 for 1.7 ounces)* contains mostly clay, tea water, water-binding agent, almond meal, sesame butter, plant oil, lactic acid, and vitamin E. The almonds can be a bit rough on dry skin, but because of the sesame butter, which can clog pores, it's hard to recommend it for oily skin either.

☺ **Lip Care Balm** *($14.99 for 0.3 ounce)* is a good, rather standard emollient lip balm for dry lips. It contains castor oil, plant oils, thickeners, and fragrance.

Kiehl's (Skin Care Only)

How did this very expensive, obscure skin-care line become so well known? Especially when you consider that the company doesn't advertise (although it does have a PR firm that handles its press relations that net a lot of attention in fashion magazines). Kiehl's has definitely gotten value out of their attention-getting media mentions.

As the company's name implies, the line has been around for quite some time; it has its origins in a family-owned pharmacy. Still, the products hardly warrant excitement or even mild enthusiasm. Most of them are surprisingly ordinary, with a dusting of natural ingredients almost always at the very end of the ingredient list, well past the preservatives. That amounts to little more than a token attempt to make the products appear more natural to consumers, who want to believe a plant or vitamin must somehow be better for the skin than something that sounds more chemical. Nevertheless, that token amount is enough to allow Kiehl's to brag about how its products nourish the skin or are more environmentally friendly, even though that may only be true for less than 1 percent of the product's content.

Of course, those who know better understand that vitamins can't nourish the skin; that using nonfat milk and plant extracts means the amount of preservative in a product must be increased to prevent deterioration; and that while plant oils may be moisturizing, they are not wonder ingredients.

The company's most interesting claim is that its products are all made by hand, just the way they were when the original Kiehl's pharmacy began selling cosmetics in 1851. Today, given the wide distribution of Kiehl's products—they are available at Bergdorf Goodman, Neiman Marcus, Barney's, Harrods, and many other stores— that claim is extremely hard to swallow. The person I talked to at Kiehl's said each product is made the way I would make a cake. But I've never baked thousands of cakes at once, or baked one cake that could serve thousands of people. I can't stir 100 pounds of flour and water; how can someone stir 100 pounds of water and waxes? Yes, it is all hand-stirred, she insisted. Even if that were true, which I strongly doubt, what extra benefit is there to hand-stirring a cosmetic anyway? It's just more personal, she said; there's better control. It may *sound* more personal, but the possibility of error or contamination is much greater.

Regardless of how the products are processed, the bottom line is, Can they do what they claim and are they worth the money? In this case, the products consist of totally ordinary ingredients, despite the fact that they are called special or natural. Many ingredients are questionable for sensitive skin types and in some instances would be irritating for any skin type. For more information about Kiehl's call (800) KIEHLS-1.

☹ **Foaming Non-Detergent Washable Cleanser** *($13.50 for 8 ounces)* is not in the least a nondetergent cleanser: the second ingredient is sodium C14-16 olefin sulfate, a cleansing agent in shampoos that is known for stripping hair color. I would call this a standard detergent facial cleanser that can dry out the skin.

☺ **Gentle Foaming Facial Cleanser for Dry to Normal Skin Types** *($13.50 for 8 ounces)* is a standard detergent-based cleansing agent, that also contains a small amount of plant oils. The plant oils in here can leave a greasy film on the skin so this would only be appropriate and worth considering for someone with very dry skin.

☺ **Oil-Based Cleanser and Makeup Remover** *($10.50 for 4 ounces)* at least has an honest name. This very greasy cleanser needs to be wiped off like cold cream and can leave a film on the face. The second ingredient is isopropyl myristate, notorious for causing breakouts. The cleanser also contains lanolin oil, which is emollient but can be a problem for sensitive skin types. If you like grease this product is an option.

☹ **Rare-Earth Oatmeal Milk Facial Cleanser #1 (Mild)** *($17.50 for 8 ounces)* doesn't contain any earth that is remotely rare, just standard kaolin and bentonite, better known as clay. But I guess if you want to charge this kind of money for clay and standard detergent cleansing agents, you have to call it rare. The minuscule amounts of vitamins, nonfat milk, and oat flour are included to boost the natural appearance of a completely unnatural product.

☹ **Rare-Earth Oatmeal Milk Facial Cleanser #2 (Medium Strength)** *($17.50 for 8 ounces)* is very similar to the facial cleanser above, only much more drying.

☹ **Rare-Earth Foaming Cleanser #2 (Medium Strength)** *($17.50 for 8 ounces)* contains both sodium lauryl sulfate and TEA-lauryl sulfate as the main detergent cleansing agents, both of which are extremely drying and irritating. I definitely would not recommend this for the face. The standard natural ingredients are listed well after the preservatives, and they won't make this cleanser any less irritating.

☺ **Ultra Moisturizing Cleansing Cream** *($16.95 for 8 ounces)* contains mostly water, thickeners, plant oil, more thickeners, preservatives, and plant oil. This is a very ordinary, somewhat greasy wipe-off cleanser that can leave a film on the skin.

☹ **Washable Cleansing Milk A Moisturizing Cleanser for Dry or Sensitive Skin** *($13.50 for 8 ounces)* is not what I would consider a "washable" cleanser. It contains oils that can leave greasy film on the skin. Protein, nonfat milk, and other "natural ingredients" are at the very end of the ingredient list, well after the preservatives, so there aren't enough of them to make this product even vaguely milky.

☺ **Milk, Honey, and Almond Scrub** *($18.50 for 6 ounces)* is a standard scrub that uses ground almonds. It also contains talc and flour, which can be hard to rinse off and can be irritating when rubbed into the skin. The nonfat milk, plant oils, and vitamins are at the end of the ingredient list. The oils may leave a greasy residue.

☺ **Ultra Moisturizing Buffing Cream with Scrub Particles** *($16.50 for 4 ounces)* is a scrub that uses a synthetic scrub ingredient; it also contains thickening agents and oils. It would be suitable for someone with very dry skin.

☹ **Pineapple and Papaya Facial Scrub Made with Real Fruit** *($26.50 for 4 ounces)* does contain pineapple and papaya, but they are potent skin irritants. (Ever get pineapple on abraded skin or in your eyes? It hurts.) This is a standard detergent cleanser with cornmeal as a scrub. You can use plain cornmeal if you want a scrub similar to this for a lot less money and without the irritation from the other ingredients.

☹ **Rare-Earth Foaming Cleaner #1 (Mild) with Scrub Grains** *($18.50 for 8 ounces)* uses sodium lauryl sulfate, which can be extremely drying and irritating, and is not recommended.

☹ **Blue Astringent Herbal Lotion** *($12.50 for 8 ounces; $22 for 16 ounces)* contains mostly water, alcohol, camphor, menthol, and aluminum chlorohydrate. Yes, that's right, the stuff used in *antiperspirants*. Not only is the alcohol drying and irritating, but the aluminum chlorohydrate can cause infection of the hair follicle. What were the chemists who made this product thinking?

☺ **Calendula Herbal Extract Toner Alcohol-Free** *($18.50 for 4 ounces)* contains plant extracts (tea) and preservatives. If you aren't allergic to the plants this tea water can be OK, but there is nothing in here particularly helpful for skin.

☹ **Cucumber Herbal Alcohol-Free Toner for Dry or Sensitive Skin** *($13.95 for 8 ounces)* is alcohol-free, but not irritant-free. It contains balm mint, pine needle, camphor, and sulfonated oils, all of which can be serious irritants. There is nothing about this product appropriate for sensitive skin.

☺ **French Rosewater** *($10.50 for 8 ounces)*, as the name implies, is mostly rose water, which is merely fragranced glycerin, not particularly helpful for skin.

☹ **Herbal Toner with Mixed Berries and Extracts** *($19.95 for 8 ounces)* does have berries but it also has peppermint and lemongrass, which can be irritating for skin.

☹ **Rosewater Facial Freshener-Toner** *($11.50 for 8 ounces)* is mostly alcohol with rose fragrance. It can be irritating and drying.

☺ **$$$ Creme d'Elegance Repairateur Superb Tissue Repairateur Creme** *($25.50 for 2 ounces)* contains mostly water, plant oil, thickeners, slip agent, more thickeners, lanolin oil, more thickeners, petrolatum, lanolin, and preservatives. Regardless of what language you say it in, this cream will not repair skin. It would be a good moisturizer for someone with very dry skin.

☺ **Kiehl's Original Formula Eye Cream, Ultra Nourishing** *($10.50 for 0.5 ounce)* contains mostly plant oil, thickeners, emollients, and preservatives. It isn't even vaguely nourishing, but it is a very good, though ordinary, moisturizer for someone with dry skin.

☺ **Panthenol Protein Moisturizing Face Cream** *($22.50 for 4 ounces)* contains mostly water, thickeners, glycerin, water-binding agents, vitamins, and preservatives. This is a good basic moisturizer for someone with dry skin. The really interesting ingredients are listed way after the preservatives and are hardly worth mentioning.

☺ **Sodium PCA Oil-Free Moisturizer** *($22.50 for 4 ounces)* contains mostly water, silicone, thickeners, water-binding agent, and preservatives. This would be a good moisturizer for someone with normal to dry skin. There are thickening agents here that can be a problem for someone with oily skin.

☹ **Superb Total Dermal Protection Face Cream with SPF 8** *($22.95 for 2 ounces; $39.99 for 4 ounces)* is exaggerating when it claims to provide "total dermal protection" with an SPF of only 8, plus it doesn't contain any UVA protecting ingredients, and is absolutely not recommended.

☺ **$$$ Light Nourishing Eye Cream** *($15.95 for 0.5 ounce)* uses a film-forming agent as a way to smooth the skin and keep water in. Other than that, it is a good ordinary moisturizer for normal to dry skin. The so-called nourishing ingredients, vitamins A and E, can't nourish the skin, but there are enough so that they could be considered antioxidants.

☺ **$$$ Moisturizing Eye Balm with Pure Vitamins A & E** *($14.50 for 0.5 ounce)* contains mostly plant oils, thickeners, vitamins E and A, more plant oil, lanolin oil, cocoa butter, and preservatives. This is a very good moisturizer for dry skin. The vitamins can be considered antioxidants.

☺ **$$$ Moisturizing Masque** *($35 for 2 ounces)* contains mostly water, plant oils, thickeners, and preservatives. It is indeed moisturizing and good for someone with dry skin. All of the fancy natural-sounding ingredients are at the end of the ingredient list, but even if there were more, they still couldn't repair skin as this mask claims.

☹ **All-Day Masque Oily-Acne** *($12.50 for 1 ounce)* contains more ingredients that can cause problems for acned oily skin than any other product I've ever reviewed. This product deserves dozens of unhappy faces. What were the formulators of this product thinking?

☹ **Rare-Earth Facial Cleansing Masque** *($16.50 for 5 ounces)* is mostly water, clay, and plant oils. There is nothing rare about the clay in here. It also contains cornstarch, which can be a skin irritant.

☻ **Rare-Earth Face Masque (Gently Astringent for Oily-Acne Skin)** *($13.50 for 4 ounces)* is a sulfur-based clay mask. There is nothing gentle about sulfur, though it is a disinfectant. That wouldn't be all that bad, but there are several thickening agents in this mask that can clog pores and cause breakouts.

☺ **$$$ Soothing and Cleansing Algae Masque for Balancing Skin Types** *($39.95 for 4.5 ounces)* contains nothing that can balance skin and is certainly not suitable for all skin types, particularly not for someone with oily or combination skin. It contains mostly slip agent, thickeners, algae, more thickener, plant oils, and preservatives. This can be a good mask for someone with dry skin.

☻ **Treatment and Concealing Stick for Blemishes** *($14.50 for 0.5 ounce)* contains more ingredients problematic for breakouts than you can imagine, including zinc oxide, lanolin oil (can you believe lanolin oil in a product for acne), isopropyl palmitate, and carnauba wax (that's car wax).

☻ **Ultra Facial Moisturizer with SPF 13** *($27 for 4 ounces)* doesn't contain avobenzone, titanium dioxide, or zinc oxide, and is not recommended.

☻ **Ultra Protection Moisturizing Face Gel with SPF 15** *($29.95 for 1 ounce)* has a good SPF number, an intolerable price, and doesn't contain avobenzone, titanium dioxide, or zinc oxide; it is not recommended.

☻ **Dermal Protection Eye and Throat Cream with SPF 6** *($27.95 for 2 ounces)* does not provide dermal protection with an SPF of only 6 and does not contain avobenzone, zinc oxide, or titanium dioxide, and is absolutely not recommended.

☻ **Ultra Moisturizing Eye Stick with SPF 18 and Vitamin E** *($15.95 for 0.5 ounce)* doesn't contain avobenzone, titanium dioxide, or zinc oxide, and is not recommended.

☻ **Ultra Protection Face Cream and Sunscreen SPF 18 PABA-free** *($40 for 2 ounces)* doesn't contain avobenzone, titanium dioxide, or zinc oxide, and is not recommended.

☹ **$$$ Ultra Moisturizing Concealing Stick with SPF 26 and Vitamin E (Matte) #1** *($19.50 for 4 grams)* is a part titanium dioxide–based sunscreen that also works as a concealer, but not a very good one. This is a fairly greasy concealer that can crease into the lines around the eyes. If you are already using a sunscreen on your face, using another one in your makeup is completely unnecessary and can cause undue irritation.

☹ **$$$ Ultra Moisturizing Concealing Stick with SPF 26 and Vitamin E (Matte) #3** *($19.50 for 0.5 ounce)* is similar to the one above and the same review applies.

☻ **Ultra Protection Moisturizing Eye Gel with SPF 18** *($28.50 for 0.5 ounce)* does not contain avobenzone, titanium dioxide, or zinc oxide, and is not recommended.

The Reviews K

☺ **$$$ Heidegger's All-Sport Water-Resistant Skin Protector with SPF 30** *($17.95 for 4 ounces)* is a good in-part titanium dioxide–based sunscreen that would be good for someone with normal to slightly dry skin.

☹ **Sun Screen—Tan Creme, "Tan Smart—Not Fast," SPF 15** *($15.95 for 8 ounces)* doesn't contain avobenzone, zinc oxide, or titanium dioxide, and is not recommended; so much for a smart sunscreen.

☺ **Sun Shield Sunblock with SPF 15** *($23.50 for 8 ounces)* is a very good nonchemical sunscreen for someone with dry skin.

☹ **Ultra Protection Water-Based Sunscreen Lotion, SPF 24** *($44 for 8 ounces)* doesn't contain avobenzone, zinc oxide, or titanium dioxide, and is not recommended.

☹ **Water-based Sunscreen Lotion With SPF 16** *($35 for 8 ounces)* doesn't contain avobenzone, zinc oxide, or titanium dioxide, and is not recommended.

☺ **Lip Balm #1** *($4.95 for 0.7 ounce)* is a very emollient lip gloss that contains mostly petrolatum, plant oils, lanolin, and preservatives.

☹ **Liquid Body Scrub and Cleanser with Natural Scrub Particles** *($18.50 for 8 ounces)* is mostly TEA-lauryl sulfate and cornmeal. Like sodium lauryl sulfate, TEA-lauryl sulfate can be drying and irritating. If you want to use cornmeal as a scrub, buy it at the grocery store and save your money as well as your skin.

La Prairie

Most all of the products in this line are called "Cellular Treatment." After a while it starts sounding silly. Even the mascara is called "Cellular Treatment Intensified Mascara." It's all incredibly gimmicky and overpriced. Even if your skin could remarkably improve with these products, the prices might kill you. So what do the few women who can afford these prices get for their money? The prestige of knowing they can afford the imperial price tag, period. High-priced skin-care lines attract women who think that the dollars they spend will buy them something special most other women can't afford. To some extent, they're right: they get an immense amount of hype. If you could read and understand the ingredient lists, you would find the prices as ludicrous as I do. Many of La Prairie's claims are based on the use of ingredients such as placental protein, flower and herb extracts, marine collagen, and amino acids. There is no research that indicates any of these ingredients can alter the skin, and product lines in all price ranges contain them, but that doesn't stop La Prairie from trying to convince you that its versions are worth the sky-high prices. In retrospect, despite how marvelous those previous ingredients were supposed to be for the skin, that didn't stop La Prairie from jumping onto the vitamin C, AHA, or licorice extract craze. One should wonder, if placental extract was supposed to be the fountain of youth, what are these other products and ingredients for? For more information about La Prairie call (800) 821-5718.

La Prairie Skin Care

☺ **$$$ Essential Purifying Gel Cleanser** *($50 for 7.3 ounces)* contains mostly water, detergent cleanser, thickener, slip agent, more thickener, more detergent cleanser, and preservative. There are some herb extracts, but they are at the end of the ingredient list, in too minuscule an amount to matter. This cleanser does rinse off, and can be good for someone with dry skin, but it doesn't work to remove makeup without the help of a washcloth. The price is a joke, right?

☺ **$$$ Foam Cleanser** *($50 for 4 ounces)* is a standard detergent-based cleanser that is about as ordinary as they come. It does contain some petrolatum (Vaseline) and silicone to cut the drying effect of the cleansing agents, as well as some anti-irritants, but those are nothing special either and it would just be better if this product didn't contain such drying detergent cleansing agents.

☺ **$$$ Purifying Creme Cleanser** *($50 for 6.8 ounces)* is meant to be rinsed off, but it actually requires a washcloth. This cleanser contains emollient thickening agents, as well as mineral oil and petrolatum, which means it leaves a film on the skin. This is merely a very expensive cold cream.

☺ **$$$ Cellular Eye Make-Up Remover** *($40 for 4.2 ounces)* is a silicone-based wipe-off cleanser that contains some plant extracts and anti-irritants. That's nice, but I wonder if the executives for these companies laugh about the women who believe they're getting something special when they spend this kind of money for such an ordinary product.

☺ **$$$ Essential Exfoliator** *($50 for 7 ounces)* is a standard facial scrub that contains mostly water, mineral oil, thickener, apricot powder, more thickeners, detergent cleanser, and preservative. This is a good scrub for dry skin, but it doesn't rinse off very well and, to say the least, is overpriced for what you get.

☹ **Cellular Purifying Lotion** *($55 for 8.2 ounces)* is a standard alcohol-based toner with a small amount of placental protein thrown in, but that can't compensate for the irritation and dryness caused by the alcohol. Besides, at best, protein extracted from the placenta does what all proteins do for the skin: it acts as a good water-binding agent.

☺ **$$$ Cellular Refining Lotion** *($55 for 8.2 ounces)* is an irritant-free toner that contains mostly water, slip agents, water-binding agents, plant extracts, glycerin, soothing agent, and preservatives. This would be a good toner for most skin types if they aren't allergic to the plant extracts in here, but either way the price tag is preposterous.

☺ **$$$ Age Management Balancer** *($65 for 8.4 ounces)* contains mostly water, several slip agents, plant extracts, water-binding agents, silicone, a tiny amount of AHA (less than 2%), anti-irritant, and preservatives. This is a good, irritant-free toner, but hardly worth the price tag. There is nothing in here that will manage age.

☹ **Age Management Cream Natural with SPF 8** *($125 for 1.7 ounces)* isn't a natural for this kind of money, and you don't even get an SPF 15! This is an embarrassing product and offensive in defining itself as a skin protector.

☹ **Age Management Intensified Emulsion with SPF 8** *($100 for 1.7 ounces)* is similar to the one above and the same review applies.

☺ $$$ **Age Management Eye Repair** *($100 for 0.5 ounce)* contains mostly water; film former; glycerin; thickeners; plant extract; AHAs; more thickeners; plant oil; pH balancer; slip agents; silicone oil; water-binding agents; vitamins A, E, and C; anti-irritant; more water-binding agents; more thickeners; and preservatives. Like most eye creams, this one contains a film former that can help skin look smooth, but it isn't unique to La Prairie. This is a good moisturizer with about 3% AHAs, which can have minor exfoliating properties.

☺ $$$ **Age Management Intensified Serum** *($140 for 1 ounce)* contains about 8% AHAs, which is fine for an exfoliant, but a lot of other 8% AHA products can do the same thing for a *lot* less money. It contains mostly water, AHAs, pH balancer, slip agents, silicone, thickeners, plant extract, more AHAs, water-binding agent, more plant extracts, anti-irritant, and preservatives.

☺ $$$ **Age Management Line Inhibitor** *($100 for 0.5 ounce)* is similar to the Age Management Intensified Serum above, and the same review applies.

☺ $$$ **Age Management Night Cream** *($125 for 1 ounce)* contains mostly water; AHAs; slip agent; pH balancer; film former; thickeners; plant extracts; more thickeners; petrolatum; silicone; more AHAs; anti-irritant; water-binding agents; more thickeners; more plant extracts; vitamins A, E, and C; and preservatives. This 8% AHA product in a moisturizing base would be good for someone with dry skin. But this endless ingredient list looks as if La Prairie just threw everything in, including the kitchen sink. There are a lot of interesting ingredients, but mostly just a dusting of each.

☺ $$$ **Age Management Serum** *($125 for 1 ounce)* is similar to the product above, and the same review applies.

☺ $$$ **Age Management Stimulus Complex PM (Delicate)** *($150 for 1 ounce)* contains mostly water, thickeners, silicone, water-binding agents, vitamins, anti-irritant, and preservatives. Unbelievable, a completely standard product, with one interesting water-binding agent for a ridiculous amount of money. I know there are women out there buying this stuff, and I just find it disheartening that they get sucked into the distortion about what a product like this can do for the skin. It's a good moisturizer for someone with dry skin, that's it.

☺ $$$ **Age Management Stimulus Complex PM (Normal)** *($150 for 1 ounce)* is almost identical to the one above, and the same review applies.

☺ $$$ **Cellular Balancing Complex** *($65 for 1.7 ounces)* contains mostly water, silicone, thickener, slip agent, sunscreen, more silicone, glycerin, several thickeners, water-binding agents, vitamins A and E, and preservatives. This is a good lightweight emollient moisturizer for normal to dry skin. There isn't enough sunscreen to protect skin from sun damage, though.

☺ $$$ **Cellular Brightening System Day Emulsion with SPF 15** *($125 for 1 ounce)* is a good sunscreen with titanium dioxide for an absurd amount of money. How much of this is someone really going to apply liberally at this price, which is the only way to get reliable sun protection? There is nothing in this product that can lighten skin (though any effective sunscreen can improve the appearance of sun damage spots). This product contains licorice extract but I have seen no real evidence that supports its effect on melanin production.

☺ $$$ **Cellular Defense Shield with SPF 15** *($95 for five 0.22-ounce vials)* has an impressive hook, similar to Avon's Anew Formula C Treatment Capsules. The crux of the matter for this product is what vitamin C can do for the skin. Like Avon's Anew, the vitamin C for this product is encapsulated, or, as the La Prairie brochure explains, hermetically sealed. A powdered form of vitamin C is kept separate from the SPF 15 moisturizer. You mix the first of the five tiny vials with the vitamin C and so on, and, violà, you have a stable antioxidant with SPF 15. Even if vitamin C were that exciting of an ingredient (it's not) the ascorbic acid La Prairie uses is considered to be one of the more irritating and least effective.

☺ $$$ **Cellular Defense Shield Eye Cream, SPF 15** *($100 for 0.5 ounce)* is a good titanium dioxide–based moisturizer with lots of emollients and vitamins. Yet given the ingredient listing this is an absurdly overpriced sunscreen. If used correctly it wouldn't even last two days.

☺ $$$ **Cellular Defense Shield Vitamin C Cream** *($125 for 1 ounce)* contains mostly silicone, Vaseline, alcohol, vitamin C, thickeners, emollients, water-binding agents, and preservatives. This is a good, fairly emollient, incredibly overpriced moisturizer for dry skin. Vitamin C is a good ingredient, but the type in here is considered to be one of the more irritating and least effective.

☺ $$$ **Cellular Eye Contour Creme** *($80 for 0.5 ounce)* comes in at $2,560 per pound, yet it is nothing more than a petrolatum-based moisturizer. It is a good emollient moisturizer for someone with dry skin, but the seemingly exciting ingredients you think you're buying come after the preservatives and don't amount to anything more than a dusting.

☺ $$$ **Cellular Neck Cream** *($105 for 1 ounce)* contains mostly water, thickeners, Vaseline, slip agents, water-binding agents, and preservatives similar to the one above, and the same review applies.

☺ **$$$ Cellular Day Creme** *($100 for 1 ounce)* contains mostly water, thickeners, slip agent, plant oil, petrolatum, glycerin, more thickeners, water-binding agent, plant extracts, and preservatives. This is a lot of money for a product that is mostly thickeners and Vaseline, but I think La Prairie was hoping you wouldn't notice, plus without a sunscreen it is a definite no-no for daytime.

☺ **$$$ Cellular Night Cream** *($105 for 1 ounce)* is a rather rich moisturizer for dry skin; it contains mostly water, petrolatum, thickeners, slip agent, more thickeners, glycerin, standard water-binding agent, silicone, and preservatives. This rather boring petrolatum-based moisturizer would be good for someone with dry skin, if she could survive the damage to her budget.

☺ **$$$ Cellular Skin Conditioner** *($70 for 4 ounces)* contains mostly water, thickeners, glycerin, pH balancer, more thickeners, water-binding agents, plant extract, and preservatives. This is a fairly ordinary but good moisturizer for someone with dry skin.

☺ **$$$ Cellular Wrinkle Cream** *($105 for 1 ounce)* contains mostly mineral oil, water, petrolatum, thickeners, slip agent, more thickeners, placental protein, and preservatives. This standard mineral oil–based moisturizer is very emollient and would be good for someone with dry skin, but calling this product ordinary is an understatement. Please don't fall for the notion that placental protein can somehow restore youth to your skin. It can't. And if this one is a wrinkle cream what are all these other products doing here?

☺ **$$$ Essence of Skin Caviar Cellular Eye Complex with Caviar Extract** *($85 for 0.5 ounce)* contains mostly water, slip agents, thickener, water-binding agents, soothing agent, thickener, and preservatives. This is a good lightweight moisturizer for someone with dry skin. It does contain 0.04% caviar, which amounts to half an egg—now, isn't that exciting?

☺ **$$$ Extrait of Skin Caviar Cellular Face Complex with Caviar Extract** *($85 for 1 ounce)* contains mostly water, silicones, glycerin, thickeners, water-binding agents, vitamins A and E, plant extracts, soothing agent, and preservatives. This is a good lightweight moisturizer for someone with dry skin.

☹ **$$$ Skin Caviar** *($100 for 2 ounces)* is mostly silicone, some water, slip agents, and water-binding agents contained in small gelatin pellets that break open when you rub them on the skin. It's a cute idea, but paying $100 for a cute idea isn't all that cute.

☹ **Time Management Moisturizer with SPF 15** *($75 for 1.7 ounces)* doesn't contain avobenzone, titanium dioxide, or zinc oxide, and is not recommended.

☺ **$$$ Soleil Suisse Cellular Anti-Wrinkle Sun Cream SPF 15** *($100 for 1.7 ounces)* is a titanium dioxide–based sunscreen that would be good for someone with dry skin. It is as ordinary as sunscreens come.

☺ $$$ **Soleil Suisse Cellular Self Tan for the Body Spray Auto-Bronzant** *($75 for 5 ounces)* contains, like all self-tanners, the active ingredient dihydroxyacetone. It will turn skin brown exactly the same way a $6 self-tanner will.

☺ $$$ **Soleil Suisse Self Tanner for Face** *($75 for 1.7 ounces)* has the same review as the one above.

☹ $$$ **Cellular Balancing Mask** *($110 for six 0.12-ounce ampoules)* is a two-part mask that you mix together. The liquid is mostly water, citric acid (an astringent and possible skin irritant), aloe vera, and preservatives. The powder contains mostly sodium bicarbonate (yes, baking soda), clay, thickeners, talc, placental protein, collagen, and fragrance. Minuscule amounts of aloe vera and baking soda are not going to balance anyone's skin, and the placental protein is a water-binding agent, nothing more.

☺ $$$ **Cellular Moisture Mask** *($65 for 1 ounce)* is a good mask for someone with dry skin. It contains water, plant oil, film former, thickeners, plant extracts, water-binding agents, and preservatives.

☹ $$$ **Cellular Purifying Clay Mask** *($65 for 1 ounce)* is a standard clay mask that contains plant oils and plant extracts. Clay can be drying, but the emollients can make up for that. This mask does contain menthol which can be a skin irritant.

☹ $$$ **Cellular Cycle Ampoules for the Face** *($275 for seven 0.1-ounce treatments)*. This one prices out to about $5,700 a pound! They can't be serious. This two-part self-mixed treatment contains the most ordinary assembly of ingredients you could imagine. The liquid contains water, slip agent, water-binding agent, plant extracts, thickeners, fragrance, and preservatives. The powder contains thickener, water, water-binding agents, and more thickener. This isn't even as interesting as a lot of other La Prairie products. Are there really women willing to buy this?

La Prairie Makeup

☹ $$$ <u>FOUNDATION:</u> **Cellular Perfection Flawless with SPF 8** *($75)* has a beautiful soft, smooth, creamy thick texture that feels wonderful on dry skin, but the SPF 8 isn't much and there is no UVA protection. **These colors are the best:** 200, 300, 500, and 600. **These are the colors to avoid:** 100, 400, 700, and 800.

☹ $$$ **Cellular Oil-Free Matte Foundation with SPF 8** *($55)* is a liquid foundation with a decent matte texture and it blends on soft and even. The limited color selection is impressive, but the SPF 8 is unimpressive and there is no UVA protection. **These colors are the best:** 15, 20, 30, 50, 70, and 80. **These are the only colors to avoid:** 40 and 60.

☹ $$$ **Cellular Treatment Foundation Satin with SPF 8** *($55)* offers only a handful of colors, and most are terrible, plus the SPF 8 isn't worth it, and there is no UVA protection. **These are the best colors:** 4, 4.5, and 5.5. **These colors are too peach, pink, or rose:** 1, 3.2, 3.5, 5.7, and 6.7.

☺ $$$ Cellular Treatment Perfecting Primer *($50)* is a sheer light moisturizer that is white and, not surprisingly, leaves a white finish on the skin. If you think giving your face a white cast will "perfect" your look, this is for you, but I think it's an inane waste.

☺ $$$ <u>POWDER:</u> **Translucent Pressed Powder** *($36)* isn't protective but it is a good standard talc-base powder with a soft powdery finish. **Foundation Finish Loose Powder** *($40)* is a standard powder with a very soft satiny finish.

☹ <u>BLUSH:</u> **Cellular Treatment Powder Blush** *($35)* has a small selection of soft and pretty colors. The texture is satiny smooth with a silky finish. **Cellular Treatment Creme Blush** *($35)* has a soft but dry finish, which isn't bad, but all the colors are shiny.

☹ <u>EYESHADOW:</u> **Cellular Treatment Eye Colour Singles** *($32)* are all slightly shiny to very shiny. That way, after you've spent a fortune on La Prairie's skin-care products to get rid of wrinkles, you can buy its makeup that helps the eye area look more wrinkly.

☺ $$$ **Cellular Treatment Ensemble de Colour** *($50)* are eyeshadows that come combined with an eyeliner color. These are minimally shiny and of the six shades Les Brun, Les Chocolate, Les Herbes, and Les Platines are great, just overpriced.

☺ $$$ <u>EYE AND BROW SHAPER:</u> **Eye Pencils** *($25)* and **Brow Pencils** *($25)* are just standard pencils; the Brow version has a mascara wand on one end. There are a handful of OK colors, but it is foolish to spend this kind of money on something so ordinary.

☺ $$$ <u>LIPSTICK AND LIP PENCIL:</u> **Matte Lipstick** *($27)* isn't what you and I would call matte, but it does go on rather thick and creamy. **Sheer Lipstick** *($27)*, as the name implies, is more gloss than lipstick. **Moisturizing Tint** *($27)* is fairly sheer, and is more gloss than lipstick. **Lasting Lipstick** *($27)* is a very glossy lipstick except that all of the shades have a strong tint that keeps the color around longer than most. **Lip Pencils** *($25)* are extremely standard pencils with a smooth, slightly dry finish and a handful of good colors, but there is no reason to spend this kind of money other than foolishness or a misguided concept of prestige.

☺ $$$ <u>MASCARA:</u> **Cellular Treatment Intensified Mascara** *($25)*, at this price, should be amazing. It isn't, but it is a good mascara that makes the lashes long, thick, and soft, and doesn't smudge.

Lac-Hydrin (Skin Care Only)

These were the original AHA products sold anywhere! They have been on the market in drugstores for years, and much of what we know about how AHAs behave is a result of these formulations. Lac Hydrin Five (stands for 5% lactic acid) and Lac-

Hydrin Twelve (this one is prescription-only and represents 12% lactic acid) are in the right pH to be effective exfoliants. These aren't elegant formulations but they are some of the best AHA exfoliants available. For more information about Lac Hydrin call Westwood Squibb Pharmaceutical (800) 333-0950.

☺ **Lac-Hydrin Five** or **Lac-Hydrin Twelve** *($9.12 for 7 ounces)* are good 5% or 12% AHA products in a standard petrolatum-based moisturizer. Either of these are only appropriate for someone with dry skin.

Lancome

Lancome remains a very popular line among baby boomers. Prices are steep but relatively reasonable (I use the term "reasonable" loosely) given Lancome's place at the high end of the cosmetics world. This very French line maintains a more casual air, at least when compared to the other European lines sold at the department stores such as Yves St. Laurent, Orlane, or Chanel, whose elitist airs are so thick you can cut them with a knife.

I still like the Lancome display units very much. They are accessible and easy to use, particularly if you want to experiment on your own. I do wish, however, that Lancome would follow the trend of the other makeup lines and divide its blushes, eyeshadows, lipsticks, and lip liners into color groups. Still, their foundation colors and formulations are some of the best around. They are divided into three groups: D for golden, N for neutral, and R for Rose (which isn't all that rose—it's really more peach). There are many superb colors for a wide range of skin tones, from light to dark (including several suitable for African-American skin tones). A few stores in selected cities now sport "supercounters" that take up an entire island and are incredibly user-friendly. The blushes are wonderful and the eye products diverse and interesting, and some of the eyeshadows have a satiny smooth matte finish.

Lancome's skin care is a vast group of products with all the latest bells and whistles. Before you jump into a Lancome product, always check the L'Oreal reviews; you'll find astounding similarities if not identical duplicates for one-fifth the price (the same is true for the makeup products). You did know L'Oreal owns Lancome and BioTherm, right? L'Oreal also recently bought Maybelline, but that's another story. For more information about Lancome call (212) 984-4444.

Lancome Skin Care

☺ **$$$ Ablutia Fraicheur Purifying Foam Cleanser** *($21.50 for 6.4 ounces)* is a very standard detergent-based cleanser that can be drying for some skin types.

☺ **$$$ Clarifiance Oil-Free Gel Cleanser** *($21.50 for 6.4 ounces)* is a very good water-soluble cleanser that takes off all the makeup without irritating the eyes or drying out the skin.

☺ **$$$ Galatee Douceur Milky Creme Cleanser** *($37.50 for 13.5 ounces)* is supposed to be a splash- or tissue-off cleanser for all skin types. It is a standard mineral oil–based wipe-off cleanser that can leave a greasy film on the skin. It also contains isopropyl myristate (the third ingredient), which can cause blackheads. However, it may be good for extremely dry skin, though it needs to be wiped off to get the makeup and the cleanser off.

☺ **$$$ Respectee Extremely Gentle Creme Gel Cleanser** *($23.50 for 6.8 ounces)* is similar to the one above only less greasy. It still needs to be wiped off to get the face clean.

☹ **Pur Controle Cleanser for Oily and Normal to Oily Skin** *($18 for 4.1 ounces)* is a very drying detergent cleanser that contains several cleansing agents known for their harsh effect on the skin, including potassium hydroxide, rather high up on the ingredient list. This cleanser would be quite drying and irritating for most skin types, creating more problems than it would help.

☺ **$$$ Bi-Facil Double-Action Eye Makeup Remover** *($18.50 for 4 ounces)* is a silicone-based wipe-off cleanser, nothing more. The price is very steep for this very basic eye-makeup remover.

☺ **$$$ Effacile Gentle Eye Makeup Remover** *($17.50 for 4 ounces)* is a detergent-based eye-makeup remover that isn't all that gentle, but it will take off eye makeup.

☺ **$$$ Eau de Bienfait Cleanser Water with Vitamins for Face and Eyes** *($23.50 for 6.8 ounces)* is a good but remarkably ordinary toner that contains mostly water, lightweight detergent cleansing agents, slip agent, tiny amounts of vitamins, fragrance, and preservatives. As an extra cleansing step it is just fine.

☺ **$$$ Exfoliance Delicate Exfoliating Gel** *($21 for 3.5 ounces)* is an OK detergent-based exfoliator that uses synthetic particles as the scrub. It's rather standard and can be drying for some skin types.

☺ **$$$ Clarifiance Alcohol-Free Natural Astringent** *($18.50 for 6.8 ounces)* contains mostly water, alum (a powdered astringent), preservatives, and slip agent. It is alcohol-free, but alum isn't the best for the skin, at least not in terms of oily skin or acne.

☹ **Tonique Controle Toner for Oily and Normal to Oily Skin** *($18.50 for 6.8 ounces)* is basically just alcohol and a small amount of zinc. The zinc will absorb oil, but the alcohol is likely to cause more oil, so it creates a vicious cycle for your face.

☺ **$$$ Tonique Douceur Non-Alcoholic Freshener for Dry/Sensitive Skin** *($27.50 for 13.5 ounces)* is indeed alcohol-free; it contains mostly water, glycerin, pH balancer, soothing agents, and preservatives. It's good, but the price is steep for this very basic ingredient listing.

☺ **$$$ Tonique Eclat** *($18.50 for 6.8 ounces)* is an OK irritant-free toner with glycerin and water-binding agents. It contain sugar cane extract, but that isn't an AHA ingredient; besides, the pH isn't low enough for it to work as an exfoliant even if it were.

☹ **Bienfait Total SPF 15** *($35 for 1.7 ounces)* doesn't contain avobenzone, zinc oxide, or titanium dioxide, and is not recommended.

☹ **Bienfait Total Fluide SPF 15** *($55 for 3.4 ounces)* doesn't contain avobenzone, zinc oxide, or titanium dioxide, and is not recommended.

☺ **$$$ Clarifiance Oil-Free Hydrating Fluide** *($35 for 2.5 ounces)* contains mostly water, silicone, glycerin, thickeners, and preservatives. This is a good, though fairly ordinary, moisturizer for someone with normal to slightly oily or slightly dry skin.

☺ **$$$ Expressive Eye Contour Age Treatment Fluide** *($42.50 for 0.5 ounce)* contains mostly water, glycerin, plant extract, thickeners, vitamin E, water-binding agents, and preservatives. This is a good moisturizer for normal to dry skin, but there is nothing in here that warrants the price tag.

☺ **$$$ Hydra Controle Hydrating & Matifying Long-Lasting Treatment Oil-Free Fresh Gel** *($30 for 1 ounce)* contains mostly water, silicone, glycerin, several thickeners, film former, vitamin B, more thickeners, and preservatives. It does contain a few unusual plant extracts, but they are at the end of the ingredient list and so almost nonexistent. A film former won't control oil, but this is a good lightweight moisturizer for someone with slightly dry skin.

☺ **$$$ Hydrative Continuous Hydrating Resource** *($42.50 for 1.75 ounces)* contains mostly water, shea butter, glycerin, standard water-binding agents, mineral oil, thickeners, a small amount of sunscreen, more thickeners, fragrance, vitamin E, and preservatives. This is a good emollient moisturizer for very dry skin.

☺ **$$$ Hydrix Hydrating Creme** *($36.50 for 1.9 ounces)* is a traditional petrolatum-based moisturizer. It contains mostly water, petrolatum, mineral oil, lanolin, thickeners, plant oil, more lanolin, and preservative. It's a good moisturizer for very dry skin, but this is a lot of money for Vaseline and lanolin.

☺ **$$$ Niosome + Perfected Age Treatment** *($60 for 2.5 ounces)* is an OK lightweight moisturizer that contains mostly water, glycerin, silicone, plant oil, water-binding agents, thickener, fragrance, and preservatives. There are some antioxidants in it, but in such negligible amounts that they don't count for much. It's a good moisturizer, but "perfected age treatment"? They've got to be kidding.

☺ **$$$ Nutribel Nourishing Hydrating Emulsion** *($38 for 2.5 ounces)* is a good, very emollient moisturizer that contains mostly water, plant oil, glycerin, mineral oil, more plant oils, thickeners, water-binding agents, fragrance, more thickeners, and preservatives.

☺ **$$$ Nutriforce Double Nutrition Fortifying Nourishing Creme** *($40 for 1.7 ounces)* contains mostly water, plant oil, silicone, thickeners, plant extracts, fragrance, and preservatives. This is a good basic (but ordinary) moisturizer for someone with dry skin.

☺ **$$$ Nutrix Soothing Treatment Creme** *($32 for 1.9 ounces)* contains mostly mineral oil, water, petrolatum, lanolin, thickeners, water-binding agents, fragrance, protein (way down at the end of the ingredient list, too little to even notice), and preservatives. This is a lot of money for mineral oil and Vaseline, but it would be good for someone with very dry skin.

☹ **$$$ Primordiale Visible Revitalizing Solution** *($67.50 for 1.7 ounces)* is, according to Lancome, not a moisturizer, but should be worn under a moisturizer (preferably one of Lancome's, I imagine) to "insulate skin from premature aging factors so it's free to repair itself." Another product to get rid of wrinkles—what a surprise. It is basically an AHA and BHA product, but the pH is not high enough to be an effective exfoliant. This ends up just being an overpriced, mineral oil–based moisturizer for dry skin.

☺ **$$$ Primordiale Nuit** *($75 for 2.5 ounces)* contains mostly water, thickener, silicone, glycerin, mineral oil, plant oil, Vaseline, vitamins, plant extracts, water-binding agents, and preservatives. This is a good emollient moisturizer for someone with dry skin.

☺ **$$$ Primordiale Yeux Visibly Revitalizing Eye Treatment** *($42.50 for 0.5 ounce)* is similar to the one above minus the oils, so it is less emollient, but the same basic review applies.

☺ **$$$ Progres Counter des Yeux Eye Creme** *($37.50 for 1.5 ounces)* is a thick eye cream that contains mostly water, thickeners, petrolatum, more thickeners, glycerin, water-binding agent, and preservatives. This is a good emollient moisturizer for dry skin around the eyes or anywhere on the face.

☺ **$$$ Renergie Double Performance Treatment** *($72.50 for 2.5 ounces)* contains mostly water, silicone, thickeners, petrolatum, more thickeners, water-binding agents, fragrance, vitamin E, and preservatives. This is a good emollient moisturizer for dry skin.

☹ **$$$ Renergie Emulsion Oil-Free Lotion** *($57.50 for 1.7 ounces)* isn't in the least oil-free. It contains plenty of silicone and very little of anything interesting or special for the face. It contains mostly water, silicones, glycerin, thickeners, more silicone, preservatives, fragrance, and a host of water-binding agents and vitamins that come well after the preservatives and fragrance. In many respects this is a very ordinary moisturizer that might be OK for someone with normal to slightly dry skin, but at best this is a why bother.

☺ **$$$ Renergie Serum Instant Lift Concentrate** *($75 for 1.7 ounce)* contains mostly water, glycerin, silicone, thickeners, and acrylates. This simple, extremely lightweight, gel-like moisturizer won't lift the skin anywhere (although your wallet will feel much lighter), but it can be good for someone with normal to slightly dry skin—at night only, of course, because it doesn't have a sunscreen.

☺ **$$$ Renergie Yeux** *($40 for 0.5 ounce)* is similar to many of the more emol-lient moisturizers in this collection. It is a good petrolatum-based moisturizer for very dry skin.

☺ **$$$ Trans-Hydrix Multi-Action Hydrating Creme** *($36.50 for 1.9 ounces)* contains mostly water, plant oil, shea butter, mineral oil, several thickeners, slip agents, fragrance, preservative, water-binding agents, and more preservatives. This is a good standard emollient moisturizer for dry skin.

☺ **$$$ Vitabolic Deep Radiance Booster** *($45 for 1 ounce)* is another addition to the vitamin C bandwagon. Vitabolic contains mostly water, glycerin, silicone, slip agent, vitamin C (ascorbic acid), more silicone, plant oils, plant extract, and preser-vatives. There is definitely vitamin C in this standard, lightweight moisturizing base, but the research (discussed elsewhere in this book) indicates that ascorbic acid is not the most effective or stable form. Ginseng and ginkgo extracts are also part of the mix in here. According to Lancome, ginseng is supposed to help the skin's resistance to stress and fatigue, and ginkgo is supposed to improve skin tone. I'm not sure what "toning the skin" means, but smearing plants on the surface of the skin can't relieve stress or fatigue. However, *Ginkgo biloba* does stimulate blood circulation, which can make the skin look rosier, but that may cause capillaries to surface and make existing ones more noticeable. While this can be a good moisturizer for someone with normal to somewhat dry skin, a lot of other details about the ingredients just aren't known.

☹ **$$$ After Sun Tan Prolonger Refreshing Gel** *($25 for 5 ounces)* is a bit of a confusing product; it is basically a self-tanner (it contains dihydroxyacetone like all self-tanners do), but the marketing makes it sound like a soothing product for sun-damaged skin. It isn't; the chemical that makes skin turn brown isn't a soothing agent in the least.

☺ **$$$ SPF 15 Face and Body Lotion with Pure Vitamin E** *($21 for 5 ounces)* is a truly excellent avobenzone-based sunscreen for someone with normal to dry or slightly oily skin! The price is high, but not terrible.

☺ **$$$ SPF 25 Face and Body Lotion with Pure Vitamin E** *($21 for 5 ounces)* is similar to the one above and the same review applies.

☺ **$$$ SPF 15 Water-Light Spray** *($21 for 5 ounces)* is a very good avobenzone-based sunscreen that is mostly slip agents, film former, and plant oil. It should work well for someone with normal to slightly dry skin.

☺ **$$$ SPF 30 Face Creme with Pure Vitamin E** *($23 for 1.7 ounces)* is similar to the one above, except that this one would be better for someone with normal to dry skin.

☹ **$$$ Empreinte de Beaute Deep Cleansing Clay Masque** *($21 for 2.5 ounces)* is a basic clay mask that contains mostly water, clay, water-binding agents, more clay, thickeners, protein, more thickener, and preservatives.

☺ **$$$ Masque No. 10 Hydrating Masque** *($21.50 for 2.2 ounces)* contains mostly water, thickeners, and preservatives. There isn't much moisture in this mask; it is just a gel that dries on the face. Not very impressive, but your skin will feel smooth when you take it off (that's true for most masks). One of the thickeners is a potential skin irritant.

☺ **$$$ Viveclat Revitalizing Smoothing Masque** *($26 for 2.6 ounces)* isn't the best of masks; the third ingredient is an acid-balancer (triethanolamine) that is best found in smaller amounts than this. It also contains alcohol and about a 2% concentration of AHA, and that's OK, but not effective as an exfoliant. There are some water-binding agents and emollients in here, but the irritating ingredients leave much to be desired.

☺ **$$$ Stick Nutrix Levres, Lip Balm** *($16.50 for 0.13 ounce)* is a very emollient but standard lip balm that contains mostly plant oil, lanolin oil, petrolatum, thickeners, and preservatives. It's good for dry lips, but very overpriced, given its similarity to products at one-third the price.

☹ **Extra Controle Anti-Imperfections Acne Treatment Matifying Solution** *($30 for 1 ounce)* is a BHA product in an alcohol-base. Alcohol can increase breakouts from the irritation it causes as well as dry out the skin and cause redness; also, the pH of this product negates the effectiveness of the BHA.

☹ **Masque Controle, Peel-Off Purifying Mask** *($22.50 for 2.5 ounces)* is an alcohol and film former–based mask, and both these ingredients can cause skin irritation and dry out the skin.

☺ **$$$ T. Controle Oil-Free Powder Gel Instant T-Zone Matifier** *($22.50 for 1 ounce)* is an interesting product made of silicone and film former, period; there is no powder in here. It will put a silky film over the skin, but don't count on this to help your oily skin. There is nothing in this product that can hold back oil. It is a decent lightweight silicone moisturizer but that's about it. Definitely test this one before you even consider this misleading product. If anything, it will make someone with oily skin feel more oily!

☹ **Spot Controle Acne Treatment** *($15 for 0.5 ounce)* contains a good amount of alcohol, which won't spot-control anything, though it can cause redness, dryness, and irritation.

Lancome Makeup

☺ <u>FOUNDATION:</u> Lancome has quite a large, almost overwhelming, array of foundations to choose from, all of which are excellent. There is even an impressive range of colors for darker skin tones. **MaquiVelour Hydrating Foundation** *($30)* is for normal to dry skin and has a soft, light texture with even coverage. **These colors** are great: Clair II, Dore Clair II, Pale Clair II, Beige III, Beige Naturel III, Beige Sable III, and Beige Bisque III. **These colors are too peach, pink, or ash:** Porcelain Delicate I, Bronze IV, Rose Clair II, and Beige Rose III.

☺ **MaquiControle** *($30)* is one of the best matte foundations around. It provides light to medium coverage and feels great on the skin. It goes on very matte and truly dry. It is one of the better choices for someone with truly oily skin. **These colors are excellent:** Porcelain I, Porcelain d'Ivoire I, Porcelain Delicate I, Clair II, Pale Clair II, Dore Clair II, Beige III, Beige Naturel III, Beige Camee III, Beige Sable III, Bronze IV, Amande Bronze IV, and Miel Bronze IV. **These colors are too pink or peach:** Beige Rose III, Beige Bisque III, Beige Rose III, Rose Clair II, and Epice Bronze IV.

☺ $$$ **Teint Idole** *($32.50)* joins the "stay-put" makeup craze. It is an excellent foundation for someone with normal to oily skin. It is quite similar to the other "stay-put" foundations in this new but growing foundation category. Teint Idole is a very good matte foundation with a soft, smooth finish that indeed has great staying power; it doesn't easily rub off. It is also tricky to blend, because once it's in place, it doesn't move. The color selection is superior: nary a bad one in the bunch.

☺ $$$ **Eau de Teint** *($25)* has almost an identical finish to Teint Idole, only more sheer, and that makes it an excellent lightweight, matte finish foundation with great colors for someone with normal to oily skin, quite similar to the other "stay-put" foundations on the market. Like Revlon's ColorStay or Maybelline Great Wear, it doesn't easily rub off. It is also tricky to blend because once it's in place, it doesn't move. Eau de Teint provides only light coverage, which for lots of women is the preferred way to go.

☹ **MaquiLibre SPF 15** *($30)* comes in the typical excellent assortment of Lancome color choices. It has a great light texture that goes on evenly and relatively sheer; regrettably, the SPF doesn't include avobenzone, titanium dioxide, or zinc oxide, and it is not recommended.

☺ **Dual Finish Powder** *($27.50)* is more like a compact powder than a foundation. It comes in an excellent assortment of colors, can be used wet, and is an option for someone with normal to slightly oily skin. It also makes a great finishing powder. You may find this one to be identical to L'Oreal's Dualite for less than half the cost at the drugstore.

☺ $$$ **Imanance Matte SPF 15 Tinted Oil Absorbing Cream** *($30)* and **Imanance Tinted Cream SPF 15** *($30)* are both great, in-part titanium dioxide–based sunscreens. Both Imanance formulations are lightweight, more like moisturizing tints, but they do provide some amount of coverage. The textures of both are wonderful, appropriate for the indicated skin types, and the colors properly neutral for most lighter skin tones. The only problem is there are no shades for darker skin tones, an unfortunate oversight. Don't expect the Imanance Matte to absorb or control oil, because it won't. Yet, all in all, Imanance is a great option for daily sun protection and minimum foundation coverage.

☺ **$$$ Cool Finish Foundation** *($46 for the foundation insert and $2.50 for the compact)* definitely has a cool finish. This liquid-to-powder finish is a unique way to apply foundation. Basically the foundation goes on the skin slightly damp and then dries to a soft powder finish. It also doesn't have a greasy after-feel like many cream-to-powder foundations do. But it tends to stick and is hard to blend, plus it tends to crumble.

☺ **$$$ Stick Express Teint Idole Foundation** *($32.50)* is a twist-up stick foundation that has a cream-to-powder finish but is far less creamy than you might suspect from looking at the applicator. The smooth application dries to a solid powder base, providing excellent medium to heavy coverage. But be forewarned: once you blend this one out, which you must do quickly, it really stays put. In fact you may find it hard to remove! The 12 shades available are for the most part terrific—the only one to watch out for is Pale, which can be too pink for most skin tones.

☺ **$$$ CONCEALER: Ombre Perfecteur Eyeshadow Base and Waterproof Eye Colour Base** *($18.50)* can both help to hold eyeshadow in place. The Eyeshadow Base has a cream-to-powder finish, and the Waterproof Eye Colour is quite waterproof, which means it must be removed with an oil-based cleanser. Actually, both of these bases help to tone down the shine of Lancome's iridescent eyeshadows and eyeshadow pencils. As a rule, I rarely recommend using eyeshadow bases. Your foundation on the lid with a powder over it can essentially do the same thing. But I should mention that there are women who prefer this step to the foundation and powder route, so you may want to give this one a try.

☺ **$$$ Effacernes Waterproof Anti-Cernes Waterproof Protective Undereye Concealer** *($17.50)* comes in four shades: Porcelain, Clair II, Beige III, Bronze IV. This has a creamy soft application with a soft, even finish. It doesn't crease and provides light to medium coverage. It isn't all that waterproof so don't worry about getting it off at night. Porcelain can be too pink for some skin types but the others are just fine. The squeeze tube container isn't the best; you tend to squeeze out more than you need. **MaquiComplet** *($17.50)* comes in a wand, provides wonderful matte coverage and doesn't crease into the lines even a little. **These colors are wonderful:** Porcelaine I, Beige III Neutral, and Bronze IV. **These colors should be avoided:** Beige III Rose, which can turn peach, and Correcteur, which is very, very yellow.

☹ **Palette Pro Complexion Perfecting Kit** *($26.50)* is a puzzling group of products. The kit contains one concealer and three color correctors: yellow to cover blue-red discolorations; green to cover ruddiness; and mauve to cover yellow. When I asked why *three* color correctors, I was told that a person might have more than one color problem on her face. What a parade of colors this kit gives you to blend over your face and keep from running into each other. In truth, any of Lancome's wonderfully neutral or yellow-based foundations will provide enough color correction for any one face. The concealing cream in the Palette Pro Kit comes in three excellent shades, but it is just a concealer. It's fairly decent, creases minimally, and would be very good for someone with dry skin, but, regrettably, it isn't sold separately.

☺ **$$$ Face Perfecting Pencil** *($15)* is a standard chubby pencil that comes in five shades. Much like concealers, these pencils are meant to cover problem areas and fill in lines by lightening them. Any concealer can do this job for you, and who needs another pencil that has to be sharpened?

☺ **$$$ POWDER: Poudre Majeur Pressed Powder** *($26.50)* is a pressed powder without talc. It goes on smoothly, with a soft even finish. **The only color to avoid is** Matte Peche.

☺ **$$$ Poudre Majeur** *($30)* is a loose powder that has shine. Setting powder that has shine seems like an oxymoron.

☹ **$$$ Powder Pro Complexion Perfecting Powder** *($20)* is a selection of four standard talc pressed powders that have a dry, silky finish. The powders mirror the color correctors of the Perfecting Kit, with one addition—a shiny shade of white (I wonder what that's supposed to correct). I am not a fan of color correctors, but if you do choose to do this step, please, use correctors that go under the makeup. Dusting mauve, green, or yellow powder on top of foundation would give the foundation a strange hue, especially out in daylight. The Pearl shade of powder can add a nice halo of shine over the face, neck, and shoulders, but shine is appropriate for nighttime only, right?

☺ **$$$ BLUSH: Blush Subtil** *($22.50)* colors are indeed subtle; they are all beautiful and have a soft, silky, sheer finish, but they are also slightly shiny. **Pommette** *($22.50)* is a cream blush that comes in six beautiful, soft, matte shades. The texture is silky, with a smooth, soft, slightly matte finish. With the resurgence of cream blushes, this is one of the better ones, but it still takes fairly flawless skin and a talent for blending for this type of blush to look convincing.

☺ **$$$ EYESHADOW:** Many of the **MaquiRiche Singles** *($10)*, **Duos** *($22.50)*, **Trios** *($35)*, and **Personal Eyes** *($22.50)* eyeshadow colors are shiny, with only a handful of matte selections. The texture is wonderful, so if you don't mind shine there are options here. Personal Eyes is a group of colors from which you can choose two and create your own duo compact. It is a good idea, but matte singles are just as convenient, and you don't have to buy two if you like only one of the colors. **La Palette de Couleur** *($35)* is a set of three eyeshadows and an eyeliner. Of the six sets, three are fairly shiny but three are fairly matte and worth a consideration if you find this concept convenient. **Eternal Eyes** *($16)* are intensely shiny eyeshadow colors in a tube. There is little reason to use this kind of cream-to-powder finish and there is even less reason for all this glitter.

☺ **L'Ombre Stylo Duo** *($23)* is an eyeshadow pen with different colors at each end, so you can pick and choose for yourself which two colors you want from a selection of eight. The idea and possible convenience, especially for touch-ups, would be worth checking out if the color choices were not so poor. **These colors are worth considering:** Matte Fumee (black), Matte Plum, and Matte Violet (which is best for darker skin tones only). Most of the rest are too shiny or too blue.

☺ **La Brosse Precise** *($15)* is a compact of two eyeshadows and one eyeliner. These fine assortments of mostly matte colors are nicely color coordinated. The only one to stay away from, due to an abundance of iridescence, is Les Granites.

☺ **EYE AND BROW SHAPER: Le Crayon Kohl** *($14)* is an assortment of good (though not exceptional) eye-lining pencils; they come in a nice range of colors, but they are no better than others I've found for less money. The claim that they don't smudge once they're on is not entirely accurate; smudging is caused by several factors, not just the pencil itself. **Le Crayon Brow Definer** *($16.50)* is a standard pencil with a comb at one end so you can brush through the line and soften it. **Avoid these colors:** Taupe, which is too shiny, and Brunette, which can be too red for many skin tones.

☺ **Maquiglace Liquid Liner** *($18.50)* and **Precision Point Artliner Automatic Eye Lining Felt Pen** *($23.50)* make very definite lines that do not blend, although the felt pen goes on softer than the liquid liner. These can be good for some eye designs. The felt pen is an interesting way to put on eyeliner. Some of these colors are fairly shiny.

☺ **Le Kohl Poudre** *($14)* is a unique pencil that goes on like a powder. It is difficult to sharpen and some of the colors are shiny, but this is quite a good option for lining the eyes softly. **Le Crayon Poudre for the Brows** *($16.50)* is a pencil; one end has a powder finish, while the other is a mascara wand meant to be combed through the brow to soften the look. It's a great idea, and not one of the colors is shiny. The color selection is limited, but if you find a match, give it a try.

☻ **Le Crayon Waterproof** *($13.50)* is a fairly waterproof pencil that comes in 15 colors. Unfortunately, most are shiny, though some of the darker shades, such as Brown and Black, are not. The pencil is hard to get off without using a wipe-off makeup remover, and I never suggest doing that; it is also fat and hard to sharpen; and because they are not 100 percent waterproof, these come off unevenly while you are in the water (although the darker colors are more waterproof than the lighter ones). **Wet Dry Liner** *($22.50)* doesn't work very well dry once it is used wet. For the money there are lots of eyeshadows that can double, dry or wet, as an eyeliner without this overpriced extra product. **L'Ombre Stylo Duo Eye Powder Pen Duo** *($23)* is an eyeshadow pen that dispenses the color from a sponge-tip applicator. The idea and possible convenience, especially for touchups, would be worth checking out, except that the color choices are so poor. Most of the colors are either too shiny or too blue. The only ones worth considering are Matte Fumee (black), Matte Plum, and Matte Violet (which is best for darker skin tones only). Not exactly what I would call an exciting collection.

☺ **Tinted Brow Groomer Modele Sourcils** *($16)* comes in only four shades: one each for redheads, brunettes, and ash blondes and one clear color to just hold brows in place. The color selection is limited, but the real potential problem is the brush, which can be too large and awkward to make application reliable.

☹ **Le Crayon Glace** *($15)* is a short, fat pencil that comes in—oh, no!—shiny, sparkly colors. These pencils are hard to sharpen, they tend to be greasy despite the powder finish, and the shiny colors are unforgivable.

☺ **LIPSTICK AND LIP PENCIL:** Lancome's lipsticks are mostly very good, the colors are beautiful, and they all have a bit of a stain, which helps the lipstick wear somewhat longer. **Rouge Absolu Matte Lip Colour** *($16)* goes on somewhat creamy and opaque but it isn't really all that matte. It is fairly creamy and does tend to bleed. **Rouge Sensation Lip Colour** *($16)* is more like a gloss than a lipstick. All are worth checking out, though I didn't find their claims about long-lasting color or reduced feathering to be true. **Rouge Absolu Hydrating Lip Colour** *($16)* is mostly a creamy lipstick that is only slightly less glossy than the Rouge Sensation. **Le Lipstique Lip Colouring Stick** *($17.50)* is a surprisingly waterproof lip liner that goes on rather thick and heavy but stays on through thick and thin, leaving a stain after it has worn off. Lancome recommends wearing it all over the lips and applying lipstick over it, which is a fine option, but you can do that with any lip pencil for a longer-lasting look. However, because of the stain, the color can last somewhat longer than other lip liners. **Lip Brio** *($18.50)* is nothing more than a standard though pricey lip gloss in a beautiful, unique package. The appearance is intriguing, but the application is just gloss with some color. **Rouge Idole** *($16.50)* is identical in every way to L'Oreal's Endure—except for the price. Endure is *$4.95*. These are both part of the ultra-matte lipstick bandwagon and they are both equally good. And despite the salespeople at the Lancome counter insisting there's a difference, I can't find one. **Le Crayon** *($15)* is a standard, automatic lip pencil that never needs sharpening. It's convenient to use and comes in a beautiful array of colors. **Lip Perfecting Pencil** *($17.50)* is supposed to perfect lips. It's just a nice name for a standard, chubby lip pencil with a glossy cream finish.

☺ <u>MASCARA:</u> Lancome is known for its great, reliable mascaras that usually don't smudge. The best are the **Defincils** and **Intencils** *($16.50)*. Defincils builds the thickest lashes and is by far my favorite, but the others are equally excellent. **Eternicils** *($17)* is a waterproof mascara that builds thick, dense lashes as well as any of their other mascaras, and, as I have stated before, I have rarely met a Lancome mascara I didn't like. Eternicils is a decent waterproof mascara that holds up under water, but does tend to chip off. It's worth a try, but don't rub your eyes when you have this one on or it will easily roll off. **Aquacils Waterproof Mascara** *($16.50)* is an excellent mascara. It builds very quickly, makes lashes long and thick without any clumps, and holds up very well in water.

☺ $$$ **Extencils** *($18)* is as good as any of the Lancome mascaras, though it won't curl your lashes as claimed. Despite my review, if you are just dying of curiosity to find out if a mascara can replace your eyelash curler, then check out **Le Grand Curl** *($5.39)* by L'Oreal, Lancome's big sister—it has the same claims and the same formulation for far less money.

☹ $$$ **Tendercils Sensitive Eyes Mascara** *($16.50)* surprised me—I had an allergic reaction to the stuff. Though I never base my reviews of a cosmetic's performance on my skin's sensitivities (because what I am allergic to may have nothing to do with what your skin is sensitive to), the very notion of having this kind of immediate reaction to a product made for sensitive eyes seemed like a bad joke. Essentially, nothing in this product makes it more appropriate for someone with sensitive eyes than any other mascara, including others from Lancome. To make matters worse, although I usually rave about Lancome's mascaras, this one isn't very good. It doesn't build very thick lashes, and it takes a long time to apply. It doesn't smear, but it still doesn't hold a candle to a lot of other mascaras on the market. **Forticils** *($15)* is a clear mascara that is supposed to be a lash conditioner. There is no way to condition or feed lashes to make them grow or be thicker, however. This product is a waste of time and money.

☹ $$$ **Hair Streaks** *($15)* are Lancome's version of hair mascara, in case you want green, purple, amber, or golden streaks of color over your hair. I do think hair mascara products are a kick, and all perform equally well. Given that this is really more a fun product than anything to take seriously, and, more important, because the products from all the lines I've tested perform almost identically, I recommend saving money by selecting the ones from Prestige and Revlon that are sold at drugstores.

Laura Mercier Classique (Makeup Only)

By many standards Laura Mercier is considered one of the finest makeup artists in New York. She doesn't get as much attention as Bobbi Brown or Kevyn Aucoin, but her work is admired by insiders and her name graces photographs in myriad fashion magazine layouts. Mercier's line has some interesting parts, but it isn't as much fun as, say, Stila, or as intriguing and versatile as Bobbi Brown's, or as extensive as M.A.C. Yet there are still some things to check out here when you happen to be in a makeup frame of mind. Foundation is a strong point for Mercier. These colors are beautifully neutral, and the same is true for the powders. The blushes are beautiful, and there are a handful of matte eyeshadows worth checking out. For more information about Laura Mercier call (888) MERCIER.

☺ $$$ <u>FOUNDATION:</u> **Foundation Primer** *($24)* is a very thin, lightweight clear gel of silicone and film former. Although the Mercier collection offers only makeup products, for some reason Mercier did decide to throw in this product, which feels soft on the skin but truly serves no purpose. It can be a good simple moisturizer for someone with normal to slightly dry skin, but more essential than this is would be a reliable sunscreen, since Mercier's foundations don't have an SPF.

☺ $$$ **Moisturizing Foundation** *($35)* features a small but beautiful array of colors in a soft, velvety foundation. If there is one thing Mercier does extremely well, it's foundations. This one is worth testing if you have dry skin and are looking for medium coverage. Enough said!

☺ $$$ **Oil-Free Foundation** *($35)* has a wonderful, smooth texture that goes on like a glove and wears beautifully. The color choice is superlative.

☹ <u>CONCEALER:</u> **Secret Camouflage** *($21)* won't be a secret to anyone. Packaged in a compact offering two shades, this is a thick, relatively dry, hard-to-blend concealer. It pulls at the skin and takes forever to blend out. Even the salesperson commented on how difficult the concealer is to use and that the colors were rather peach.

☺ $$$ **Secret Concealer** *($18)* comes in three great shades in a small pot, and has a very creamy smooth texture. It covers beautifully and creases minimally.

☺ $$$ <u>POWDER:</u> The **Pressed Powder** *($25)* and **Loose Powder** *($28)* are very good but very standard talc-based powders that have a smooth, satiny feel with a dry finish, which means they would work best for someone with normal to oily skin. The colors for both are excellent (only the Loose Powder Star Dust is shiny, which can be great for a special evening look; in the Pressed Powder, only one is a shiny Bronzing Powder).

☺ $$$ <u>BLUSH:</u> **Cheek Colour** *($18.50)* are a small group of colors that have a soft smooth finish, but be careful, because most have some amount of shine.

☺ $$$ <u>EYESHADOW:</u> The very attractive neutral matte **Eye Colour** *($15)* shades go on easily, if not a bit too softly. They are worth a peek, but you won't notice much difference between these and any of the other designer lines with matte shades.

☺ $$$ <u>EYE AND BROW PENCIL:</u> Although Mercier recommends lining the eye or filling in the brows with eyeshadow and a thin squared-off brush, she has very standard **Eye and Brow Pencils** *($15)*. I agree that powder is the way to go for almost all kinds of eyelining and brow shaping. The meager selection of pencils is probably to satisfy consumers who are stuck in their ways.

☺ $$$ <u>LIPSTICK AND LIP LINER:</u> **Lip Pencils** *($15)* is a very standard but good selection of lip pencils. There is only one type of lipstick, a standard **Creme** *($15)* with a more glossy than creamy finish, but it comes in a nice range of colors.

☹ <u>MASCARA:</u> This **Mascara** *($16.50)* not only doesn't build any length, but it almost seemed to somehow make my lashes look shorter.

☺ $$$ <u>BRUSHES:</u> This collection features some very good **Brushes** *($20 to $38)* made with varying types of animal hair. They are soft and lovely, and most are very usable.

Le Mirador (Skin Care Only)

Le Mirador is created by the American owner of the Le Mirador Resort and Spa in Geneva, Switzerland. These products were supposedly the winners of the first (and, by the way, only) International Skin Care Competition. Not surprisingly, we are never given the results of that competition. Aren't you curious who else was in the running? I'd love to know who came in second or third, or even in tenth place. Plus, how was the winner determined? Did a group of women end up looking 10, 20, or 30 years younger, or were there some other determining factors, and who judged those results? None of this information is available anywhere in the world—strange for a competition don't you think? Usually contestants are part of the news. As it turns out, the competition was created, funded, and overseen by the owner of Le Mirador. There was no scientific process or protocol involved, and the winner was an arbitrary decision of the owners, not some independent, unbiased group of judges as the infomercial for these products claims. While the misinformation regarding these products is disturbing, that doesn't mean there aren't some interesting products in this line to consider. Just ignore the ad, and consider whether or not these products suit your skin type. For more information about Le Mirador call (800) 345-1515.

☺ $$$ **Dual Action Facial Cleanser** *($19 for 6 ounces)* is a standard detergent-based water-soluble cleanser for most skin types. It contains a small amount of AHAs, but the pH isn't low enough for them to work as an exfoliant so they shouldn't be a problem. There are hosts of vitamins in this product, but even if they did have an effect on the skin, they would be rinsed down the drain before they had a chance.

☺ $$$ **Revitalizing Eye Cream** *($22 for 0.5 ounce)* is a lightweight moisturizer that contains mostly water, silicones, thickeners, and preservatives. This is a lot of money for a fairly ordinary eye product. It would be good for normal to dry skin.

☺ **$$$ Triple Action Revitalizing Moisturizer SPF 15** *($21.71 for 2 ounces)* was launched on QVC the day avobenzone was approved by the FDA for preventing UVA sun damage. Le Mirador bounded onto the airwaves claiming they were the first to offer this latest development to the consumer. They weren't. Shade UVAGuard from Schering-Plough has been available at drugstores for quite some time and for about a fifth of the price. Triple Action Revitalizing Moisturizer is still a good day-time moisturizer, and the UVA protection is state-of-the-art, but the other claims are exaggerated. For example, just because this product contains "marine-origin collagen" (and not that much of it) doesn't mean it will have any effect whatsoever on the collagen in your skin.

☹ **$$$ Anti-Oxidant Night Cream with AHA and Pycnogenol** *($24.53 for 2 ounces)* is a very good emollient moisturizer for someone with dry skin, and it definitely contains antioxidants including pycnogenol. That's all fine and good, but pycnogenol is no more impressive than lots of other antioxidants being used in cosmetic lotions these days. The product also doesn't contain enough AHA to have an effect as an exfoliant. One word of warning: this product contains a host of irritating plant extracts, including spearmint, clove, dandelion, ivy, and witch hazel. This is a risky concoction for someone with plant allergies or sensitivities.

Lip Ink (Makeup Only)

☺ **$$$ Lip Ink** is supposed to guarantee indelible lip color, or as close to it as you can get anywhere in the cosmetics world. It lasts 50 percent longer than any other lipstick, according to their ads. Well, hold on to your lips, because this product delivers, maybe not as well as the ad claims, but it is impressive. Despite the name, it's not ink, just a very strong, semipermanent lip stain that doesn't rub off or easily wear off. Mine lasted a full day and a half—through meals, a shower, bedtime, and past the next morning, but readers of my newsletter have complained that it didn't last quite that long for them. Basically, Lip Ink is a quick-drying liquid lip color that feels very wet when applied, and after it dries—and you must let it dry—it feels like nothing on the lips. What is left behind are fully colored, dyed lips!

Unfortunately, Lip Ink doesn't add a drop of moisture, so if you have dry, cracked lips, using Lip Ink will give you fully colored, dyed, dry, cracked lips. To that end, the ☺ **$$$ Lip Ink Starter Kit** *($45)* includes **Lip Ink Shine**, which is just an emollient lip gloss, to keep the lips from drying out. Surprisingly, that gloss doesn't compromise the staying power of the lip color, but it will rub off on anyone you are snuggling up to! By the way, Lip Ink claims that Lip Ink Shine contains light reflectors to reduce signs of aging. Any gloss can provide a dewy, moist surface that looks smoother; they make theirs sound unique, and it isn't.

I know this all sounds great, but I have a few warnings about this product that you should know about. First and foremost, it isn't that easy to use. Here are some excerpts from the instructions that come with the kit: "Always start with clean, dry lips. Then, before applying Lip Ink Color, massage a small amount of Lip Ink Shine into the lips until the shine disappears. [This isn't really necessary if your lips aren't dry, and it can make the color bleed.] Shake the vial three times against the palm of your hand before using. When open, always keep the vial vertical and remove the applicator slowly. [If you don't, it will spill or splatter and make a mess.] Apply with long, smooth strokes in one direction only, not back and forth. Allow 20 seconds between layers for drying. Keep your lips apart and do not blot or pucker your lips during this time. After each application you will feel a refreshing mint-like tingle on your lips. [It felt like burning, not tingling, to me, and caused my lips to feel swollen and irritated.] After the third layer is dry, apply a small amount of Lip Ink Shine to your lips. Once every two weeks, take a paper towel and wipe the Lip Ink applicator tip free of any oil, wax, or food particles that may have accumulated." Like I said, this product definitely takes work! You have to be careful about applying it perfectly or your mistakes will be semipermanent.

Lip Ink also insists that you are not to combine their product with any other lipstick products because they are not compatible. I did not find that to be true in the least. If anything, I found that it helped provide a lasting base, and I could experiment with other colors over it. Of course, those colors came off, but the Lip Ink did last.

I was also disturbed by a few of Lip Ink's claims, such as its being hypoallergenic, which is a completely meaningless, unregulated term, especially given the burning sensation they warn about (but play down by calling it "tingling"). They also claim their products are "93% formulated from natural herbs and botanicals" but they aren't in the least: these products have a preponderance of synthetic ingredients and dyes, including everything from aluminum lakes (a synthetic dye) to alcohol (lots of alcohol), propylene glycol, phenoxyethanol, and on and on.

The Lip Ink Kit contains two **Lip Ink Colors** *($15 each)*; one **Lip Ink Shine** *($15)*; one **Lip Ink Off Vial** *($5)*, for carrying a transportable version of the lip color remover; one **Lip Ink Off Refill Bottle** *($10)*; and one **Purse Carrying Case** *($15)*. For more information on Lip Ink, call (310) 796-0595.

Lip Last (See English Ideas)

Lorac by Carol Shaw

Lorac is Carol spelled backward. Now that you're in on the secret, you kind of wonder why she didn't just leave out the "Lorac," which isn't all that clever or interesting, but then, what's in a name anyway? In many ways Carol Shaw's line is most disappointing. The foundations are unimpressive, the concealers are greasy and tend to crease, the color selection is almost too small. Lorac is one of the few makeup-artist lines that also includes skin-care products, but there are only five, which is ridiculously limited. Women with oily skin and women with very dry skin should not be using the same cleansing products. For more information about Lorac Cosmetics and where to find them in your area, call (800) 845-0705.

Lorac by Carol Shaw Skin Care

☹ **Face Wash** *($20 for 8 ounces)* is a standard detergent-based cleanser that can be drying for most skin types. This one also isn't the easiest on the eye area.

☺ **$$$ Makeup Remover** *($15 for 4 ounces)* is a fairly standard eye-makeup remover that will indeed take off eye makeup. Of course, I never recommend wiping off makeup on any part of the face, *especially* not the thinner, unsupported skin around the eye.

☹ **Toner** *($18 for 4 ounces)* contains menthol, which makes it too irritating for all skin types.

☺ **$$$ Moisturizer** *($37.50 for 2 ounces)* contains mostly water, glycerin, a long list of thickeners, water-binding agent, more thickeners, plant extracts, anti-irritant, vitamin E, and preservatives. This remarkably ordinary and almost boring moisturizer would be good for someone with normal to dry skin, but for this money it should contain something unique or state-of-the-art.

☺ **$$$ Vitamin E Stick** *($16 for 0.15 ounce)* contains almost no vitamin E to speak of. It is just a basic, greasy, Chapstick-like product made of castor oil, waxes, and petrolatum. It's good for dry lips but the price is absurd.

Lorac by Carol Shaw Makeup

☹ **FOUNDATION:** Shaw's line has two types of foundation: **Satin Makeup** *($35)* and **Oil Free Makeup** *($30)*. The Satin Makeup comes in eight colors, and half are either too yellow (we're talking jaundice) or ashy green. **Stay away from** M4, M5, M7, and M8. The Oil Free foundation doesn't have the same color problem, but it tends to blend on somewhat streaky and the color separates. (As this book went to press the Oil Free Makeup was being reformulated to correct for the separation problem.)

☹ **CONCEALER: Coverup** *($14)* is very greasy concealer, and though it blends on smoothly, it can crease under the eye, plus most of the colors are too ashy or peach to recommend.

☺ **$$$ POWDER:** Both the loose and pressed powders have a dry, smooth texture and a good color selection. **Face Powder** *($22.50),* the loose version, comes in a large tub that isn't all that easy to use. **Perfect Powder** *($32)* is a pressed powder that is supposed to contain a "unique botanical formula to reduce pores." It does have minuscule amounts of plant extracts, but they won't change the appearance of pores, and it contains more silicone than plant extracts, but Shaw forgot to mention that. Both the loose and pressed powder have a very dry, sheer finish and mostly good colors. **Avoid** CP4.

☺ $$$ <u>BLUSH:</u> The attractive selection of matte **Blushes** *($14)* is a strong point of this line. There aren't many to choose from, but what's there is great.

☺ $$$ <u>EYESHADOW:</u> The shades of mostly matte neutral **Eyeshadows** *($16)* are virtually indistinguishable from those of M.A.C., Bobbi Brown, and philosophy.

☺ $$$ <u>EYE AND BROW PENCIL:</u> **Standard Eye Pencils** *($12)* are, well, standard. There is nothing else to say. **Eye Pencil** *($12)* is just a standard pencil with only two colors to choose from.

☺ $$$ <u>LIPSTICK AND LIP PENCIL:</u> The lipsticks and glosses claim to contain a "lip rejuvenator." They don't. They contain exactly the same lipstick and gloss ingredients found in a million other lipsticks and glosses. The **Lipstick** *($17.50)* is rather creamy and smooth. The **Lip Tint** *($13.50)* are pots of heavily pigmented glosses that have some amount of stain. The **Lip Gloss** *($15)* is just that. **Lip Pencil** *($12)* is just a standard pencil with a great color selection.

☺ $$$ <u>MASCARA:</u> Lorac's **Mascara** *($17)* is a decent mascara that builds good length though not much thickness.

☺ $$$ <u>BRUSHES:</u> This nice assortment of brushes *($12 to $30)* is just fine, with some great options. The Blush and Powder brushes tend to be stiff and are not recommended.

Lord & Berry (Makeup Only)

Along the aisles of your local drugstore are a handful of small cosmetic lines specializing in a modest array of inexpensive color items. Wet 'n' Wild, Jane, M Professional, Nat Robbins, Naturistics, and Prestige are a few of the ones you may have seen and lines I've reviewed in the past. All of them have some exceptional products that are worthy of your attention, not only for your pocketbook but for creating beautiful makeup elegance. For some reason, I kept overlooking Lord & Berry. That was a mistake. While this isn't an exciting line, it does have some excellent inexpensive options for lipstick, lip pencil, and eyeliner that you may want to consider. The only significant negative in this line is the lack of testers for any of the products; even the actual color of the product is hidden from sight. Plus, the color swatch provided is a poor facsimile of the real color you get, I've noticed, from all the products I tested. Though at these prices you can afford to make a mistake or two.

☹ **Conceal-It** *($3.37)* comes in a thick pencil and the colors are all either too pink or peach to recommend.

☺ **Ultimate Matte Lipstick** *($3.37)* isn't ultimate but it is a rather good lipstick in pencil form. It is supposed to be a cream-to-powder formula, but it applies just like any other lipstick pencil. I would rather not have to sharpen my lipsticks, but for those who find this an easy way to put on a lip liner and lipstick without changing products this one is as good as any. **Satin Intense Lipstick** *($3.37)* isn't all that intense, but is an excellent cream lipstick with decent staying power. **Sheer Lipstick** *($3.37)* is accurately described; it is simply a glossy lipstick, and as good as they come. **Brilliance Lip Gloss** *($3.37)* is a standard but very emollient lip gloss. **Kiss Proof Lipstick** *($3.37)* is much like any of the ultra-matte lipsticks available from Revlon ColorStay or Maybelline Budgeproof. This one has a good matte finish that doesn't budge, and it doesn't chip or roll off. **Kiss Proof Lip Liner** *($2.52)* has as much staying power as any lip pencil, but it conveniently twists up and has a great smooth texture. **Waterproof Ultimate Matte Lip Liner** *($2.52)* isn't any more waterproof than any other pencil, it's just a good standard lip pencil that you have to sharpen.

☺ **Powder Liner** *($3.37)* is a pencil that gives a surprisingly soft, powdery finish. It is an attractive look for lining. What a shame you can't see the colors of these pencils, or test them for yourself. One end of the pencil has a smudge tip that can help soften the line. **Luxury Liner** *($3.37)* is just an automatic sharpening pencil, but it has a much softer application than the Line 'N' Shade below and works quite well. **Ink Well** *($3.37)* is a standard liquid liner that goes on solid, but it dries well (meaning it doesn't look shiny), and it doesn't chip or peel during the day.

☹ **Smudgeproof Liner** *($3.37)* has a great soft application. It goes on almost wet and smoothly, and then dries to a solid, almost sticky finish—but that doesn't keep it from smearing.

☺ **Natural Brow** *($3.37)* is a standard brow pencil that has a smooth finish and decent color choices. One end of the pencil is a brush that can soften up lines that get drawn on looking too harsh.

☺ **Line 'N' Shade Waterproof Eye Liner** *($3.37)* isn't any more waterproof than other pencils. This one has a fairly greasy, opaque application. It goes on easily but can slide into lines if used along the lower lashes.

☹ **Dramatic Eyes Defining Mascara** *($3.37)* doesn't clump as badly as the thickening version, but it also doesn't build much length or define lashes in the least. **Dramatic Eyes Thickening Mascara** *($3.37)* easily clumps, builds minimal length, and is just a very poor mascara overall.

☺ **Dramatic Eyes Waterproof Mascara** *($3.37)* builds nice definition and length and stays on quite well in water.

L'Oreal

It is fitting that L'Oreal follows Lancome so closely in my alphabetical listing, because both are owned by the same parent company in France. As a result, many products present in both lines are essentially indistinguishable, like L'Oreal's Sensitique Mascara and Lancome's Tendercils Mascara. Skin care has its share of copycats too. L'Oreal Hydra Renewal is almost ingredient by ingredient the same as Lancome Hydrative. When L'Oreal was about to launch Colour Endure Mascara (to accompany its Colour Endure Lipstick) I said in my newsletter that I would be willing to bet that, much the way L'Oreal's Colour Endure Lipstick was identical to Lancome's Rouge Idole Lipstick, L'Oreal's Colour Endure Mascara would be identical to Lancome's Eternicil Mascara, and it was! What a shame no one took me up on my bet. Of course not every product is duplicated, but enough of them are so you'd be wise to check out the drugstore line before the department-store version.

Despite the similarities between Lancome and L'Oreal, there are also glaring differences. Foundation colors for L'Oreal are mediocre to poor, while Lancome excels in foundation colors and textures. Lancome has wonderful, not to say sublime blush textures while L'Oreal's, though good, are just standard. Same for the lipsticks and the pressed powders (plus L'Oreal has pressed and loose powders that are shiny, and that just makes no sense). When it comes to skin care though, especially for moisturizers, I think you would find more similarities between these two sister lines than contrasts. For more information about L'Oreal call (800) 322-2036.

L'Oreal Skin Care

☹ **Plentitude Hydra Fresh Foaming Face Wash with Beta Hydroxy** *($4.99 for 6.5 ounces)* is a water-soluble cleanser with some potent detergent cleansing agents that can leave the face dry. It does contain BHA, but the pH is too high for it to be effective as an exfoliant and even if it wasn't, in a cleanser it would just be rinsed down the drain; as it is, the BHA could get in the eye, a real problem.

☹ **Plentitude Shine Control Foaming Face Wash with Pro-Vitamin B5** *($4.99 for 6.5 ounces)* is virtually identical to the cleanser above, minus the plant oil. That is helpful for oily skin, but the cleansing agents are still fairly drying for most skin types. Causing dry skin does not help oily skin in the least.

☺ **Plentitude Refreshing Eye Makeup Remover** *($4.99 for 4.2 ounces)* contains mostly water, slip agent, detergent cleanser, and preservatives. It does take off eye makeup, but why pull at the eye area, causing it to sag, if you don't have to?

☹ **Plentitude Hydra Fresh Toner with Beta Hydroxy** *($4.99 for 8.5 ounces)* is an alcohol-based toner with a small amount of salicylic acid. There is never a reason to use alcohol on the skin, never.

☺ **Plentitude Shine Control Double-Action Toner Oil Free** *($4.99 for 8.5 ounces)* is an interesting product that suspends zinc oxide in a solution that's mostly alcohol and glycerin. Zinc oxide doesn't offer great oil absorption, at least not as good as clay or magnesium, but it is thought to have some healing properties. Without the alcohol, which can irritate skin and prevent it from healing, this would be worth checking out. Zinc oxide can block pores, but in this version that seems unlikely.

☺ **Plentitude Active Daily Moisture Lotion Oil-Free with Vitamide Complex, for Normal to Oily Skin** *($5.99 for 4 ounces)* contains mostly water, silicone (so it obviously is not oil-free), glycerin, several thickeners, vitamin E, more thickeners, and preservatives. It also contains small amounts of balm mint and salicylic acid; both can be skin irritants, but there's probably not enough to affect the skin. This would be an OK lightweight moisturizer for someone with normal to slightly dry skin.

☺ **Plentitude Active Daily Moisture Lotion SPF 15, with UVA/UVB Sunscreen, for All Skin Types** *($7.39 for 4 ounces)* contains mostly water, thickener, silicone, glycerin, plant oils, more silicones, slip agent, more thickeners, fragrance, and preservatives. It does contain antioxidants, but they are at the very end of a long ingredient list, which means they can't keep even a puff of air off the face. This sunscreen wouldn't be very good for someone with normal to oily skin because of the oils, or for someone with sensitive skin because it contains aluminum starch, which can be a skin irritant and cause breakouts.

☺ **Plentitude Active Daily Moisture Lotion with Vitamide Complex for Normal to Dry Skin** *($5.99 for 4 ounces)* contains mostly water, plant oils, glycerin, thickener, silicone, more thickeners, vitamin E, more thickeners, fragrance, and preservatives. It also contains small amounts of salicylic acid and balm mint; both can be skin irritants, but there's probably not enough to affect the skin. The amount of vitamin E is also insignificant. This could be a good emollient moisturizer for someone with dry skin but not for someone with sensitive skin.

☺ **Plentitude Advanced Overnight Replenisher** *($9.92 for 1.7 ounces)* contains mostly water, silicone, plant oil, thickeners, petrolatum, more plant oil, more water-binding agent, and preservatives. This would be a good emollient moisturizer for someone with dry skin.

☺ **Plentitude Excell-A3 Alpha Hydroxy Cream SPF 8 with Triple Fruit Acid** *($9.99 for 1.7 ounces)* contains mostly water, silicone, thickeners, glycerin, water-binding agent, plant oil, fruit extracts, fragrance, and preservatives. SPF 8 is OK for limited sun protection, but this isn't an AHA product, at least not if you want the benefits of exfoliation. You can't tell what kind of fruit extracts are in it, and they probably have nothing to do with real AHAs such as glycolic or lactic acid, or they would be listed as such. Nevertheless, this is a good emollient moisturizer for someone with dry skin.

☺ **Plenitude Hydra Renewal Daily Dry Skin Cream with Pro-Vitamin B5** *($5.99 for 1.7 ounces)* is a very good emollient moisturizer for dry skin; it contains mostly water, glycerin, thickener, silicone, slip agent, mineral oil, plant oil, water-binding agents, a long list of other thickeners, and preservatives. There is a tiny amount of vitamin E, but too little to have much effect.

☺ **Plenitude Revitalift Anti-Wrinkle Firming Cream with Pro-Retinol A & Par-Elastyl, for Face and Neck** *($9.99 for 1.7 ounces)* contains mostly water, silicone, glycerin, mineral oil, thickeners, vegetable oil, water-binding agent, more thickeners, vitamin A, and preservatives. It won't change a wrinkle on your face or firm anything, but it is a good emollient moisturizer.

☹ **Plentitude Shine Control Moisturizer Oil-Free for Combination to Oily Skin** *($5.99 for 4 ounces)* contains mostly water, silicone, glycerin, film former, thickeners, fragrance, and preservatives. This could be OK as a lightweight moisturizer, but it contains balm mint, which is an unnecessary skin irritant.

☹ **Excell-A³ Alpha Hydroxy Moisturizer SPF 8 with Triple Fruit Acids** *($9.99 for 4 ounces)* falls short on several counts: it has an SPF 8 instead of an SPF 15, no avobenzone, titanium dioxide, or zinc oxide, and no AHAs. What a waste of your time and money.

☺ **Eye Defense with Liposomes** *($9.99 for 0.5 ounce)* is a good emollient moisturizer for dry skin. It contains mostly water, plant oil, slip agents, water-binding agents, thickeners, and preservatives.

☻ **Future E Moisture + A Daily Dose of Pure Vitamin E** *($8.99 for 4 ounces)* is just an OK moisturizer with a tiny amount of vitamin E and BHA. The pH isn't low enough to make the BHA effective for exfoliating, and the ingredients are extremely ordinary for someone with normal to slightly dry skin. Almost all of the other L'Oreal moisturizers are a better choice than this or the one below.

☹ **Future E Moisture + A Daily Dose of Pure Vitamin E for Your Skin SPF 15** *($8.99 for 4 ounces)* does contain a tiny amount of vitamin E, which isn't great but also isn't bad. What is bad is that this SPF 15 product doesn't include avobenzone, titanium dioxide, or zinc oxide.

☺ **Wrinkle Defense** *($10.44 for 1.4 ounces)* contains mostly water, silicone, thickeners, plant oil, water-binding agents, vitamins, fragrance, and preservatives. This won't change or fight off a wrinkle but it is a good moisturizer for dry skin.

☺ **Overnight Defense** *($11.99 for 1.7 ounces)* is a very good emollient moisturizer for dry skin. It contains mostly water, silicone, plant oil, thickeners, water-binding agents, fragrance, and preservatives.

☺ **Revitalift Eye Anti-Wrinkle and Firming Cream** *($9.99 for 0.5 ounce)* is similar to the one above, and the same review applies.

☹ Revitalift Oil-Free Anti-Wrinkle + Firming Lotion *($10.69 for 1.7 ounces)* contains mostly water, silicone, thickeners, water-binding agents, fragrance, and preservatives. This is just an OK moisturizer, with a rather ordinary formulation for dry skin.

☺ **Revitalift Night Anti-Fatigue + Recovery Complex** *($9.99 for 1 ounce)* is more of a lotion that contains mostly water, silicone, glycerin, thickener, vitamin A, plant oil, fragrance, and preservatives. It would be good for someone with normal to slightly dry skin.

L'Oreal Makeup

FOUNDATION: L'Oreal is one of the few drugstore lines to sometimes make foundation tester units available, but it isn't consistent from store to store and their foundation colors for the most part are shockingly poor.

☹ **Hydra Perfecte Protective Hydrating Makeup SPF 12** *($7.45)* is a lightweight foundation with a wonderful texture for normal to dry skin. However, the SPF doesn't have UVA protection, and the colors aren't the best. Only Sand Beige and Nude Beige are neutral skin tones.

☺ Visible Lift Line Minimizing Makeup *($9.37)* is an excellent foundation for someone with normal to dry skin. While I wouldn't say it gets rid of wrinkles, it does help smooth out skin to some degree by virtue of its soft, sheer coverage (heavier coverage tends to make any amount of wrinkles look more evident). It looks great if you want minimal coverage, but be careful with this one—it can settle into imperfections such as scars and make them more noticeable. Of the 12 colors, the only ones to look out for are Golden Beige (too peach), Sun Beige (too peach), and Cappuccino (too ash). One of the ways I tested this foundation was to apply Chanel Teint Lift Eclat SPF 8 to one side of my face and the L'Oreal Visible Lift to the other. Everyone I asked thought the L'Oreal side looked far less wrinkled. You may want to test this one for yourself—it's worth it to just see how much better looking a $10 foundation can be than a $50 foundation with the same claims.

☹ **Mattique Matte Oil-Free Makeup** *($8.75)* has a good, fairly matte texture, but it also has a slightly sticky feel. Someone with oily skin might not like it. **All of the colors are too pink or peach** to recommend.

☹ **Feel Perfect Foundation SPF 15** *($7.86)* has no reliable UVA protection, the amount of silicone in this product makes it difficult to blend evenly, and the colors are ghastly. Maybe L'Oreal should run next door and take a look at Lancome's foundation shades: nary a pink or a peach in the lot.

☹ **Visuelle Invisible Coverage Cream-Powder Makeup** *($7.45)* has an incredibly smooth, almost nonexistent finish, although there is a small amount of shine that goes with the application. Only four of the eight colors are reliable; **be sure to avoid** Pale, Beige Blush, Sand Beige, and Deep Beige.

☹ **Colour Endure Stay-On Makeup** *($8.95)* might indeed stay, but why would you want it to? The colors in this group of products are almost embarrassing. Except for one (Sand Beige), they are all either too pink, too orange, or too yellow.

☺ <u>CONCEALER:</u> **Mattique Conceal Oil-Free Cover-Up** *($4.73)* is a very good stick concealer that goes on quite sheer and smooth, although it does have a slight tendency to crease into the lines around the eyes. **Feel Perfecte Concealer** *($5.89)* comes in three fairly neutral shades with a smooth, flawless finish! It is a great concealer for sheer to medium coverage.

☹ **Hydra Perfecte Concealer SPF 12** *($4.73)* is a good, lightweight, sheer concealer that provides even coverage. It has a slight tendency to slip into the lines around the eyes and the SPF has no UVA-protecting ingredients.

☺ <u>POWDER:</u> **Visuelle Pressed Powder** *($6.20)* has a beautiful, soft, translucent finish and some great colors—not a problem shade in the bunch. It does contain wheat starch (second on the ingredient list), which can cause allergic reactions for some skin types.

☹ **Mattique Oil-Free Softly Matte Pressed Powder** *($6.94)* is supposed to be for someone with oily skin, and the product label exults that it is oil-free and oil-absorbing and controls shine, but what they don't tell you is that this powder is iridescent. It doesn't control shine, it puts more on! **Hydra Perfecte Perfecting Loose Powder** *($8.89)* is also iridescent, but it doesn't make any claims about controlling shine or oil. However, it seems contradictory to apply a powder to set makeup and reduce shine, only to end up adding sparkles.

☺ **Feel Perfecte Powder** *($8.46)*. While I'm not fond of the Feel Perfecte foundation (a rather dismal choice of colors and a poor "stay-put" finish), this powder gets high marks. This standard talc-based powder also comes in three shades: Light, Medium, and Deep. Again, Deep isn't all that deep, but all three have a light, soft, dry finish. Sadly, the packaging is such that you can't see the color unless you open the box.

☺ <u>BLUSH:</u> **Visuelle Softly Luminous Powder Blush** *($6.94)* has a wonderful soft, easy-to-blend texture and a great color selection, with some perfect contour shades as well. **Blushesse** *($6.10)* feels very similar to the Visuelle Blush, only with a slight amount of shine, but it goes on just as smoothly and evenly. **Quick Shimmer Face & Body Blush** *($7.89)* is a creamy twist-up spread of color that disappears into a faint hint of tint, leaving behind a lot of shine.

☺ <u>EYESHADOW:</u> **Soft Effects Singles** *($4.75)* have a handful of very good neutral shades that are mostly matte; some of the colors are labeled as perle and are easy to avoid, but some of the mattes also have some shine. **The best matte shades are:** Sand, Terra, Buff, and Blush. **The "matte" shades to avoid because they have some amount of shine are:** Sable, Bark, Eggplant, and Marine. Definitely avoid all of the **Trios** *($4.75)*, and **Quads** *($5.50)*; either they come in strange combinations, or one or more of the colors are shiny.

☺ **EYE AND BROW SHAPER:** Le Grand Kohl Perfectly Soft Liners *($5.29)* are extra-long pencils in fairly muted colors that go on smooth without being too greasy, and blend well without streaking. **Pencil Perfect Automatic Eye Liner** *($5.10)* isn't what I would call perfect; if anything, it tends to go on creamier than most, and that means a greater chance of smearing, but at least it doesn't need sharpening. **Lineur Intense** *($5.47)* is a traditional liquid liner in a tube; it goes on like the name says—intense—and stays that way all day. **Super Liner** *($5.68)* is a very liquidy liner with a soft pen applicator tip. It takes awhile to dry and then never quite sets which means you can smooth out the line making the line less than dramatic, but it also smears easily. **Brow Elegance** *($4.13)* is a standard brow pencil, slightly greasier than most.

☺ **Brow Colourist** *($6.73)* is a two-sided pencil. One end is a very standard pencil with decent brow colors (the cap has a stiff brush for combing through the brows), the other is a sponge tip that dispenses a very shiny whitish eyeshadow. **EyeColour Brightener** *($6.73)* is a very creamy, almost greasy eye pencil; one end has a sponge tip for blending, which would be useful, but all the shades are exceedingly shiny. **Eye Smoker** *($6.73)* is a chubby pencil that goes on creamy but all the colors are shiny.

☺ **LIPSTICK AND LIP PENCIL:** Sheer Colour Riche SPF 15 *($6.28)* is true to its name: it goes on sheer, more like a gloss than a lipstick, but it is very moist and the SPF 15 is in part titanium dioxide. **Colour Riche Hydrating Creme and Perle Lip Colour** *($7.79)* is a fairly glossy lip color that comes in both shiny and nonshiny finishes. These are more gloss than lipstick. **Colour Supreme Matte, Creme, or Perle** *($7.79)* seems redundant, because it's so similar to the Colour Riche. The Supreme Creme and Perle feel the same as the Riche versions. However, the Supreme Matte, while not matte in the least, is a great creamy, opaque finish lipstick. **Endure Stay-On Lip Colour** *($6.39)* is strikingly similar to Revlon's ColorStay Lipstick. They are both very matte, go on thickly, and stay in place. However, they both feel very dry, and regardless of Endure's claim about containing oil, there is no real emollient feel. **Rouge Pulp** *($5.39)* is a fairly standard lip gloss that comes in vivid colors. It's got a great name, and there really isn't much else to say.

☺ **Crayon Petite Automatic Lip Liner** *($5.50)* is a standard twist-up lip pencil that is slightly more creamy than most. It comes in a nice array of colors. **Crayon Grande** *($4.95)* is a cute dual-function, stocky pencil that is supposed to be a lip liner and lipstick in one. It is awfully cute, and the marketing sales pitch makes them sound convenient, but they aren't. They are hard to sharpen and the lipstick part is just an OK lipstick.

☺ **Rouge Virtuale** *($7.29)* is a group of Perle, Creme, and Matte lipstick shades that seem about as standard a group of lipsticks as any in the L'Oreal lineup (not including their Endure Color Stay-On lipstick which is an ultra-matte lipstick). Rouge Virtuale Matte lipsticks aren't matte in the least; in fact they're rather creamy and have poor staying power. The Creme is more like a gloss and the Perle is nicely iridescent and sheer. As a whole, they are rather unimprssive.

☺ **MASCARA: Lash Out Extending Mascara** *($5.39)* is excellent, but I prefer a shorter wand. It does build long, thick lashes and non-clumped lashes, with no chance of smearing. **Le Grand Curl** *($5.39)* is supposed to lift and curl as you apply it, which it does, but no more so than any other great mascara I've tested. Le Grand Curl is just that: a great reliable mascara. **Voluminous Mascara** *($4.99)* always went on long and thick, but it used to smudge and smear easily, making it an unreliable mascara to recommend. That seems to have changed. Voluminous Mascara also comes in shades of Blue, Gold, and Auburn, with matching shiny eyeshadows. Quite a concept. **Accentuous Precisely Defining Mascara** *($4.14)* goes on easily building long, beautiful lashes.

☹ **Colour Endure Stay-On Mascara** *($5.39)* builds decent length, but minimal to no thickness, and it takes a long time get anywhere. It doesn't smudge or smear and it isn't waterproof—it washes off with a water-soluble cleanser—but it is somewhat water-resistant so you may need an eye-makeup remover to get every last trace off. **Formula Riche** *($5.39)* has the same problems, although both separate lashes nicely without making them look spiked. **Sensitique Hypoallergenic Mascara** *($3.99)* is merely a cheaper version of Lancome's Tendercils Sensitive Eyes Mascara. Did Lancome think no one would notice that their parent company, L'Oreal, had come out with an identical product? Tendercils is an OK mascara, but little about it guarantees you won't be allergic to it. The same is true for Sensitique. Sensitique goes on well, building long lashes without clumping; it doesn't smear, and it doesn't have the odor problem the Tendercils mascara has. You may or may not be allergic to the Sensitique, but in general it is a good mascara.

☹ **Lash Out Waterproof Mascara** *($5.39)* is just a very mediocre mascara; it can take 15 coats before you see any length or thickness, and then not much and it can clump slightly. However, it does hold up under water, which may make up for its drawbacks.

☺ **Voluminous Waterproof** *(5.39)* is great in all departments. It builds decent length in just a few coats, doesn't clump, and it stood up under a good amount of water pressure.

Lubriderm (Skin Care Only)

☹ **Body Bar** *($2.79 for 4 ounces)* is a standard detergent-based cleansing bar that contains tallow. Tallow can cause breakouts and allergic reactions, and the detergent cleansing agent can be quite drying. The bar also contains some petrolatum and mineral oil to soften the blow, but they aren't much help.

☹ **Loofa Bar** *($2.79 for 4 ounces)* is similar to the bar above, only with scrub particles, and the same review applies.

☹ **One Step Facial Cleanser** *($8 for 8 ounces)* would be a great cleanser if it were really water-soluble; unfortunately, it isn't. Your skin is likely to feel greasy once you're done rinsing. This may be an option for someone with dry skin, but it would require a washcloth to get it all off.

☺ **Dry Skin Care Lotion Fragrance Free** *($6.59 for 10 ounces)* contains mostly water, mineral oil, petrolatum, thickener, lanolin, more thickeners, and preservatives. This is a very good emollient, though boring, moisturizer for someone with dry skin.

☺ **Dry Skin Care Lotion Original Fragrance** *($6.59 for 10 ounces)* is identical to the lotion above, only with fragrance, and the same review applies.

☹ **Moisture Recovery Creme** *($6.79 for 4 ounces)* is nice but nothing to get excited about. It contains 4% AHAs, but the pH isn't low enough to allow them to work as exfoliants.

☺ **Moisture Recovery Lotion** *($10 for 8 ounces)* is similar to the cream above, but with no more than 2% AHAs, which means it is an OK moisturizer but a poor AHA product.

☺ **Moisture Recovery Gel Creme** *($4.29 for 4 ounces)* contains mostly water, thickener, glycerin, mineral oil, silicone, thickeners, and preservatives. You won't recover from anything with this product, but it is a good emollient moisturizer for someone with dry skin.

☺ **Skin Therapy Moisturizing Lotion for Normal to Dry Skin** *($6.99 for 16 ounces)* contains mostly water, mineral oil, petrolatum, lanolin, thickeners, silicone, and preservatives. This is a very good, though ordinary, moisturizer for very dry skin.

☺ **Skin Therapy Moisturizing Lotion Fragrance-Free, for Normal to Dry Skin** *($6.99 for 16 ounces)* is similar to the one above, only fragrance-free.

☺ **Advanced Therapy Gel Cream for Rough, Dry Skin** *($5.23 for 7.5 ounces)* is similar to the one above, and the same review applies.

☺ **Seriously Sensitive Lotion for Extra Sensitive Skin** *($6.59 for 10 ounces)* contains mostly water, slip agent, glycerin, mineral oil, petrolatum, thickeners, silicone oil, and preservatives. Nothing about this product makes it better for someone with sensitive skin. It is a good ordinary emollient moisturizer for someone with dry skin.

☺ **Seriously Sensitive Lotion for Extra Sensitive Dry Skin** *($6.59 for 10 ounces)* is almost identical to the lotion above, and the same review applies.

☹ **Daily UV Lotion with Sunscreen Moisturizer & Sun Protection SPF 15** *($5.68 for 10 ounces)* doesn't contain avobenzone, titanium dioxide, or zinc oxide, and is not recommended.

M Professional (Makeup Only)

If you are in the market for new eyeshadows, blushes, lip pencils, eye pencils (even though I don't recommend them, there are some great ones here), lipsticks, or mascara, then you must absolutely consider taking a look at this inexpensive drugstore line of makeup products! Almost every selection from M Professional gives Bobbi Brown, Philosophy, M.A.C., Nars, Lorac by Carol Shaw, and Stila a run for their money. If all these companies, including M Professional, aren't buying most of their makeup from the same contract manufacturer or using almost identical formulations, I'll eat every page of this book.

Between M Professional, Black Opal, Physicians Formula, Revlon, Almay, and L'Oreal, is there really any reason to shop for makeup at a department store (except maybe to try on foundations)? By the way, M Professional adds a cute gimmick to their packaging that is a bit silly but definitely fun. Each product has an insert with the company's idea of good makeup advice and tips. For example, their blush insert says, "Use of this product may cause interesting looks"; and an eye pencil insert explains not to "make wrinkle lines in your forehead with this pencil; it may not create a desirable look." If you want to find where M Professional is sold call (800) 662-6776.

☺ **Eyeshadows** *($1.83)* and ☺ **Blush** *($2.29)* are smooth and soft and go on effortlessly. Every shade I've seen is beautifully matte with a good basic neutral-tone base. There isn't an obnoxious color in the bunch to avoid, although that doesn't mean you still shouldn't be careful, because they can always stick a blue or shiny green in when I'm not looking!

☺ **Moisture Lipstick** *($3.27)* is just a standard cream lipstick with a creamy (as opposed to glossy) light coverage. **Matte Lipstick SPF 15** *($2.99)* doesn't have a reliable sunscreen formulation either, but it is exceptionally matte with solid opaque coverage and no smearing or bleeding. A poor SPF in an opaque-covering lipstick like this one is less of a worry than some others, because the blanket of color offers some amount of protection on its own—though don't count on it for a day out in the sun. **Lip Liner** *($2.39)* is just some very good standard lip liners. **Lipgloss** *($2.68)* is a very good standard lip gloss in a nice range of neutral colors. **Duo Lip Liner and Lip Gloss** *($3.99)* is a two-sided product; one end is a standard lip liner, the other a tube lip gloss. If this sounds convenient to you, then this is a fine option if you want gloss and lip liner. **Sheer Lipstick SPF 15** *($2.99)* is a poor sunscreen formulation, but it is a good sheer, glossy lipstick.

☺ **Eyebrow Powder and Brush** *($2.25)* are just matte eyeshadows in shades that can work for eyebrows. Powder is a great way to fill in brows and this product comes with a very decent soft brush. **Eye Liner** *($2.39)* is just some very good standard eyeliners. **Duo Eye Liner and Mascara** *($3.99)* is a two-sided product, one end is a standard eyeliner, the other a mascara. The M Professional Mascara is great and the pencil is decent so if this sounds convenient to you, then this is an option to consider.

☺ **Duo Brow Pen and Brow Gel** *($3.99)* is a two-sided product, one end is a standard eye pencil in colors suited to the brow, and the other end is a brow gel with a matching color to the pencil. The Brow Gel goes on almost too wet, making the brows look more lacquered than you may want.

☺ **Mascara** *($2.82)* is a good mascara that creates long, unclumped lashes, but tends to smear.

☺ **Brushes.** These brushes are very inexpensive and may be fine for your purse to have around for touch-ups, but don't count on them for a reliable application. The bristles aren't as soft or as nicely packed (meaning dense) as they could be to blend colors on evenly.

M.A.C.

Once the new kid on the block as a start-up cosmetics company with attitude, M.A.C. (which stands for Makeup Art Cosmetics) is now a serious contender in the prestigious world of department store cosmetics. This Toronto-based company was purchased by Estee Lauder not too long ago and the line is now well distributed throughout the United States and Canada in upscale department stores and free-standing boutiques. The name of this company is actually quite accurate. M.A.C. claims its products are used by many professional makeup artists, and in my experience that is true. Most professional makeup artists prefer matte eyeshadows and blushes, and this line has a generous offering. The color selection for everything from blush to lipstick and foundations is exceptional too. Also, most of the makeup brushes are beautiful, full, and soft, as well as properly sized to fit the contours of the face and eyes. You will find this color line a pleasure to shop—at least for the most part.

Unfortunately, M.A.C.'s skin-care line is in another category altogether. These products are supposed to be filled with vitamins, antioxidants, and oxygen boosters, and are purportedly pH-balanced. Those claims are all rather exaggerated, and the products aren't worth the steep prices, but that's to be expected—after all, this is the world of cosmetics. M.A.C. claims that these products are "based on dermatologically advanced moisturization concepts [using] noncomedogenic compounds." Although these products don't contain mineral oil, lanolin, or isopropyl myristate, they have plenty of other ingredients that could make you break out or irritate your skin. M.A.C.'s advanced moisturizing ingredients aren't so advanced anymore; in fact, lately they've become fairly standard. By the way, the lactic acid listed in most of the M.A.C. products is there only in small concentrations, which makes it a good moisturizing ingredient but not an exfoliating ingredient.

A stand-up-and-notice feature of the M.A.C. line is their recycling program. If you bring in six empty M.A.C. plastic packages (no glass, pencils, or brushes) you get a free lipstick. That's a great marketing strategy that is good for the company and good for the environment! For more information about M.A.C. call (800) 387-6707.

M.A.C. Skin Care

☹ **Exfoliating Cleanser** *($14 for 4 ounces)* will indeed take off some skin, but potassium hydroxide and the other cleansing agents are skin irritants.

☹ **Foaming Cleanser for Normal to Oily Skin** *($12 for 4 ounces)* is similar to the one above and the same review applies.

☺ **$$$ pH Balanced Cleanser for All Skin Types Especially Normal to Dry** *($16 for 8 ounces)* is an OK water-soluble cleanser that can clean off all your makeup without burning your eyes, but it can be somewhat drying. It has a long list of water-binding ingredients that can help soothe the skin, but most will be washed away before they have a chance to do any good.

☺ **Eye Makeup Remover** *($15 for 4 ounces)* should be gentle and effective, although the detergent cleanser, listed among the first items on the ingredient list, can be irritating for some skin types.

☹ **PA-1 Phyto-Astringent Purifying Toner for Normal to Oily Skin** *($15 for 4 ounces)* is basically water, alcohol, cucumber extract, and witch hazel. The alcohol and witch hazel can be quite irritating, making oily skin worse.

☹ **PA-2 Phyto-Astringent Purifying Toner for Normal Skin** *($15 for 4 ounces)* is almost identical to PA-1, with some orange and papaya extract added. Both can cause skin irritations, and the alcohol and witch hazel only add fuel to the fire.

☺ **PA-3 Phyto-Astringent Purifying Toner for Dry Skin** *($15 for 4 ounces)* is a very good irritant-free toner for dry skin, although it won't purify anything.

☹ **PA-S Phyto-Astringent Purifying Toner for Sensitive Skin** *($15 for 4 ounces)* would be a great toner if it didn't contain grapefruit, which is hardly appropriate for sensitive skin or any skin type for that matter.

☺ **$$$ CR-1 Night Emulsion Cellular Recovery for Normal to Oily Skin Types** *($28 for 2 ounces)* contains mostly water, silicone, thickeners, water-binding agents, vitamins, preservatives, and antioxidants. This is a good emollient moisturizer for someone with dry skin but completely inappropriate for someone with oily skin.

☺ **$$$ Night Emulsion CR-2 Cellular Recovery for Normal to Dry Skin Types** *($28 for 2 ounces)* is almost identical to CR-1. It is a very good moisturizer, but it can't help your cells recover from anything.

☺ **$$$ CR-S Night Emulsion Cellular Recovery for Sensitive Skin Types** *($28 for 2 ounces)* is a good lightweight moisturizer for normal to dry skin, but there is nothing in here that makes it more appropriate for sensitive skin types.

☺ $$$ EP-1 Environmental Protective Day Emulsion for Oily Skin *($24 for 1.6 ounces)* contains mostly water, thickeners, pollen extract, plant oils, and preservatives. This is a very good, although overly expensive, emollient moisturizer for someone with dry skin; it would only cause problems for someone with oily skin.

☺ $$$ EP-2 Environmental Protective Day Emulsion for Normal Skin *($24 for 1.6 ounces)* is almost identical to EP-1, and the same review applies.

☺ $$$ EP-3 Environmental Protective Day Emulsion *($24 for 1.6 ounces)* is almost identical to EP-1 and EP-2, and the same review applies.

☺ $$$ EP-S Environmental Protective Day Emulsion for Sensitive Skin Types *($24 for 1.6 ounces)* doesn't include sunscreen, and without sunscreen this is not a product you can wear during the day, though this it is a good moisturizer for normal to dry skin.

☺ $$$ EP-T Environmental Protective Day Emulsion for All Skin Types *($24 for 1.6 ounces)* is similar to the one above, and the same review applies.

☺ $$$ EZR Day/Night Emulsion for All Skin Types *($28 for 1 ounce)* is a good moisturizer for someone with normal to dry skin; it's similar to most of the other M.A.C. moisturizers.

☺ NMF-Natural Moisturizing Factors for All Skin Types *($18 for 4 ounces)* contains many of the same ingredients as the other moisturizers and is fine for normal to dry skin.

☹ VM-1 Vitamin and Mineral Hydrating Mask, for Normal to Oily Skin *($14 for 2.5 ounces)* contains sodium lauryl sulfate as the fourth ingredient as well as menthol, and both are strong potential skin irritants.

☹ VM-2 Vitamin and Mineral Hydrating Mask, for Dry and Dehydrated Skin *($14 for 2 ounces)* contains water, clay, glycerin, sesame oil, standard slip agents, more clay, thickeners, vitamins A and E, and preservatives. This is a standard clay mask with some oil added to reduce the dryness caused by the clay. If you want a clay mask, this one is OK for some skin types.

M.A.C. Makeup

☺ FOUNDATION: Matte Finish *($20)* isn't all that matte. Someone with oily skin would not be pleased with this formulation; it's best for someone with normal to dry skin. **These colors are great:** N1, N3, N4, N9, N10, C2, C3, C4, C5, and Brunette. **These colors are too pink, peach, or ashy:** N5, C6, and C7.

☺ Satin Finish *($18)* has a lovely emollient feel and provides medium coverage for normal to dry skin (it is surprisingly similar to the Matte Finish). **These colors are great:** N1, N2, N3, N4, N6, N7, N9, C2, C3, C4, C5, C6, and C7. **These colors are too peach for most skin tones:** Copper and N5.

☺ Studio Fix Pressed Powder Foundation *($19)* is a silky-smooth powder foundation that provides medium coverage; although M.A.C. recommends it for normal to oily skin, it's really best on normal skin. **Most all of the shades are impressive.** ☺ **The only ones to watch out for are:** C-6, C-7, C-8, N-8, N-9, and N-10. These can be slightly peach or ash for some skin tones.

☺ **EP-T Day Emulsion Moisturizer** *($28)* is a lightweight, soft-finish, sheer foundation. It is an option for someone with dry skin who wants only a hint of foundation, but it would be far better if this had an SPF 15 with UVA protection so it wouldn't require a sunscreen underneath. Most of the colors are excellent, only C-5, C-6, N-1, N-5, and N-7 are either slightly too peach, pink, or ash for some skin tones.

☺ <u>CONCEALER:</u> **Concealer** *($10)* goes on rather heavy and thick, but it provides excellent coverage and stays on well without much slippage. M.A.C. recommends mixing it with the foundation or a little moisturizer before you apply it, probably to soften the thickness of the concealer, which can be a problem for someone who wants a more sheer application.

☹ **Correcting Tint** *($10)* is an assortment of cream concealers meant to correct skin tone. Colors of olive, red, mauve, green, and brown are supposed to even out uneven skin color. They end up leaving a strange shade on the skin that doesn't camouflage the underlying color, and it interacts even more strangely with the foundation you apply over it.

☺ <u>POWDER:</u> **Pressed Powder** *($18)* is a standard talc-based compact powder with a soft but slightly dry finish. N-9, N-10, C-7, and C-9 can be either too peach or too ash. **Loose Powder** comes in a shake-it bottle *($14)* or a traditional tub *($17)*. Both are good, but the tub is easier to use. The shake-it bottle gets shaken all over the place, making it messy; the tub ends up being more convenient. Be careful with C-3, C-5, C-7, and C-6, which can be slightly ash on some skin types, and N-5, which can be slightly peach. **Blot Powder** *($12)* has a translucent, dry finish. It works well.

☺ <u>BLUSH:</u> M.A.C.'s **Blushes** *($13)* are packaged just like the eyeshadows, in round see-through containers. The colors are fine—they go on true, and there is a large matte assortment—but fairly standard, nothing exceptional. $$$ **Creme Color for Eyes, Lips, Cheeks** *($14)* is just a very nice cream-based range of colors that can be used all over the face—well not all the colors, unless you are interested in having grayish-tan colored lips. I find the consistency too greasy for the eyes and the color too sheer and short-lasting for the lips, but for the cheeks it works great if you are looking for a cream blush. One caution: These do have a touch of shine.

☺ <u>EYESHADOW:</u> The **Eyeshadows** *($11.50 and $13)* have a large neutral matte selection. There are several shiny eyeshadows to wade through, but for the most part these are displayed separately, readily identified, and easily avoided or tolerated depending on your preferences. M.A.C. has one of the best neutral color palettes in the business. Warning: Some of the colors can be a bit on the heavy (greasy or grainy) side, and they go on more intense than they look.

☺ <u>EYE AND BROW SHAPER:</u> The **Eye Pencils** *($9.50)* are like almost every other eye pencil on the market. **Creme Liner** *($9.50)* is an ultra-dramatic liner that comes in a pot for a very thick matte look. Avoid the Aluminum shade.

☺ **LIPSTICK AND LIP PENCIL:** Most of M.A.C.'s lipsticks are excellent. **Matte Lipstick** *($13.50)* doesn't bleed and doesn't require a sealer, which always thrills me. The only problem is that it can be somewhat drying and make the lips peel or feel caked by the end of the day. **Satin Lipstick** *($13.50)* is wonderful and nicely creamy without being thick. It's supposed to be semi-matte; I don't see it, but maybe you will. **Sheer Lipstick** *($13.50)* is more a gloss than a lipstick; it contains a lot of vitamin E, which is a big selling point but not all that essential for the lips. An SPF 15 with UVA protection would be more impressive and worth the expense. **Liptone** *($13.50)* is a tint that goes on like a gloss, dries, and then becomes sort of a color stain on the lips. If you can get used to the texture, it's an interesting option for lip color that has some staying power. **Cream Lipstick** *($13.50)* is fairly standard but has a good smooth finish. The color selection for all of these lipstick groupings is pretty impressive. **LipGlass** *($9)* is a very emollient, tenacious lip gloss. The **Lip Pencils** *($9.50)* are like almost every other lip pencil on the market.

☹ **MASCARA:** The **Mascara** *($12)* is just OK and tends to smear slightly.

☺ **BRUSHES:** M.A.C. has one of the best selections of brushes you'll find anywhere *(38 different brushes ranging from $6 to $65)*. The big brushes are a little pricey, but they last forever if you take good care of them. Though there are indeed great inexpensive brushes to be found, if you're going to splurge, this is one area where the extra expense won't be wasted. Be sure to check out M.A.C.'s #142 brush. It is an excellent versatile eyeshadower. The only brushes to really avoid are #12, a sponge tip that comes free in most eyeshadow compacts; #13, a fantail brush that I'm sure has some function, but that is truly unnecessary for daily makeup application; and #24, a mascara spool that is easy to duplicate by washing out an old mascara wand.

Make Up For Ever—Paris

This extensive line of eyeshadows, foundations, powders, pencils, and concealers was originally created for use in the theater. Of course, the fact that a color line is used on stage does not mean it has what your face needs for daytime or even evening wear. There is much about Make Up For Ever—Paris that makes it difficult for me to recommend. Many of the hues, shades, textures, and products are inappropriate or just too heavy for most skin types or for a soft, natural look. Even the salesperson had a rough time making this line sound tempting.

Make Up For Ever's primary and significant strength is its vast selection of colors for most skin tones, especially medium to darker skin tones, and that is assuredly a welcome addition at the cosmetics counters.

The skin care for this line is an afterthought and is hardly worth a first much less a second look. As this book goes to print it is no longer being sold through Nordstrom and exactly where it will settle is not known for certain. For more information about Make Up For Ever, call (800) 757-5175.

Make Up For Ever—Paris (Skin Care)

☹ **Cleansing Milk** *($30 for 6.6 ounces)* is a standard mineral oil–based wipe-off cleanser that also contains lanolin. This is a very expensive emollient cold cream and can leave a greasy film on the skin.

☹ **Cleansing Oil** *($30 for 3.3 ounces)* is mostly silicone and mineral oil. This is one of the most overpriced products in this book and there is absolutely no reason to recommend it.

☹ **Eye Make-Up Remover** *($27 for 3.38 ounces)* is almost identical to the one above and the same review applies.

☹ **Tonic Lotion** *($30 for 6.6 ounces)* contain plant extracts and alcohol.

Make Up For Ever—Paris (Makeup)

☹ **FOUNDATION: Pre-Makeup Base** *($19)* is a tinted moisturizer that, like other color correctors, comes in lavender, green, orange, yellow, blue, white, and transparent. Color correctors come and go, and mostly, I believe, they should go. This unnecessary step builds up too much product and often mixes badly with the foundation.

☺ **Soft Modeling Film** *($24)* is an emollient liquid foundation that would be best for someone with normal to dry skin. It provides light to medium coverage and has an impressive selection of colors. **Most of the colors are excellent. These colors should be avoided:** 1, which is too rose; 5, 7, and 13, which are very orange; 6 and 14, which can be too ash; and 12, which can be too yellow.

☹ **Pan Stick** *($27)* contains mostly petrolatum, carnauba wax, lanolin, and castor oil. It is a greasy mess of a foundation, impossible to recommend. Just as bad, the wide range of colors displays strong tones of pink, orange, ash, rose, and peach. There are a few good colors, but why bother?

☹ **Pan Cake** *($27)* is, as the name implies, a cake of pressed powder that you can apply wet or dry. There are 16 colors, almost all too peach, orange, or ash. If the theater is your goal, these can be useful; otherwise, they are better left behind the counter.

☹ **CONCEALER: Eye Concealer Stick** *($16)* is a lipstick-style concealer that comes in only one shade; it is slightly pink, which is inappropriate for most, if not all, skin tones. Although it goes on rather sheer, the texture is quite greasy, and it can crease into the lines around the eye. **Pot Concealers** *($17)* are waterproof and come in an excellent array of colors for medium to darker skin tones. They provide serious coverage, but you have to put up with a dry, thick appearance. **Eye Concealer Pencil** *($17)* is a standard thin pencil that comes in two colors, one for Caucasian skin and one for darker skin tones. Each of the two pencils has a different color at each end, but the colors aren't the best, particularly the one for darker skin tones, which is strongly orange. You also have to get used to applying a concealer with a texture so dry that it feels like you're poking yourself.

☺ POWDER: **Poudre Libre** *($27)* is a standard talc-based loose powder with a soft texture. **Almost all of the colors are very good and neutral. These colors should be avoided:** 114 (hot pink), 2 (lavender pink), 6 (lavender), and 4 (green). **Compact Powder** *($27)* is a standard talc-based powder with a great color selection. Although nothing exceptional, it is a good powder with a nice texture.

☺ EYESHADOW AND BLUSH: Referred to as **Colors** *($14)*, these versatile items come in more than a hundred shades, and a good number of them are matte. The colors are strongly pigmented, so even the softest-looking pink goes on red, and the palest taupe goes on deep brown. (This is a definite drawback for those with lighter skin tones, but a strong plus for women with darker or African-American skin tones.) There are shiny colors in this mix, and several blues and greens, so pay attention. (Avoid. Avoid.) Just for the record, these colors don't hold a candle to M.A.C.'s, and M.A.C.'s cost less. Make Up For Ever also offers something called **Star Powders** *($17)*, little pots of loose iridescent powder in a fun range of colors. If you're feeling impetuous or are under 30 and want a sparkling effect, they could make an interesting splash of color somewhere, or everywhere.

☺ EYE AND BROW SHAPER: **Demographic Pencils** *($15)* are standard, everyday pencils for the eyes, brows, and lips. They come in an attractive collection of colors, except for the blues and greens, and they go on easily. The lip-pencil colors are much more vivid than you would imagine from just looking at them, so try them on before buying.

☺ LIPSTICK AND LIP PENCIL: While color choice seems to be Make Up For Ever's strong point, the three lipsticks, **Matte**, **Transparent**, and **Nacre** *(all $16)*, offer a surprisingly small selection. The Matte lipsticks go on thick and matte and stay on well, with little to no bleeding. The Transparents are simply sheer, greasy lipsticks. The Nacres are standard creamy, iridescent lipsticks, something I never recommend. The Demographic Pencils, reviewed above, include lip pencils.

☺ MASCARA: The **Mascara** *($16)* goes on easily, builds long thick lashes, and stays on well without smearing.

☺ BRUSHES: This line features more than 15 brushes, and a few are quite usable, but the quality (the bristles are supposed to be sable and pony, but they are too soft and loose) and the price (around $25 for even the tiniest brush) may be hard to swallow. While the bristles have a wonderfully soft texture, they are too sparse to hold color well or offer good control on the cheeks or eyes.

Marcelle (Canada Only)

This reasonably priced drugstore line has some good products that perform well and look great. The packaging is simple, and some of the products are fragrance-free. Sad to say, this isn't an exciting line; the foundations have an incredibly poor color selection, the eyeshadows all have some amount of shine, the blushes do too, and the pressed powders are fairly peach or pink. However, the lipsticks and pencils are worth investigating.

The skin-care products boast that they are hypoallergenic, but they aren't; there's no way any company can know what your skin may be allergic to. Also, many of these products contain ingredients that have a rather high potential for irritation or breakouts, such as witch hazel, several sunscreen ingredients, plant extracts, menthol, alcohol, and isopropyl myristate. For more information about Marcelle products call (800) 387-6707. **Note:** All prices listed for Marcelle products are in Canadian dollars.

Marcelle Skin Care

☺ **2 In 1 Face and Eye Cleanser** *($10.95 for 170 ml)* is a standard wipe-off cleanser that will remove makeup, but the pulling and tugging at the skin can worsen sagging.

☺ **Aquarelle Aqua-Pure Cleansing Bar Oil-Free** *($5.38 for 125 g)* is a standard bar soap that can be quite drying for almost all skin types. It contains tallow, which can cause breakouts.

☺ **Aquarelle Oil-Free Purifying Cleansing Gel for Oily Skin** *($10.58 for 170 ml)* is a good, standard detergent cleanser for most skin types. It won't purify anything, but it can clean the skin without irritation or dryness, and it won't irritate the eyes.

☺ **Cleansing Cream** *($7.98 for 240 ml)* is a very heavy, mineral oil–based detergent cleanser that can leave a greasy film on the skin. Calling this product hypoallergenic is stretching the facts; it contains sodium lauryl sulfate, an ingredient well known for being a skin sensitizer.

☺ **Cleansing Milk Combination Skin** *($9.89 for 240 ml)* is a standard detergent-based, water-soluble cleanser. It contains a tiny amount of lactic acid that probably isn't enough to be a problem for the skin or eyes, but there are several waxes in here that could clog pores. This cleanser can be a problem for many skin types.

☺ **Cleansing Milk Oily Skin** *($10.50 for 240 ml)* is similar to the one above and the same comments apply.

☹   **Cleansing Milk for Dry to Normal Skin** *($9.88 for 240 ml)* is a mineral oil–based cleanser that must be wiped off. It can leave a greasy film on the skin.

☺   **Gentle Foaming Wash All Skin Types** *($8.98 for 170 ml)* isn't all that gentle, but it is a good standard detergent-based, water-soluble cleanser that can be drying for most skin types.

☺   **Hydractive Water Rinseable Cleansing Lotion for Dehydrated/Normal to Dry Skin** *($11.95 for 180 ml)* is a wipe-off cleanser that isn't all that rinseable, and isn't very good at removing makeup either. You have to use a washcloth, and that isn't a great way to remove makeup because it can be irritating and pulls at the skin. It could be OK for someone with very dry skin who doesn't wear much makeup, but it can leave a greasy film.

☹   **Hydractive Hydra-Pure Cleansing Bar for Dehydrated/Normal to Dry Skin** *($6.38 for 125 g)* is a standard tallow-based bar cleanser; the cleansing agents can be drying to the skin and the tallow can clog pores.

☹   **Soap** *($2.68 for 100 g)* is similar to the bar cleanser above and the same review applies.

☹   **Creamy Eye Make-Up Remover** *($6.58 for 50 ml)* is basically just mineral oil, some thickeners and slip agents, and petrolatum. It will wipe off makeup and leave a greasy film on the skin, but this isn't much different from the mineral oil–based face cleansers above.

☹   **Eye Make-Up Remover Pads** *($6.98 for 60 pads)* are mineral oil–soaked pads. Wiping off makeup is a problem, and this is an expensive way to do it when a bottle of mineral oil and some cotton would have the same effect for a fraction of the price.

☺   **Eye Make-Up Remover Lotion Oil-Free** *($7.48 for 120 ml)* contains detergent cleansing agents, slip agent, and preservatives. It will remove makeup, but wiping off makeup is a problem for skin.

☹   **Scrub Wash for All Skin Types** *($8.98 for 100 ml)* is a clay cleanser that also contains witch hazel, zinc oxide, alcohol, detergent cleanser, thickener, and preservatives. Not only is it *not* hypoallergenic, but the clay and zinc oxide make it hard to rinse off.

☹   **Aquarelle Oil Normalizing Toner Alcohol-Free for Oily Skin** *($9.98 for 240 ml)* contains mostly water, witch hazel, slip agents, aloe, film former, and preservatives. Technically, it is alcohol-free, but the witch hazel contains a small amount of alcohol and can be a skin irritant.

☺   **Hydractive Reviving Toner, Dehydrated and Normal to Dry Skin** *($11.25 for 180 ml)* contains mostly water, slip agent, water-binding agents, glycerin, aloe, film former, anti-irritant, and preservatives. This would be a very good nonirritating toner for most skin types.

The Reviews M

☹ **Skin Freshener, Combination Skin** *($8.98 for 240 ml)* is mostly just alcohol and glycerin and is not a good idea for any skin type I can think of. Calling alcohol hypoallergenic is someone's idea of a joke, right?

☹ **Skin Freshener, Normal to Dry Skin** *($8.98 for 240 ml)* is similar to the product above, and the same review applies. This product also contains aluminum chlorohydrate, a key ingredient in underarm deodorant, which can cause breakouts and allergic reactions.

☹ **Skin Toner, Combination Skin** *($7.95 for 240 ml)* is similar to the Skin Freshener for Combination Skin above, and the same review applies.

☹ **Skin Toner for Oily Skin** *($8.98 for 240 ml)* is similar to the Skin Freshener for Combination Skin above, only it contains even more alcohol and the same review applies.

☺ **Alpha-Radiance Cream Normal to Dry and Sensitive Skin** *($14.38 for 60 ml)* doesn't contain more than 3% AHAs, and that isn't enough to make it effective as an exfoliant. It won't renew skin, although it could be an OK moisturizer for someone with dry skin.

☺ **Alpha-Radiance Lotion, Combination to Oily and Sensitive Skin** *($14.38 for 120 ml)* is similar to the cream above, and the same review applies.

☺ **Aquarelle Aqua-Matte Hydrating Fluid** *($12.58 for 120 ml)* contains mostly water, several thickeners, fragrance, more thickeners, aloe, silicone, and preservatives. There are some good water-binding agents and antioxidants here, but in amounts too minuscule to have value for the skin. This is an OK but ordinary moisturizer for someone with normal to slightly dry skin.

☹ **Formula 24 Cream for Oily Skin** *($7.48 for 60 ml)* contains mostly water, slip agent, thickeners, sulfur, and preservatives. Sulfur is a disinfectant that may have an effect on acne, but it doesn't make sense to put it in a cream base that contains thickeners that can cause breakouts.

☺ **Hydractive Eye Contour Gel** *($11.95 for 15 ml)* contains mostly water, glycerin, water-binding agent, film former, thickener, and preservatives. This is a good lightweight moisturizer for normal to slightly dry skin.

☺ **Hydractive Hydra-Repair Night Treatment for All Skin Types** *($17.95 for 60 ml)* contains mostly water, plant extracts, thickeners, silicone, plant oil, water-binding agent, and preservatives. Of the ingredients mentioned in the name of the product on the label, only hyaluronic acid (a good water-binding agent) comes well before the preservatives. All the others are at the end of the list, in amounts barely worth mentioning. This is a good emollient moisturizer for someone with dry skin, but more because of the standard ingredients than the fancy-sounding ones.

☺ **Hydractive Hydra-Replenishing Cream** *($15.25 for 40 ml)* is a very ordinary, boring moisturizer for dry skin that contains mostly water, glycerin, thickeners, film former, water-binding agent, silicone, and preservatives.

☹ **Oil-Free Multi-Defense Lotion Daily Moisturizer SPF 15** *($13.48 for 120 ml)* doesn't contain avobenzone, zinc oxide, or titanium dioxide as the active ingredients, and is not recommended.

☹ **Multi-Defense Cream Daily Moisturizer SPF 15** *($12.95 for 60 ml)* doesn't contain avobenzone, zinc oxide, or titanium dioxide as the active ingredients, and is not recommended.

☺ **Moisture Cream** *($8.58 for 40 ml, $11.98 for 60 ml)* contains isopropyl myristate, which is known for causing breakouts, as the third ingredient; so much for hypoallergenic. Other than that, this is a good, ordinary emollient moisturizer for someone with dry skin. It does contain AHAs, but only about 2%, not enough to make it an exfoliant.

☺ **Moisture Lotion** *($9.88 for 90 ml, $12.58 for 120 ml)* is similar to the cream above, but without the AHAs, and the same review applies.

☺ **Night Cream** *($8.58 for 40 ml)* is almost identical to the Moisture Lotion above, but it's a cream, and the same review applies.

☺ **Anti-Aging Cream** *($11.95 for 40 ml)* contains mostly water, thickeners, water-binding agents, plant oil, and preservatives. This is a very good moisturizer for someone with dry skin, but there is nothing anti-aging in this product whatsoever. The collagen and elastin here are nothing more than water-binding agents; they have no effect on the collagen and elastin that are part of your skin.

☹ **Clay Mask** *($8.98 for 100 ml)* contains mostly water, witch hazel, clay, glycerin, thickener, and preservatives. This is a standard clay mask, but I wouldn't call clay or witch hazel hypoallergenic.

☺ **Dry Skin Lubricating Cream** *($9.95 for 120 ml)* is a very heavy, thick moisturizer for someone with exceptionally dry skin. It contains mostly mineral oil, petrolatum, wax, and thickeners.

☺ **Eye Care Cream, Ultra-Light** *($7.68 for 15 ml)* contains mostly water, several thickeners, glycerin, aloe, film former, water-binding agents, vitamin E, silicone, and preservatives. This is a good moisturizer for someone with normal to dry skin.

☺ **Eye Cream Ultra Rich** *($6.78 for 15 ml)* is just mineral oil, petrolatum, wax, and preservatives. It is about as close to Vaseline as you can get, which makes it greasy and good for very dry skin.

☺ **Gentle Purifying Mask** *($10.25 for 50 ml)* is a standard clay mask that also contains some plant oil and water-binding agents to help reduce the drying effect of the clay. This can be good for someone with normal to dry skin.

☹ **Time Release Hydrating Mask** *($8.95 for 50 ml)* is just a moisturizer that is left on the face, meaning wiped off instead of washed off; it will keep moisturizing, just like any other moisturizer. This one contains mostly water, thickeners, silicone, water-binding agents, fruit extracts, and preservatives. The fruit extracts have nothing to do with AHAs, and there aren't enough in here even if they did. What is a problem for this product is that it contains menthol, a skin irritant, which is a shame, because the moisturizing ingredients here are good ones.

☹ **Self-Tanning Lotion with Alpha-Hydroxy Acid Moisturizing Formula for Face** *($8.98 for 50 ml)* is a standard dihydroxyacetone-based self-tanner. It contains about 4% AHA, but the pH is too high for it to work as an exfoliant.

☺ **Protective Block No Chemical Sunscreen Cream SPF 25** *($12.95 for 50 ml)* is an excellent sunscreen for dry skin. It contains both titanium dioxide and zinc oxide as the active ingredients.

☺ **Protective Block No Chemical Sunscreen Lotion SPF 25** *($12.95 for 120 ml)* is an excellent sunscreen for dry skin. It contains both titanium dioxide and zinc oxide as the active ingredients.

☺ **Protective Block No Chemical Sunscreen Spray SPF 15** *($12.95 for 120 ml)* is an excellent sunscreen for dry skin. It contains titanium dioxide as the active ingredient.

☹ **Sun Block Cream SPF 8** *($7.95 for 90 ml)* doesn't contain avobenzone, zinc oxide, or titanium dioxide as the active ingredients, and the SPF number is dismal.

☹ **Sun Block Cream, SPF 15** *($6.78 for 90 ml)* doesn't contain avobenzone, zinc oxide, or titanium dioxide as the active ingredients, and is not recommended.

☹ **Sun Block Cream, SPF 20** *($7.95 for 90 ml)* doesn't contain avobenzone, zinc oxide, or titanium dioxide as the active ingredients, and is not recommended.

☹ **Sun Block Lotion SPF 8** *($7.95 for 120 ml)* doesn't contain avoben-zone, zinc oxide, or titanium dioxide as the active ingredients, and the SPF number is dismal.

☹ **Sun Block Lotion SPF 15** *($6.78 for 120 ml)* doesn't contain avobenzone, zinc oxide, or titanium dioxide as the active ingredients, and is not recommended.

☹ **Sunblock Lotion, SPF 20** *($7.95 for 120 ounces)* doesn't contain avobenzone, zinc oxide, or titanium dioxide as the active ingredients, and is not recommended.

☺ **After Sun Lotion, All Skin Types** *($7.95 for 120 ml)* is a good basic moisturizer for dry skin. It contains mostly water, thickeners, mineral oil, petrolatum, silicone, and preservatives.

Marcelle Makeup

☹ <u>FOUNDATION:</u> **Moisture Rich Foundation for Dry/Normal Skin** *($8.25)* would be a good foundation if the colors weren't so pink and peach. **Matte Finish Oil-Free Foundation** *($8.25)* and **All Day Protection with SPF 8** *($8.75)* both have a very poor color selection. The All Day Protection with such a low SPF is a terribly misleading name, especially since this one doesn't include UVA protection. **Sheer**

Tint Moisturizer *($10.25)* comes in three shades of which only Creme Beige resembles any known skin tone.

☺ <u>CONCEALER:</u> **Cover-Up Stick** *($6.25)* is a lipstick-type concealer with a terrible selection of colors, none of which I recommend. **Concealer Crayon** *($6.25)* is a fat pencil that comes in three OK shades: Light, Beige Cameo, and Dark (which isn't all that dark). The texture is workable, but it tends to crease into the lines around the eye.

☹ <u>POWDER:</u> **Pressed Powder** *($9.75)* and **Face Powder Loose** *($9.75)* are most all too peach or pink to recommend. The only passable shade for both is Translucent. **Pressed Bronzing Powder** *($9.75)* comes in two shades, and both are too peach or red for most skin tones.

☺ <u>BLUSH:</u> **Velvety Powder Blush** *($6.95)* does have a very soft, smooth finish, but the colors are all shiny and the application too soft and sheer for darker skin tones.

☹ <u>EYESHADOW:</u> **Eyeshadow Singles** *($7.75)* are all fairly shiny and not recommended unless you have to wear shine; then these colors do go on soft and even, with a great range of neutral shades.

☺ <u>EYE AND BROW SHAPER:</u> **Kohl Eye Liner** *($6.75)* is similar to many other pencils on the market though this one has a slightly drier texture than most. **Waterproof Eye Liner** *($6.75)* is a standard eye pencil that goes on creamy soft; it does stay on well when wet, but so do most eye pencils.

☹ **Powder Eye Liner** *($6.75)* is not all that powdery, it's really just a pencil that goes on somewhat choppy and tends to roll off.

☺ <u>LIPSTICK AND LIP PENCIL:</u> Marcelle has a good but limited selection of lipsticks. **Hydra Rouge Lipstick** *($7.95)* has a slightly glossy finish. **Impeccable Lip Color** *($7.95)* has a great creamy, soft matte application. **Sheer Lip Color** *($7.25)* is just that, a sheer, glossy-finish lipstick. The fairly standard **Lip Definition Crayon** *($5.95)* is a standard pencil with a nice range of colors.

☹ <u>MASCARA:</u> **Superlash Mascara** *($8.50)* takes a long time to build definition and even then it doesn't build very much. It would be OK if you just want a lightweight makeup look, but this is more a why bother than anything else. **Ultimate Lash Mascara** *($8.50)* does build length and thickness but it also clumps and makes lashes look stiff and unnatural.

Mariana Chicet (Skin Care Only)

While some of Chicet's products are interesting, particularly for dry skin, and the philosophy of the line is fascinating, it is based on so much erroneous, inaccurate, and unsubstantiated information that I almost don't know where to begin. For example, Chicet claims that she has "analyzed the effects of AHAs and found that the adverse effects far outweigh the benefits." Amazing statement. All of the studies I've read concerning AHAs indicate just the opposite. Yes, using AHAs may cause skin irritation and there are still many unknowns, but the reason they have become so intensely popular in such a short period of time is because they work so well to smooth skin and unclog pores. Chicet also states that AHAs clog pores. If anything, AHAs' ability to unglue dead skin cells and slough them from the surface of the skin means they can *prevent* pores from becoming clogged.

Chicet's brochure proudly states that none of her products contain mineral oil, petrolatum, artificial colors, or perfumes, but instead use natural emulsifiers and emollients derived from animals and plants. It is standard practice for so-called "natural" skin-care lines to eschew mineral oil and petrolatum as being problematic, yet no cosmetics researcher (even from the natural side of the world) has ever shown that mineral oil and petrolatum are anything but good moisturizing agents and completely benign. On the other hand, Chicet's products contain jojoba oil and lanolin, which are known to be comedogenic according to every report I've seen published in *Cosmetics & Toiletries,* the industry's foremost magazine. She also describes mineral oil and petrolatum as not being absorbed by the skin, which happens to be beneficial; if everything is absorbed, what's left on the surface to prevent dehydration? Moreover, several of the ingredients touted in her line are also not absorbed well by the skin, such as sodium hyaluronate and collagen. That's not bad; in fact, they are great for the skin because they prevent the air from taking moisture out of the skin, but no better than mineral oil or petrolatum do.

There is also much fuss made about milk and apple juice in Chicet's products. As always, when food is used in cosmetics, the amount of preservatives being used has to increase proportionately. That can cause problems for the skin. Also, food makes the bacteria living on and in your skin very happy and creates a great environment for them to thrive in. Milk and apple juice are great foods, but terrible skin-care agents.

I could go on, but you get the picture. That doesn't mean there aren't some interesting products in this line, but it takes a lot of effort to get beyond the distortions and misleading information. You can call the Marianna Chicet company at (800) 995-4490.

☺ **$$$ Emollient Cleanser** *($16.50 for 4 ounces)* is nothing more than a standard-issue cold cream that needs to be wiped off and can leave the face feeling greasy. I never recommend wiping off makeup because it pulls the skin, and over time that can cause sagging, especially around the eyes.

☺ **$$$ Nutrient Milk Cleanser** *($15.50 for 8 ounces)* is similar to the cleanser above but in lotion form.

☹ **Apple Milk Cleanser and Toner** *($8.50 for 8 ounces)* contains mostly water, apple juice, milk, alcohol, and preservatives. This is just a toner that contains alcohol, juice, and milk. Food on the face can cause problems by being a wonderful food source for bacteria, and alcohol is irritating.

☹ **Apple Milk Cleanser and Toner for Very Sensitive Skin** *($8.50 for 8 ounces)* is identical to the product above but minus the alcohol. The lack of alcohol is nice, but the other ingredients are completely useless for the skin.

☹ **Gommage for Oily Skin** *($11 for 0.25 ounce)* is a powder to which you add water to make a paste. It contains mostly oatmeal, wheat bran, egg white, spearmint, milk, and preservatives. It is a lightweight scrub, but the food is a feast for the bacteria on the surface of the skin and spearmint can be a skin irritant.

☹ **Gommage for Combination Skin and for Oily Sensitive Skin** *($11 for 0.25 ounce)* is virtually identical to the product above, and the same review applies.

☹ **Gommage for Dry and Sensitive Skin** *($11 for 0.25 ounce)* is almost identical to the product above, minus the spearmint. At least someone knew spearmint is a problem for sensitive skin, but I feel strongly that it is a problem for all skin types.

☺ **$$$ Clay and Fresh Sea Plant Mask for Oily Sensitive Skin** *($13 for 2 ounces)* contains mostly zinc oxide, egg white, clay, magnesium, and preservatives. Zinc oxide can clog pores and can be a problem for someone with oily skin, but this can be an OK mask for someone somewhere I'm sure.

☺ **$$$ Fresh Nourishing Mask for Dry Skin** *($15 for 2 ounces)* contains mostly oat protein (emollient), egg yolk, and preservatives. Oats and egg yolk won't feed the skin from the outside in, but this mask may feel OK on the skin.

☺ **$$$ Day and Night Revitalizing Concentrate** *($45.50 for 1.15 ounces)* contains mostly water, 33% natural soluble collagen solution, 29% hydrolyzed elastin, 15% hyaluronic acid solution, 10% conjugated glycopeptides, 6% glycosaminoglycans, 6% saccharide isomerate, 100% plant extracts from Switzerland (do the Swiss have better plants than anyone else?), and preservatives. The percentages are nice, but they aren't accurate, or at the very least they're confusing. The percentages add up to 199%, and content can only be 100%. Even if we say 100% refers to the plants and not to the content of the product, we're still at 99%, and there is no way the water and preservatives add up to only 1% of the product. If that were true, this would not be something you would want to put on your face. It is a good moisturizer for dry skin, with fairly standard water-binding agents, but that's about it.

☺ **$$$ Maximum Moisturizing Complex** *($38 for 1 ounce)* contains mostly water-binding agent, thickener, more water-binding agent, thickener, and preservatives. This is a good moisturizer for someone with dry skin.

☺ **$$$ Moisturizing Mist Complex** *($8.50 for 4 ounces)* is similar to the product above but with less water-binding agent.

☺ **$$$ Bone Marrow Cream** *($29 for 1.35 ounces)* contains mostly plant oil, bone marrow oil (from cattle), several thickeners, water-binding agents, and preservatives. This would be a good, very emollient moisturizer for dry skin, but don't expect anything special from bone oil (which is essential beef fat, similar in nature to tallow).

☺ $$$ **Revitalizing Cream** (*$30.50 for 2 ounces*) is almost identical to the product above but minus the bone oil, and the same review applies.

☺ $$$ **Ideal Moisturizer** (*$25.50 for 2 ounces*) is almost identical to the product above, and the same review applies.

☺ $$$ **Revitalizing Lotion Concentrate** (*$28.50 for 2 ounces*) contains mostly water, plant oils, bone oil, thickeners, water-binding agents, more thickeners, and preservatives. This is a very good, emollient moisturizer for someone with dry skin.

☺ $$$ **Rich Moisturizer** (*$27.50 for 2 ounces*) contains mostly plant oil, water, lanolin, thickeners, and preservatives. This is indeed rich, and would be good but heavy for someone with very dry skin.

☺ $$$ **Oil-Free Moisturizer** (*$25 for 2 ounces*) contains mostly water, thickeners, water-binding agent, and preservatives. It is oil-free, and that's nice, but some of the thickening agents such as vegetable wax and glyceryl stearate can be a problem for oily skin. Still, it should be fine over somewhat dry areas.

☹ $$$ **Melanin Sunscreen for Dry Skin** (*$11 for 0.5 ounce*) is a titanium dioxide–based sunscreen that contains mostly water, plant oils, melanin, thickeners, and preservatives. This would be just fine but—it has no SPF rating. If you use a sunscreen without an SPF rating, you are gambling with the health of your skin. One salesperson at Mariana Chicet said it had a rating of about SPF 10, while another said around 18. Yet, another one mentioned the more you put on the more protection you get, which means it could be as high as you want. None of that is true. The standards for SPF ratings are very specific and tightly regulated by the FDA. This kind of misinformation is as irresponsible and unethical as a cosmetics company can get.

☹ $$$ **Melanin Sunscreen Oil Free** (*$11 for 0.5 ounce*) has much in common with the sunscreen above, and the same review applies.

Marilyn Miglin (Skin Care Only)

I have a great deal of affection for the name Marilyn Miglin. My first experience with makeup artistry was with an extremely talented (though completely condescending) salesperson at Marilyn Miglin's first store in downtown Chicago's prestigious Oak Street area. I was a mere 18 years old at the time. I came in sporting white eyeshadow under the eyebrow, brown in the crease, and, yes, blue eyeshadow on the eyelid. After acting completely annoyed at my request for a spontaneous makeup appointment right then and there, even though there were no other appointments waiting, she finally agreed to do a quick makeup application. With a great deal of disinterest that I would never stand for today, this woman inadvertently but deftly taught me the art of contouring under the cheekbone and the temple area, layering eyeshadows to create depth and shape for the eye, and creating perfectly lined lips (start in the middle and work your way out; place the line along the inside of the lip, not the outside). No blue eyeshadow, she dictated, adding that I should never use white under the eyebrow unless I wanted to look like I had swollen eyes. She carried on at length about the horrors of pink eyeshadow, but delighted in using a shiny white powder to accent the top of my cheekbone, the center of my lips, and the center of my forehead to add beguiling highlights. I left in awe of her work and with several products in tow, including a pot of that shiny white powder.

Time went on and I learned other techniques from a variety of makeup artists I worked with, but I never forgot my first real initiation into my newfound (and clearly lasting) career choice. Thank you, Marilyn Miglin.

Miglin made many attempts to go national with her skin-care and makeup line, but that kind of department-store distribution never worked well for her. She finally found her niche in the world of television home shopping. Her name has become well known to a wide range of consumers. But what about her products, which she claims are the be-all and end-all for skin care? I would love to say that I find them as enthralling as I found my first makeup experience at the Marilyn Miglin counter, but that just isn't the case. The line Miglin is most often showcasing is her **Perfect Balance P.D.S.** (P.D.S. stands for patented delivery system), accompanied by the **Iolight Facial Enhancer**. I only wish the products were even half as miraculous as the brochure descriptions. Alas, most of the emphasis is on the marketing language and not the products.

A patented delivery system sounds interesting, but lots and lots of different cosmetics companies, from Lauder to L'Oreal, offer lots and lots of patented delivery systems. Delivery systems are how a product delivers its ingredients to the skin. Almost any mixture of ingredients placed on the skin, say water and oil, has its own delivery system of sorts. Delivering any skin-care ingredient into the skin, however, has no effect on the skin's health. Skin-care ingredients cannot regenerate skin cells or skin structures, although that's the claim you are asked to believe about Miglin's Perfect Balance P.D.S. products. Still, it is interesting to point out that Miglin's delivery system is supposed to be an advanced form of liposomes. Liposomes are the patented delivery system from L'Oreal. How she improved on their formula is not explained, and no one at Miglin's company seemed to know either. Liposomes are a good way to hold moisturizing ingredients in the skin, but that's about it.

Miglin has a handful of impressive-sounding ingredients that supposedly perform all kinds of wonders. Oxygen is one of the more notable, but of course there isn't enough oxygen in these products to blow out a candle, let alone revitalize the skin. A group of water-binding agents called TCN-NA is supposed to be a biological activator. It may be when it's broken down via digestion internally, but externally this is nothing more than a large group of amino acids forming polypeptide polymers that have way too large a molecular structure to be absorbed into the skin. They're fine for binding water in the skin, but that's all.

The products are sold in tandem with the ⊗ **Iolight Facial Enhancer** *($99 when sold alone or $89 with the five Perfect Balance P.D.S. products)*, an infrared light/heat source as well as a vibrating facial massager. Scientifically speaking, when it comes to wavelength frequency infrared light is just beyond visible light radiation. That means you get heat without light, and that's about it. This little lamp warms up the skin and the massage action vibrates the skin, which can definitely increase blood flow, but it can cause more problems than benefits. Artificially heating up the skin and vibrating it can cause surface capillaries to break, or risk creating a network of spider capillaries all over the face.

An unattributed quote in Miglin's product brochure is "Dermatologists tell us that only 20% of the changes we see in our skin are the natural result of the aging process ... fully 80% are the direct result of neglect." What kind of neglect? The quote doesn't tell us. All the dermatologists I've ever interviewed, as well as the Skin Cancer Association, say that the only neglect that damages the skin is unprotected sun exposure, and Miglin doesn't include a sunscreen in her skin-care regime. Can you believe it? She's selling five basic skin-care products, plus two more that make the standard inflated claims about the miracle of vitamin C. That makes seven products, and no sunscreen! If you are interested in finding out more about Miglin's skin-care system, call (800) 284-3900 or (800) 662-1120.

⊗ **Clean Tone** *($25 for 4 ounces)* is a wipe-off makeup remover that contains a long list of vitamins and water-binding agents. You are still just wiping off makeup, which can pull at the skin, causing it to sag, and the vitamins and water-binding agents are being wiped away as well.

⊗ **Liquid Veil** *($25 for 4 ounces)* is an alcohol-based facial mask that contains a hairstyling agent. It dries into a plastic-like layer over the skin that you then peel off. Both of the main ingredients can dry and irritate the skin. The brochure says, "The tingling tells you it is working." All the tingling communicates is irritation and dryness.

☺ **$$$ Energy** *($22.50 for 4 ounces)* contains mostly water, thickener, aloe, water-binding agents, vitamins, plant extracts, silicone, plant oil, minerals, more thickeners, and preservatives. This is a good toner-like moisturizer for someone with normal to dry skin, but don't expect the vitamins to feed your skin. The brochure copy explains that "surface cells get a metabolic boost, taking in nutrients and eliminating waste and toxins." How absurd. Surface skin cells are dead and are incapable of taking in or excreting anything.

☺ **$$$ Perfect Balance Oxygen 600** *($37.50 for 4 ounces)* contains a minuscule amount of oxygenated water (though all water is oxygenated. After all H_2O means two hydrogen molecules with an oxygen molecule). It would be a good moisturizer for someone with dry skin. It contains mostly water, aloe, slip agent, thickeners, silicone, more thickeners, water-binding agent, lactic acid (about 2% to 3%), more water-binding agents, vitamins, plant oil, more water-binding agents, and preservatives. This product claims to be super-oxygenating for the skin, amplifying the skin's oxygen intake. Even if it were possible to improve the skin's appearance by delivering oxygen to it, there isn't enough oxygen in here to serve that function. The skin's aging process is very complicated, and there is no single cause of aging that can be bandaged up with a cosmetic. If extra oxygen were the answer, we would all live in oxygen tents and no one would wrinkle. But it isn't just oxygen, or free-radical damage (which requires the presence of oxygen), or the depletion of many other components of the skin's structure. All it takes to stop most of the skin's wrinkling is a sunscreen. Too bad that isn't part of Miglin's skin-care routine.

☺ **$$$ Restore** *($40 for 4 ounces)* is fairly similar to the product above, minus the oxygen. It would be a good moisturizer for someone with normal to dry skin.

☺ **$$$ Perfect C Firming Creme** *($30 for 2 ounces)* contains mostly water, thickeners, aloe, more thickeners, slip agent, silicone, thickener, vitamin C, water-binding agent, more thickeners, silicone, fragrant oils, and preservatives. This is a good moisturizer for someone with normal to dry skin, but don't count on the vitamin C lasting very long given how unstable an ingredient it is.

☺ **$$$ Perfect C Serum** *($35 for 0.85 ounce)* is identical to the product above, minus the emollient thickening agent. The same comments apply.

Mary Kay

Mary Kay had some rough waters to get through in 1998. I have to admit, it was a bit of a shocking story. Here is the gist of the report that appeared on television and in newspapers across the country: "A former star saleswoman for Mary Kay Cosmetics says the firm took away her job and her company car after she failed to make her sales quota because she was ill with breast cancer and pregnant. In a wrongful-firing lawsuit filed last week in Contra Costa County [California] Superior Court, Claudine Woolf, 28, said that when her twin medical issues left her unable to work last year, Mary Kay first towed away her company car, a shiny red Pontiac Grand Am. Then the company told her it could make 'no exceptions' on sales quotas—not even for a woman simultaneously battling to save her own life and that of her unborn child. What galled her the most, Woolf said in an interview, is that the $1 billion direct-sales firm boasts that it has shown what it calls 'a commitment to bettering the lives of women around the world' by donating millions of dollars to support breast cancer research. . . . 'It was beyond me that they wouldn't make an exception for one of their own people who had it.' "

According to the story that appeared on *NBC Dateline,* Mary Kay wasn't commenting on the lawsuit, and a spokeswoman said Ms. Woolf has kept her status all along. Woolf's lawyer said that the reinstatement came after they heard the lawsuit was coming.

I have not been able to get a response from anyone at Mary Kay Inc. regarding this story, except that they insist that all their sales representatives are self-employed and not employees of the Mary Kay company. My attorney says legally the Mary Kay company appears to be well within their rights, but I have to agree to a certain extent with Woolf; if Mary Kay can donate money to cancer clinics surely it can have some charity left over for its own representatives, despite the technicalities of employment status.

Despite the legal morass, Mary Kay is one of the original home-sales cosmetics companies. Since beginning her firm in 1963, Mary Kay Ash (with her son's help) has built herself quite an empire. There are now more than 300,000 Mary Kay salespeople. As impressive as this all sounds, and it is impressive, the average salesperson's income is more like $5,000 to $10,000 a year. Obviously, the ability to sell does not come naturally to every member of the sales force.

The strong points of Mary Kay products are the great blushes, very good foundations, and reasonably priced eye and lip pencils. The colors are conveniently divided into Cool, Warm, and Neutral. But there are lots of pitfalls to watch out for, such as a huge selection of blue eyeshadows, a cream concealer that easily creases into the lines around the eyes, lipsticks that tend toward the greasy side, and a skin-care system (including foundation) that often forces you to buy all or none of it, although that usually depends how stalwart a position the line rep you're with takes.

Another potential problem arises from the way the products are marketed. Each salesperson buys her products and samples from the company and sells them directly to the consumer, and so, because of the logic of cash flow, not everyone can afford to stock all of the colors. What tends to happen is that the consumer is shown only what the salesperson has in stock. For more information about Mary Kay call (800) 627-9529.

Mary Kay Skin Care

☹ **Creamy Cleanser** *($10 for 6.5 ounces)* is indeed a creamy cleanser, but it can't be rinsed off without the aid of a washcloth. It can also leave behind traces of makeup.

☺ **Deep Cleanser** *($10 for 6.5 ounces)* is a water-soluble detergent cleanser that can be too drying for most skin types.

☹ **Gentle Cleansing Creme** *($10 for 4 ounces)* is a traditional, greasy cold cream containing mostly mineral oil, water, petrolatum, beeswax, glycerin, and other waxes. It might be gentle, but it is also quite heavy, and wiping off makeup is not good for the skin.

☹ **Purifying Bar** *($12 for 4.2 ounces, $10 for refill)* is a standard bar soap that won't purify anything, but it may dry out the skin and clog pores.

☺ **Oil-Free Eye Makeup Remover** *($14 for 3.75 ounces)* contains water, silicone, slip agents, and preservative. This very simple product will remove eye makeup, but it takes wiping, and that isn't good for the skin.

☹ **Hydrating Freshener** *($11 for 6.5 ounces)* contains mostly water, slip agent, preservative, and a small amount of arnica and peppermint, which can irritate the skin.

☹ **Blemish Control Toner** *($11 for 6.5 ounces)* contains mostly water, alcohol, slip agent, more alcohol, menthol, and eucalyptus oil. This is too irritating to even be considered an option for any skin type.

☹ **Purifying Freshener** *($11 for 6.5 ounces)* contains mostly water and alcohol, which can irritate the skin.

☺ **Balancing Moisturizer** *($16 for 4 ounces)* is a good basic moisturizer for normal to dry skin, containing mostly water, mineral oil, water-binding agents, thickeners, plant oil, and preservatives.

☺ **Enriched Moisturizer** *($16 for 4 ounces)* isn't all that enriched or all that different from the moisturizer above, and the same comments apply.

☺ **Extra Emollient Moisturizer** *($16 for 4 ounces)* is a very rich, somewhat heavy moisturizer for dry skin; it contains mostly water, wax, plant oils, water-binding agents, thickeners, and preservatives.

☺ **Extra Emollient Night Cream** *($11 for 2.5 ounces)* is a very rich, extremely heavy moisturizer for someone with severely dry skin. It contains mostly petrolatum, mineral oil, several thickeners, and preservatives.

☺ **Oil-Control Lotion** *($16 for 4 ounces)* is a lightweight moisturizer that contains mostly silicone, thickeners, film former, and preservatives. Nothing in this product can control, change, or affect the amount of oil your skin produces. It is just an OK moisturizer for slightly dry skin and that's about it.

☺ **$$$ Advanced Moisture Renewal Treatment Cream** *($19 for 2.5 ounces)* is a good, rich moisturizer for dry skin, but it's nothing special; it contains mostly water, mineral oil, thickeners, petrolatum, plant oil, and preservatives. Some vitamin E and water-binding agents are in this product, but they come well after the preservatives, so there isn't enough to matter or make it very interesting.

☺ **$$$ Instant Action Eye Cream** *($15 for 0.65 ounce)* contains mostly water, thickeners, vitamins, anti-irritant, water-binding agents, silicone, and preservatives. This is a good moisturizer for dry skin.

☹ **Triple-Action Eye Enhancer** *($15 for 0.65 ounce)* claims to have more benefits in one little product than almost any other I've ever seen. According to the company's magazine, it has much more than just triple action; I lost count after six benefits. It has free-radical scavengers, AHAs, and light-diffusing ingredients; it can be used as an eyeshadow base or as an under-eye concealer; it reduces puffiness and increases skin firmness; and, finally, it reduces the appearance of wrinkles. What's in this little miracle? Mostly silicone, film former, clay, several thickeners, and preservatives. There are tiny amounts of vitamins E and A, but they are at the end of the ingredient list and are completely insignificant. Then what about those benefits? Well, there aren't enough AHAs in this product to exfoliate skin, which is actually good, because you wouldn't want that on your eyelids. It doesn't have light-diffusing properties. The film-forming ingredients can form a tight layer over the skin, giving the illusion of smoother skin. This product is a poor under-eye concealer. It would probably work well as an eyeshadow base, although for most women an eyeshadow base is unnecessary.

☺ **$$$ Triple Action Lip Enhancer** *($15 for 0.5 ounce)* contains mostly water, silicone, film former, thickeners, plant oils, lanolin, petrolatum, water-binding agents, and preservatives. This is a very good emollient moisturizer for the lips, but the amount of AHA is minimal and the triple benefit it should have contained is sunscreen.

☹ **Skin Revival System** *($40 when purchased together)* is a two-part product consisting of **Skin Revival Cream** or **Skin Revival Cream Oil-Free** *($25 for 1.5 ounces)* and **Skin Revival Serum** *($25 for 1.5 ounces)*. This is Mary Kay's answer to the AHA and BHA craze. The claims are just short of miraculous, yet it is overpriced and neither part contains much AHA. One of the salespeople told me it contains about 5% AHAs, but I couldn't get a firm number from the company. You're supposed to apply the serum, let it dry, then apply the cream, then add an additional moisturizer if you want. That's more complicated than it needs to be. The Skin Revival Serum is an alcohol-based gel lotion that makes it unnecessarily irritating and drying for most skin types. It does seem to contain about 5% AHA and a form of BHA that doesn't exfoliate (it is the alkaline form not the acid form) and a pH of 3, but the alcohol is a problem for skin. The Skin Revival Cream is mostly a rich moisturizer with less than 1% AHA and a form of BHA that doesn't exfoliate. Don't waste your time with this; there are plenty of products that contain 8% AHAs in a good pH that don't include alcohol or salicylic acid, both of which can irritate the skin.

☺ **Acne Treatment Gel** *($6 for 1.25 ounces)* contains mostly water, slip agent, and benzoyl peroxide (5%). The active ingredient is the benzoyl peroxide, and it could work great as a disinfectant for acne.

☺ **Clarifying Mask** *($12 for 4 ounces)* is a standard clay mask that can definitely dry the skin, but for a clay mask it's OK.

☺ **Moisture Rich Mask** *($12 for 4 ounces)* is a very emollient cream that contains mostly water, thickeners, plant oil, water-binding agent, plant oils, petrolatum, and preservatives. It also contains an insignificant amount of vitamin A. This should feel very good on dry skin.

☹ **Revitalizing Mask** *($12 for 4 ounces)* is a standard clay mask that also contains a lightweight abrasive that is fairly rough on skin. It is thicker than most because it also contains carnauba (as in car) wax, so it can also clog pores and be difficult to rinse off.

☹ **Indulging Soothing Eye Mask** *($15 for 4 ounces)* contains mostly water, slip agent, film former, witch hazel, plant extracts, thickeners, and preservatives. This isn't indulging as much as it is potentially irritating.

☹ **Sun Essentials Ultimate Protection Sunblock SPF 30** *($9.50 for 4.5 ounces)* doesn't contain avobenzone, zinc oxide, or titanium dioxide, and is not recommended.

☹ **Sun Essentials Sensible Protection Sunblock SPF 15** *($9.50 for 4.5 ounces)* doesn't contain avobenzone, zinc oxide, or titanium dioxide, and is not recommended.

☹ **Sun Essentials Intense Protection Sunblock SPF 20** *($9.50 for 4.5 ounces)* doesn't contain avobenzone, zinc oxide, or titanium dioxide, and is not recommended.

Mary Kay Makeup

☺ FOUNDATION: Day Radiance Formula I Foundation for Dry Skin SPF 8 *($11 for refill, $8 for compact)* is a thick creamy foundation that comes in pancake form. It goes on somewhat heavy but can blend out smooth. It can be good for someone with very dry skin. The SPF number is disappointing but it is a titanium dioxide–based sunscreen. **These colors are excellent:** Pure Ivory, Soft Ivory, Antique Ivory, Buffer Ivory, Dusty Beige, Almond Beige, True Beige, Fawn Beige, and Mahogany Bronze. **These colors are too peach, pink, ash, yellow, or copper for most skin tones:** Rose Petal Ivory, Blush Ivory, Delicate Beige, Mocha Bronze, Bittersweet Bronze, Rich Bronze, Toasted Beige, and Cocoa Beige.

☺ **Day Radiance Formula II for Normal to Dry Skin SPF 8** *($11)* has a beautiful texture with a smooth, light finish and is great for someone with normal to dry skin. The SPF number is disappointing, but it is a titanium dioxide–based sunscreen. **These colors are excellent:** Pure Ivory, Antique Ivory, Buffed Ivory, True Beige, Fawn Beige, Almond Beige, Toasted Beige, and Cocoa Beige. **These colors are too peach, pink, ash, yellow, or copper for most skin tones:** Rose Petal Ivory, Soft Ivory, Blush Ivory, Delicate Beige, Dusty Beige, Mocha Bronze, Rich Bronze, Walnut Bronze, Bittersweet Bronze, and Mahogany Bronze.

☺ **Day Radiance Formula III Oil-Free for Oily and Combination Skin** *($11)* is a lightweight foundation that works great for oily skin types, but it would be better with an SPF like the other foundations. **These colors are excellent:** Fawn Beige, Toasted Beige, True Beige, Almond Beige, Antique Ivory, Buffed Ivory, Pure Ivory, Soft Ivory, Cocoa Beige, and Mahogany Bronze. **These colors are too peach, pink, ash, yellow, or copper for most skin tones:** Delicate Beige, Dusty Beige, Blush Ivory, Rose Petal Ivory, Mocha Bronze, Bittersweet Bronze, Walnut Bronze, and Rich Bronze.

☺ **Cream-to-Powder Foundation** *($11 for refill, $8 for compact)* has a great, smooth soft finish without feeling greasy or thick. There are only a handful of colors but for the most part they are all excellent; only Bronze 1 and Bronze 2 are too orange for most skin tones.

☺ **CONCEALER: Full Coverage Concealer** *($9.50)* is a tube concealer with a soft, creamy application that provides good, smooth coverage. Unfortunately, it tends to crease and continue creasing long after it's applied. **Full Coverage Neutralizing Concealer** *($9.50)* is a group of lavender, mint, and yellow tints that just add strange colors to the face. These types of products never really help even out skin tone.

☺ **POWDER: Powder Perfect Loose Powder** *($12.50)* and **Powder Perfect Pressed Powder** *($7.50)* are talc-based powders with a soft, dry consistency. They go on sheer, and three of the four colors are quite good; only Bronze can be too peach for most skin tones.

☹ **BLUSH: Powder Perfect Cheek Color** *($8)* is sold in separate tins that can be placed in a refillable compact. You buy the compact *($7)* separately and fill it with the colors of your choice. In a way, it's very convenient: you don't have to keep paying for a compact. Unfortunately, most all of the blush colors are very shiny; only Nutmeg is a matte shade. What a shame, because these do have a soft, silky-smooth finish. **Creamy Cheek Color** *($6)* is a standard cream blush that comes in two shades. These are OK, but they tend to be greasier and to slide off rather than blend on smooth.

☹ **EYESHADOW: Powder Perfect Eye Color** *($5 for each eyeshadow, $15 for the compact)* is sold in separate tins that can be placed in a refillable compact. You buy the compact separately and fill it with the colors of your choice. The only negative is that all of the eyeshadows, even the matte ones, have some amount of shine. There is also an incredible range of pastel blues, green, and pinks—an incredibly long-out-of-date eye color selection.

☺ **EYE AND BROW SHAPER:** The **Eye Defining Pencils** *($6.50)* are standard pencils that have a smooth finish and a reasonable price.

☹ The **Eyebrow Pencils** *($7)* have a slightly slick texture, which can make for a shiny brow.

☺ **LIPSTICK AND LIP PENCIL: Signature Color Moisturizing Lipstick** *($10)* has a creamy, slightly glossy finish with a good range of colors, though there need to be more neutral tones—the large group of vivid shades is dated. **Lip Liner Pencil** *($7)* is a small but good group of standard lip pencils.

☹ MASCARA: **Flawless Mascara** *($8)* and **Conditioning Mascara** *($8)* have different brush sizes but end up applying identically. They build no length or thickness and are a complete disappointment. **Waterproof Mascara** *($8)* doesn't hold up well under water, it tends to chip and peel off after a few dunks. **Endless Performance Mascara** *($8.50)* just doesn't perform up to any standard. It doesn't build any length or thickness. If you wanted a mascara that didn't do anything, this would be one to choose.

Dr. Mary Lupo (Skin Care Only)

Dr. Lupo is a dermatologist with an impressive list of credentials. She has created her own skin-care line that has some interesting AHA products and a handful of overblown claims. Her sunscreen boasts UVA protection, but one doesn't contain any UVA protecting ingredients. Her conditioning cleanser uses sodium lauryl sulfate (SLS), known for being one of the most irritating detergent cleansing ingredients around. Surely as a dermatologist Lupo would have known SLS is used as the irritation standard against which other ingredients are judged.

Still, there are some good AHA products in here, particularly lightweight ones. They're pricey for what you get, but they are well-formulated. For more information about Dr. Mary Lupo's products, call (800) 825-1998.

☹ **Conditioning Cleanser** *($22 for 6 ounces)* is an OK water-soluble cleanser, but the detergent cleansing agents are sodium lauryl sulfate and potassium hydroxide, both of which can be quite drying. There probably aren't much of them in here, but I am always concerned when I see them listed in a product designated as gentle.

☺ $$$ **Gentle Purifying Cleanser** *($22 for 7 ounces)* is a fairly standard detergent-based water-soluble cleanser that is, in many respects, quite good for most skin types, except dry. But it's not worth $22.

☺ $$$ **AHA Renewel Gel I** *($25 for 3.5 ounces)* is a good 8% gel AHA product containing lactic acid. It contains no other irritants and should work well to exfoliate the skin without clogging pores. Given the extremely limited selection of AHA liquids or gels that contain no irritants, this one is pretty good.

☺ $$$ **AHA Renewal Gel II** *($25 for 3.5 ounces)* is similar to the one above, and the same review applies.

☺ $$$ **AHA Renewal Lotion I** *($25 for 3.5 ounces)* is an 8% AHA lotion in a standard moisturizing base. This is pretty pricey and is just as effective as Alpha Hydrox at the drugstore for far less.

☺ $$$ **AHA Renewal Lotion II** *($25 for 3.5 ounces)* is similar to the one above, and the same review applies.

☺ **Daily Age Management Moisturizer, SPF 15** *($23 for 2 ounces)* does not contain avobenzone, titanium dioxide, or zinc oxide, and is not recommended.

☺ $$$ **Daily Age Management Oil Free Moisturizer SPF 15** *($23 for 2 ounces)* is a titanium dioxide–based sunscreen with a great SPF. It is a good sunscreen that goes on light, but it would be best for someone with normal to slightly dry skin.

☺ $$$ **Intensive Target Moisturizer** *($38.50 for 1 ounce)* contains mostly water, glycerin, silicones, vitamins, thickeners, water-binding agents, more thickeners, plant oil, and preservatives. If you want to spend this kind of money on a fairly standard moisturizer with vitamin E, it's up to you, but this is as overpriced as it gets for a simple product.

☺ $$$ **Vivifying Serum C** *($39.95 for 1 ounce)* is just fine if you want a vitamin C in a lightweight gel.

Matrix Essentials Skin Care

Matrix has had a bit of a rocky road, being sold and resold. Clairol was its most recent owner, but it has now been turned over to Bristol-Myers Squibb as a new acquisition. How this will affect all of the Matrix line of products, ranging from Matrix Essentials Skin Care to their primary focus, hair care, including Systeme Biolage, Vavoom, and Logics International, is yet to be seen.

If you've been at a hair salon lately you may have encountered the Matrix Essentials Skin Care products. Perhaps you noticed them while you were waiting for your appointment. I would suggest that you not get too excited about this rather pricey assortment of products and go back to reading your magazine while you wait. These aren't bad, just nothing special, and surprisingly overpriced for what you get. Matrix makes much ado about something they call Si-Complex. It turns out that Si-Complex is an ingredient called methylsilanol mannuronate, a form of silicone. It is a good skin-care ingredient, as most silicones are, but it is not special or rare, simply a rather standard cosmetic compound. There are no coloring agents in these products, which is nice, but the claim made about it being fragrance-free (that's what the stylist at the salon I was at told me) isn't true. There are plant extracts in here that provide plenty of fragrance. For more information about Matrix skin care, call (800) 6-MATRIX.

☻ $$$ **Foaming Face Wash, for All Skin Types** *($18 for 5.3 ounces)* is a standard detergent-based cleanser that can be drying for some skin types.

☺ $$$ **Gentle Cleansing Wash, for Normal, Dry, or Sensitive Skin** *($18 for 5.3 ounces)* is a standard detergent-based water-soluble cleanser that contains fewer detergent cleansing agents and more emollients than the one above. This would be better for someone with normal to dry skin. The plant extracts in here make the claim about this being good for sensitive skin highly questionable.

☺ **$$$ Gentle Eye Makeup Remover** *($15 for 5.3 ounces)* is a standard detergent-based wipe-off makeup remover. It actually contains more detergent cleansing agents than most eye-makeup removers, so be careful with this one, it could irritate the eyes. Not that I recommend wiping off makeup, but if you're into this step, you might find this version sensitizing.

☺ **$$$ Daily Moisture Lotion for Normal, Dry, and Sensitive Skin** *($22 for 2 ounces)* is a very good moisturizer for someone with dry skin. It contains mostly plant water, water-binding agents, thickeners, plant oils, vitamin E, and preservatives.

☹ **$$$ Firming Eye Creme** *($30 for 0.5 ounce)* is a rather ordinary moisturizer for dry skin that contains mostly water, a long list of thickeners, emollients, vitamins, film-former, and preservatives. This would be a good moisturizer for someone with dry skin, but the Daily Moisture Lotion is far more interesting and less expensive.

☹ **$$$ Hydrating Lotion, Oil Free, for Combination/Oily Skin** *($32 for 2 ounces)* contains several ingredients that could be a problem for someone with oily skin, including jojoba wax and emulsifying wax. This could be a good lightweight moisturizer for someone with normal to dry skin, but someone with oily skin would not want to use this all over their face.

☹ **$$$ Nourishing Age Defying Eye Cream** *($35 for 0.5 ounce)* won't firm anything, but the fourth ingredient, aluminum starch octenylsuccinate, could be a problem for some skin types.

☺ **$$$ Nourishing Night Cream** *($30 for 1 ounce)* is a very good moisturizer for someone with dry skin. It contains mostly plant water, thickeners, plant oils, water-binding agents, vitamins, emollients, and preservatives.

☹ **$$$ Sebo-Control Gel Masque** *($20 for 3.3 ounces)* is mostly witch hazel with some interesting water-binding agents. It's hard to get around the irritation that witch hazel can cause, despite some of the other interesting ingredients in this mask.

Max Factor (Makeup Only)

Max Factor, *the* makeup artist for the rich and famous in the 1920s, is credited with developing the first mass-produced makeup products that were more than heavy powders or tints for the cheeks and lips. He made the men and women in films look exotic, sweet, masterful, wicked, or seductive in a way that was less obvious than on the stage, and he did it with unprecedented flair and creativity. Pancake Makeup and Erase, which have survived to this day, were the first foundation and coverstick. (I don't recommend pancake foundation for anyone, but it's nice to recognize the roots of the makeup we are all wearing.)

In recent years Max Factor has attempted to bring its image into the '90s with an array of products called High Definition and Lasting Definition. Unfortunately, in comparison to lots of other lines, there isn't much to look at here. The eyeshadows and blushes are all shiny, which is a shame because they have a velvety soft finish. The foundations have some pretty terrible color choices, and the application for most leaves a lot to be desired. The pencils and lipsticks are good, but then it's hard to make a bad pencil or lipstick. All in all, his line is dull, drab, and dreary. The dark navy packaging makes identifying the names and colors of the products difficult and not very inviting. For more information about Max Factor, call (800) 862-4222.

☺ <u>FOUNDATION:</u> **Pan-Cake Makeup** *($6.76)* and **Pan-Stick Makeup** *($6.76)* are both packaged in sealed plastic wrap that prevents you from viewing the colors. For that reason alone these are difficult for me to recommend, but in addition the textures of both the Pan-Cake and the Pan-Stick are too heavy, thick, and greasy and **almost all of the colors are too peach or pink.**

☺ **Whipped Creme Makeup** *($6.76)* has the most awful array of foundation colors I have ever seen. Who is buying this stuff? **High Definition Compact Makeup** *($6.24)* also has terrible colors.

☺ **Lasting Performance Stay Put Makeup** *($7.75)* does stay put, and the colors for the most part are pretty good, but it has a very powdery finish that makes the skin look grainy and rough, and it feels terrible on the skin.

☺ **Rain All Day Hydrating Makeup** *($8.79)* and **Balancing Act Skin Balancing Makeup** *($8.79)* both have a fairly smooth, even texture but also a poor range of colors that tend to be too peach or pink for most skin tones. The formulas are almost identical, so the names are completely irrelevant. There is nothing hydrating about Rain, and nothing balancing about Balancing Act. Both would be appropriate for someone with normal to slightly oily or slightly dry skin who wants a matte finish.

☺ **Powdered Foundation** *($7.75)* works better as a pressed powder than a foundation. The colors are actually quite good, but this foundation tends to be powdery and can cake on the skin.

☺ **Skin Perfecting Liquid to Powder Makeup** *($6.66)* has a dreadful selection of colors.

☺ <u>CONCEALER:</u> **Erase Colour Precise** *($3.75)* is a creamy liquid that provides good medium coverage and has great colors. This concealer really hides dark circles, but it does tend to crease into the lines around the eyes.

☺ **Erase Secret Cover-Up** *($3.99)* concealer stick was the staple of my youthful days. The coverage is good, the consistency is creamy without being greasy, and the colors are actually quite good. It is not the best on dry skin, it can easily crease into the lines around the eyes, and the fragrance is too pungent for my taste.

☺ <u>POWDER:</u> **Lasting Performance Pressed Powder** *($6.24)* has a sheer, soft finish but all the shades are shiny.

☺ <u>BLUSH:</u> **Natural Blush-On** *($5.99)* is a soft, exceedingly smooth blush in a subtle range of pastel colors. All of the shades have some amount of shine.

☹ <u>EYESHADOW:</u> **Eyeshadow Singles** *($2.46),* **Duos** *($2.64),* and **Quads** *($3.73)* are all either too shiny or come in too poor combinations of colors to recommend.

☺ <u>EYE AND BROW SHAPER:</u> **Pen Silks** ($4.91) is a standard twist-up pencil with a somewhat creamy application. The **Brush & Brow Eyebrow Color** *($5.25)* is a powder shadow that colors the brow with a hard brush. The powder works beautifully, but the firm brush is a throwaway and shouldn't be used. A soft brush would be better. **Brow Tamer** *($4.99)* is a clear gel that can keep brows in place. It works well, but you can get the same effect by spraying hair spray on a toothbrush and combing it through your brows. **Eyeliner Pen** *($4.13)* is a liquid eyeliner that is applied with a felt-tip pen applicator; it works well, although it tends to dry slightly sticky.

☺ **Kohliners** *($4.16)* are a good assortment of standard eye pencils that are a bit on the greasy side; one end is a sponge tip. **Eyebrow and Eyeliner** *($3.20)* is a standard pencil that's almost identical to the Kohliner.

☺ <u>LIPSTICK AND LIP PENCIL:</u> Except for the fragrance, which has a strong waxy odor, Max Factor has some good lipsticks. **Lasting Color Lipstick** *($5.69)* has an extremely creamy finish, but you won't find it lasting longer than any other creamy finish lipstick. **LipSilks** *($6.49)* is just a lipstick with a glossy sheer application. **Lip Color Palette** *($6.69)* is a fairly emollient lipstick. The **Lip Liner** *($5.36)* pencil is great; one end is a lipstick brush, which can be convenient.

☹ **Stay Put Anti-Fade Lip Foundation** *($4.50)* does prevent lipstick from feathering, but it also tends to make the lipstick cake and dries out the lips.

☺ <u>MASCARA:</u> **2000 Calorie Mascara** *($4.95)* goes on easily, doesn't smear, and makes lashes thick and long. It tends to flake if you overbuild the lashes. Don't overdo, and it should last the whole day. **S-T-R-E-T-C-H Mascara** *($4.95)* builds decent length and some amount of thickness.

☹ **Super Lash Maker** *($4.95)* is a terrible mascara with a strange tiny brush that is difficult to use and builds no length or thickness.

Maybelline (Makeup Only)

Early in 1996 Maybelline was purchased by L'Oreal. As this book went to press, the purchase had not affected the displays or many of the products available, but it is hard to believe that things won't change; although Maybelline already has its act together in many aspects of makeup, it was also lacking in many areas. There are some impressive products, particularly pressed powders (these have improved a lot), mascaras, concealers, pencils, blushes, and inexpensive brushes, and the prices are wonderful. With a little caution, you can come away from the Maybelline section of the drugstore with some great bargains and a beautiful look. For more information about Maybelline call (800) 944-0730.

☺ <u>FOUNDATION:</u> **True Illusion Liquid to Powder Makeup SPF 10** *($5.76)* is not a liquid-to-powder in the least, rather it is a very standard, though very good, cream-to-powder makeup with a great sunscreen (well, almost great—SPF 15 would be great, this one is only an SPF 10). The colors are excellent, and if you like this style of foundation it is one to consider. Remember that cream-to-powder foundations work best for someone with more normal skin than for other types, because the cream part can be too emollient and greasy for oily or combination skin and the powder part too drying for dry skin.

☹ **Moisture Whip Liquid Makeup** *($3.88)* has a terrible selection of foundation tones. **Revitalizing Liquid Makeup** *($6.37)* is supposed to be both a good AHA product and a good sunscreen. That combination might be possible, but in this case the AHA ingredient isn't an effective exfoliant; also, the colors are some of the worst you'll see anywhere. **True Illusion Makeup SPF 10** *($4.99)* closely resembles Lancome's packaging for their foundations. As attractive as the packaging is, and despite the sheer, smooth application of the foundation, the active ingredients do not include avobenzone, zinc oxide, or titanium dioxide, and this product is therefore not recommended unless you are willing to wear a reliable sunscreen underneath. What a shame, because the colors are great, the texture impressive and sheer, and the price—well, it's cheap!

☺ **Natural Defense Makeup with SPF 15 (Nonchemical Sunscreen)** *($4.24)* is definitely worth checking out. The SPF is great and the nonchemical sunscreen-base is a nice option. Some of the colors are surprisingly good. This wonderfully lightweight foundation offers soft, subtle coverage. It is best for someone with normal to dry skin. The colors are generally neutral, but there isn't much for darker skin tones. **These colors are excellent:** Light Ivory, Ivory, Light Beige, Soft Beige, Deep Beige, and Golden Beige. **These colors are too peach or rose:** Medium Beige and Rose Beige. It would be a mistake not to give this one a closer look, but it is still a guess when you can't test before you buy.

☺ **Maybelline Great Wear Makeup** *($4.72)* is great! This foundation goes on incredibly smoothly in a matte finish, and works best for someone with normal to oily skin. And the color selection is wonderful: a wide range of neutral, natural color tones! **The only two colors to beware of are:** Fair Ivory, which can be slightly too pink, and Sand, which can be slightly too peach. The rest are superior. It would be a mistake not to give this one a closer look but it is still a guess when you can't test before you buy.

☺ **Long-Wearing Liquid Makeup** *($3.29)* and **Shine-Free Oil-Control Liquid Makeup** *($3.95)* both have some good colors to choose from, and good textures, but since you can't test the colors it makes these a risky purchase.

☺ <u>CONCEALER:</u> **Maybelline Great Wear Concealer** *($4.19)* gets the same raves as the foundation. This excellent, noncreasing concealer goes on in a matte finish, but smoothly, without looking dry or crinkly. It comes in four superb shades. It is best for someone with normal to oily skin, but it can work for dry skin types too, depending on the texture of the skin. **Undetectable Creme Concealer** *($3.65)* goes on easily and dries to a matte, smooth finish; it stays in place and really covers. I wouldn't exactly call it undetectable, but it does come in three good shades—Light, Medium, and Dark Medium (which isn't all that dark)—and doesn't crease.

☹ **Shine-Free Oil-Control Cover Stick** *($3.65)* won't control oil in the least, but although the colors have improved the concealer goes on very dry, and then melts and easily creases into lines around the eyes. **Coverstick** *($3.68)* is packaged so that you can't see the color, although most of the colors are quite good; still, this one has a very greasy consistency and easily creases. **Revitalizing Coverstick** *($4.99)* comes in three reliable shades, but it easily creases in the lines around the eyes.

☺ <u>POWDER:</u> **Shine-Free Oil-Control Translucent Pressed Powder** *($3.35)* won't control oil, but it is a wonderful soft, dry powder that goes on smooth and sheer and is indeed oil-free. **Finish Matte Pressed Powder** *($3.29)* is also exceptional, with beautiful colors and a silky, even texture. It does contain a tiny bit of mineral oil but not enough for your skin to notice one way or the other. **Moisture Whip Translucent Pressed Powder** *($3.36)* has a slightly peach assortment of colors but a smooth, soft finish.

☺ <u>BLUSH:</u> **Natural Accents Blush** *($2.69)* comes in ten attractive, subtle (and I mean subtle) shades; all of them are fairly matte and worth a closer look. **Great Wear Blush** *($4.19)* is a cream blush that has a soft, matte, slightly staining finish; once this product dries, it's on till you put some effort into getting it off. I'm not one to be fond of cream blushes, but this one does work well for a sheer effect. It comes in a nice range of fairly matte colors.

☹ **Brush/Blush I** *($3.05)*, **II** *($3.23)*, and **III** *($3.39)* come in single, duo, and trio compacts. They are all somewhat shiny—not awful, just not great. They go on rather choppy and have poor staying power.

☹ <u>EYESHADOW:</u> **Expert Eyes Eyeshadows Single, Duo, Trio, and Quad** *($2.32 to $4.09)* mostly have a large amount of shine or dreadful colors, and cling unreliably. They go on choppy and have minimal staying power. **Natural Accents Eyeshadow** *($2.62)* comes in a M.A.C.-like compact, but all the colors have some amount of shine; even the "matte" shades are iridescent. They cling poorly and blend unevenly.

☺ **Maybelline Great Wear Eyecolor** *($4.20)* are lipstick-type applicators that go on like a cream, blend easily, and dry to a matte finish. None of these eyeshadow colors stays all that well, and it's hard to control blending with this kind of texture

The Reviews M

and applicator. Still, if you've got the technique down for cream eyeshadows, these are an option. Just don't give up your powder eyeshadows yet.

☺ **EYE AND BROW SHAPER: Expert Eyes Brow and Eye Liner Pencil** *($3.09)* is an automatic pencil that can be sharpened to a finer point than most, but other than that it is just a standard pencil with a dry texture, which means less smudging. **Ultra-Brow Brush-On Brow Color** *($3.42)* is a great standard brow powder. It comes with the standard hard brush that needs to be tossed away and replaced with a good soft professional brush. **Smoked Kohl Liner** *($4.20)* is a standard pencil that has a smudge tip at one end. It's as reliable as any. **Great Line Waterproof Eye Liner** *($4.88)* is a standard twist-up eyeliner that has a smooth, soft texture. It is slightly more waterproof than other pencils, but only slightly.

☺ **Lineworks Liquid Liner Washable** *($3.29)* is a standard liquid liner that dries to a smooth, flat finish. Unfortunately it applies a bit unevenly, and it's hard to correct for mistakes. It does wear well during the day, and that's a plus. **Lineworks Felt-Tip Eye Liner** *($3.94)* is just like a felt-tip pin, but it delivers a liquid liner that dries to a smooth, flat finish. It doesn't budge once in place, which makes application tricky and unforgiving. This is a serious looking line, no softness for this one. It doesn't chip or flake during the day.

☹ **Maybelline Eye Express Easy Eyelining Pen** *($4.24)* does go on easily, but it takes a while to dry. Actually, it never did seem to quite set up the way I was expecting. It stayed tacky to the touch for quite awhile. Later in the day, if you accidentally touch it, a chunk of the line can come off. This is an express line to pass up. **Expert Eye Twin Brow and Eye Pencil** *($1.87)* is a very greasy pencil dating back to the '40s. This has to be the way Joan Crawford drew on her eyebrows! The same is true for **Linework Ultra-Liner Waterproof Liquid Liner** *($3.75)*, a standard liquid liner that has good staying power under water, but that tends to peel or smudge if accidentally rubbed.

☺ **LIPSTICK AND LIP PENCIL: MoistureWhip Lipstick** *($3.99)* is supposed to have an SPF 8 but it doesn't list any UVA protection and is not recommended for that purpose; however, in terms of application, MoistureWhip and **LongWearing Lipstick** *($3.99)* both have a rich, creamy, slightly glossy texture; it's hard to tell the two apart. LongWearing isn't all that long wearing but it is a good basic lipstick if you don't have a problem with lipstick bleeding into the lines around the mouth. **Budgeproof Lip Color** *($4.72)* now has a large range of colors to choose from and they provide ultra-matte competition for Revlon's ColorStay. It doesn't bleed, it stays on at least as well as any other matte lipstick, and the price is great. **Moisture Whip Gloss** *($3.76)* is a standard gloss in a small but pretty group of colors. **Precision Lip Liner** *($3.77)* and **Budgeproof Lip Liner** *($4.12)* both work equally well, and are good choices for lip liners.

☺ **Maybelline Lip Express** *($3.99)* is an oversized (at least in width, not in height) lip pencil that is supposed to double as a lip liner and lipstick. To some extent, that's exactly what it does, but not very well. Like all chubby lip pencils, these are difficult to sharpen, and the color part is so soft that it is impossible to keep a tip on the end, so it's tricky to create a smooth, even line around the mouth, and that means you have to sharpen often because the tip keeps disappearing. And after all that, the lipstick part is, well, just lipstick.

☺ **Maybelline Lip Polish** *($3.72)* provides a somewhat creamy, somewhat powdery textured spread of sheer colored glitter over the lips. What can I say? It does sparkle (the glitter can fill into the lines on the mouth and look messy after a while), and it isn't as greasy and smeary as most glosses, but it isn't as smooth either.

☹ **MASCARA:** **Great Lash Mascara** *($4.20)* does go on well and builds some amount of length, though it takes effort; it definitely doesn't build thickness, and it has a tendency to smear. **Magic Mascara** *($3.95)* has an awkward curved brush, and the mascara doesn't build much length or thickness and wears poorly. **Perfectly Natural Mascara** *($3.25)* is OK, but it doesn't build up much thickness. **Lash by Lash Mascara** *($3.49)* took forever to build any definition, it smeared later in the day, and the two products I purchased were practically dried up from the very first time I tested them.

☺ **Great Lash Pro Vitamin** *($4.72)* is a good lengthening and thickening mascara that may clump slightly but doesn't smear. The "pro vitamin" (a combination of vitamin Bs) won't do anything for your lashes, though. **Illegal Lengths Mascara** *($4.55)* is an excellent mascara without being too thick or clumpy, and it doesn't smear or flake. And, yes it does build lots and lots of length, almost too much! **Volum' Express** *($4.16)* has its strong points. It builds thick, long lashes and doesn't smear. A word of warning: It can go clumpy and thick, a definite problem for some, but the thick and long application can make it worth the struggle. **Extremely Gentle Mascara** *($3.99)* isn't gentle, but it does build nice long lashes without clumping or chipping.

☺ **Wonder Curl Mascara** *($4.34)* doesn't perform any better in the arena of making lashes curl than the others. While this is a good mascara in terms of length and performance, it isn't as impressive as the L'Oreal or Lancome versions.

☺ **Volum' Express Waterproof Mascara** *($4.16)* builds quickly and thickens with no clumps and stays on underwater. **Illegal Lengths Waterproof Mascara** *($4.55)* definitely lengthens but don't count on getting any thickness out of this one. It does stay on just fine in water. **Great Lash Waterproof Mascara** *($3.99)* thickens, lengthens, and doesn't clump, and you can swim for most of the day without a smudge!

☹ **Ultra-Big Ultra-Lash Waterproof** *($3.99)* is an ultra disappointment. I've never tested a mascara before that I thought made my lashes look shorter until I put this one to the test.

☺ **BRUSHES:** The **Eyeshadow Brush** *($3.05)*, **Blush Brush** *($3.46)* and **Face Brush** *($7.06)* are extremely soft but firm, and work surprisingly well. The **Eye Contour Brush** *($4.29)* is an option for brows or eyelining but it is too small for eyeshadow, and the **Retractable Lip Brush** *($5.06)* is a standard lip brush.

Maybelline Shades of You

Maybelline's Shades of You is a limited group of color products for African-American skin tones. It excels in blush and lipstick but falls woefully short in the foundation, concealer, and pressed-powder arena. For more information about Maybelline Shades of You call (212) 818-1500.

☹ **Shades of You 100% Oil-Free Compact Creme Makeup SPF 9** *($4.29)* has a soft, smooth, matte finish. Technically this product is oil-free, but there are several ingredients that could be problematic for oily or blemish-prone skin. All of the colors are either too peach, orange, or ashy to recommend. The SPF 9 with titanium dioxide is OK, but even for women of color, to prevent skin discoloration caused by sun damage, an SPF 15 would be far better.

☹ **Shades of You Oil-Free Liquid Water-Based Makeup** *($4.25)* has a few good colors to consider (primarily Café Au Lait, Honey, and Amber), and a light smooth texture. Strangely, this "oil-free" makeup has some amount of sparkle in it, which makes the skin look shiny, just the opposite of what you would expect from an oil-free foundation.

☹ **Shades of You 100% Oil Free Coverstick** *($2.95)* has a fairly greasy application and some amount of noticeable shine. I'm not sure why Maybelline feels darker skin tones need to shine, but they don't. Plus, the colors are all fairly peach.

☹ **Shades of You 100% Oil-Free Pressed Powder** *($3.36)* and **Shades of You Oil Control Loose Powder** *($3.36)* both have a lovely assortment of colors, but they are all shiny! Why would anyone make an oil-free, oil-control powder shiny? You may absorb oil, but you would still be shining! Isn't that negating the entire purpose of a pressed powder?

☺ **Shades of You 100% Oil-Free Powder Blush** *($3.36)* has a mostly soft, somewhat dry, matte finish. It goes on soft without being heavy or grainy and there are some wonderful colors to consider.

☺ **Shades of You Lipstick** *($3.52)* has a great color selection with remarkably appropriate shades for women of color. They have a nice moist feel that tends to be more greasy than creamy. All the colors have some amount of tint that keeps the shade around longer. **Shades of You Lasting Finish Long-Wearing Matte Lipstick** *($3.52)* is virtually identical to Maybelline Budgeproof Lip Color only in deeper shades. This is an excellent option for a matte-finish lipstick. **Shades of You See**

Through Colors *($4.72)* is a lipstick with a glossy finish. **Shades of You Lip Liner** *($2.73)* is a very standard, ordinary group of lip pencils. They work just fine.

M.D. Formulations (Skin Care Only)

In the area of serious AHA products, M.D. Formulations far surpasses its competition, offering some of the highest-percentage glycolic acid–based AHA products on the market. Not only do most of its products have over 12% AHAs (8% to 10% is the standard percentage in most other good AHA products, available from such lines as Alpha Hydrox, Avon, Pond's, and my own line of skin-care products, among others), but M.D. Formulations also has a line of AHA products, called Forte, with up to 20% glycolic acid. If you're of the opinion that more is better, then look no further. However, let me warn you that I do not encourage or recommend over 10% AHAs for the skin on a daily or even semi-regular basis. At this time, there have been no long-term studies that have established the effect of higher concentrations of AHA products on the skin. In fact, this much irritation of the skin on a daily basis theoretically can be harmful, and could actually cause skin to wrinkle (because repetitive irritation damages skin tissue). They have also included some BHA, as salicylic acid, in their formulations. It is my opinion that there is no need to combine these in a single product. BHA is better for exfoliation in the pore, and AHAs for sun-damaged skin on the surface. If you don't have clogged pores you don't need the BHA, and if you have both sun-damaged skin and clogged pores, the BHA will do both.

M.D. Formulations makes everything from moisturizers and acne products to shampoos (considered good for dandruff or psoriasis) and foot and nail treatments. If you want to exfoliate skin on any part of your body with an AHA concentration that can really make a difference, you will be impressed by some of these products. However, M.D. Formulations makes several products that I think are problematic for skin, containing unnecessarily irritating ingredients, and its AHA moisturizers are fairly ordinary and absurdly overpriced. Other than for their AHA content, these are not elegant or even very interesting formulations, and one face can only take so much exfoliation. Despite those reservations, and the fact that these products are incredibly overpriced, if you pick and choose carefully, you stand to find some very good AHA products.

M.D. Formulations was originally sold only to physicians for retail sale, but now, to expand its market while retaining its so-called professional air, it is also sold through salons and spas. For more information about these products, or the name of a physician near you who sells these products, call 800-55-FORTE. You can also have the products shipped to you directly by calling that same number. Under the company name Herald Pharmacal, M.D. Formulations has created a line of products called **Aqua Glycolic**, sold in drugstores and priced from $8.50 to $16—they are reviewed earlier in the Product-by-Product Reviews section.

☹ **Facial Cleanser, with 12% Glycolic Compound** *($25 for 8 ounces)* is a problem for most skin types. It is overkill to put AHAs in a cleanser that could accidentally get too near your eyes or mouth when splashing and cause serious irritation. I would not recommend washing the face or other body parts with this product. This is also a lot of money for an ordinary detergent cleanser.

☺ **Facial Cleanser Basic** *($16 for 8 ounces)* is a gentle water-soluble cleanser for most skin types. Actually, this product is pretty much a knock-off of Cetaphil Gentle Skin Cleanser for about the same amount of money.

☹ **Glycare Cleansing Gel for Oily Skin with 12% Glycolic Compound** *($25 for 8 ounces)* is similar to the 12% cleanser above, and the same review applies.

☹ **Purifying Toner for Combination-Oily Skin** *($16 for 5.3 ounces)* is mostly witch hazel and a lot of alcohol, and is not recommended. This won't purify but it will irritate skin and make it red.

☺ **$$$ Advanced Hydrating Complex Cream Formula** *($40 for 1 ounce)* contains mostly water, several thickeners, water-binding agent, slip agent, thickener, and preservative. A good water-binding agent and Nayad (yeast) are at the very end of the ingredient list, so the amount of each is negligible, although there is no real evidence Nayad performs any real function for skin.

☹ **Advanced Hydrating Complex Gel Formula** *($40 for 1 ounce)* is a below-average, very expensive, non-AHA moisturizer for the eyes. It contains water, alcohol, thickener, water-binding agent, more thickeners, and preservatives. Although the moisturizer also contains a good water-binding agent and Nayad (yeast), they are at the very end of the ingredient list, so the amount of each is negligible. If the skin around your eyes is dry, this won't do much to change it, and the alcohol could make things worse.

☺ **$$$ Facial Lotion with 12% Glycolic Compound** *($55 for 2 ounces)* is just AHAs with a thickener and preservatives. This is a good basic AHA product for most skin types; however, if you have normal to dry skin, you will most likely need a moisturizer too, that is, if you can first recover from the price.

☺ **$$$ Facial Cream with 14% Glycolic Compound** *($75 for 2 ounces)* is similar to the one above, only with slightly more AHA content.

☺ **$$$ Vit-A-Plus Night Recovery Complex** *($56.25 for 1 ounce)* is mixture of AHA, BHA, and a tiny amount of vitamin A. I'm not one to recommend BHA with AHA, but this one is an option. I've written before about the overblown claims concerning vitamin A in skin-care products, but if you are interested there are products that contain this ingredient in larger amounts than this product and for far less money.

☺ **$$$ Vit-A-Plus Revitalizing Eye Cream** *($61.25 for 0.5 ounce)* is similar to the one above only in cream form, and the same comments apply.

☺ **$$$ Vit-A-Plus with Vitamin A** *($35 for 1 ounce)* is a lightweight serum version of the two Vit-A products above, which can make this one good for someone with normal to oily skin.

☺ **$$$ Vit-A-Plus2 with Alpha Retinyl Complex** *($62.50 for 0.4 ounce)* is similar to the ones above, and the same comments apply.

☹ **Sun Protector, SPF 20** *($30 for 4 ounces)* doesn't contain avobenzone, titanium dioxide, or zinc oxide, and is not recommended.

☺ **$$$ Benzoyl Peroxide 5% for Extremely Oily and Acne-Prone Skin** *($25 for 4 ounces)* is a good benzoyl peroxide disinfectant for someone with problem skin; of course you can buy similar products at the drugstore for less, but this is still a good alternative.

☺ **$$$ Benzoyl Peroxide 10% for Extremely Oily and Acne-Prone Skin** *($25 for 4 ounces)* is identical to the toner above except for the proportion of benzoyl peroxide, and the same review applies.

☹ **Glycare 5 for Extremely Oily or Acne-Prone Skin** *($40 for 4 ounces)* is an alcohol-based toner with 7% AHAs. I don't recommend using alcohol on anyone's skin, and the alcohol in combination with the AHAs can cause extreme irritation. The product also contains eucalyptus oil, another skin irritant.

☹ **Glycare 10 for Extremely Oily or Acne-Prone Skin** *($43.75 for 4 ounces)* is identical to the Glycare 5 except that it contains 12% AHAs. The same warnings about irritation apply.

☹ **Glycare Acne Gel Acne Medication** *($20 for 2 ounces)* would be an option for a combined BHA and AHA product if it wasn't for the alcohol.

☺ **$$$ Skin Bleaching Lotion** *($30 for 1.5 ounces)* is a standard 2% hydroquinone product. To make it more effective, use it in conjunction with a good AHA cream or lotion and a reliable sunscreen.

☺ **$$$ Smoothing Complex with 10% Glycolic Compound** *($35 for 0.5 ounce)* is identical to the Night Cream below except it has less AHA and does not contain a few of the thickeners. It is a good overall AHA product, though these prices are just not warranted for what you get.

☺ **$$$ Vit-A-Plus Hydra-Firming Masque** *($37.50 for 4 ounces)* is a standard clay mask with AHA. Now this is exfoliation overkill.

☹ **Forte Glycare Cleansing Gel with 15% Glycolic Compound** *($25 for 8 ounces)* is similar to the Facial Cleanser 12% above, only with more AHAs, and the same review applies.

☹ **Forte Facial Cleanser with 15% Glycolic Compound** *($25 for 8 ounces)* is similar to the Facial Cleanser 12% above, only with more AHAs, and the same review applies.

☺ **$$$ Forte I Facial Lotion with 15% Glycolic Compound** *($45 for 2 ounces)* is similar to the lotion above, only with more AHAs, and the same review applies.

☺ **$$$ Forte II Facial Lotion with 20% Glycolic Compound** *($47 for 2 ounces)* is similar to the Facial Lotion 12% above, but with more AHAs, and the same review applies. The long-term effects of this much AHA are unknown.

☺ **$$$ Night Cream with 14% Glycolic Compound** *($60 for 2 ounces)* is a simple AHA cream of water, thickeners, and preservative. The ordinary moisturizing base probably would not be sufficient for someone with very dry skin, but it is a good strong AHA product.

☺ **$$$ Forte I Facial Cream with 15% Glycolic Compound** *($32 for 1 ounce)* is similar to the cream above, but with more AHAs, and the same review applies.

☹ **$$$ Forte II Facial Cream with 20% Glycolic Compound** *($35 for 1 ounce)* is similar to the creams above, but with even more AHAs, and the same review applies. This product is pretty intense and definitely not for everyone. The long-term effects of this much AHA are unknown.

☺ **$$$ Forte Advanced Hydrating Complex Cream Formula** *($45 for 1.7 ounces)* is a very ordinary moisturizer of mostly thickeners and minimal water-binding agents.

☹ **Forte Advanced Hydrating Complex Gel Formula** *($45 for 1.7 ounces)* is a very overpriced, ordinary gel with too much alcohol content.

☺ **$$$ Vit-A-Gel with Vitamin A Propionate** *($40 for 1 ounce)* contains mostly aloe vera, slip agents, vitamin A, more slip agent, thickeners, several water-binding agents, and preservatives. If you're looking for a good dose of vitamin A, here it is, but the best part of this product is its lightweight water-binding agents. It's pricey for what you get, but it is a good lightweight moisturizer for someone with normal to slightly dry or combination skin.

☹ **Forte I Glycare with 15% Glycolic Compound** *($18 for 2 ounces)* is identical to the Glycare 5 and 10 except that it contains more AHAs. The same warnings about irritation apply.

☹ **Forte II Glycare with 20% Glycolic Compound** *($20 for 2 ounces)* is identical to the Glycare 5, 10, and 15, except that it contains more AHAs. The same warnings about irritation apply. The long-term effects of this much AHA are unknown.

☺ **$$$ Forte Skin Bleaching Gel with 2% Hydroquinone in a Base Containing 10% Glycolic Compound** *($30 for 1.5 ounces)* is what I recommended in the review above: hydroquinone with AHAs. It is worth a try, but don't expect dramatic results; these products lighten skin about 30% to 40% when used in conjunction with a reliable sunscreen.

☺ **$$$ Forte Glycare Perfection Gel, 1% Salicylic Acid in a Base Containing 5% Glycolic Compound** *($18 for 1.7 ounces)* is overpriced for what you get. According to the company, there is some evidence that this combination of salicylic acid and AHAs can be beneficial for acne; I am not convinced, especially given that this product also contains alcohol, and that can dry and irritate the skin causing breakouts, not reducing them.

Merle Norman

The Merle Norman boutiques are in dire need of serious cosmetic surgery, not just a face-lift. All of the stores I've been to have had a slightly worn, almost eerie, antiquated feel. Although some products, particularly the pencils, have been revamped, the foundation and concealer colors are some of the poorest around, these are the most awful shades of pink, peach, and orange imaginable. If you want to check out what I mean by a foundation or concealer being the wrong color, these are the products to inspect. The displays are still poorly organized and not very user-friendly; in fact, they appear almost haphazard. It would be much better if there were some color or style groupings. As it is, the colors have no relation to one another; they seem just strewn all over.

Although this all sounds pretty dismal, with some tweaking this line could really be an option. The matte blushes and eyeshadows are good and there's an extensive selection for women of all skin tones and colors, it's just that the color choice is all wrong. If Merle Norman is going to join the rest of the world going into the millennium it needs to take a good hard look at itself, preferably through more contemporary, fashionable glasses. For more information about Merle Norman call (800) 348-8889.

Please note: Merle Norman boutiques are privately owned and each one can set prices as they see fit so the prices listed below may vary store to store.

Merle Norman Skin Care

☹ **Cleansing Cream, Original Formula** *($18 for 16 ounces)* is a mineral oil–based wipe-off cleanser that contains thick waxes and cocoa butter. It's pretty much just overpriced cold cream.

☹ **Cleansing Lotion** *($18 for 14 ounces)* is similar to the cream above, but with less wax. It is still fairly greasy and contains petrolatum, lanolin, and a thickener that can cause breakouts.

☹ **Gel Cleanser** *($12 for 4 ounces)* is an alcohol-based detergent cleanser containing sodium lauryl sulfate, and these are both are very irritating ingredients. This product is absolutely not recommended.

☹ **Luxiva Collagen Cleanser** *($17 for 6 ounces)* is a mineral oil–based wipe-off cleanser that can leave a greasy film on the skin. It does contain collagen, but that serves no purpose in a cleanser.

☹ **Luxiva Skin Refining Cleanser** *($18.50 for 4 ounces)* won't refine anyone's skin. It has some synthetic scrubbing beads, which are OK for mechanical exfoliation, but it also contains a fair amount of potassium hydroxide, which can be irritating. This product tends to leave a greasy film, which is not great for someone with normal to oily skin.

☹ **Special Cleansing Bar, Soap Free** *($9.50 for 4 ounces)* is a wax-based bar cleanser that contains two problematic detergent cleansing agents (sodium lauryl sulfate and sodium C14-16 olefin sulfate); both are extremely irritating for all skin types.

☺ $$$ **Instant Eye Makeup Remover for Sensitive Eyes** *($10 for 3 ounces)* is a detergent-based cleanser that isn't what I would call good for sensitive skin. It's OK for removing makeup, but could be a problem over the eye area.

☺ $$$ **Very Gentle Eye Makeup Remover** *($10 for 2 ounces)* contains mostly mineral oil, which is gentle, but it's a lot like the wipe-off face cleansers above. Why bother with a second product if you're already wiping greasy stuff over your face to take off your makeup?

☹ **Fresh 'N Fair Skin Freshener** *($17 for 14 ounces)* is an alcohol-based cleanser that will leave the face feeling dry and irritated.

☹ **Luxiva AHA Toner** *($14.50 for 6 ounces)* is mostly alcohol and some amount of menthol, and that makes it mostly irritating for all skin types.

☺ $$$ **Luxiva Collagen Clarifier** *($14.50 for 6 ounces)* does indeed contain collagen; in fact, it is the third item on the ingredient list. Collagen is a good water-binding agent, but that's about it. This product would be fine as a toner for someone with normal to dry skin.

☹ **Refining Lotion** *($17 for 14 ounces)* is almost all witch hazel and preservatives. The minuscule amounts of other ingredients in the lotion aren't worth mentioning. Witch hazel contains a good percentage of alcohol and is a potential skin irritant.

☹ **Luxiva AHA Emulsion with Alpha Hydroxy Acids** *($31 for 1 ounce)* contains sugarcane extract, which is not the same thing as an alpha hydroxy acid, and a minimal amount of lactic acid, which is an AHA, but not enough of it to work as an exfoliant.

☺ $$$ **Luxiva Collagen Support** *($20 for 2 ounces)* contains mostly water, slip agent, collagen, elastin, water-binding agent, thickeners, preservatives, and more water-binding agents. This is a very good moisturizer for normal to dry skin types. The collagen and elastin won't change or improve wrinkles, but you already knew that, right?

☺ $$$ **Luxiva Night Creme with HC-12** *($37.50 for 2 ounces)* contains mostly water, slip agent, a long list of thickeners, silicone, shea butter, plant oils, preservatives, and plant extracts. This is a good emollient moisturizer for dry skin types, but HC-12 is just a clever marketing name for a combination of plant oils, water-binding agent, plant extracts, and vitamins.

☺ $$$ **Luxiva Day Creme with HC-12** *($21.50 for 2 ounces)* is identical to the cream above except that it contains a small amount of sunscreen—not enough to adequately protect the skin from sun damage, though as a moisturizer at night it would be just fine for dry skin.

☺ **$$$ Luxiva Energizing Concentrate** *($37.50 for 1 ounce)* contains mostly water, slip agents, silicone, plant extract, water-binding agents, and preservatives. Protein, yeast, and amino acids show up at the end of the ingredient list, which makes them barely present. This won't energize the skin, but it is a good moisturizer for normal to slightly dry skin types.

☺ **$$$ Luxiva Eye Cream** *($20 for 0.5 ounce)* contains mostly water, almond oil, a very long list of thickeners, plant oil, more thickeners, petrolatum, more thickeners, and preservative. The interesting water-binding agents are at the end of the ingredient list, meaning they're almost nonexistent. This overpriced moisturizer could be good for someone with dry skin.

☺ **$$$ Luxiva Protein Cream** *($39.50 for 4 ounces)* contains mostly water, petrolatum, a long list of thickeners, collagen, more thickeners, and preservatives. This is a good moisturizer for someone with dry skin.

☹ **Luxiva Triple Action Eye Gel** *($19 for 0.5 ounce)* contains mostly water, slip agents, aloe, witch hazel, plant extract, water-binding agent, and preservatives. Most of the plant extracts, antioxidants, and water-binding agents are at the end of the ingredient list, which means they're practically nonexistent; the witch hazel can be an irritant.

☺ **$$$ Luxiva Hydrosome Complex Advanced Hydrator** *($31.50 for 1 ounce)* contains mostly water, thickeners, aloe, slip agent, silicone, shea butter, more thickeners, more water-binding agents, and preservatives. This is a good, emollient, somewhat lightweight moisturizer for normal to dry skin types.

☺ **Intensive Moisturizer** *($15 for 1.25 ounces)* contains mostly water, mineral oil, slip agents, several thickeners, lanolin oil, more thickeners, lanolin oil, and preservatives. I would recommend this extremely rich moisturizer only for someone with extremely dry skin.

☹ **Miracol Booster Revitalizing Lotion Concentrate** *($11 for 1.25 ounces)* contains mostly water, alcohol, thickeners, and preservatives. Alcohol makes skin dry and irritated and that is bad for all skin types.

☹ **Miracol Original Formula Revitalizing Lotion** *($14.50 for 5.5 ounces)* contains mostly water, thickener, egg white, thickener, fragrance, and preservatives. By now everyone knows that egg white doesn't work miracles for the skin. It just puts a sticky film over the skin.

☹ **Miracol Creamy Formula Revitalizing Cream** *($14.50 for 6 ounces)* is almost identical to the lotion above, and the same review applies.

☺ **Moisture Emulsion** *($15.50 for 3 ounces)* contains mostly water, mineral oil, slip agent, several thickeners, and preservatives. This is an OK, standard moisturizer for someone with dry skin.

☹ **Moisture Lotion** *($12 for 3 ounces)* is similar to the moisturizer above, but more lightweight. It's an OK, rather ordinary moisturizer for someone with dry skin.

☹ **Protective Veil** *($11 for 3 ounces)* contains mostly water, thickener, slip agents, more thickeners, and preservatives. The second thickening agent is isopropyl palmitate, which can cause breakouts. The company recommends this for someone with oily skin—big mistake.

☺ **Aqua Lube** *($12 for 2 ounces)* contains mostly mineral oil, water, wax, thickener, petrolatum, lanolin, more thickeners, and preservatives. "Lube" is a good name for this extremely rich moisturizer, which I would recommend only for someone with extremely dry skin; however, the company recommends it for oily skin. The only word for that is "insane."

☹ **Super Lube** *($12 for 2 ounces)* is basically petrolatum and wax. You could use Vaseline and be just as happy, but I wouldn't recommend either. Petrolatum by itself is not hydrating or emollient enough for most skin types; it's just greasy.

☹ **Sun Defense Lip Block SPF 15** *($8 for 0.15 ounce)* doesn't contain avobenzone, titanium dioxide, or zinc oxide, and is not recommended.

☹ **Sun Defense Sunscreen for Face and Body, SPF 8** *($13.50 for 4 ounces)* has an SPF 8 and that just doesn't cut it for defending against sun damage, plus this product doesn't contain avobenzone, titanium dioxide, or zinc oxide, and is not recommended.

☹ **Sun Defense Sunscreen for Face and Body, SPF 25** *($16.50 for 4 ounces)* doesn't contain avobenzone, titanium dioxide, or zinc oxide, and is not recommended.

☺ **Sun Free Self Tanning Creme Light** *($13.50 for 4 ounces)* like all self-tanners, contains dihydroxyacetone, the ingredient that turns skin brown. It works as well as any of them.

☺ **Lip Moisture** *($8 for 0.07 ounce)* is a good, though standard, emollient lip balm.

☹ **Makeup Texturizer** *($11 for 1 ounce)* contains mostly alcohol and is not recommended.

Merle Norman Makeup

☹ **FOUNDATION:** Luxiva Liquid Makeup SPF 16 *($14.50)* is an extremely light, but emollient, foundation; however, the SPF has no UVA protection, and the colors are almost all to peach, pink, orange, or ash to recommend.

☹ **Luxiva Ultra Powder Foundation** *($18)* is a standard talc-based powder that goes on in a grainy, powdery finish that can look caked and dry. There are only a handful of decent colors to select from out of a large array.

☹ **AquaBase** *($13.50)* is an extremely creamy, rather thick foundation that is supposed to provide matte coverage. It is somewhat matte, but can feel too thick if you don't blend it carefully. If you want medium coverage and a silky feel and have normal to dry skin, this is a great foundation with some wonderful colors for a wide range of skin tones. **These colors are great:** Alabaster Beige, Ivory, Palest Porcelain (slightly pink), Champagne Beige, Delicate Beige, Cream Beige, Palest Ivory (great for light skin tones), Toasted Almond, Ecru, Maple Cream, Golden Beige, Amber Glow, Bronze Glow, Cafe Au Lait, Toffee, and Mahogany. **These colors are too pink, peach, rose, or yellow:** Translucent, Bamboo, Fawn Beige, Porcelain, Taffy Cream, Golden Birch, and Gentle Tan.

☺ **Luxiva Ultra Foundation with HC-12** *($22)* claims to "retexturize" skin with HC-12, which seems to be a combination of plant oils, water-binding agent, plant extracts, and vitamins. If you have very dry skin, they will help moisturize it; if that's what they mean by "retexturizing," this product will do that. **These colors are great, with no unnatural undertones:** Ivory, Alabaster, Creamy Beige, Simply Beige, Soft Bisque, Quiet Rose, Ecru, Pure Beige, Sun Beige, and Cafe Au Lait. **These colors are too pink, peach, or yellow for most skin tones:** Palest Porcelain, Porcelain, Sandy Beige, Golden Beige, Tan Beige, Cafe Beige, Soft Honey, Toffee, and Bronzewood.

☹ **Total Finish Compact** *($15)* is as close to greasepaint as you will ever find, but even greasepaint isn't this greasy. The salesperson confided that everyone calls this the "Tammy Faye Bakker foundation," and all the colors are as far from natural skin tone as you can get.

☹ **Oil-Control Makeup** *($15)* won't control oil in the slightest; it isn't even oil-free—it contains plant oil. It has some talc, but that won't help much given these other ingredients. The color selection is ridiculously small and most of the colors are too pink or peach to recommend.

☹ **Powder Base** *($12.50)* is more creamy, actually greasy, than powder, and has an almost sticky feel. It finally blends out quite sheer and smooth, but with almost no powder feel, so the name is confusing, plus it tends to stain the skin—it is that thick.

☹ **Luxiva Liquid Creme Foundation** *($20)* has some of the most awful colors I've ever seen, and a greasy texture too.

☹ **Color Corrector** *($9.50)* comes in four shades: White, Yellow, Mint, and Lilac (really rose). I never recommend color correctors because they are an unreliable way to affect skin color and an add unnecessary layer of makeup over the skin.

☹ **CONCEALER: Retouch Cover Creme** *($9)* has mostly peach and pink shades, and it can crease into the lines around the eyes. **Oil-Free Concealing Creme** *($9)* is oil-free but still has a fairly emollient texture. It goes on drier than the Retouch, but it also tends to crease and has a terrible assortment of colors.

☹ **POWDER:** Remarkable Finish Loose Powder *($15)* and **Remarkable Fin-**

ish Pressed Powder *($12.50)* are standard talc-based powders that go on soft and smooth. The seven colors are all fairly peach or pink. **Remarkable Finish Oil Control Loose Powder** *($15)* and **Remarkable Finish Oil Control Pressed Powder** *($12.50)* are talc-based powders that go on soft and smooth. The seven colors are all too peach or pink to recommend.

☺ **BLUSH**: **Blushing Powder** *($12.50)* textures vary a bit, but most are soft and blend on easily. There is a vast selection of blush colors for a wide range of skin tones; most have a slight amount of shine, but not enough to be a problem. **Luxiva Cream Blush** *($14)* has a soft, smooth, sheer finish and a great range of colors. While this isn't my preferred way to recommend applying blush, if you prefer cream blushes, this is a fine option.

☺ **EYESHADOW:** **Powder Rich Eyeshadows Singles** *($11)*, **Duos** *($14)*, and **Trios** *($15)* come in some very good matte shades that blend on smooth and soft. **These colors are matte and beautiful:** Taupe Suede, Cocoa, Rosy Brown, Cappuccino, Wheat, Sepia, Chestnut, Peach Blossom, Honey, Pumpkin Spice, Cashmere, Olive, Cashmere/Suede, Wine & Rose, Warm Naturals, Cool Naturals, Butternut/Spice, Sand/Wall St. Grey, Brown Velvet, Rose Taupe, Auburn, Rich Brown, and Cinnamon Spice.

☹ **Shimmer Stick** *($13)* is a cream eyeshadow in pencil form that is intensely shiny, blends out to nothing, and is hard to sharpen.

☺ **EYE AND BROW SHAPER:** **Automatic Definitive Eye Pencil** *($11)* has a soft, slightly creamy application that dries to a transfer-resistant finish. It comes in a twist-up container and does have impressive staying power. **Trim Line Eye Pencils** *($11)* are standard pencils that come in a small but good color selection. They go on soft but not greasy. **Definitive Eyelining Pen** *($10)* is a standard liquid liner with a stiff applicator. It works fine for a dramatic look, but the color selection is limited. **Automatic Eyeliner** *($10)* is a standard liquid eyeliner with a brush applicator; this one can tend to chip. **Tinted Brow Sealer** *($10.50)* is a lightweight mascara with a wand that comes in three brow-appropriate colors. This product works well to make brows look defined and natural. **Only Natural** *($9.50)* is a group of matte brow-powders that come with a stiff brush. Forget the brush, but the powders work well to create a defined brow without looking greasy or drawn on. **Definitive Brow Pencil** *($9.50)* is a standard brow pencil with a somewhat dry finish. This one works as well as any.

☺ **LIPSTICK AND LIP PENCIL:** **Lipstick** *($10.50)*, **Color Rich Lip Creme** *($10.50)*, and **Luxiva Ultra Lipcolor** *($11.50)* are practically indistinguishable. These are fairly creamy to glossy and have a small amount of stain that helps keep the color around longer than most. **Semi-Transparent Lipstick** *($8.95)* is more gloss than lipstick and has little to no staying power. **Moist Lip Color** *($9)* is a very greasy gloss that comes in a tube and, like all glosses, has limited staying power. **Automatic De-**

finitive **Lip Pencil** *($11)* has a soft, slightly creamy application that dries to a trans-fer-resistant finish. It comes in a twist-up container and does have impressive staying power. **Lip Pencil Plus** *($12)* is a fat, two-sided pencil; one end has a matte finish and works as the lip liner, the other end is creamy and has a lipstick finish. I find these kinds of products more gimmicky than useful (I hate sharpening anything), but this is a fun product to check out.

☹ **Lip Treatment Cream** *($8.95)* is supposed to prevent bleeding. It does an OK job, but it doesn't feel great and it tends to peel off.

☹ **MASCARA: Creamy Flo-Matic Mascara** *($10)* is an OK mascara. It doesn't clump, but it also doesn't build very thick lashes. **Luxiva Ultra Mascara** *($15)* isn't bad, just unimpressive for the money. It builds OK length and some thickness but it takes time. For the money you would expect more. **Ultra Thick Mascara** *($12)* goes on in a thick clumpy mess that makes lashes look unnatural and unattractive.

☹ **BRUSHES:** Merle Norman's brush selection has some great shapes and sizes but the **Powder** and **Blush** brushes bristles are too sparse and too stiff to be of much use and they don't feel very nice against the skin.

☺ The only brushes to consider in this group are the four **Eyeshadow Brushes**; these are for the most part quite nice.

Moisturel (Skin Care Only)

☹ **Moisturel Sensitive Skin Cleanser** *($7.76 for 8.75 ounces)* is a reliable skin cleanser that I've recommended for a long time. But its second ingredient is sodium lauryl sulfate, and that is too risky as a skin irritant for many skin types. With so many good water-soluble cleansers available that don't use potentially irritating detergent cleansing agents, there is no reason to chance this one.

☺ **Moisturel Cream** *($7 for 4 ounces)* is a Vaseline-based moisturizer that also contains silicone, glycerin, and thickeners. This is a good but extremely standard moisturizer for dry skin.

☺ **Lotion** *($8 for 8 ounces)* is similar to the one above, only in lotion form, and the same basic review applies.

Mon Amie

This infomercial skin-care line was endorsed by Kathy Lee Gifford. It seems to have gone the way of many infomercials and is no longer to be found. This line was difficult for many women to use and Mon Amie struggled with an overwhelming number of returns. When you see my comments about the formulations you won't be surprised why that happened. If you didn't already have dry skin, you might after trying these products. What is really a shame about Mon Amie is that the makeup products are impressive, with matte eyeshadows and blushes and good neutral skin-tone foundations. Sadly, it is always hard to buy makeup sight unseen. For example, when I bought my kit the Mon Amie phone representative asked what color my skin was; she determined from my response I had a medium skin tone. As a result I was sent a beautiful range of peach blushes and lipsticks and yellow-based eyeshadows; the only problem is that most of the time I prefer blue-tone eyeshadows and blushes, not yellow.

Please note that the prices for the skin-care products are the company's suggested retail prices, which helps make their kits look like a huge bargain in comparison (even though you get a limited amount of each product). For example, you are told that if you were buying a kit with all these skin-care and makeup products it would retail for $339, but if you get Mon Amie's kit it costs $119.85. Even if these products did retail for $339 I would suggest that would be a waste of money. If the skin-care products were better, the $119.85 would be a fair price, if you liked all the colors, cleansers, and moisturizers. As it stands, I think that is unlikely for most women who venture into this "deal." For more information about Mon Amie products call (800) 544-3300.

Mon Amie Skin Care

☹ **Gentle Facial Cleanser** *($14.95 for 6.7 ounces)* is a standard detergent cleanser; TEA-lauryl sulfate, the second ingredient and the primary cleansing agent, is very drying. This product is anything but gentle.

☹ **Moisturizing Skin Clarifier** *($14.95 for 3.5 ounces)* contains mostly water, alcohol, slip agents, salicylic acid, and preservatives. It's beyond me why anyone would even think of calling this product moisturizing when it contains mostly alcohol and 5% salicylic acid. But wait a minute: the package says it *doesn't* contain alcohol. Didn't anyone look at the ingredient list? Alcohol is right there, in black and white. Salicylic acid does exfoliate the skin, but in an alcohol base it can be a problem for even the oiliest, least sensitive complexion.

☺ $$$ **Daytime Moisturizer Replenishment Complex SPF 15** *($24.95 for 1.75 ounces)* contains mostly water, thickeners, vitamin E, water-binding agents, silicone, more thickeners, and preservatives. This is a very good sunscreen for someone with normal to somewhat dry skin.

☺ $$$ **Intensive Eye Serum** *($39.95 for 0.5 ounce)* contains mostly water, thickeners, water-binding agents, vitamin E, and preservatives. This isn't all that intensive, but it is still a very good lightweight moisturizer for someone with normal to slightly dry skin.

☺ $$$ **Nighttime Renewal Complex** *($36.95 for 1.75 ounces)* contains mostly water, thickeners, plant extract, more thickeners, silicone, sugar extracts (AHAs), more thickeners, water-binding agents, and preservatives. The amount of AHAs isn't much, maybe 4%, but given that the toner contains salicylic acid, how much exfoliation can your skin take? Only one ingredient needs to be exfoliating; two is excessive, and using both can be irritating and drying for most skin types.

Mon Amie Makeup

☺ <u>FOUNDATION:</u> The **Foundation** *($19.95)* is beautifully neutral and has a wonderful creamy texture that is fine if you have normal to dry skin. Someone with oily skin would not be pleased with the consistency, though. You get two separate colors that can be blended together to create the right shade for your skin tone. That isn't as convenient as having one foundation that matches your skin exactly, but it does reduce the chances of getting an entirely wrong shade, given that you can't try it on before you buy it.

☹ <u>CONCEALER:</u> **Concealer Stick** *($14.95)* goes on easily; it also creases easily, which is not what concealers are supposed to do.

☺ <u>POWDER:</u> **Pressed/Translucent Powder** *($19.95)* is a standard talc-based powder that has a soft texture and goes on dry.

☺ <u>EYESHADOW AND BLUSH</u>: The two **Blushes** and four **Eyeshadows** you receive in the kit *($19.95)* have wonderful textures and are perfectly matte. The eyeshadows are mostly neutral shades with no garish colors, and the blushes are soft colors that are easy to apply. You may not be thrilled with the array of colors if they don't work with your skin tone or aren't colors you want, but if they do match, the quality and colors are superior.

☺ <u>EYE AND BROW SHAPER:</u> The kit also comes with a two-sided **Brow Pencil** *($12.95)*, a two-sided **Eye Liner Pencil** *($14.95)*; the colors are fine and the texture is firm but soft, with only a slightly greasy feel.

☺ <u>LIPSTICK AND LIP PENCIL:</u> The kit includes three **Lipsticks** *($24.95)*, which seems quite generous. One is a sheer, glossy lipstick that easily feathers into the lines around the mouth and may not be of much use, but the other two have nice, somewhat creamy, matte textures. Again, the colors may not be right, but the quality is there. The two-sided **Lip Pencil** *($9.95)* is identical to the Eye Liner Pencil.

☹ <u>MASCARA:</u> This is a good **Mascara** *($12.95)* that goes on well and has decent staying power. It isn't exciting, but it is reliable.

Murad (Skin Care Only)

Like M.D. Formulations, Neostrata, Dr. Mary Lupo, and other medically oriented AHA-containing lines of skin-care products, Murad boasts an above-average AHA. After all, it's creator is Dr. Murad of infomercial fame. Most of his products contain 8% glycolic acid, which makes them very reliable AHA creams and lotions. Murad also has its share of products that contain alcohol and other irritating ingredients. I should mention that the prices are a bit excessive, at around $40 per product, especially compared with Neostrata (which has a similar AHA content) at around $16 per product. Where Murad takes a back seat to these other lines is that here every skin type has a skin-care routine calling for a total of at least eight to ten products. By most medical standards that is not only excessive, it is overkill and harmful to skin.

I've received many letters asking me about Dr. Murad's extremely successful infomercial. In my opinion, the doctor has crossed a line, and I fear this is a growing trend in the world of dermatologists-turned-cosmeticians. We all assume that a dermatologist knows everything there is to know about skin-care products in regard to their formulation, use, and effectiveness. Most important, we expect them to know, and tell us, the absolute truth about skin care. We don't expect cosmetics-counter hype from these highly trained medical professionals.

Regardless of whether dermatologists know best about lotions and potions, no scrupulous doctor would, with a clear conscience, sell products using the ludicrous claims made for the extended line of Murad products. Any doctor who is willing to sell products such as Murasome Cellular Serum, claiming it neutralizes free-radical damage (when most researchers will tell you that is only a theory that has not yet been proven true for the skin), or Murad Purifying Clay Masque, saying it provides the ideal environment for cellular repair, has sold out completely. Every product has the same hype, the same unsubstantiated claims, the same exaggeration about the beneficial effects of ingredients that are present only in the tiniest amounts, without even a mention of the standard ingredients that make up the bulk of these products. For more information about Murad call (800) 336-8723.

☹ **AHA/BHA Exfoliating Cleanser, Deep Cleansing for All Skin Types** *($23 for 6 ounces)* is a standard detergent-based cleanser that contains plant oil and about 4% AHA and 1% salicylic acid (BHA). AHAs and BHA are a problem in cleansers, because you don't want to get them in the eye and because their effectiveness is washed down the drain.

☺ **$$$ Moisture Rich Skin Cleanser** *($19.50 for 6 ounces)* is a standard detergent-based cleanser with thickening agents and a small quantity of conditioning agents. It isn't what anyone would call rich, though it is a good cleanser for someone with normal to dry skin. There is also a small amount of grapefruit extract in there that can be irritating for some skin types, so be careful.

☺ **$$$ Refreshing Skin Cleanser** *($19.50 for 6 ounces)* is an extremely standard detergent-based cleanser for someone with normal to oily or combination skin. It can be drying for someone with dry skin.

☺ **$$$ Gentle Make-up Remover** *($16.50 for 4.2 ounces)* is an extremely standard wipe-off makeup remover, extremely overpriced for a very ordinary group of ingredients. It does contain a small amount of glycolic acid, but thankfully the pH isn't low enough to make it active on the skin; that would be a huge mistake in something that might get in the eye.

☹ **Clarifying Astringent** *($14.50 for 6 ounces)* contains mostly witch hazel as well as some amount of menthol and lemongrass oil; all are completely unnecessary skin irritants.

☹ **Clarifying Gel** *($48 for 1.4 ounces)* contains mostly alcohol, which makes it too drying and irritating for all skin types.

☹ **Hydrating Toner** *($14.50 for 6 ounces)* contains mostly witch hazel, a completely unnecessary skin irritant.

☹ **Advanced Combination Skin Formula** *($48 for 3.3 ounces)* is a lightweight gel that contains about 7% AHAs and about 1% BHA. It also contain a good deal of alcohol which makes it a problem for all skin types.

☹ **Advanced Oily Prone Skin Formula** *($48 for 3.3 ounces)* is almost identical to the one above and the same review applies.

☹ **Advanced Sensitive Skin Formula** *($48 for 3.3 ounces)* is almost identical to the one above, and that makes calling it a "sensitive skin formula" a bad joke.

☺ **$$$ Advanced Sensitive Skin Smoothing Cream** *($48 for 1.7 ounces)* is about a 6% glycolic acid–based moisturizer. It's very overpriced, but good for dry skin.

☹ **Advanced Skin Smoothing Lotion** *($48 for 5 ounces)* is similar to the one above except this one contains orange, cinnamon, and grapefruit oils, all potential and completely unnecessary skin irritants.

☹ **Advanced Skin Smoothing Cream SPF 8** *($48 for 1.7 ounces)* has a low SPF. With so many good SPF 15s around, why bother with this one when it comes to protecting your skin from sun damage?

☺ **$$$ Cellular Eye Gel** *($29 for 0.5 ounce)* contains mostly water, film former, slip agent, thickeners, water-binding agents, anti-irritants, and preservatives. This is a good lightweight moisturizer for slightly dry skin.

☺ **$$$ Intensive Formula** *($48 for 3.3 ounces)* is a good 8% AHA in a lightweight moisturizing base for someone with normal to dry skin. It contains its share of anti-irritants and water-binding agents but the price is way out of proportion for what you get.

☺ **$$$ Murasome Cellular Serum for All Skin Types** *($42 for 1.4 ounces)* is a good, overpriced, lightweight moisturizer for normal to slightly dry skin. It contains mostly water, glycerin, thickeners, water-binding agents, plant extracts, silicone, and preservatives.

☺ **$$$ Murasome Eye Complex 10 SPF 8** *($50 for 0.5 ounce)* has a low SPF. With so many good SPF 15s around, why bother with this one when it comes to protecting your skin from sun damage?

☺ **$$$ Murasome Night Reform** *($52.50 for 1.4 ounces)* is a good 8%

AHA in a lightweight, slightly moisturizing base. It contains mostly water, lots of thickeners, vitamins, anti-irritant, water-binding agents, plant extracts, plant oils, and preservatives.

☹ **Perfecting Day Cream SPF 15** *($29 for 2.25 ounces)* doesn't contain avobenzone, zinc oxide, or titanium dioxide, and is not recommended. So much for the concept of "perfecting."

☺ **$$$ Perfecting Night Cream** *($31 for 2.25 ounces)* contains mostly water, plant oils, thickeners, water-binding agents, vitamins, and preservatives. This would be a good moisturizer for someone with dry skin.

☺ **$$$ Perfecting Serum** *($52 for 1 ounce)* is merely a lightweight lotion of water-binding agents, vitamins, and plant oils. It is a very good moisturizer for someone with normal to slightly dry skin.

☺ **$$$ Skin Perfecting Lotion** *($27 for 2 ounces)* contains mostly water, plant oil, glycerin, several thickeners, several water-binding agents, and preservatives. This is a good moisturizer for someone with dry skin.

☺ **$$$ Skin Soothing Formula** *($9.50 for 0.5 ounce)* is a Vaseline-based moisturizer with lanolin and a tiny amount of BHA. It isn't the right pH for the salicylic acid to be effective, and a BHA product is never considered soothing.

☹ **$$$ Murasun Daily Sunblock Bronzer SPF 15** *($16.50 for 4.2 ounces)* is a titanium dioxide–based sunscreen with a bit of color that is mostly on the peach side.

☹ **$$$ Murasun Daily Sunblock Light Tint SPF 15** *($16.50 for 4.2 ounces)* is almost identical to the one above only with less color, and the same basic review applies.

☺ **Murasun Daily Sunblock with Antioxidants SPF 15** *($16.50 for 4.2 ounces)* is a titanium dioxide–based sunscreen that would be very good for someone with normal to slightly dry skin.

☹ **Murasun Daily Sunscreen with Antioxidants SPF 15** *($16.50 for 4.2 ounces)* doesn't contain avobenzone, zinc oxide, or titanium dioxide, and is not recommended.

☹ **Murasun SPF 15 Lip/Eye/Nose Protection** *($10.50 for 0.5 ounce)* does not contain avobenzone, titanium dioxide, or zinc oxide, and is not recommended.

☺ **$$$ Murasun Waterproof Sunblock with Antioxidants SPF 30** *($19 for 4.2 ounces)* is a good in part titanium dioxide–based sunscreen for someone with normal to dry skin.

☹ **Acne Management Formula for Skin Prone to Acne** *($13 for 0.5 ounce)* is a confusing product. While it does contain sulfur as a disinfectant, and AHA and BHA for exfoliation, it also contains a range of thickening ingredients that can clog pores. There are far better ways to exfoliate and disinfect skin than this one.

☹ **Acne Management Masque** *($32 for 2.5 ounces)* is similar to the one above, except in the form of mask, but the same warnings apply.

☹ **Advanced Acne Prone Skin Formula for Acne Prone Skin** *($46 for 3.3 ounces)* is a BHA and AHA lotion that also contains a lot of alcohol. That only exacerbates the potential for breakouts from irritation.

☹ **Age Spot and Pigment Lightening Gel** *($48 for 1.4 ounces)* would be a decent skin-lightening product with its 2% hydroquinone, but it also contains a lot of alcohol which can cause unnecessary skin dryness and irritation.

☹ **Hydrating Gel Masque** *($22.50 for 2.25 ounces)* contains mostly water, film former, slip agent, plant extracts, thickeners, vitamins, water-binding agents, and preservatives. Those ingredients wouldn't be bad in a mask, but several of the plant extracts, including horsetail, pine cone, and lemon, can be irritating for most skin types.

☺ **$$$ Purifying Clay Masque** *($22.50 for 2.25 ounces)* is a standard clay mask with some water-binding agents. This is as good as any clay mask and can feel good on the skin, but don't expect it to purify anything, it just absorbs oil.

☺ **$$$ Youth Builder Collagen Supplement** *($45 for 120 tablets)* hits rock bottom: this is a doctor selling vitamins claiming to get rid of wrinkles. Isn't there an ethics board that can put a halt to this kind of nonsense?

Nars (Makeup Only)

Those of you who regularly or even occasionally scan the fashion magazines have surely noticed the plethora of new cosmetics lines created, or at least endorsed, by an assortment of relatively little-known New York and Los Angeles makeup artists (well, unknown to anyone outside of the Manhattan or L.A. fashion scene). This trend took off a few years ago when M.A.C. (Makeup Art Cosmetics), a small but thriving cosmetics company based in Toronto, specializing in color items, came on the market with a wide selection of products makeup artists really did prefer to use: matte, neutral-toned eyeshadows; soft, muted blushes; a large selection of soft but very usable brushes; and, most notably, neutral to yellow-based foundations. The notion that a makeup artist's line could find a following took off and several New York and Los Angeles–based makeup artists from Bobbi Brown to Laura Mercier joined the fray, as well as the namesake for this line, makeup artist Francois Nars.

Nars has one of the smaller color lines available, and if it didn't have any competition I would recommend taking a closer look at a few of its interesting products. But so many other lines offer a large selection of beautiful matte colors and reliable product choices that Nars' collection looks almost paltry. Also, unlike his peers, Nars offers a large number of very intense blue, green, silver, and iridescent eyeshadows. I guess that makes this line stand out, but my recommendation is to stay away, at least from the eyeshadows. For more information, call Nars Cosmetics at (212) 941-0890.

☺ **$$$ FOUNDATION:** Nars' two types of foundations come in a good though small range of colors. **Balanced Foundation** *($37)* has a smooth, soft texture, blends on easily, and has a great finish. **The colors to avoid** are Sahara, Sedona, Jamaica, and Hawaii, which are all too peach or ash for most skin tones. **Oil Free Foundation** *($37)* doesn't have the same color problems as the Balanced Foundation, and it has a great, soft matte finish. **The only colors to avoid are** Sedona, Jamaica, Hawaii, and Sahara; all of these are too peach or ash for most skin tones.

☺ CONCEALER: The texture of this **Concealer** *($16)* is rather heavy and thick, making it hard to blend, plus the colors are all fairly ash for most all skin types.

☺ $$$ POWDER: Both the **Pressed Powder** *($24)* and the **Loose Powder** *($30)* come in several very good shades, with great smooth, slightly dry textures, but they are nothing more than standard powders. The loose powder is very messy to use, with powder flying all over the place, and it does have a slight amount of shine, which isn't the best for those looking to reduce shine not add to it. **The only color to avoid** is Mountain, it is too ash for most skin tones.

☺ $$$ BLUSH: The impressive **Blush** *($20)* selection features muted neutral shades with a smooth though slightly dry texture. Silvana is the only shiny color; Desire is an ultra-pink shade that stands out like a sore thumb in the midst of the subtle blush colors.

☹ EYESHADOW: The only matte eyeshadows are the **Single Eyeshadows** *($15)*, but a lot of them are shiny and/or blue. The **Duo Eyeshadows** *($27)* are also a problem, and likewise shiny and blue.

☺ $$$ **Multiple Sticks** *($32)* is a twist-up tube of sheer, creamy, pearlescent color. For adding shine over the eyes, lips, cheeks, and face (ergo the name "Multiple"), it can be fine, though a bit greasy. The color range is impressive, ranging from a soft rose, white, and pink, to yellow.

☺ $$$ EYE AND BROW PENCIL: The four **Eyeliners** *($16)* and four **Eyebrow Pencils** *($16)* are as standard as they come (the Eyeliner pencils are slightly more creamy than the drier finish Eyebrow Pencils), and absolutely not worth the price tag.

☺ $$$ LIPSTICK AND LIP PENCIL: There is a good selection of standard **Lip liner Pencils** *($16)*. The three types of lipstick range from a standard creme **Matte Lipstick** *($19)* with a good amount of stain and opaque coverage, to **Frost Lipstick** *($19)*, which has a shiny, more glossy finish, to **Sheer Lipstick** *($19)*, a sheer lip gloss in a tube. The most confusing aspect is that the types of lipstick are not indicated. You have to test each one to find the texture you want. There is also a **Lip Gloss** *($19)* which is just a very standard gloss with a small number of colors to choose from.

☺ $$$ MASCARA: The **Mascara** *($19)* isn't terrible, it just isn't great, and for this kind of money it should be great. It does build long, thick lashes, but it takes a long time to achieve that, and you do end up with some clumping.

☺ **$$$ <u>BRUSHES:</u>** This small assortment of brushes *($17 to $30)* is exceptional and very usable, though the excessive cost is questionable.

Nat Robbins (Makeup Only)

If you've happened into your drugstore lately and perused the wall where the makeup products are displayed, you may have noticed this small and extremely inexpensive makeup line. If you've passed it by, next time be sure you stop long enough to check out a handful of extremely interesting products. I am the last person to be a snob about price when it comes to the cosmetics industry, but I was really surprised how much I liked several of these lip products, eyeshadows, and eyeliners. For more information on this line, call (800) 444-0563.

☺ **Mechanical Definer Eyeshadow** *($2.95)* is a twist-up eyeliner pencil with a thick point. It goes on smoothly and easily with no drag. This is an excellent way to line the eye. It would not be my choice for applying eyeshadow, but it could be a quick, easy way to do touch-ups during the day. This is definitely a unique find for shaping the eyes, and one I will keep in my makeup bag. **Cream Eyeshadow** *($2.95)* is a thick pencil that goes on smooth and creamy and blends out to a soft matte finish. Some of the colors are slightly shiny, and sharpening can be troublesome, but it is a clever option for creating a fast eye design and competes with any I've seen at the department stores.

☹ **Cream to Powder Shadow Plus Base** *($2.03)* is just what it says: a cream-to-powder shadow. It goes on very sheer, leaving only a hint of color and a slight amount of shine. Once it's blended, it doesn't budge. This can create an especially soft look if you have a knack for controlling this kind of eyeshadow, but the shine will displease those with wrinkles.

☺ **Perfect Liquid Eyeliner** *($2.49)* isn't exactly perfect, but it is a very good liquid eyeliner that goes on evenly and doesn't chip or flake.

☻ **Stay-Put Liquid Liner** *($2.99)* is a mess of a product. It is difficult to apply, the brush is stiff and applies the color in strange streaks, it tends to chip, and while you might be hoping it's waterproof, it isn't. Stay-put products should stay put and not chip, don't you think?

☺ **ColorMatte Lipstick** *($1.89)* is an excellent soft matte lipstick. It goes on smooth, without feeling thick or heavy, and stays slightly creamy the entire time it's on. It didn't feather or bleed, and it has a strong stain, so the color lasts longer than most. What a find! **Everlasting Matte Lipstick** *($2.95)* is a lipstick in the form of a pencil, but it can be used either as a lip liner or a lipstick. It goes on smooth and creamy, with a soft matte finish, and stays that way for quite a while. If you didn't have to sharpen this one, I could see getting used to this kind of product. **Stay-Put Lipcolor** *($2.99)* is as good as any of the new ultra-matte lipsticks. It is less drying than some and doesn't chip or wear off in clumps. Most important, it doesn't bleed and it stays on quite well. **Color Matte Lip Liner** *($2.36)* is a very good standard lip liner. **Mechanical Definer Lip Liner** *($2.76)* is an excellent standard lip liner that doesn't have to be sharpened. **Stay-Put Lip Liner** *($2.99)* is a good, standard, twist-up lip pencil, but it's no more waterproof than any other lip pencil. All lip and eye pencils stay fairly well, though they do easily budge when they come in contact with any creamy face or lip product.

☺ **Everlasting Moisture Rich LipColor SPF 15** *($1.89)* is an extremely glossy lipstick with a stain. That helps keep the color around longer, but the greasy look is distracting. **Mega Color Lipstick** *($1.42)* is an OK lipstick that is more glossy than creamy. It does have a stain, which helps keep the color around longer. **Lip Lacquer** *($2.32)* is similar to the lip gloss, but with more pigment concentration. It is too greasy for a daytime look. **Color Wand Lip Gloss** *($2.32)* is a standard, extremely emollient gloss with shine.

☺ **Hydrawear Lip Gloss** *($2.99)* is an incredibly emollient lip gloss with decent staying power for a gloss, but the applicator takes some getting used to. You squeeze the tube, which then brings the gloss to the tip connected to the tube. It isn't the easiest method of getting gloss on the lips, and the tube isn't easy to squeeze, but once you get it on it's just fine.

☺ **Lash Building Mascara** *($2.32)* doesn't build that much length, but it does build thickness without clumping. It isn't the best mascara I've ever tried, but it ranks up there with some of the good ones.

☹ **Stay-Put Mascara** *($2.99)* doesn't stay put all that well either, and no matter how long you spend applying it, it doesn't build any length or thickness. Did anyone try this mistake of a mascara before putting it on the market?

☹ Nat Robbins also offers an assortment of **brushes** *($2.50 to $11)*, but they are all of poor quality and not recommended. The bristles are too stiff, the density too sparse, and the texture too floppy to offer much control or feel nice on the skin.

Natura Bisse (Skin Care Only)

For those of you who have heard of or sampled Natura Bisse, I assume that must mean you've been hanging out at the Neiman Marcus makeup counters where this overpriced, pointless line is sold. It is hyped (and I mean overhyped), as a high-concentration AHA product line. It is supposed to provide the highest concentration of AHAs you can buy. Natura Bisse's Glyco Peeling Plus 50% AHA and Glyco Peeling 25% AHA aren't anywhere near as potent as those percentages imply. If they were, after you had applied the stuff your face would start burning, and after a few minutes it would feel as if it were falling off. Actually, if it was an effective AHA, your skin *would* start falling off after a few minutes, and you would be a peeling, oozing, red mass of skin. But you have nothing to worry about from these products, because they are all buffered to a pH of over 4.5 (a fact the company extols on their brochures), which means they can't perform as serious exfoliants and pose little to no risk to your skin, though they do pose a serious risk of wasting your money. This is because AHAs, in order to be effective, need to be in a pH of 3 to 3.5; much over 4 and they just don't work that well. At a pH over about 3.5, the acid becomes a salt and no longer works to improve cell turnover. I know this sounds like a fine line to cross, but when it comes to pH there is a huge difference between 3.5 and 4.5. Consider that 7 is water but 8 can be an alkaline shampoo or cleanser.

Aside from the AHA claims, there are a host of other gimmicks lurking in this line that range from thymus extract to amniotic fluid, horse protein serum, and a handful of plant extracts. None of those things benefit skin in any substantial way. There are also products claiming to add oxygen to the skin, but none of them contain enough to give air to one skin cell. This line may have an elite air about it, but many of the products, particularly the sunscreens and acne products, are poorly formulated, while the moisturizer is more contrivance than substance. For more information about Natura Bisse, call (800) 7-NATURA.

☺ **China Clay Cleanser Purifying and Cleansing Paste** *($35 for 4.2 ounces)* contains clay, and is hard to rinse off. This is a standard detergent-based cleanser with clay, that's it, but is this any way to clean the skin and for this kind of price tag?

☺ **$$$ Dry Skin Milk Cleanser** *($24 for 6.5 ounces)* contains mostly thickeners, egg oil, plant extracts, and preservatives. It is an OK cleanser for dry skin but it can leave a greasy film on the skin. There is nothing about egg oil that is more beneficial for the skin than any other form of oil.

☹ **Facial Cleansing Gel Foaming Cleanser** *($28 for 7 ounces)* is a standard detergent-based cleanser that also contains a fairly potent film former, styrene, which is irritating for all skin types.

☹ **Oxygen Cream for All Skin Types** *($54 for 2.5 ounces)* contains hydrogen peroxide, which can release oxygen, but once this product is opened, the oxygen is used up (because hydrogen peroxide is a very unstable ingredient). Plus, isn't this an absurd amount of money for what you could get just as well from an 89-cent bottle of hydrogen peroxide at the drugstore?

☹ **Oxygen Concentrate for All Skin Types** *($72 for 1 ounce)* is similar to the Oxygen Cream above and the same review applies.

☺ **$$$ Sensitive Cleansing Cream for All Skin Types** *($27 for 7 ounces)* is a standard detergent-based cleanser that would be good for most skin types. It contains a small amount of papaya extract, which can be a skin irritant, but there probably isn't enough to negatively affect the skin.

☺ $$$ **Eye Make-up Remover Hypo-Allergenic Lotion** *($23 for 3.3 ounces)* is just water, a detergent agent, and plant extracts. It will take off makeup, but there are more effective products than this available.

☺ $$$ **Dry Skin Toner Moisturizing Toner** *($24 for 6.5 ounces)* is an OK, ordinary toner that contains water, slip agent, water-binding agents, plant extracts, and preservatives. There is a small amount of witch hazel in here that shouldn't be a problem for most skin types.

☹ **Oily Skin Toner, Astringent** *($24 for 6.5 ounces)* is mostly alcohol and is not recommended for any skin type.

☺ $$$ **Sensitive Toner for All Skin Types** *($22.50 for 6.5 ounces)* is a good irritant-free toner for most skin types.

☹ **Glyco-Eye, Eye Contour Exfoliater Gel Cream Vitalizer, with Glycolic Acid** *($56 for 0.8 ounce)* isn't in a low enough pH to make it effective. At this price, and for this minuscule amount of product, all the right components should be in place.

☹ **Glyco-Face, Exfoliating Night Cream with Glycolic Acid, for Normal to Dry Skin** *($64 for 2.5 ounces)* is similar to the one above, and the same review applies.

☹ **Glyco-Peeling 25% Glyco-Peeling Plus 50%** *($95 for 12 0.1-ounce ampoules)* is similar to the one above, and the same review applies.

☹ **Action Complex Facial Fluid, with Vitamin A+C+E** *($84 for 1 ounce)* contains way too much alcohol amidst a bunch of gimmicky ingredients (ranging from amniotic fluid to thymus extract) to be recommended.

☹ **Basics-Eye Contour Cream SPF 10** *($52 for 0.8 ounce)* doesn't contain avobenzone, titanium dioxide, or zinc oxide, and while SPF 10 isn't terrible, this product is not recommended.

☹ **C+C Vitamin Complex Concentrated Serum with Double Vitamin C** *($110 for four ampoules at 0.2 ounce each)* is an inanely overpriced product that uses ascorbic acid as the form of vitamin C. Without getting into the discussion about whether or not vitamin C is worth it for the skin, ascorbic acid is thought to be one of the worst ways to deliver vitamin C to the skin.

☹ **C+C Vitamin Cream Refirming Cream SPF 6** *($66 for 2.5 ounces)* has a SPF 6, and that's bad enough, but it doesn't contain avobenzone, titanium dioxide, or zinc oxide, and is not recommended.

☹ **Cytokines Eye Contour Cell Renewal Gel SPF 10** *($65 for 0.8 ounce)* doesn't contain avobenzone, titanium dioxide, or zinc oxide, and is not recommended.

☹ **Cytokines Facial Day Cream Cell Renewal Day Cream SPF 6** *($72 for 1.7 ounces)* doesn't contain avobenzone, titanium dioxide, or zinc oxide, and is not recommended.

☹ **Cytokines Top Ten Fluid, Cell Renewal Complex, Skin Growth Factor** *($110 for 1 ounce)* not only can't renew skin, but it contains a good deal of alcohol which kills skin; I imagine that would put you back at the beginning, as well as create irritation and dryness.

☹ **Double Action Hydroprotective Day Cream for Dry Skin SPF 6** *($52 for 2.5 ounces)*, at SPF 6, is bad enough, but this product also doesn't contain avobenzone, titanium dioxide, or zinc oxide, and is not recommended.

☺ **$$$ Elastin Refirming Night Cream for Deeply Dry Skin** *($56 for 2.5 ounces)* contains mostly water, thickeners, lanolin, water-binding agents, and preservatives. This is a very good, but extremely standard, overpriced moisturizer for very dry skin.

☹ **Essential Shock Concentrate for Mature Skin** *($142 for 12 0.1-ounce ampoules)* is a two-part product, with the ampoules containing amniotic fluid and alcohol, and the bottle containing water-binding agents. If this seems like it's worth $142 for less than an ounce of product, nothing I can say will stop you.

☺ **$$$ Essential Shock Night Cream for Dry Aged Skin** *($74 for 2.5 ounces)* is similar to the Elastin Refirming Night Cream above, and the same review applies.

☺ **$$$ Hydroprotective Concentrate for Dry Skin** *($78 for 1.2 ounces)* is just thickeners with lanolin and a small amount of amniotic fluid. It would be good for dry skin, but the amniotic fluid is not the reason this moisturizer works for dry skin.

☺ **$$$ Rose Mosqueta Oil for Dry Aged Skin** *($32 for 1 ounce)* is, as the name implies, rose hip oil with some thickening agents. It can be good for dry skin, but so can any pure oil.

☺ **$$$ Sensitive Concentrate Calming Concentrate for All Sensitive Skin Types** *($108 for 1.2 ounces)* contains mostly water, plant extracts, thickeners, water-binding agents, and preservatives. This would be a good lightweight moisturizer for someone with normal to slightly dry skin, if the price tag doesn't make you dry up first.

☺ **$$$ Sensitive Eye Gel Calming Gel for the Eyes** *($52 for 0.8 ounce)* is similar to the Concentrate above and the same basic review applies.

☺ **$$$ Sensitive Gel Cream Soothing Gel Cream for All Skin Types** *($48 for 2.5 ounces)* is similar to the Concentrate above only in cream form, and the same basic review applies.

☺ **$$$ Sensitive Night Cream Soothing Night Cream for All Skin Types** *($58 for 2.5 ounces)* is similar to the Cream above, and the same basic review applies.

☹ **Special Lift Immediate Firming Concentrate** *($42 for 0.6 ounce)*. What can I say about a product that contains horse serum proteins, amniotic fluid (from who knows where), and alcohol? Just this: What a complete waste of money.

☹ **Stabilizing Concentrate, for Oily Skin** *($74 for 12 0.1-ounce ampoules)* is similar to the one above, and the same warning applies.

☹ **Stabilizing Gel Cream for Oily Skin** *($46 for 2.5 ounces)* contains mostly alcohol, which won't stabilize anyone's skin, though it can be extremely irritating and drying.

☹ **Titian, Neck and Chest Firming Serum** *($74 for 1.7 ounces)* is similar to the Stabilizing Gel and Concentrate above, and the same review applies.

☹ **Vital Gel Cream for Mature Skin SPF 6** *($70 for 2.5 ounces)* has an SPF 6; that's bad enough, but this product doesn't contain avobenzone, titanium dioxide, or zinc oxide, and is not recommended.

☺ **$$$ Sun Protector SPF 30 Hydrating Sun Block for All Skin Types** *($53 for 4.2 ounces)* is an in-part titanium dioxide–based sunscreen. It has a slightly moisturizing base, which makes it good for someone with slightly dry skin.

☹ **Sun Shield, SPF 20 Refirming Cream for Dry Skin** *($53 for 4.2 ounces)* doesn't contain avobenzone, titanium dioxide, or zinc oxide, and is not recommended.

☺ **$$$ Ananas Finishing Mask, for Mature Skin** *($38 for 4.2 ounces)* includes anana, a fancy name for pineapple extract, which can be a skin irritant, though there's not much of that in here so it probably isn't a problem. Other than that, it is just a bunch of thickening agents, which makes it a do-nothing kind of product.

☹ **Glyco-Spot, Exfoliating Gel for Hyperpigmentation with Glycolic Acid** *($60 for 1.7 ounces)* would be a decent hydroquinone-based skin-lightening product except this one contains a lot of alcohol, which makes it too irritating and drying for all skin types.

☹ **Oxygen Finishing Mask for All Skin Types** *($32 for 4.2 ounces)*. See the review for the Oxygen Cream above; the same comments apply for this product.

☺ **$$$ Sensitive Mask Soothing Mask for All Skin Types** *($32 for 2.5 ounces)* is just thickening agents and film former, with some plant extracts. It does contain a tiny bit of papaya extract, which can be a skin irritant for most skin types, but probably not enough to affect the skin. This is just a do-nothing mask that won't do anything good or bad for the skin.

☺ **$$$ Treatments-Splendid Finishing Mask for Dry Skin** *($34 for 4.2 ounces)* is similar to the mask above minus the plant extracts, and the same basic review applies.

☺ **$$$ Thermal Mud Finishing Mask for Oily Skin** *($36 for 4.2 ounces)* contains way too many thickening agents that can clog pores or make skin feel oilier. This mask is not recommended.

☹ **Slim Wrap Body Cover** *($7.50 for 98 feet)* compresses the skin for an hour or two and then back to normal. Saran wrap comes cheaper than this and would work the same.

☹ **Bust Beauty Cream Daily Firming Cream** *($50 for 5.3 ounces)*. I thought I would include this and the next few products just to make the point that at any price women are willing to believe that a cosmetic can add inches in one area but take off inches in another. None of these products can come close to doing one iota of what they claim, though they are all decent moisturizers and that is helpful, but they won't erase a dimple on your thighs or a stretch mark anywhere on your body.

☹ **Cell-u-lite Cream Daily Diminishing Cream** *($56 for 5.3 ounces)* gets the same comments I make for the Bust product above.

☹ **Cell-u-lite Concentrate Diminishing Concentrate** *($112 for 12 ampoules at 0.3 ounce)* gets the same comments I make for the Bust product above.

☹ **Erase Cream Stretch Mark Prevention and Repair** *($58 for 5.3 ounces)* gets the same comments I make for the Bust product above.

☹ **Slim Body Concentrate Reducing Concentrate** *($118 for 12 at 0.3 ounce)* gets the same comments I make for the Bust product above.

☹ **Slim Body Cream Daily Reducing Cream** *($60 for 5.3 ounces)* gets the same comments I make for the Bust product above.

Natural Glow from Naturistics (Makeup Only)

This is a small line of color cosmetics found at the drugstore that boasts about their natural ingredients. Natural ingredients? I'm incredulous. How does a company with the preponderance of ingredients listed on their products such as polybutene, quaternium-22, sorbitan sesquioleate, and D&C Red No. 30 dye rationalize calling themselves natural? Most companies do rationalize this and they also rationalize that everything natural is good and wonderful for the skin, yet there are lots of natural ingredients I wouldn't want you putting on your skin (you've heard me say this before). What counts now is whether or not the Natural Glow products perform well, and indeed there are a handful of decent products, just not many. The shadows are all shiny and powdery (meaning they don't cling well), the foundations have terrible colors and poor SPFs, and the lipsticks are just passable. The strengths? The blushes are pretty and soft, the pencils are as good as any, the mascara is exceptionally thickening (though clumpy), and the brushes soft and workable. For more information about Natural Glow products call (516) 293-7070.

☹ **Natural Matte Oil-Control Liquid Makeup** *($3.16)* has a very poor selection of colors. All of them are too peach or pink to recommend. **Sheer Liquid Powder Makeup SPF 15** *($3.16)* has terrible colors and no UVA protection.

☹ **Natural Cover Concealer** *($2.61)* has only two shades, and both are too peach or pink to consider.

☹ **Natural Matte Pressed Powder** *($2.81)* does have a soft, smooth texture but you can't tell the color through the container so there is no way to know if you are getting the right color.

☺ **Sheer CheekColor Powder Blush** *($2.81)* and **Naturally Matte Powder Blush** *($2.81)* have a wonderful, though small selection of soft neutral blush colors, and the application is soft and smooth. The Sheer CheekColor does have a slight amount of shine but not enough to show.

☺ **Long Wearing Sheer Eyeshadow Plus Eyeshadow Base Duos and Trios**

($2.81) or **Singles** (without Eyeshadow Base) *($2.81)* are all shiny and fairly powdery, though the Eyeshadow Base works OK to hold eyeshadow. Some of the color combinations are nice, but these aren't the best for application.

☺ **Soft Look Eye Pencil** *($2.20)* is a standard eye pencil in a handful of decent shades that work as well as any. It has a slightly drier texture than most.

☹ **Naturally Matte Lip Color** *($3.16)* is Natural Glow's attempt at an ultra-matte finish that goes on creamy and dries to an unmovable finish. It does work; it's actually drier than most, but it also tends to easily pill and chip almost immediately after putting it on. **Longer Wear Lipcolor SPF 15** *($3.16)* has no UVA protection. It is just a fairly glossy lipstick.

☺ **Glossy Lip Balm** *($2.81)* is just what the name implies, a good emollient lip gloss. **Lip Treat Lip Balm** *($2.81)* is pretty similar to the previous one. **Natural Fruit Flavor Roll-On Gloss** *($2.81)* is a fun, very emollient, tasty gloss. **Soft Look Lip Definer** *($2.36)* is a standard eye pencil in a handful of decent shades that work as well as any. It has a slightly drier texture than most.

☺ **Soft and Full Thickening Mascara** *($2.81)* does build incredibly long, thick lashes, but unfortunately it does tend to clump, giving a slightly Tammy Faye Bakker look to the lashes. For me, I like thick and full lashes like this and don't mind working through the clumps, but this kind of look isn't for everyone.

☹ **Powder Blush** *($4.76)* and **Blush Brush** *($3.99)* are decent brushes that feel soft on the skin. They tend to be a little floppy, and so don't control the color as well as I would recommend, but these are still an inexpensive option.

Nature's Cure

Nature's Cure is a two-part acne treatment system, with supposedly homeopathic pills that are supposed to treat acne, and an acne medication cream. There is one group of pills for women and one for men; both are ☹ **Natural Homeopathic Acne Tablets** and **Acne Medication Cream** *($10.10 for 60 tablets and 1 ounce of cream)*. I can't speak to the tablets other than to say I have yet to see any research supporting the notion that plant extracts and minerals of any kind can somehow change a blemish, or why one formula would work for men versus women. I am even more puzzled that these pills include lactose, when so many people are lactose intolerant and lactose can be a source of allergic reactions. What I can review more specifically is the 5% benzoyl peroxide cream (really a gel) that can be a decent though hardly natural disinfectant for breakouts. It is only part of an acne treatment, however, because you would still need an exfoliant, gentle cleanser, and an oil-absorbing mask, but this isn't a bad option.

Neostrata (Skin Care Only)

Aquaglycolic, Murad, Alpha Hydrox, M.D. Formulations, Exuviance, Neostrata, and Avon's Anew all sell products with effective AHA concentrations and pH levels. Actually, Neostrata owns Exvuiance, with Exvuiance being the more upscale line, but only in appearance, not formulation.

What are the differences between all these AHA lines? Although the sales pitches vary, with each one waxing poetic about the quality of their particular company's AHA complex or compound, or their added vitamins or plants, the truth is that the results of all these products are the same. Well-formulated AHAs, meaning the concentration and pH are effective, provide good, consistent exfoliation that reduces the thickness of the skin's outer layer, which in turn can solve many skin problems, including dryness, blemishes, sun damage, and skin discolorations. Which product line should you choose? Good question. Alpha Hydrox, Aquaglycolic, Neostrata are the most reasonably priced of this group, but other products, such as Avon's Anew, also contain a good percentage of AHAs. Basically they are all options, and this is where your personal preference plays a major role.

Neostrata products are not all that easy to obtain; they are available mostly through physicians. Call (800) 628-9904 to find a physician in your area who carries the products, or (609) 520-0715 to find out which drugstores in your area carry the products.

☹ **Sensitive Skin AHA Facial Cleanser** *($12.95 for 4 ounces)* is a standard detergent-based, water-soluble cleanser that contains 4% AHAs. Although that isn't much, AHAs are wasted in a cleanser and can be a problem if you get the product in your eyes.

☺ **Skin Smoothing Cream** *($12.95 for 1.75 ounces)* contains 8% AHAs as well as water, several thickeners, silicone, more thickeners, and preservatives. This is a good AHA product in an ordinary but emollient moisturizing base.

☺ **Skin Smoothing Lotion** *($16.95 for 6.8 ounces)* contains 10% AHAs and is quite similar to the cream above, but in lotion form. This is a good AHA product in an ordinary base for slightly dry skin.

☹ **$$$ NeoStrata-15 AHA Body and Face Lotion** *($26.95 for 6.8 ounces)* is similar to the one above, only with a higher concentration of AHAs. I do not recommend concentrations of AHAs over 10%. The skin does not require that much exfoliation, and after all you only have so many skin cells, so the extra irritation that increased AHAs create may be damaging to skin.

☹ **$$$ NeoStrata-15 AHA Face Cream** *($25.95 for 1.75 ounces)* is similar to the one above and the same comments apply.

☺ **$$$ Polyhydroxy AHA Eye Cream** *($22.95 for 0.5 ounce)* uses the same mix of AHAs as found in the Exuviance line. This still exfoliates the skin with about an 8% concentration of AHAs in a standard moisturizing base for normal to dry skin.

☺ **$$$ Polyhydroxy AHA Ultra Moisturizing Face Cream** *($22.95 for 1.75 ounces)* is similar to the one above, and the same comments apply.

☹ **Daytime Skin Smoothing Cream, SPF 15** *($21.95 for 1.75 ounces)* doesn't contain avobenzone, zinc oxide, or titanium dioxide, and is not recommended.

☹ **Polyhydroxy Daytime Protection Cream Special Care SPF 15** *($22.95 for 1.75 ounces)* doesn't contain avobenzone, zinc oxide, or titanium dioxide, and is not recommended.

☹ **Solution for Oily and Acne Skin** *($16.50 for 4 ounces)* contains 8% AHAs as well as alcohol, slip agents, and preservatives. The alcohol is too irritating and drying for most skin types.

☹ **Gel for Age Spots and Skin Lightening** *($11 for 1.6 ounces)* is a standard 2% hydroquinone skin-lightening product that also contains 10% AHAs. This would be a good product to try on age (sun-damage) spots, except that the second item on the ingredient list is alcohol, which can be drying and irritating to most skin types.

☺ **Sensitive Skin AHA Face Cream** *($17.50 for 1.75 ounces)* contains mostly water, plant oil, thickener, AHAs, more thickeners, glycerin, silicone, and preservatives. This is a good emollient moisturizer with about 4% AHAs. It would indeed be good for someone with sensitive skin interested in trying an AHA product.

☺ **Sensitive Skin AHA Eye Cream** *($16.95 for 0.5 ounce)* is almost identical to the cream above, which means it is completely unnecessary.

☹ **AHA Lip Conditioner** *($3.95 for 0.1 ounce)* doesn't contain avobenzone, zinc oxide, or titanium dioxide, and is not recommended.

Neutrogena (Skin Care Only)

Neutrogena has been around since 1954, when that first clear amber bar of soap was manufactured. How well I remember discovering it when I was a teenager. It didn't leave quite the same soapy film as most bar soaps, and the amber color just radiated purity and a deep clean that could get rid of blemishes. I just knew that my acne would go away if I diligently washed my face with this little gem. Of course, that wasn't the case. It didn't change my acne one little bit, and it dried my skin just the way other bar soaps did. Oh well, so much for amber clarity.

Since then, Neutrogena has created a skin-care line with some products worth considering for all skin types, although the emphasis is still on women who worry about breakouts; ironically, that is where the products really are a disappointment. One major point of contention: While several of these products are promoted as being noncomedogenic and being good for acne-prone skin, many of them contain either seriously irritating ingredients or pore clogging ingredients that are at best offensive for a company to be selling these days. Neutrogena should know better. For more information about Neutrogena call (800) 421-6857.

☹ **Antiseptic Cleanser for Acne-Prone Skin Alcohol- and Fragrance-Free** *($3.78 for 4.5 ounces)* contains a large number of ingredients that are too irritating for all skin types, including camphor, peppermint oil, eucalyptus oil, and benzalkonium chloride. It's nice that it doesn't contain alcohol or fragrance, but these other things are just as irritating to the skin, if not more so. While the label directs you to avoid using the product on the eye area, as it will burn the skin there, it is likely to burn the skin anywhere on the face.

☹ **Antiseptic Cleanser Alcohol Free Sensitive Skin Formula** *($3.78 for 8 ounces)* contains the same irritating ingredients as the cleanser above, which makes the name Sensitive Skin Formula unconscionable.

☺ **Cleansing Wash for Skin Irritated by Drying Medications or Facial Peels** *($6.99 for 6 ounces)* is an ironic product, given how irritating and drying many of Neutrogena's products are for the skin. This is a standard, detergent-based, water-soluble cleanser that isn't as gentle as the name implies. It can be drying for some skin types.

☹ **Deep Clean for Normal to Oily Skin** *($5.20 for 6 ounces)* contains sodium C14-16 olefin sulfonate as the detergent cleansing agent, which is too irritating for all skin types. This product also contains BHA, and that's a waste in a cleanser both because its effectiveness is washed away and because of the risk of getting it in the eyes.

☹ **Deep Clean Cream Cleanser** *($5.18 for 6 ounces)* contains BHA, which is a waste in a cleanser both because it's effectiveness is washed away and because there's a risk of getting it in the eyes, plus this one also contains menthol, a skin irritant.

☺ **Extra Gentle Cleanser** *($6.06 for 6.7 ounces)* is indeed gentle, using one of the less irritating detergent cleansing agents. It doesn't remove makeup very well, but it can be an option for someone with dry skin.

☹ **Oil-Free Acne Wash Gentle Yet Effective Cleanser for Acne Treatment** *($6.75 for 6 ounces)* is similar to the Deep Clean cleanser above except with more BHA; this product is not recommended.

☺ **Fresh Foaming Cleanser Soap-Free Cleanser for Combination Skin** *($6 for 5.5 ounces)* is a very good detergent-based, water-soluble cleanser for most skin types.

☺ **Liquid Neutrogena Facial Cleansing Formula (Available in Fragrance or Fragrance-Free)** *($7.50 for 8 ounces)* is a fairly drying water-soluble cleanser that can thoroughly clean the face but that would be a problem for anyone with sensitive, dry, or combination skin. Even someone with oily skin may find this irritating.

☺ **Non-Drying Cleansing Lotion** *($6 for 5.5 ounces)* is an OK water-soluble cleanser for someone with dry skin, but it doesn't take off makeup all that well and tends to leave a slight film unless it's used with a washcloth (which can be quite irritating to the face).

☹ **Transparent Facial Bar Acne-Prone Skin Formula** *($2.20 for 3.5 ounces)* is a standard tallow-based bar cleanser. Tallow can clog pores and the detergent cleansing agents in here are fairly drying.

☹ **Transparent Facial Bar Dry Skin Formula** (Available in Fragrance or Fragrance-Free) *($2.20 for 3.5 ounces)* is similar to the bar cleanser above, and the same review applies.

☹ **Transparent Facial Bar Oily Skin Formula** (Available in Fragrance or Fragrance-Free) *($2.20 for 3.5 ounces)* is similar to both bar cleansers above, and the same review applies.

☹ **Transparent Facial Bar Original Formula** (Available in Fragrance or Fragrance-Free) *($2.20 for 3.5 ounces)* is similar to the bar cleansers above, and the same review applies.

☺ **Alcohol-Free Toner** *($6 for 8 ounces)* is a very good and irritant-free toner that would be quite soothing for most skin types.

☹ **Clear Pore Oil-Controlling Astringent Salicylic Acid Acne Medication** *($3.78 for 8 ounces)* would be a decent BHA toner except that it is almost 50% alcohol, and that makes it exceedingly drying and overly irritating for all skin types.

☺ **Combination Skin Moisture Oil-Free** *($9.50 for 4 ounces)* contains mostly water, silicone, thickener, glycerin, more thickeners, plasticizing agent (hair spray), water-binding agents, vitamin E, and preservatives. Supposedly this moisturizer can "put moisture in dry areas [and] take shine out of oily areas." There is no way this product can hold back its moisturizing agents for some areas and absorb oil in oily areas. Everything gets deposited all over. It's a good, standard, lightweight moisturizer for someone with normal to slightly dry skin, and that's about it.

☺ **Healthy Skin Eye Cream** *($9.46 for 0.5 ounce)* contains mostly water, thickener, glycerin, more thickeners, plant extract, vitamins, glycolic acid, anti-irritant, silicone, thickeners, and preservatives. The little bit of glycolic acid in here and the high pH make this a moisturizing cream, not an exfoliant, so it is just fine for the eye area. This isn't an exciting product, but it is a good moisturizer for someone with normal to slightly dry skin.

☺ **Healthy Skin Face Lotion Delicate Skin** *($10.10 for 2.5 ounces)* is identical to the original Healthy Skin Face Lotion in almost every way except that the Delicate Skin version contains about a 5% concentration of glycolic acid. It has a good pH which makes this an option for a more gentle AHA product that still has some effectiveness for exfoliation. It is best for someone with normal to dry skin.

☹ **Healthy Skin Face Lotion with SPF 15** *($9.46 for 2.5 ounces)* doesn't contain titanium dioxide, zinc oxide, or avobenzone, and is not recommended.

☺ **Healthy Skin Face Lotion** *($10 for 2.5 ounces)* is a decent 8% AHA moisturizer containing glycolic acid.

☺ **Healthy Skin Anti-Wrinkle Cream with Retinol** *($10.89 for 1.4 ounces)* climbs aboard the retinol bandwagon and is identical in many ways to Avon's Retinol Recovery Complex or Lauder's Diminish. It can be good as a lightweight but standard moisturizer for someone with normal to dry skin, but that's about it. There is no substantiating research indicating that retinol can behave like Retin-A.

☹ **Intensified Day Moisture SPF 15** *($10.50 for 2.25 ounces)* doesn't contain titanium dioxide, zinc oxide, or avobenzone, and is not recommended.

☺ **Intensified Eye Moisture 12-Hour Hydration** *($7.57 for 0.5 ounce)* contains mostly water, glycerin, thickener, film former, more thickeners, water-binding agents, plant extracts, anti-irritants, and preservatives. This is a good moisturizer for normal to dry skin.

☺ **Light Night Cream Won't Clog Pores** *($10.50 for 2.25 ounces)* contains mostly water, glycerin, plant oil, thickeners, petrolatum, more thickeners, silicone, and preservatives. Many of the thickeners in this moisturizer could indeed clog pores, and the oils would make the skin feel greasy. This is a good emollient moisturizer for someone with normal to dry skin, but I wouldn't call it light.

☺ **Moisture Non-Comedogenic Facial Moisturizer for Sensitive Skin** *($9.50 for 2 ounces)* contains mostly water, glycerin, thickener, silicone, petrolatum, more silicone, more thickeners, and preservatives. This is probably great for someone with dry, sensitive skin, but the thickeners could cause breakouts for someone with blemish-prone skin.

☹ **Moisture Non-Comedogenic Facial Moisturizer SPF 15 Sheer Tint** *($9.50 for 4 ounces)* doesn't contain titanium dioxide, zinc oxide, or avobenzone, and is not recommended.

☹ **Moisture Non-Comedogenic Facial Moisturizer SPF 15 Untinted** *($9.50 for 4 ounces)* doesn't contain titanium dioxide, zinc oxide, or avobenzone, and is not recommended.

☹ **Glow Sunless Tanning Lotion SPF 8 Deep Glow Non-Streaking Formula** *($9 for 4 ounces)* doesn't contain titanium dioxide, zinc oxide, or avobenzone, and is not recommended for outdoor use, but as a self-tanner it works as well as any. (By the way, all self-tanners can streak, but that has to do with application not the formulation).

☹ **Glow Sunless Tanning Lotion SPF 8 Light/Medium Natural-Looking Color Non-Streaking Formula** *($7.19 for 4 ounces)* is similar to the one above and the same comments apply.

☹ **Kids Sunblock, SPF 30** *($7 for 4 ounces)* doesn't contain titanium dioxide, zinc oxide, or avobenzone, and is not recommended.

☹ **Oil-Free Sunblock, SPF 30** *($9 for 4 ounces)* doesn't contain titanium dioxide, zinc oxide, or avobenzone, and is not recommended.

☺ **Sensitive Skin Sunblock SPF 17 No Irritating Chemical Sunscreen Ingredients** *($7.20 for 4 ounces)* is one of the few pure titanium dioxide–based sunscreens available at the drugstore. It does leave a white film on the skin, but if that doesn't bother you this is a very good sunscreen for someone with sensitive dry skin.

☹ **Sunblock SPF 30** *($5.50 for 2.25 ounces)* doesn't contain titanium dioxide, avobenzone, or zinc oxide, and is not recommended.

☹ **Sunblock Spray SPF 20** *($7.20 for 4 ounces)* doesn't contain titanium dioxide, avobenzone, or zinc oxide, and is not recommended.

☹ **Sunblock Stick, SPF 25** *($5.30 for 0.42 ounce)* doesn't contain titanium dioxide, avobenzone, or zinc oxide, and is not recommended.

☹ **Waterproof Sunblock, SPF 15** *($7.30 for 2.25 ounces)* doesn't contain titanium dioxide, avobenzone, or zinc oxide, and is not recommended.

☹ **Deep Pore Treatment** *($7 for 2 ounces)* does contain BHA, but the pH is above 5 and that means it isn't reliable as an exfoliant.

☹ **Clear Pore Treatment Nighttime Pore Clarifying Gel Salicylic Acid Acne Treatment** *($6.75 for 2 ounces)* is similar to the one above, and the same review applies.

☺ **Oil-Absorbing Acne Mask Natural Clay Mask 5% Benzoyl Peroxide** *($5.70 for 2 ounces)* contains benzoyl peroxide, and that's a great way to disinfect blemish-prone skin, but it would be far better in an irritant-free gel or liquid than in a clay mask someone only uses occasionally.

☹ **Maximum Strength Oil-Controlling Pads, Salicylic Acid Acne Medication** *($3.80 for 50 pads)* contains almost 50% alcohol, which is too irritating and drying for all skin types.

☹ **Multi-Vitamin Acne Treatment** *($5.12 for 2.5 ounces)* is a lotion with 1.5% salicylic acid along with 4% to 5% glycolic acid. That would be an interesting combination of AHA and BHA to try, given the potential effectiveness of each, but the pH is too high for this to have any exfoliating benefit for the skin. There is also no evidence anywhere that vitamins taken internally or applied externally have any effect whatsoever on acne.

☹ **Oil Absorbing Drying Gel for Oily Skin Control** *($3.50 for 0.75 ounce)* contains mostly alcohol, slip agents, and preservatives. Alcohol won't control oil, and it is definitely drying. In fact, all this product can really do is dry and irritate the skin.

☹ **On-the-Spot Acne Treatment Tinted Formula 2.5% Benzoyl Peroxide** *($6.75 for 0.75 ounce)* contains benzoyl peroxide and that's a great way to disinfect blemish-prone skin, but it would be far better in product that didn't have such a strange peach-colored tint.

☹ Lip Moisturizer, SPF 15 with PABA-free Sunblock Protection *($3.29 for 0.15 ounce)* doesn't contain titanium dioxide, avobenzone, or zinc oxide, and is not recommended.

Nivea Visage (Skin Care Only)

For more information about Nivea call (800) 233-2340.

☹ Foaming Facial Cleanser Deep-Cleansing Formula *($5.49 for 6 ounces)* is a standard detergent-based, water-soluble cleanser that can be quite drying and that contains some potentially pore-clogging ingredients.

☹ Gentle Facial Cleansing Lotion, Moisturizing Cleanser *($5.49 for 6 ounces)* is a standard mineral oil–based cleanser that doesn't rinse off very well and doesn't take off all the makeup without the aid of a washcloth, which isn't very gentle on the skin at all.

☺ Visage Hydro-Cleansing Gel *($5.07 for 5.5 ounces)* is a standard detergent-based cleanser that can be quite good for someone with normal to oily skin. It can also remove eye makeup without irritation.

☺ Alcohol Free Moisturizing Facial Toner *($5.49 for 6 ounces)* is a soothing, lightly moisturizing, fairly irritant-free toner. It contains mostly water, slip agents, several water-binding agents, preservative, and fragrance.

☺ Eye Contour Gel with Liposomes *($7.97 for 0.5 ounce)* contains mostly water, slip agents, thickener, glycerin, more slip agents, water-binding agents, and preservatives. It is a good lightweight moisturizer for normal to dry skin.

☹ Facial Nourishing Creme Essential Daily Moisturizer SPF 4 *($5.39 for 1.7 ounces)* with its low SPF 4 is an embarrassment for Nivea, plus it doesn't contain avobenzone, titanium dioxide, or zinc oxide, and is absolutely not recommended.

☹ Facial Nourishing Lotion Essential Daily Moisturizer SPF 4 *(6.39 for 3 ounces)* has the same review as the one above.

☹ New Improved Anti-Wrinkle and Firming Creme with Vitamins A and E SPF 4 *($9.39 for 1.7 ounces)* has the same review as the Facial Nourishing Creme above.

☹ Inner Beauty Daytime Renewal Treatment Natural AlpHA Complex *($10.45 for 1 ounce)* doesn't contain enough AHA or the right pH for it to work as an effective exfoliant. It is merely a good lightweight moisturizer for someone with dry skin.

☹ Inner Beauty Nighttime Renewal Creme Natural AlpHA Complex *($8.99 for 1.7 ounces)* is similar to the moisturizer above, only more emollient, and the same review applies.

☹ New Optimale Cumulative Care Creme, Multi-Vitamin and Co-Enzyme Complex SPF 6 *($9.69 for 1.7 ounces)* doesn't have enough sunscreen to make it worthwhile for day wear even though it does have a part titanium dioxide base. What a shame the SPF number is so out of line, because this product has a very good emollient base for dry skin.

☹ **New Triple Benefit Moisture Lotion, SPF 15** *($9.39 for 3 ounces)* doesn't have much going for it. It may be a decent moisturizer, but it doesn't contain avobenzone, titanium dioxide, or zinc oxide to protect against UVA damage, and is not recommended.

☹ **Optimale Eye Cumulative Care Creme, with Vitamins C, E, and Provitamin B5, SPF 6** *($7.97 for 0.5 ounce)* with its SPF 6 is a waste for your skin, plus this product doesn't contain avobenzone, titanium dioxide, or zinc oxide, and is absolutely not recommended.

☹ **Shine Control Mattifying Fluid Oil-Absorbing Moisturizer SPF 4** *($6.39 for 3 ounces)* contains several ingredients that could be problematic for someone with oily skin, and the SPF 4 is too low for anyone to consider wearing during the day.

Noevir (Skin Care Only)

When this Japanese in-home-sale, multilevel-marketed skin-care line first came to the United States, its sales representatives seemed to be more assertive than those from, say, Nu Skin or Mary Kay. That has been toned down a great deal, but some of the company's more outlandish claims continue. I was told that Noevir is special because Dr. Suzuki (creator of the Noevir product line) was "one of the few scientists with a Ph.D. in cosmetics research." Actually, the area of cosmetics research is filled with Ph.D.s from all sorts of disciplines: medical, chemical, and cosmetics research. Suzuki hardly stands alone. Another quote from the literature: "The medical profession supports Noevir's belief that products with mineral oil and other petroleum-based products are not beneficial to the skin." Well, plenty of studies indicate that mineral oil and petrolatum are just fine and quite useful for the skin, and I have never seen any studies indicating the opposite.

Another problem is that Noevir doesn't have a sunscreen as part of its daily skin-care routine. This philosophy is almost prehistoric. In addition, the brochure announces that Noevir products contain no preservatives or fragrances, even though those substances are listed in black and white on the labels.

Almost every Noevir product has an assortment of collagen, placental protein, vitamin E, spleen extract, thymus extract, umbilical extracts, DNA, plant extracts of every kind, and a host of water-binding agents. I explain in the introduction why these ingredients are a waste, but if you want to believe that a hunk of dead spleen or thymus can create healthy skin cells ("almost like a transplant," I was told), I have a bridge I'd like to sell you.

Noevir has six different product groupings and a host of specialty items that are very difficult to tell apart because many of the product names are the same. Only two categories are organized according to skin type; the others seem to be all-purpose. The main distinctions seem to be price and implied quality, because the individual products are not that different from one another. This system of product classification reminds me strongly of Shiseido, another Japanese line; I imagine Noevir began as a way to compete with Shiseido's successful department-store line.

To order products or get more information about Noevir, call (800) 437-2258 or (800) 872-8888. Don't believe anything the salespeople tell you, though, because as long as they are being trained by this company, they are not being told the truth and therefore can't give you straight information.

☺ **$$$ 003 Line (For All Skin Types) Deep Cleansing Cream** *($18 for 3.5 ounces)* is a fairly standard wipe-off cleanser that doesn't clean all that deeply, nor is it the least bit water-soluble. It can leave a film, and wiping off makeup pulls at the skin and can cause sagging.

☺ **$$$ 003 Simple Cleansing Foam** *($18 for 3.8 ounces)* is a standard detergent-based, water-soluble cleanser that can possibly leave a slight film on the skin because of the few oils that appear at the end of the ingredient list. The detergent cleansing agents are fairly strong and can dry out the skin.

☻ **003 Perfect Toning Rinse** *($18 for 4.3 ounces)* is a standard alcohol-based toner that can irritate and dry the skin. It contains its share of plant extracts, including balm mint and mistletoe; both can cause skin irritation.

☻ **003 Gentle Moisturizing Lotion** *($18 for 4.3 ounces)* is not what I would call gentle. The second ingredient in this product is alcohol, which dries out the skin and has no place in any product that claims to moisturize.

☺ **$$$ 003 Protecting Cream** *($25 for 1.2 ounces)* is a good moisturizer that contains mostly water, slip agent; thickener; plant oil; more thickeners; witch hazel (can be a skin irritant); plant extracts (including balm mint and mistletoe, which can be skin irritants); more plant oils; vitamins E, D, and A; and preservatives. The plant oils and vitamins are too far down on the ingredient list to be of any significance, and some of the plant extracts can cause problems.

☺ **$$$ 95 Herbal Cleansing Massage Cream** *($30 for 3.5 ounces)* is a fairly greasy wipe-off cleanser that is almost identical to several cleansers in this line. Massaging it around the face may feel good, but you can do that with almost any oil-based moisturizer, most of which cost a lot less. Some of the plant extracts can be skin irritants.

☺ **$$$ 95 Herbal Facial Cleanser** *($30 for 3.5 ounces)* is a standard detergent-based, water-soluble cleanser that can be somewhat drying for many skin types. Who thought up these prices?

☹ **95 Herbal Cleansing Rinse** *($20 for 5 ounces)* is a standard alcohol-based toner that also contains some water-binding agents, but they won't counteract the drying and irritating effects of the alcohol.

☹ **95 Herbal Skin Balancing Lotion** *($30 for 4 ounces)* is a standard alcohol-based toner that also contains some good water-binding agents, but they won't counteract the drying and irritating effects of the alcohol.

☹ **95 Herbal Enriched Moisturizer** *($36 for 3.3 ounces)* would be a good moisturizer for normal to dry skin types except that the second ingredient is alcohol, which has no place in a moisturizer.

☺ **$$$ 95 Herbal Skin Cream** *($40 for 1 ounce)* is a good emollient moisturizer for dry skin; it contains mostly water, slip agent, several thickeners, plant oils, several water-binding agents, placental protein (animal), plant extracts, and preservatives. One sales rep explained that using this cream would be like getting baby cells transplanted onto your skin. Nothing could be further from the truth.

☺ **$$$ Series 4 Deep Cleanser** *($30 for 3.5 ounces)* is virtually identical to many of the other wipe-off cleansers Noevir sells. Why this one has a different name is anyone's guess. Wiping off makeup is always a problem for the skin. The price is ridiculous, but that's standard for this line.

☺ **$$$ Series 4 Light Cleansing Foam** *($30 for 3.5 ounces)* is virtually identical to many of the other detergent-based, water-soluble cleansers Noevir sells. It can be drying for most skin types, and it contains tallow, which can cause breakouts, high up on the ingredient list.

☹ **Series 4 Enriched Toner** *($30 for 4 ounces)* is virtually identical to all the other alcohol-based toners Noevir sells; they all dry and irritate the skin, and are a waste of your hard-earned money.

☺ **$$$ Series 4 Protective Moisturizer** *($40 for 1 ounce)* contains mostly water, plant oil, several thickeners, more plant oil, water-binding agents, vitamin E, plant extracts, preservatives, and fragrance. This would be a good emollient moisturizer for someone with dry skin. One of the thickeners is tallow, which is high up on the ingredient list and can cause breakouts.

☺ **$$$ 105 Herbal Cleansing Massage Cream** *($70 for 3.5 ounces)* is virtually identical to many of the other wipe-off cleansers Noevir sells. Wiping off makeup is always a problem for the skin. The price is even more ridiculous than prices for the other cleansers.

☹ **105 Herbal Cleansing Rinse** *($32 for 4 ounces)* is a standard alcohol-based toner that also contains some water-binding agents, placental protein, and plant extracts, but they won't counteract the drying and irritating effects of the alcohol.

☺ **$$$ 105 Herbal Facial Cleanser** *($56 for 3.5 ounces)* is virtually identical to many of the other detergent-based, water-soluble cleansers Noevir sells. It can be drying for most skin types, and it contains tallow, which can cause breakouts. That anyone would charge (or spend) this much money for a cleanser is shocking.

☹ **105 Herbal Skin Balancing Lotion** *($62 for 4 ounces)* is virtually identical to all the other alcohol-based toners Noevir sells, with the same list of water-binding agents. Alcohol dries and irritates the skin no matter what else you put in with it. But if you are willing to waste your money on animal placenta, who am I to stop you?

☺ **$$$ 105 Herbal Enriched Moisturizer** *($70 for 2.6 ounces)* is virtually identical to the other moisturizers Noevir sells; the only real difference is that this one is even more expensive.

☺ **$$$ 105 Herbal Skin Cream** *($70 for 0.7 ounce)* is virtually identical to the other moisturizers Noevir sells; the only real difference is that this one is even more expensive. It contains tallow, which can cause breakouts, rather high up on the ingredient list.

☹ **505 Herbal Skin Balancing Lotion/Skin Lotion** *($88 for 5 ounces)* is another outrageous product. Surely there can't be anyone willing to lay out this kind of money for some alcohol and water-binding agents? Most of them sound pretty nifty, but they can't change, feed, or do much of anything else for your skin.

☹ **505 Herbal Enriched Moisturizer/Milk Lotion** *($132 for 3.3 ounces)* is insulting: it is incredibly overpriced and incredibly similar to the other moisturizers in this line, and alcohol is the third item on the ingredient list.

☺ **$$$ 505 Herbal Skin Cream** *($220 for 1 ounce)* is even more insulting than all of the other products combined. It is a good moisturizer, but so overpriced that it seems like a bad joke.

☹ **Medicated Skin Care Formula Cleansing Treatment** *($14 for 2.6 ounces)* is a fairly strong detergent cleanser that also contains salicylic acid, which should never be used near the eyes or lips because of its potential to irritate and burn mucous membranes.

☹ **Medicated Skin Care Clarifying Toner** *($14 for 2.3 ounces)* is an alcohol-based toner that also contains salicylic acid (see the previous review). This toner contains some soothing agents, but they won't help the irritation caused by the alcohol and the salicylic acid.

☹ **Medicated Skin Care Blemish Cream** *($16 for 0.7 ounce)* contains mostly water, clay, alcohol, more clay, sulfur, and preservatives. It won't get rid of acne or blackheads, and the clay and sulfur can be very drying and irritating.

☺ **$$$ Special Night Cream** *($35 for 0.7 ounce)* contains mostly thickeners, plant oils, more thickeners, fragrance, vitamin E, mink oil, and preservatives. This is a very thick, rich moisturizer for someone with very dry skin. If you are expecting a miracle from mink oil, you would want a product that contains more of it than this one does.

☺ **$$$ Eye Treatment Stick** *($30 for 0.19 ounce)* isn't much of a treatment, but it is a good lubricating emollient for dry skin.

☺ **$$$ Eye Treatment Gel** *($65 for 0.52 ounce)* contains mostly water, slip agent, water-binding agents, vitamin E, more water-binding agents, thickeners, fragrance, and preservatives. This is a good moisturizer for someone with normal to dry skin. But it's probably your head that needs treatment if you pay this kind of money for a moisturizer.

☹ **$$$ Eye Makeup Remover** *($16 for 3.3 ounces)* is a standard detergent-based wipe-off makeup remover. It does take off eye makeup, but wiping is never good for the skin.

☹ **Suspension** *($80 for 1 ounce)* contains mostly water, plant oil, glycerin, alcohol, slip agent, thickeners, water-binding agents, plant extracts, more thickeners, preservatives, and fragrance. Alcohol is fourth on the list. Need I say more? I think not.

☹ **Recovery Complex** *($45 for 1 ounce)* contains mostly water, silicone, alcohol (irritant), thickeners, slip agent, fruit extracts, more thickeners, plant oils, water-binding agents, vitamins A and E, plant extracts, and preservatives. Fruit extracts are not the same thing as AHAs, because there is no way to know exactly what has been extracted.

☹ **Advanced Moisture Concentrate** *($65 for 0.83 ounce)* contains all the trendy water-binding agents and alcohol. You already know what I'm going to say, except at these prices I feel like screaming.

☹ **Moisturizing Formula Concentrate** *($35 for 1 ounce)* is similar to the product above, and the same review applies, except that the price is slightly more tolerable.

☹ **Revitalizing Essence** *($60 for 0.24 ounce)* comes in four separate vials, which combined have a very interesting ingredient list, but alcohol comes before all of the fun stuff on the list, and it is drying and irritating for most skin types.

☹ **Night Recovery Complex** *($50 for 1 ounce)* contains all the trendy water-binding agents and alcohol. You already know what I'm going to say: "Save your money."

☹ **Ultimate Peel-Off Masque** *($35 for 2.4 ounces)* places a layer of plastic over your face; after it dries you peel it off. That can make the skin feel smooth, but this product also contains alcohol, which can dry and irritate the skin.

☹ **Clay Masque** *($23 for 3.5 ounces)* contains mostly water, glycerin, alcohol, clay, thickeners, water-binding agents, vitamin E, plant extracts, and preservatives. This line puts alcohol in almost everything. I'm getting tired of warning against it. Except for the alcohol, this could be a very good clay mask.

☺ **$$$ Sun Defense SPF 15** *($24 for 4.2 ounces)* is a good, partly nonchemical-based sunscreen. It doesn't contain any of the gimmicky ingredients all these other Noevir products do, but, ironically, it is the only one that can really protect the skin and stop wrinkles.

Noxzema (Skin Care Only)

☹   **Original Skin Cream** *($4.31 for 10 ounces)* is one of the most irritating skin-care products around. It contains lye, camphor, menthol, phenol, clove oil, and eucalyptus oil. It hurts my skin just thinking about it.

☹   **Plus Cleansing Cream** *($3.67 for 10 ounces)* is just as caustic as the cream above.

☹   **Plus Cleansing Lotion** *($3.81 for 10.5 ounces)* is just as caustic as the two above, and is not recommended for any skin type.

☺   **Sensitive Cleansing Cream** *($3.67 for 10 ounces)* just isn't a very effective cleanser, but at least they took the irritating ingredients out of this one. It can be an option to clean sensitive, dry skin, if you aren't wearing makeup.

☺   **Sensitive Cleansing Lotion** *($3.25 for 10.5 ounces)* is similar to the Sensitive Cleansing Cream above, and the same review applies.

☹   **Normal Astringent Balanced Deep Cleansing** *($3.19 for 8 ounces)* is mostly alcohol and menthol and is just pure irritation and dryness, nothing more.

☹   **Oily Astringent Salicylic Acid Acne Medication** *($3.19 for 8 ounces)* contains menthol, which is unnecessarily irritating for all skin types.

☹   **Sensitive Toner** *($3.79 for 8 ounces)* is mostly alcohol and fragrance and that would be a problem for all skin types, especially someone with sensitive skin!

☹   **2 in 1 Pads Regular Strength** *($3.67 for 90 pads)* contains a host of irritating ingredients that are damaging to skin, including camphor, menthol, and eucalyptus.

☹   **2 in 1 Pads Maximum Strength** *($3.67 for 90 pads)* is very similar to the Pads above, and the same review applies.

Nu Skin (Skin Care Only)

First I want to say how impressed I was at Nu Skin's forthcoming provision of information to the consumer about their ingredient listing. Without hesitation the company supplied all the information I requested. I wish all companies made their ingredient listings this accessible, but alas only a handful do. In direct contrast to this consumer-thoughtful assistance, the Nu Skin salespeople were so over-the-top in their presentation that I was left speechless and for me that is rare. The pressure I experienced to recruit me as a salesperson was intense. Plus, I left with the distinct impression from the salesperson that Nu Skin was busy curing cancer and AIDS and saving the rain forest at the same time.

It is far beyond the scope of this book to investigate every claim this company makes for their products, but at least as far as skin care is concerned I can assure you Nu Skin is not a miracle, a cure, the total answer, or even part of the answer for every woman's skin-care needs. Nevertheless, the people who sell this line want you to believe it can alter your life as well as your skin. Like all of the other lines I've reviewed, this one contains some very good products, some useless ones, and some that are simply overpriced and a waste of money.

What sets Nu Skin apart is its intense direct-marketing strategy and its problems with the law. According to the March 1992 issue of *Drug and Cosmetic Industry* magazine, Nu Skin International has responded to complaints and lawsuits in Ohio, Illinois, Michigan, Florida, and Pennsylvania by voluntarily consenting to change some of its marketing and sales policies. One of the problems was that sales reps, in order to keep their commission percentage up, would overbuy cosmetics and then be stuck with them. After signing agreements with the attorney generals' offices in these states, Nu Skin was supposed to refund up to 90 percent of the money its distributors paid for products that went unsold. According to another report in the October 1997 issue of *Cosmetic Dermatology*, Nu Skin International agreed to pay a $1.5 million civil penalty to settle Federal Trade Commission (FTC) charges over claims it made for some of its products. "The FTC alleged that Nu Skin could not produce adequate substantiation for the claims, and that Nu Skin violated a 1994 FTC order requiring the firm to have competent and reliable scientific evidence to support benefit claims for any product they sell." But when you have Christy Brinkley as your new spokesperson, who cares about shoddy business practices?

When it comes to claims. Nu Skin's brochures state that their products have "All of the good and none of the bad," but that depends on how you define "bad." The products contain peppermint oil, spearmint oil, witch hazel extract, grapefruit extract, camphor, sulfur, sulfuric acid, and fragrance, all of which are very irritating and known skin sensitizers. I would consider those not just bad, but very bad.

The skin care presentation I received for the Nu Skin skin-care products was one of the most peculiar I've experienced anywhere. For example a Clinique toner was set on fire and then compared to the Nu Skin toner that would not light. Of course the reason the Clinique toner was flammable is because it contains alcohol and the Nu Skin one did not ignite because it didn't contain alcohol. But there are lots of skin-care products besides Nu Skin that don't contain alcohol and also aren't flammable. Regardless, flammability doesn't indicate irritation potential anyway. Paper is flammable but it isn't irritating. Camphor doesn't ignite but it is definitely irritating and shows up in one of Nu Skin's products. I was also shown a pH demonstration indicating that the pH of most bar soaps and cleansers, including expensive ones, was over 8, and most were over 9, but that Nu Skin's bar cleanser was about a pH of 5.5. High pH is definitely a problem for drying and irritating skin. So Nu Skin's bar cleanser is definitely less irritating when it comes to pH, but there are factors besides pH that can cause irritation. The cleansing agent in Nu Skin's bar cleanser is sodium cocoyl isethionate and that can be irritating. Additionally, the ingredients that keep

Nu Skin's bar in its bar form can clog pores. I could go on, but this was about as misleading a demonstration as I've seen anywhere in the cosmetics industry.

Another difficulty is that this product line includes almost every gimmick in the book. Some are good for the skin, but most are just for show, to cover all the necessary bases of "natural" skin care: royal bee jelly, human placenta extract, aloe vera, vitamins, wheat germ oil, walnut husks, collagen, jojoba oil, and herbal extracts. As you may have already guessed, the first ingredients—the primary components of the products—are fairly standard ones, such as water, thickeners, water-binding agents, and plant oils.

There are some good products in the line, but they are not the miracles the company would like you to believe they are. For more information about Nu Skin call (800) 345-1000.

☺ **Cleansing Lotion** *($10.50 for 4.2 ounces)* contains mostly water, aloe, thickener, and oils. It needs to be wiped off and can leave a greasy feeling on the skin. Wiping off makeup pulls at the skin, which can cause sagging.

☺ **Facial Cleansing Bar** *($10.30 for 3.5 ounces)* is a standard detergent-based bar cleanser. It can be drying for most skin types.

☺ $$$ **Nu Color Eye Makeup Remover** *($13.15 for 2 ounces)* is a silicone- and plant oil–based wipe-off cleanser that can leave a greasy feel. It will remove makeup, but wiping off makeup is always a problem for skin.

☹ **Clarifex pH Scrub Acne Medication Cleansing Scrub** *($13.30 for 2.65 ounces)* contains too many irritating ingredients, including sulfur, sulfuric acid (yes, sulfuric acid), and salicylic acid, to make it an option for any skin type. Irritation hurts the skin's healing process.

☺ $$$ **Exfoliant Scrub Extra Gentle** *($11.95 for 2.5 ounces)* contains mostly water, aloe, glycerin, seashells (as an abrasive), and thickeners. The sea shells can be rough on the skin, so calling this product gentle is a stretch.

☺ **Facial Scrub** *($11.45 for 2.5 ounces)* is by far more gentle than the one above, despite the name difference. This one uses walnut-shell powder that does work as a scrub, and it can be good for someone with normal to dry skin.

☹ **MHA Revitalizing Toner** *($10.30 for 4.2 ounces)* could be considered an option for a lightweight AHA and BHA toner except that it contains camphor, which makes it unnecessarily irritating for all skin types.

☹ **pH Balance Facial Toner** *($8.45 for 4.2 ounces)* contains mostly, water, aloe, witch hazel (a skin irritant), glycerin, slip agent, water-binding agents, camphor, and preservatives. The witch hazel and camphor cause irritation, making this toner a problem for all skin types.

☺ $$$ **MHA Revitalizing Lotion** *($18 for 1 ounce)* is supposed to be a combination AHA and BHA lotion; thankfully, this one doesn't have a low enough pH to make it an effective exfoliant. If this product could exfoliate the skin, and you used it along with the other AHA and BHA combination products in the MHA grouping, you would have a seriously irritated face.

☹ **MHA Revitalizing Lotion with SPF 15** *($19.95 for 1 ounce)* doesn't contain avobenzone, titanium dioxide, and zinc oxide, and is not recommended.

☺ **$$$ Celltrex Skin Hydrating Fluid** *($26.75 for 0.5 ounce)* is a lightweight moisturizer for normal to dry skin that contains mostly water, aloe, slip agent, water-binding agents, thickener, vitamin E, and preservatives. The collagen in this product won't affect the collagen in your skin.

☺ **$$$ Enhancer Skin Conditioning Gel** *($9.15 for 2.5 ounces)* is a lightweight gel that contains mostly water, aloe, slip agents, glycerin, water-binding agents, soothing agent, fragrance, and preservatives. These ingredients can nicely retain moisture in the skin, but they won't heal anything. The amounts of RNA and royal jelly are too minute to talk about, but at any amount they are strictly gimmicks and offer nothing for the skin.

☺ **$$$ HPX Hydrating Gel** *($49.95 for 1.5 ounces)* contains mostly water, plant oil, slip agent, human placental protein (whose idea was this?), vitamin E, water-binding agent, and preservatives. The placenta doesn't deserve comment, and the rest just makes this a good moisturizer for normal to slightly dry or combination skin.

☺ **$$$ Ideal Eyes Vitamins C&A Eye Refining Creme** *($28.60 for 0.5 ounce)* is a vitamin C wannabe. It does contain vitamin C, some thickeners, vitamins, and water-binding agents, which make it a good moisturizer, but it won't heal skin or cause wrinkles to disappear.

☺ **$$$ Intensive Eye Complex Moisturizing Cream** *($40 for 0.75 ounce)* contains mostly water, aloe, thickeners, plant oils, water-binding agents, vitamins, soothing agent, and preservatives. For the most part this is a very good moisturizer for dry skin that is exceedingly overpriced, but one of the ingredients is sulfur, and that can be too irritating for many skin types.

☺ **$$$ NaPCA Moisture Mist** *($19.80 for 8.4 ounces)* is a lightweight toner of water, slip agent, and water-binding agents. It would be good for most skin types. It does contain about 1% lactic acid, but at that percentage it is a water-binding agent, not an exfoliant.

☺ **$$$ NaPCA Moisturizer** *($19.80 for 2.5 ounces)* is a good lightweight moisturizer for normal to dry skin that does contain sodium (Na) pca, which is just one of many good water-binding agents; it's not the best, nor essential, just good. This product also contains water, slip agent, water-binding agents, vitamins, thickeners, fragrance, and preservatives.

☺ **$$$ Rejuvenating Cream** *($28.45 for 2.5 ounces)* won't rejuvenate the skin, although it can be a good moisturizer for normal to dry skin. It contains mostly water, aloe, slip agent, several thickeners, vitamins, water-binding agents, and preservatives. You're supposed to believe that the tiny amounts of royal jelly, algae, and RNA can rejuvenate your skin; they can't, and there are so little of them in this cream that it's almost silly.

☺ $$$ **Sunright 15 Maximum Protection Sunscreen** *($17.15 for 3.4 ounces)* is a good in-part titanium dioxide–based sunscreen that can be good for someone with dry skin.

☺ $$$ **Sunright 23 Face and Hands Ultimate Sunscreen Protection** *($13.85 for 4 ounces)* is similar to the one above and the same review applies.

☺ $$$ **Sunright 28 Ultimate Sunscreen Protection** *($17.45 for 3.4 ounces)* is similar to the sunscreens above, and the same comments apply.

☺ $$$ **Sunright Lip Balm 15** *($5.65 for 0.25 ounce)* is a very emollient lip balm that is a very good in-part titanium dioxide–based sunscreen.

☹ **Sunright Spray 10** *($20.75 for 4.2 ounces)* doesn't contain avobenzone, titanium dioxide, or zinc oxide, and is not recommended.

☺ $$$ **Sunright Prime Pre and Post Sun Moisturizer** *($16.10 for 5 ounces)* is just a good lightweight moisturizer for dry skin. It has no sunscreen, so you would never apply it before going outside in the sun.

☺ $$$ **Sunright Tan Sunless Tanning Lotion** *($17 for 3.4 ounces)* is a standard dihydroxyacetone-based self-tanner that would work as well as any, though there are far cheaper and as-effective versions at the drugstore.

☹ **Clarifex pH Mud Acne Treatment Mud** *($13.30 for 5 ounces)* is basically just clay and sulfur. It can be drying and irritating for most skin types.

☺ $$$ **Clay Pack** *($13.60 for 2.5 ounces)* is a standard clay mask that contains mostly water, standard water-binding agents, clay, thickeners, and preservatives. Again, the vitamins and royal bee jelly are at the end of the ingredient list, meaning you get only a tiny amount. Besides the clay, this product contains no other irritants or drying agents, so it could be a fairly gentle clay mask, or at least as gentle as clay can be on the skin.

☹ **Face Lift with Activator Original Formula** and **Sensitive Skin Formula** *($33.30 for 2.6 ounces of the Face Lift Powder and 4.2 ounces of the Activator)* is really two separate items you mix together to get the results implied by the name. Basically, the Face Lift Powder is egg white, cornstarch (a possible irritant), and silica (sand). The Activator contains water, benzethonium chloride (a possible skin irritant), aloe vera, soothing agent, and water-binding agent. The Activator swells and irritates the skin, and the egg white and cornstarch in the Face Lift Powder temporarily dry it in place, which supposedly makes it look smoother. It doesn't, at least not for long. Irritation around the eyes can be a problem and might cause more wrinkles.

☺ **$$$ Interim MHA Diminishing Gel** *($18.40 for 1 ounce)* is just water, slip agents, film-former, water-binding agents, silicone, and preservatives. This is a good lightweight moisturizer for someone with normal to slightly dry skin.

☹ **$$$ Skin Brightening Complex** *($17.80 for 0.5 ounce)* uses licorice extract and kojic acid to lighten the skin, but without hydroquinone I am not convinced that research shows these ingredients are effective by themselves (particularly the licorice extract). Still, at this amount it wouldn't last more than a few days if you were to use it anywhere but on your face. If you do want to give this product a try anyway, please keep in mind that skin lighteners only work in conjunction with a sunscreen.

Dr. Obagi (Skin Care Only)

I've written about the controversy surrounding Dr. Obagi and his skin-care products before. I finally found time to review a few of his products and discuss my thoughts with several dermatologists, and the findings make for some interesting, though debatable, reading. For those of you who aren't familiar with Dr. Zein E. Obagi, he is a dermatologist who created his own skin-care line, to be used in conjunction with his Blue Peel and a prescription for Retin-A. His anti-aging program took off as dermatologists and plastic surgeons alike started to sell his skin-care products and perform his Blue Peel. The Obagi Nu-Derm products are as far from being "dermatologic" as you can imagine, and are considered quite controversial among dermatologists. For the most part, there is nothing in these products that cannot be found elsewhere for far less money. In contrast, the Blue Peel is completely different and can be used only by dermatologists.

Dr. Obagi's Blue Peel is a standard trichloroacetic acid (TCA) peel that has been performed by dermatologists and plastic surgeons for years. TCA is used for peeling the face, neck, hands, and other exposed areas of the body. It causes fewer pigment problems than other doctor-only peels such as phenol, and is considered excellent for "spot" peeling of specific areas. It can be used for medium or light peeling, depending on the concentration and method of application. AHA and BHA peels are considered light peels, and are often done in a series of six. TCA peels are best for fine lines and can be somewhat more effective on deeper wrinkling, but are performed only once every couple of years. Many of the dermatologists I spoke to feel a TCA peel is a viable option for many skin types, despite consumers' fascination with AHA peels. But Obagi doesn't like AHA or BHA peels for most any reason, though he doesn't really explain why.

As for the Obagi products, they are sold exclusively through dermatologists' offices and are given the marketing affectation of being "prescribed" by the doctor. But except for the 4% hydroquinone products in this line, these items are strictly cosmetic and not prescription in the least. There are many reasons why a woman should see a dermatologist. As Obagi states in his brochure, a professionally applied peel, Retin-A, and an effective skin-lightening product can be the best game plan for reducing the effects of sun damage. The rest of the products, however, are just cosmetics—and are no better or worse than other products being sold today in an array of venues. Obagi's customer service number is (800) 636-SKIN.

☺ $$$ **Nu-Derm, Cleanser I** *($24 for 8 ounces)* isn't all that gentle, but it is gentler than Nu-Derm Cleanser II. This could be a good detergent-based cleanser for someone with normal to oily skin.

☹ **Nu-Derm Cleanser II** *($24 for 8 ounces)* is supposed to remove dead skin cells, impurities, and excess oils without damaging the skin's moisture content. Given that the detergent cleansing agent (the third ingredient after the water content) is TEA-lauryl sulfate, one of the most notorious skin irritants in cosmetics, the chances are it will not only hurt the skin's moisture content but also hurt the skin. This product is not recommended.

☺ $$$ **Nu-Derm Toner I** *($24 for 8 ounces)* is supposed to restore the skin's natural pH balance, which shouldn't be necessary if the Obagi cleanser didn't damage or change it. However, this is a good irritant-free toner for most skin types, similar to the one below but minus the irritants.

☹ **Nu-Derm Toner II** *($24 for 8 ounces)* is supposed to restore the skin's natural pH balance, which shouldn't be necessary if the Obagi cleanser didn't damage or change it. The toner contains mostly water, aloe, slip agent, detergent cleansing agent, soothing agent, water-binding agent, plant extracts, fragrance, and menthol. If it weren't for the witch hazel, arnica, and menthol, this could be a decent toner, but these three ingredients add unnecessary irritation without any benefit whatsoever for the skin.

☺ $$$ **Nu-Derm, Clear I** *($60 for 2 ounces)* is the same as the Clear II below, but in a moisturizing base and without the SLS.

☹ **Nu-Derm Clear II** *($64 for 2 ounces)* contains 4% hydroquinone. This type of product is a standard way to treat darkened, sun-damaged areas of the face if a 2% hydroquinone product doesn't work. However, I am concerned that the second ingredient in this product is sodium lauryl sulfate (SLS), a fairly potent skin irritant. Why anyone would want to add more potential irritation to an already irritating product is anyone's guess, but it makes this an unacceptable formulation. Other, less expensive 4% hydroquinone products are available without SLS. Also, using 4% hydroquinone can produce either hyperpigmentation (darker areas) or hypopigmentation (lighter patches of skin).

☺ $$$ Nu-Derm Exfoderm *($60 for 2 ounces)* is a well-formulated AHA product.

☹ **Nu-Derm Sunfader I** *($50 for 2 ounces)* is a standard 2% hydroquinone product that also contains a sunscreen with SPF 20. That is an intriguing concept:

mixing a skin-lightening agent with sunscreen. However, this sunscreen doesn't contain titanium dioxide, zinc oxide, or avobenzone, and therefore provides inadequate protection. Also, lots of 2% hydroquinone products are available for a lot less money than this one.

☹ **Nu-Derm Sunfader II** *($50 for 2 ounces)* is basically identical to the product above, but with 4% hydroquinone and an SPF of 15. The same basic review applies, except that 4% hydroquinone can cause pigmentation problems.

☺ **$$$ Nu-Derm Tolereen** *($40 for 2 ounces)* is a 0.5% hydrocortisone moisturizer. There are many reasons to use a product that contains hydrocortisone. Minor irritations, skin rashes, allergic reactions, dermatitis, and some inflammations can be calmed quite effectively with an over-the-counter hydrocortisone lotion or cream. For years I have been recommending Lanacort and Cortaid, both found in the drugstore at a 1% strength for less than $5 an ounce, to deal with minor skin problems. Lanacort and Cortaid work so well that most irritations and rashes are eliminated in a day or two with just a few applications. Charging $40 for the same thing at half the strength is unconscionable. Keep in mind that hydrocortisone is for sporadic, infrequent usage only. The base shouldn't make that much difference, because you will be using it only for a short time.

☺ **$$$ Nu-Derm Action** *($30 for 2 ounces)* is a standard emollient moisturizer that can be good for dry skin.

☺ **$$$ Nu-Derm Action Plus** *($30 for 2 ounces)* is a standard emollient moisturizer that can be good for dry skin.

☺ **$$$ Nu-Derm Eye Cream** *($50 for 1 ounce)* is a standard emollient moisturizer that can be good for dry skin, but it is incredibly overpriced.

Oil of Olay (Skin Care Only)

"Oil Olay" (or "Oil of Ulay" in parts of Canada) must be a very convincing name, because the line's popularity remains strong. For the longest time I wondered if people really thought it was some kind of oil derived from an exotic plant. It's not a very exciting line, lacking any state-of-the-art moisturizing ingredients, interesting water-binding agents, or plant oils; in fact, many of these formulations are so boring they are hard for me to recommend, but for a basic moisturizer they aren't bad.

The three new products in the Oil of Olay Age Defying series all contain salicylic acid (beta hydroxy acid, or BHA) and are not all that new. They are really a reintroduction and slight revamping of the Oil of Olay Visible Recovery series, which also contained salicylic acid but was pulled from the market by Procter & Gamble in February 1995 because of numerous complaints regarding irritation. Using some secret change in formulation, Oil of Olay claims it has eliminated the irritation problem. Maybe, but in the long run, as is true with any exfoliant, that depends on your skin type. Much as the AHAs are, BHA is effective as an exfoliant only in a low pH base. For BHA, the preferred pH is around 3, with a concentration of 1% to 2%. That's fairly acidic, and can be quite irritating to the skin, but it is what makes the BHA work.

Strangely, enough despite the research accompanying the press release for these products substantiating the pH of 3, only two of this line's Age Defying products have a pH of 3, while the sunscreen has a pH of 6, which makes it incapable of exfoliation. Also, there is no information on the label about percentages. Moreover, I only recommend BHA for someone with blemish-prone skin, because BHA can penetrate into a pore. (Someone with sun-damaged skin doesn't need that kind of penetration.) To that end, these BHA products are in emollient bases inappropriate for someone with blemish-prone skin.

ProVital is a line of skin-care products Oil of Olay is aiming at "mature" women. Grouping women of a certain age into one grand, indefinite bunch euphemistically called mature is insulting. I've said this more times than I can count: age does not determine skin type. There are 50-, 60-, and 70-year-old women with all sorts of skin conditions ranging from breakouts, whiteheads, oily skin, and rosacea to sun damage and blackheads; dry skin is not the only skin type for older women and they should not all be using the same products. For more information about Oil of Olay call (800) 285-5170.

☹ **Daily Renewal Cleanser Age Defying Series with Gentle Microbeads and Beta Hydroxy Complex** *($4.60 for 6.78 ounces)* is a standard detergent-based water-soluble cleanser that also contains salicylic acid. There is no reason to risk splashing salicylic acid into the eyes, and any exfoliation potential is rinsed off and washed down the drain.

☺ **Facial Cleansing Lotion** *($3.87 for 6.78 ounces)* is a lightweight cleanser that doesn't quite rinse off without the aid of a washcloth; it can leave a residue on the skin, but it could be OK for someone with dry skin.

☺ **Foaming Face Wash** *($3.87 for 6.78 ounces)* is a standard detergent-based, water-soluble cleanser that cleans the face well and can be good for most skin types.

☺ **Sensitive Skin Foaming Face Wash** *($3.87 for 6.78 ounces)* is similar to the one above and the same review applies.

☹ **Refreshing Toner** *($3.35 for 7.2 ounces)* contains mostly alcohol and is not recommended.

☺ **Daily Renewal Cream Age Defying Series Beta Hydroxy Complex** *($8.91 for 2 ounces)* contains mostly water, thickener, glycerin, BHA, more thickeners, vitamin E, silicone, more thickeners, fragrance, and preservatives. It isn't an exciting formula, but it does have a good pH to make it a good exfoliator, although the amount of salicylic acid is a mystery. If you are interested in trying a BHA product instead of an AHA, this is a reasonable one to consider, though only for someone with normal to dry skin.

☹ **Daily UV Protectant Beauty Fluid Daily Care Series Moisture Replenishment Lotion SPF 15** *($7.99 for 6 ounces)* doesn't contain avobenzone, zinc oxide, or titanium dioxide, and is not recommended.

☹ **Daily UV Protectant Cream Daily Care Series SPF 15** *($15.76 for 2 ounces)* doesn't contain avobenzone, zinc oxide, or titanium dioxide, and is not recommended.

☹ **Sensitive Skin Daily UV Protectant Beauty Fluid SPF 15** *($6.58 for 4 ounces)* doesn't contain avobenzone, zinc oxide, or titanium dioxide, and is not recommended.

☺ **Moisture Replenishing Cream Daily Care Series** *($5.76 for 2 ounces)* contains mostly water, glycerin, thickener, petrolatum, silicones, more thickeners, and preservatives. It is a good, but very ordinary, moisturizer for someone with dry skin.

☺ **Night of Olay Night Care Cream** *($5.76 for 2 ounces)* contains mostly water, glycerin, thickeners, silicone, more thickeners, more silicone, and preservatives. This is a good, but extremely ordinary, moisturizer for normal to dry skin.

☺ **Oil-Free Beauty Fluid Daily Care Series** *($7.99 for 6 ounces)* contains mostly water, glycerin, thickeners, silicone, more thickeners, and preservatives. This is an ordinary moisturizer that contains more thickeners than anything else, but it can be good for dry skin.

☺ **Oil-Free Replenishing Cream, Daily Care Series** *($5.76 for 2 ounces)* contains mostly water, glycerin, thickener, silicone, more thickener, more silicone, fragrance, and preservatives. It won't replenish anything, and the thickening agents can clog pores, but it is a good, albeit extremely ordinary, moisturizer for normal to dry skin.

☺ **Original Beauty Fluid, Moisture Replenishment Lotion** *($7.99 for 4 ounces)* is a very ordinary moisturizer that contains only water, mineral oil, and thickeners. There is nothing beautiful about this one, but it can be good for dry skin.

☹ **Age Defying Series Protective Renewal Lotion Beta Hydroxy Complex SPF 15** *($8.91 for 4 ounces)* does not contain avobenzone, titanium dioxide, or zinc oxide, and is not recommended.

☹ **Revitalizing Eye Gel Age Defying Series** *($8.91 for 0.5 ounce)* contains witch hazel as the second ingredient, which is too irritating for any part of the face, and especially the eye area.

☺ **Sensitive Skin Beauty Fluid** *($6.58 for 4 ounces)* contains mostly water, thickeners, glycerin, mineral oil, petrolatum, silicone, and more thickeners. This would be good for dry skin, but it is such a dated, boring formula.

☺ **Sensitive Skin Replenishing Cream Daily Care Series** *($5.76 for 2 ounces)* is similar to the one above, only somewhat more emollient, and the same review applies.

☺ **ProVital Perfecting Moisturizer Lightly Tinted Cream** *($8.99 for 1.7 ounces)* is a one-tint product which just can't translate to a variety of different skin tones. It is a good, though ordinary, emollient moisturizer for skin, but that's about it.

☺ **ProVital Night Cream** *($8.99 for 2 ounces)* is similar to the one above only without the tint and slightly less emollient.

☹ **ProVital Protective Moisture Lotion SPF 15** *($8.99 for 4 ounces)* doesn't contains avobenzone, zinc oxide, or titanium dioxide, and is not recommended.

Ombrelle (Sun Care Only)

The world of sunscreens has changed dramatically over the past two years. Information about UVA protection versus UVB protection has completely changed what we need to consider when buying sunscreens. In the section on sunscreens in Chapter Two I discuss at length why certain UVA ingredients are essential when considering which sunscreen to buy. Ombrelle is a small line of sunscreen products that includes avobenzone as one of its active ingredients. That makes these products a great option for daily sun protection. For more information about Ombrelle call (800) 582-8225.

☺ **Ombrelle Spray Mist SPF 15** *($10 for 4 ounces)* is a great sunscreen for both UVA and UVB protection. Unfortunately, it is in an alcohol base, and that can be drying and irritating for the skin when used on a regular basis.

☺ **Ombrelle Sunscreen Lotion SPF 15** *($10 for 4 ounces)* is a great sunscreen for both UVA and UVB protection in a standard, lightweight, moisturizing base. It would be good for someone with normal to slightly dry skin.

☺ **Ombrelle Sunscreen Lotion SPF 30** *($10 for 4 ounces)* is similar to the lotion above only with a higher SPF.

Organic Essentials from Linda Chae
(Skin Care Only)

Organic Essentials boasts that Linda Chae, the creator of the line, is a leading skin nutritionist. I have never run across her name in any of the interviews and research I've done on various issues concerning antioxidants, plant extracts, and vitamins, and I've seen no published research from her. However, I am very skeptical when someone refers to themselves as an expert in skin care and doesn't offer a reliable sunscreen as part of their daily skin-care routine. I can't say this enough: any skin-care routine that doesn't include a sunscreen is leaving your face unprotected against the major cause of skin damage.

Having said all that, I'm afraid Linda Chae's products are very difficult to review. On one hand they are incredibly simple, once you get through the cornucopia of flowers, trees, fruits, and vegetables on the ingredient lists—but the lists themselves are mind-boggling. Several standard cosmetic ingredients can be found in the midst of all the vegetation, but the hope and hype built into natural botanical mayhem and vitamin overkill are impossible for me to decipher. Every plant and vitamin is accompanied by seven or eight claims about rejuvenating, fighting wrinkles, firming the skin, reducing stress, fending off free-radical damage, increasing circulation, and on and on. If you took the claims seriously, you would think that using just one product should bring you perfect health not to mention perfect skin. I've discussed at length the lack of evidence about natural ingredients and their benefit for skin, but clearly women can't get enough of them despite the lack of evidence that they provide benefits, because practically everyone is sticking whole farms and forests in their products.

Here is the best I can provide in terms of evaluating these products; the belief in plants is up to you. According to my research, many of the plants in these products, including grapefruit, lavender oil, geranium oil, peppermint, jojoba oil (can cause breakouts), and many other flowers, weeds, trees, fruits, and vegetables, can be problematic for the skin. For more information about Organic Essentials, call (800) 882-7240.

☺ **$$$ Clarifying Facial Cleanser** *($15 for 4.2 ounces)* contains lots of plant extracts, several thickening agents, emollients, standard detergent cleansing agents, plant oils, and preservative. Many of the plant oils can be possible sensitizers, but basically this is just a good water-soluble cleanser.

☹ **Gentle Cleansing Pads** *($14 for 80 pads)* is similar to the cleanser above only you have to wipe at the face to clean the skin, and that pulling can cause the skin to sag.

☺ **$$$ Herbal Exfoliating Scrub** *($22.50 for 2.5 ounces)* contains lots of plant extracts, thickeners, ground-up walnuts, emollients, water-binding agents, plant oils, and preservative. This standard scrub (remember the days of honey and almond pits?) isn't the least bit energizing, but it is a good old-fashioned exfoliant for someone with dry skin.

☹ **Energizer Purifying Gel** *($22.50 for 4 ounces)* contains mostly plant water, glycerin, more plant extracts, plant oils, vitamins, water-binding agents, and preservative. The tingle you feel when applying this product is from the peppermint and orange oil, which can irritate the skin.

☺ **$$$ Sheer Moisture Lotion** *($31 for 1.7 ounces)* contains mostly aloe, plant water, lots of plant extracts, glycerin, thickeners, silicone oil, water-binding agents, more plant extracts, plant oils (mostly fragrant), vitamins, and preservatives. It is supposed to be an effective defense against daily environmental stresses. Without a sunscreen, it can't combat environmental stress during the day. At night it can be a very good moisturizer for someone with normal to dry skin.

☺ **$$$ Rich Moisture Cream** *($35.50 for 1.7 ounces)* is similar to the lotion above but in cream form, and the same review applies.

Origins

Estee Lauder started off the 1990s with a new cosmetics line called Origins, and what a concept it has! A quote from one of the brochures sums it up quite nicely: "Origins marries the forces of nature with the vigor of modern science to make provocative differences in the way you experience cosmetics." To put it in my own words, "Origins uses all of the current fads on the market to create one of the most gimmicky makeup and skin-care collections around." The brochures, like most of the packaging, are made of recycled paper. The ad copy is loaded with exotic-sounding botanicals, herbs, and oils. References to ancient Egyptian and Roman know-how are frequent. No other department-store line makes a more persuasive case for the glory of natural products (except maybe Clarins, but only maybe). Origins even sells sensory-therapy oils and gels that are "thousands of years old." Of course, the oils and gels aren't that old, but the idea is that whoever was around thousands of years ago and used these concoctions must have known what they were doing.

While the skin care leaves me somewhat unexcited, I am very impressed with the color presentation at the Origins counter. The lipsticks, eyeshadows, blushes, and lip pencils are all divided into three color groupings: Peach to Rust, Beige to Tan, and Ivory to Pink. All of the colors have minimal or no shine, and most are soft and muted and therefore extremely easy to use. The textures are wonderful, and the application is almost flawless. Although I like the eyeshadows, be aware that a few have some shine; many of the salespeople insisted that all the colors are matte, but they are not. The amount of flower extract in many of the Origins products is also cause for concern. If you have any hay fever-type allergies, these extracts will cause you problems. "Natural" ingredients are not necessarily the best for all skin types.

Origins (like Aveda and The Body Shop) offers skin-care systems based on every fad in the book and then some, including botanicals, essential oils, recycled packaging (including a recycling service at its counters for the empty bottles and compacts), products that aren't tested on animals, "ancient" skin-care treatments, anti-stress formulas, and aromatherapy. The recycling efforts and animal-free testing are praiseworthy examples. However, the ancient and natural stuff is the real bait that hooks women. The ingredients are so obscure that it's difficult, even for me, to see beyond the plants and herbs. Even the salespeople I interviewed didn't know "what all those herbs were about." As you might expect, juxtaposed around the "special" oils and herb extracts are standard skin-care ingredients. Also, many of the "good" ingredients are at the far end of the ingredient lists, meaning they are practically nonexistent.

Origins' basic skin-care theory is that all skin wants to act normal, the way it did when we were young. As we grow up, our skin gets confused or behaves badly, not because it wants to, but because it lacks something. If skin is supplied with the correct plants and oils, according to Origins, "nature's memory" can "retrain" your skin to function the way all skin wants to function—normally. What an enticing concept. Of course, the ingredients that supposedly retrain your skin are derived from the "ancient science of essential oils," which assumes that people who lived long ago had great skin because of this special knowledge. It does sound convincing, but, alas, there aren't any ancient people around to prove or disprove those claims. Moreover, you can't retrain the skin; that claim sounds like something the FDA should take a closer look at. But I have to admit that this is one of the most creative skin-care ploys I've ever seen, and that is saying a lot.

In order to review this line without writing an entire book about it, I have summarized most of the plant extracts (which are little more than plant tea) by listing them as just that: plant extracts or plant water. Keep in mind that once a plant has been put in a cosmetic and preserved, it has little, if any, benefit, regardless of whether it had any in the first place. Having said all that, I still think Origins offers some good products; you just have to read between the lines to find out what they are. For more information about Origins call (800) 723-7310.

Origins Skin Care

☹ **Cream Bar** *(9.50 for 5.2 ounces)* is a standard bar cleanser with fairly drying detergent cleansing agents, but this one also contains some very irritating and sensitizing plant extracts, including clove, wintergreen, and spruce needles.

☹ **Liquid Crystal Extra Gentle Cleanser** *($14 for 6.7 ounces)* contains mostly thickeners and plant oils; it can leave a greasy film on the face, and you have to use a lot of cleanser to remove all your makeup without the aid of a washcloth.

☹ **Mint Wash** *($14 for 6.7 ounces)* includes mint, a skin irritant, as are the spearmint, orange zest, and lemon peel in this product. This cleanser can burn the eyes and irritate the skin, and is not recommended.

☹ **Pure Cream Rinseable Cleanser You Can Also Tissue Off** *($14 for 6.7 ounces)* contains peppermint, lime, and tangerine oils, which can burn the eyes and are skin irritants.

☺ **Well-Off Fast and Gentle Eye Makeup Remover** *($11 for 3.4 ounces)* is a standard detergent-based eye makeup remover. It works, but there is nothing particularly gentle about it.

☹ **Never A Dull Moment Age Erasing Skin Polisher with Fruit Enzymes** *($22.50 for 3.5 ounces)* has a great name, but it's an ordinary product. It contains mostly plant extracts, slip agents, thickeners, plant extracts, walnut shells, more thickeners, papain (an enzyme) and preservatives. I've written before about the problems of enzymes in cosmetics: they just aren't stable enough or mild enough (they don't have the water-binding properties of AHAs) to exfoliate the skin very well, if at all. Plus there are several ingredients in this product that pose a definite concern about irritation, including eucalyptus, mint, grapefruit, pine, and mango.

☺ **Swept Away Gentle Slougher for All Skins** *($15 for 3.4 ounces)* is a fairly gritty exfoliant that also contains peppermint and grapefruit, both useless as skincare ingredients, but that can irritate and hurt skin.

☹ **Swept Clean Special Sloughing for Oily-Acting Skin** *($15 for 3.4 ounces)* is almost identical to the one above except for the addition of menthol, which only makes it more irritating for the skin.

☺ **Comforting Solution If Your Skin Acts Sensitive** *($17 for 5.7 ounces)* is supposed to help sensitive skin defend itself against the environment. It can't protect against the environment; however, it is a soothing toner of sorts that contains aloe vera, plant oils, soothing agent, vitamin E, water-binding agent, and preservatives. This product contains far too many potentially sensitizing ingredients to be considered reliable for someone with sensitive skin.

☺ **Drenching Solution** *($17 for 5 ounces)* contains mostly plant water, aloe, plant oils, water-binding agent, plant extract, thickener, vitamin E, preservative, more thickeners, and preservatives. It is a good toner of sorts, but it won't teach skin to retain water, and several of the plant extracts in here are potential skin sensitizers.

☹ **Managing Solution** *($17 for 5 ounces)* is a toner that is supposed to normalize oil production, but its ingredients—plant water, essential oil, aloe vera, vitamin E, slip agents, and preservatives—won't change oil production. Actually, the oil content and irritating ingredients (including peppermint and lemon) are a problem for all skin types.

☹ **Mending Solution** *($17 for 5 ounces)* is almost identical to the product above, only this one is supposed to energize the skin's "look-young systems." No one's skin has "look-young systems." But isn't it amazing that such similar products are supposed to do such disparate things for the skin?

☺ **Sprinkler System** *($13.50 for 6.7 ounces)* is a great name for a rather standard toner that contains mostly plant water, slip agent, detergent agent, minerals, essentials oils (fragrance), and preservatives. It's OK for someone with normal to slightly dry skin, but the plants in here, including coriander and cinnamon, can be problematic for some skin types.

☹ **Tuning Solution** *($17 for 5 ounces)* is supposed to rebalance the oily and dry areas of your face. It doesn't contain anything capable of doing that, but it does contain lemon and eucalyptus, among other extracts that can be irritating for the skin.

☹ **Starting Over** *($22.50 for 1 ounce)* is supposed to improve cell renewal, and while the sugarcane extract is supposed to make you think you are getting an AHA product you aren't. Even if you were, there isn't enough of the extract at the right pH for this moisturizer to work as an exfoliant.

☺ $$$ **Constant Comforter** *($22 for 1.7 ounces)* contains mostly plant water; slip agent; thickener; plant oils; several thickeners; plant extract; anti-irritant; vitamins; water-binding agent; more plant oils, and preservatives. This is a good emollient moisturizer for normal to dry skin, but it won't calm anything; in fact, many of the plant oils are potential skin sensitizers.

☺ $$$ **Eye Doctor** *($25 for 0.5 ounce)* is similar to the Constant Comforter above and the same basic review applies.

☹ **Fine Tuner If Your Skin Acts Confused** *($22 for 1.7 ounces)* is supposed to even out combination skin. None of its ingredients can change oily skin, although some of them can make oily skin feel oilier, including plant oils and shea butter, both of which can be a problem for someone with any amount of oily skin.

☺ $$$ **Line Chaser Stop Sign for Lines** *($25 for 0.5 ounce)* can't stop wrinkles, but it is a good lightweight moisturizer for normal to slightly dry skin. It contains mostly plant water, thickeners, slip agent, water-binding agents, vitamins, and preservatives.

☺ $$$ **Night-A-Mins** *($27.50 for 1.7 ounces)* is named and packaged to look like oral vitamins. Night-A-Mins definitely contain a group of vitamins, but as you now know, they are more gimmicky than effective and not the least bit nutritious for the skin. This product contains mostly fossilized water (meaning water with minerals, but all water contains minerals), silicones, thickeners, slip agents, vitamin C, B vitamins, water-binding agents, plant oil, plant extracts, more thickeners, and preservatives. This would be a good moisturizer for someone with normal to dry skin, but that's about it.

☹ **Oil Manager If Your Skin Acts Oily** *($22 for 1.7 ounces)* contains nothing that can stop oil or close pores. It does contain some plant oils, as well as thickening agents that can clog pores, which would be a problem for someone with oily skin. What was Origins thinking?

☺ $$$ **Steady Drencher If Your Skin Acts Dry** *($22 for 1.7 ounces)* is a good emollient moisturizer for someone with dry skin. It contains mostly plant water, plant oils, aloe, slip agent, several thickeners, more plant oil, vitamins A and E, anti-irritants, more vitamins, plant oils, water-binding agents, and preservatives.

☺ $$$ **Time Mender** *($22 for 1.7 ounces)* contains mostly plant water, thickener, slip agent, more thickeners, anti-irritant, more thickeners, vitamin E, silicone, preservatives, and a long list of plant oils. This is a very good moisturizer for dry skin. The company claims that this product can firm the skin, but all the plant oils and water-binding agents in the world can't do that.

☺ $$$ **Urgent Moisture** *($25 for 1.7 ounces)* contains mostly plant water, glycerin, thickeners, slip agent, water-binding agents, more thickeners, silicone, and preservatives. This is a good lightweight moisturizer for normal to dry skin. It is supposed to perform best in super-dry weather, but it doesn't contain enough emollients to protect the skin from serious dehydration.

☺ **Let the Sunshine SPF 14** *($13.50 for 5 ounces)* is one of the better titanium dioxide–based sunscreens on the market.

☺ **$$$ Silent Treatment Instant UV Face Protector SPF 15** *($15 for 1.7 ounces)* is a nonchemical (titanium dioxide–based) sunscreen suspended in a silicone base. It is a great idea, but it can leave a slightly white cast on the skin. I was very concerned to see that this product contains lavender oil, which can cause photosensitivity (if you go out in the sun wearing lavender oil, you can get an allergic reaction). Given the frequency of application needed to protect the skin adequately (including the chest and the back of the hands), this is a pricey little sunscreen.

☺ **Summer Vacation: The Natural-Looking Self Tanner** *($17.50 for 5 ounces)*, like all self-tanners, uses dihydroxyacetone to turn the skin brown. This works as well as any of them.

☹ **Clear Improvement Active Charcoal Mask to Clear Pores** *($16.50 for 3.4 ounces)* is a standard clay mask that contains mostly plant water, clay, slip agent, thickeners, standard water-binding agent, charcoal, more thickeners, and preservatives. The charcoal is supposed to lift impurities out of the pores, but it can't do that; also, there is hardly any charcoal in this product. Otherwise, this is an OK clay mask.

☺ **Drink Up 10 Minute Moisture Mask** *($17.50 for 3.4 ounces)* contains mostly plant water, thickeners, plant oil, slip agents, more thickeners, essential oils (fragrance), algae, more plant oils, and preservatives. It definitely contains oils and should feel nice as a mask if you have dry skin, but no more so than applying a regular moisturizer over the skin and letting it stay in place for ten minutes.

☹ **$$$ No Puffery** *($20 for 0.64 ounce)* claims it can release trapped fluids and toxins from the skin, but that is not possible. It contains mostly plant water, slip agent, water-binding agent, plant extracts, and preservatives.

☹ **Out of Trouble** *($17.50 for 3.4 ounces)* is meant to be a way to solve blemishes and blackheads. I wish it could, but this formulation is what's in trouble. It contains mostly water, thickeners, zinc oxide, titanium dioxide, more thickeners, camphor, BHA, sulfur, and clay. Zinc oxide and titanium dioxide can clog pores and cause breakouts, camphor and sulfur can cause irritation and redness, and there isn't enough BHA at the right pH to have an impact on exfoliating the skin.

☹ **Spot Remover to Clear Up Acne Blemishes** *($10 for 0.3 ounce)* is a standard salicylic acid and alcohol solution. Without the alcohol this product may have been an option.

☹ **Zero Oil Instant Matte Finish for Shiny Places** *($10 for 0.64 ounce)* cannot stop oil production, but it can absorb some amount of oil. It contains mostly plant water, sodium magnesium silicate (which can absorb oil, the way talc or magnesium can), camphor (which can be a skin irritant), slip agents, and preservatives. This is pretty much a modified version of Phillips' Milk of Magnesia, which can do the same sort of thing, only better. There is no reason to use camphor on skin.

☹ **Lip Remedy** *($10 for 0.17 ounce)* isn't much of a remedy. This lip product contains a long list of thickeners, plant oil, more thickeners, and preservatives. It also contains menthol and camphor, which are more irritants than anything else. There are better emollient lip balms available that can help smooth dry lips.

☺ **$$$ Mind Your Mouth** *($6.50 for 0.15 ounce)* is a very emollient, standard lip gloss. It doesn't contain sunscreen, but it is very good for dry lips any time of year, as long as it isn't daytime.

Origins Makeup

☺ <u>FOUNDATION:</u> **Original Skin** is the clever name for Origins' foundations, although it is hardly accurate. This stuff doesn't look like original skin, it looks like foundation—a nice foundation, but foundation nevertheless. The salesperson told me Original Skin would make my skin look like a baby's bottom and let it breathe the way it does without foundation. Although I thought Original Skin was pretty good, it did not make my skin look like a baby's bottom, nor was the product less opaque than other foundations. It also did not hide tiny lines (foundation almost always makes lines look more prominent, and this one is no exception). Don't expect anything unique in terms of ingredients, either; besides some plant extracts and a small amount of plant oils, this is just a good standard foundation. Please note that the names of the foundations reviewed below are perfectly accurate. Also, all of the foundations below are best for normal to oily skin (the salespeople will tell you that all skin types can use them, but they are not very emollient or moisturizing).

☺ **Some Coverage** *($14.50)* is almost watery, like a liquid, but it goes on sheer and blends more evenly than you would expect. **These shades are good to excellent:** Paperwhite, Ivory, Linen, Tawny (may turn slightly peach), Fair, Flax (may turn slightly rose), Tan, Amber (may turn slightly ash), Copper (may be too orange for some skin types), Bronze (may be too orange for some skin types), Sepia, and Mahogany. **These shades are too pink, orange, peach, rose, or ash for most skin types:** Porcelain, Blushing, Beige, Rosy, Golden, and Sable.

☺ **More Coverage** *($14.50)* provides just that: more coverage than the Some Coverage foundation above. **These shades are good to excellent:** Ivory, Linen, Paperwhite, Blushing (can turn pink), Fair, Flax (can turn pink), Tan (can turn orange), Sable, Copper (can turn peach), Amber (can turn ash), Sepia, Bronze, Mahogany, and Tawny (can turn peach). **These shades are too pink, orange, peach, rose, or ash for most skin types:** Porcelain, Rosy, and Golden.

☺ **Most Coverage** *($14.50)* ups the coverage another notch and is fairly opaque. These shades are good to excellent: Ivory, Linen, Paperwhite, Blushing (can turn pink), Fair, Flax (can turn pink), Tan (can turn orange), Sable, Copper (can turn peach), Amber (can turn ash), Sepia, Bronze, Mahogany, and Tawny (can turn peach). These shades are too pink, orange, peach, rose, or ash for most skin types: Porcelain, Rosy, and Golden.

☹ <u>CONCEALER:</u> **Original Skin Concealer** *($10)* has a smooth, light texture, and some OK colors, but all of the shades are shiny, which isn't best for under the eye when it comes to smoothing out lines or helping the area to look even with the foundation (unless your foundation is shiny). This is a definite problem waiting to happen.

☺ <u>POWDER:</u> **Original Skin Pressed Powder** *($13.50 for the powder refill and $4 for the compact)* and **Original Skin Loose Powder** *($16)* are soft and sheer powders. All of the colors are beautifully neutral and natural.

☺ <u>BLUSH:</u> **Brush-On Color** *($11 blush refill, $4 compact)* tends to go on a bit dry, but it is very attractive and would work well for someone with normal to oily or combination skin. **All 15 colors are superb. Pinch Your Cheeks** *($10)* is a tiny tube of liquid blush that tints the cheek. It is best for someone with smooth, flawless skin that is neither oily nor dry. That limits who can use it, but it is a good cheek tint. **Slip Cover Comfortable Cover for Cheeks** *($12)* is a good, fairly easy-to-apply cream blush that comes in three somewhat shiny shades. They are an option for someone with smooth, even skin and a knack for blending color with the fingers or a sponge.

☺ <u>EYESHADOW:</u> Origins has a superb array of matte **Eye Accent Eyeshadows** *($11)*. Most of the colors in this line are wonderfully neutral or earth-toned, and worth a try. One small warning: Not all of these colors are matte; a very few have a small amount of shine, but not enough to show up on the skin.

☺ **Kohl Mine** *($9.50)* is a fat eye pencil that goes on creamy and dries to a powder. It is an interesting way to apply one color, but difficult to blend over the eye with other shades. I prefer powders, but this is a fun option; however, pencils are always tricky to keep sharpened. **Slip Cover Comfortable Cover for Eyes** *($10)* are just creamy eyeshadows that are hard to blend unless you have the knack for this style of eyeshadow application; it is not one I recommend. The color selection, though small, is lovely, and if you like this kind of product it's worth a closer look.

☺ <u>EYE AND BROW SHAPER:</u> The very standard **Eye Pencils** *($11)* come in great colors, although the selection is limited. **Kohl Mine** *($9.50)* are very tiny amounts of creamy crayons that dry to a matte finish and can be used as eyeliners or eyeshadows. They tend to crease, so be wary of the thickness of the application. The **Brow Pencil** *($11)* has a smooth finish but is a very standard pencil. **Just Browsing** *($11)* is a brow color that you apply like mascara. This is a great way to make brows look full and filled in. **All four shades are good. Brow Fix** *($11)* is just a clear hair spray–like mascara that helps keep brows in place without adding color.

☺ <u>**LIPSTICK AND LIP PENCIL:**</u> **Lip Color** *($11)* is very glossy, and the color won't survive to your midmorning break. If you have a problem with lipstick bleeding into the lines around your mouth, you'll feel this lipstick traveling the second you put it on. **Lip Gloss** *($10)* is a standard tube gloss. **Slip Cover Comfortable Cover for Lips** *($11)* is just good old-fashioned lip gloss with a cute name. **Lip Pencil** *($11)* is a standard but good pencil that comes in a very flattering array of colors.

☺ **Origins Pick-Up-Sticks—Sheer, Matte, and Shimmer** *($12)* is a cute dual-function, stocky pencil that is supposed to be a lip liner and lipstick in one. It is awfully cute, and the marketing sales pitch makes them sound convenient, but they aren't. They are hard to sharpen and the lipstick part is just an OK lipstick. The Matte isn't all that matte, but rather creamy, the Sheer is just a gloss finish, and the Shimmer is shiny.

☺ <u>**MASCARA:**</u> **Underwear for Lashes** *($11)* is a gimmicky, completely unnecessary undercoating for the lashes that you apply before the mascara. The claim is that it helps the lashes grab more mascara. A good mascara should suffice; this is a wasted extra layer on fragile lashes.

☺ **Fringe Benefits Mascara** *($11)* is a good mascara that builds evenly and doesn't smear.

☺ **$$$** <u>**BRUSHES:**</u> Origins' brushes *($15 to $50)* are not only beautiful, but also relatively inexpensive, at least compared with those being sold at the neighboring counters, and they are 100% synthetic, something none of the other cosmetics lines at the department store have, and that is a strong point! The brushes range from $15 for eyeshadow brushes to $50 for a long-handled powder brush (I use Maybelline's $3 powder brush; it works great, and I've had it for over two years now—just thought you'd want to know). The blush and powder brushes are really too big and floppy for most faces, and the eyeliner brush is fairly thick and wouldn't work well to create a precise line, but there are good options among the other sizes, depending on what you are adept at using.

Orlane

Attracting a wealthy clientele and convincing them that what they're buying is the absolute best isn't an easy task because the issue isn't money. Women who buy Orlane products aren't wondering whether they can afford the $500- to $1,000-plus it costs to take care of their skin the Orlane way; they just want to be assured that what they're getting is the best of the best, regardless of cost. Orlane's slick, sapphire blue packaging with silver letters is stunning. Its opulent, elegant appearance communicates prestige. But there has to be more to skin care than brilliant packaging, right? How does Orlane seduce a woman into believing its cosmetic chemists know something no one else does?

Orlane's pitch is that a Nobel laureate created "anagesium," one of the ingredients in its Anagenese line of products. Now, *that* is a great angle. Of course, I haven't received any information on who the person is or was, or what the research revealed. But it definitely sounds good.

Orlane says that anagesium is a combination of proteins that are supposed to provide some outstanding benefit to the skin. However, the ingredient lists reveal the truth: there are no unique proteins, or unique anything, in any of the Orlane products. Every product contains standard ingredients just like those used by the rest of the industry. Most of Orlane's products contain proteins and amino acids, which can help keep water in the skin, but they are not the only ingredients that can do that, and Orlane is not the only cosmetics company using them.

Maybe I shouldn't say that all of Orlane's ingredients are standard. Two hard-to-miss components are brain and spleen extract. What the consumer is supposed to swallow (no pun intended) is that a hunk of dead cow brain or spleen can have some rejuvenating effect on the skin. La Prairie makes the same body-parts ingredient claims, but there is no evidence or research to support this contention.

All of Orlane's brochures feature gushing phrases such as "optimum functioning of the epidermis," "natural molecules called Oxytoners," and "creates the proper environment for the skin." It all sounds so impressive—until you take a closer look and notice that the claims just don't jibe with the accurate information on the ingredient list. No facts, no actual research, no proof is given in anything I've read from the company. It is all hyperbole. Charts for Orlane's Anagenese Total Time Fighting Care proclaim that it has produced a 52 percent reduction in wrinkles. But nowhere are there details of how that study was done, how many women were in it, what age group was tested, whether the study was double-blind, and who measured the before-and-after results. A 52 percent reduction might appeal to your emotions and hopes, but without more data it's a meaningless number.

It is hard for me to imagine that a woman could sincerely believe that spending this kind of money on skin-care products will prevent wrinkles or aging skin or make her skin more beautiful. Women who can afford the so-called best products still have to get face-lifts and eye tucks. But believe these claims they do—Orlane's sales are not hurting.

To be fair, and I always try to be, the line does have several creams and lotions that have a wonderfully silky texture. Orlane has one of the largest selection of skin-care products of any line I've ever reviewed. As I mentioned, most Orlane products contain fancy water-binding ingredients in the form of proteins and amino acids, and although they aren't unusual, they are indeed interesting. Proteins work primarily by staying on top of the skin and preventing dehydration, while amino acids are better able to penetrate the skin and protect against moisture loss a little more deeply. That's about it, though. Do I think that translates into some extraordinary benefit for the skin? No. But they do feel nice and can keep the skin moist. Orlane is principally a skin-care line; its makeup line is rather ordinary and almost inconsequential. For more information about Orlane call (800) 775-2541.

Orlane Skin Care

☺ **$$$ B21 Bio-Energic Cleansing Preparation Care for Face** *($40 for 6.8 ounces)* is a standard mineral oil–based wipe-off cleanser. It is shockingly standard given the price tag. Pulling at the skin by wiping off makeup, even at this price, can sag the skin and still leave a greasy film on the skin.

☺ **$$$ B21 Oligo Vit-A-Min, Vitalizing Cleanser for Dry or Sensitive Skin Types** *(32.50 for 8.4 ounces)* is similar to the one above only slightly less greasy. It does have a host of water-binding agents and vitamins, but they come well after the preservative and hardly amount to anything.

☺ **$$$ Hydralane Moisturizing Cleanser, Continuous Hydro-Active System** *($25 for 13.3 ounces)* is a mix of thickening agents and silicones. It is a standard wipe-off cleanser that can leave a film behind on the skin.

☺ **$$$ Normalane Foam Cleansing Gel for Mixed and Oily Skins** *($25 for 4.2 ounces)* is a very standard detergent-based cleanser that can be good for someone with oily skin.

☹ **Blue Line Eye Makeup Remover** *($19.50 for 2.5 ounces)* is a standard detergent-based wipe-off cleanser, except the second ingredient is witch hazel, and that can be unnecessarily irritating.

☹ **Blue Line Gentle Exfoliating Cream for All Skins** *($28 for 2.5 ounces)* uses synthetic particles (polyvinyl chloride) in a detergent cleanser with lots of thickening agents. It's an OK, standard scrub, but the scrub particles can be irritating.

☹ **Treatment Creme Very Gentle Exfoliating Cream** *($28 for 1.6 ounces)* is similar to the one above, and the same review applies.

☺ **$$$ B21 Bio-Energic Lotion Vivifiante Preparation for Face Care** *($40 for 6.8 ounces)* is a good irritant-free toner with slip agents and water-binding agents, but for $40, yikes!

☺ **$$$ B21 Bio-Energic Vivifying Lotion for All Skins** *($40 for 6.8 ounces)* contains mostly water, slip agent, water-binding agents, fragrance, and preservatives. This would be a good nonirritating toner for most skin types. The serum protein in this is just a fancy name for a standard water-binding agent.

☹ **Blue Line Purifying Lotion for Combination and Oily Skin** *($29 for 6.8 ounces)* is a salicylic acid-based toner. The pH is too high for the salicylic acid to work as an exfoliant.

☺ **$$$ Blue Line Soothing Lotion Alcohol-Free for Dry or Sensitive Skin** *($29 for 6.8 ounces)* contains mostly water, water-binding agents, detergent cleansing agents, and preservatives. This isn't the best for sensitive skin, but it is a good irritant-free toner.

☺ **$$$ Hydralane Moisturizing Toner, Continuous Hydro-Active System** *($25 for 13.3 ounces)* contains mostly water, slip agents, witch hazel, water-binding agents, more slip agents, and preservatives. The witch hazel can be a skin irritant, but the other standard ingredients are good for the skin and nonirritating.

☹ **Normalane Astringent Soothing Lotion for Mixed and Oily Skins** *($25 for 6.8 ounces)* contains mint and a form of phenol, and both are too irritating for all skin types. It is supposed to be a salicylic acid–based lotion, but the pH isn't low enough for it to work as an exfoliant.

☹ **Extrait Vitale Multi-Active Revitalizer with Apple Alpha-Acids** *($70 for 1.7 ounces)* contains apple extract, which is unrelated to AHA. It also contains cornstarch, which can be a skin irritant.

☺ **$$$ Anagenese Eye Contour Cream Total Time Fighting Care for All Skins** *($40 for 0.5 ounce)* contains mostly water, thickeners, plant oil, vitamins, silicone, and preservatives. It also contains something called hirudinea extract, which is an extract obtained from leeches. How that is supposed to benefit skin no one at Orlane could tell me. This is a good, though very standard moisturizer for dry skin.

☺ **$$$ Anagenese Total Time Fighting Serum** *($52.50 for 1.7 ounces)* contains mostly water, lots of thickeners, silicones, plant oils, preservatives, vitamins, and water-binding agents. This standard lightweight moisturizer is good for someone with normal to slightly dry skin.

☺ **$$$ B21 Bio-Energic Absolute Skin Recovery Care** *($130 for 1.7 ounces)* contains mostly water, silicone, several thickeners (one is cornstarch, which can be a skin irritant), water-binding agents, plant oil, plant extracts, fragrance, and preservatives. This can be a good moisturizer for someone with dry skin if the price doesn't get your first.

☺ **$$$ B21 Absolute Skin Recovery Care Eye Contour** *($75 for 0.5 ounce)* is a Vaseline-based moisturizer that also contains mineral oil, thickeners (including cornstarch, which can be an irritant), plant oils, water-binding agents, and preservatives. This is a very good but fairly ordinary moisturizer for dry skin.

☺ **$$$ B21 Bio-Energic Absolute Youth Cream Age Defense-Protective Oxytoning Care** *($130 for 1.7 ounces)* is a boring group of thickeners, silicone, preservatives, and a few water-binding agents. The tiny bit of yeast extract in here wouldn't raise a crumb or provide your skin with "Oxytoning." This is a good but standard moisturizer.

☹ **B21 Bio-Energic Absolute Youth Concentrate Age Defense Protective Oxytoning System** *($300 for 0.7 ounce)*. Excuse me, I fell off my chair. But now that I've regained my composure, let me tell you what your $4,800 a pound (that's what this stuff prices out to) will get you: mostly water, thickeners, water-binding agents, castor oil, polystyrene (like the stuff used to make plastic cups), some vitamins, cow blood, and preservatives. There is no reason to recommend this product for any skin type.

☺ **$$$ B21 Bio-Energic Anti-Fatigue Recovery Care** *($130 for 1.7 ounces)* contains mostly water, silicone, lots of thickeners, water-binding agents, and preservatives. There's also some of the leech extract in here. Basically, this is just a lightweight moisturizer for slightly dry skin.

☺ **$$$ B21 Bio-Energic Anti-Fatigue Recovery Care Eye Contour** *($75 for 0.5 ounce)* is a mineral oil–based moisturizer with thickeners, petrolatum, water-binding agents, spleen extract, and preservatives. The spleen extract is useless, but this is a good basic moisturizer for dry skin.

☺ **$$$ B21 Bio-Energic Intensive Nurturing Care Nightly Concentrate for Dry and Very Dry Skin** *($110 for 1.7 ounces)* is similar to the one above, except instead of spleen extract the gimmick here is royal bee jelly. Regardless, the same basic review applies.

☺ **$$$ B21 Bio-Energic Morning Recovery Concentrate** *($60 for 1 ounce)* is a lightweight lotion that contains mostly water, water-binding agents (in part from a protein extracted from cow blood and calfskin), plant extracts, and preservatives. It's a good, albeit strange, moisturizer for normal to minimally dry skin, though I suspect you're supposed to believe more miraculous things about this combination of ingredients.

☺ **$$$ B21 Bio-Energic Points Vulnerable Creme for All Skins** *($70 for 1 ounce)* contains mostly water, thickeners, slip agents, silicones, water-binding agents, and preservatives. This is a good, standard moisturizer for dry skin.

☺ **$$$ B21 Bio-Energic Protective and Moisturizing Base** *($75 for 1.7 ounces)* is a mineral oil–based moisturizer with thickeners, slip agents, preservatives, and water-binding agents. It's a good basic moisturizer for dry skin.

☺ **$$$ B21 Bio-Energic Protective Oxytoning System for All Skin Types** *($300 for 0.7 ounce)* contains mostly water, thickeners, water-binding agents, vitamins, and some yeast. The yeast won't provide oxygen to the skin, nor will the cow extract help anything, but this is a good moisturizer for normal to dry skin.

☺ **$$$ B21 Bio-Energic Ultra-Light Cream for the Day** *($75 for 1.7 ounces)* contains mostly water, slip agent, thickeners, aloe, spleen extract, more thickeners, water-binding agents, more thickeners, silicones, and preservatives. This is a good, average moisturizer for someone with normal to dry skin.

☺ $$$ **B21 Bio-Energic Super Moisturizing Concentrate Day and Night** *($95 for 1.7 ounces)* contains lots of thickeners, some water-binding agents, and preservatives. It's a good though exceptionally ordinary moisturizer for dry skin.

☹ **B21 Oligo Eye Balm for Sensitive, Fragile and Allergic Skin Types** *($40 for 0.68 ounce)* is a confusing group of ingredients that includes several waxes and talc. Talc can be irritating for the skin and isn't helpful for dry skin.

☺ $$$ **B21 Oligo Gentle Soothing Cream for Sensitive Fragile & Allergic Skin Types** *($63 for 1.7 ounces)* contains mostly water, thickeners, Vaseline, plant oil, silicone, water-binding agents, preservatives, and some vitamins. This is a good though standard moisturizer for dry skin.

☺ $$$ **B21 Oligo Light Smoothing Cream** *($63 for 1.7 ounces)* is similar to the one above, and the same review applies.

☺ $$$ **B21 Oligo Vit-A-Min Vitalizing Lotion for Dry and Sensitive Skin Types** *($32.50 for 8.4 ounces)* contains mostly water, slip agents, water-binding agents, and some minerals. This is a good lightweight lotion for normal to slightly dry skin.

☺ $$$ **Extrait Vital Biological Cream for Dry and Very Dry Skins** *($60 for 1.7 ounces)* contains mostly water, plant oil, slip agent, thickeners, plant extract, plant oils, more thickeners, spleen extract, water-binding agents, and preservatives. This is a good emollient moisturizer for someone with dry skin, but the minuscule amounts of spleen extract and proteins aren't enough to make a difference on the skin, even if they were somehow useful, which they aren't.

☺ $$$ **Extrait Vital Biological Emulsion** *($45 for 1.3 ounces)* contains mostly water, slip agents, thickeners, mineral oil, thickener, water-binding agents, plant oil, more thickeners, and preservatives. This is a good emollient moisturizer for someone with dry skin.

☺ $$$ **Extrait Vital Eye Contour Serum** *($42 for 0.33 ounce)* contains water, slip agent, water-binding agent, thickener, calfskin, spleen extract, more thickeners, several water-binding agents (including a tiny amount of lactic acid, but not enough to make this an AHA product), more thickeners, and preservatives. This is a very good emollient moisturizer for someone with dry skin. I don't have to discuss the spleen or calfskin extract, right?

☺ $$$ **Hydralane Eye Contour Moisture Care** *($35 for 0.5 ounce)* contains mostly water, thickeners, silicone, water-binding agents, and preservatives. This is a good moisturizer for dry skin.

☺ $$$ **Hydro-Climat Moisture Shell Multiprotective Fluid** *($48 for 1.7 ounces)* contains mostly water, silicone, thickeners, mineral oil, water-binding agents, and preservatives. This is a good lightweight moisturizer for dry skin.

☺ **Normalane Correcting Gel, Mixed and Oily Skins** *($22.50 for 0.5 ounce)* is mostly water, water-binding agents, and detergent cleansing agent. It can be quite irritating for the skin to leave detergent cleansing agent on the skin.

☹ **Normalane Night Balancing Gel** *($30 for 1 ounce)* contains several irritating ingredients that should not be left on the skin, including a detergent cleansing agent and balm mint.

☺ **$$$ Nutrilane Total Nutrition System for Dry or Delicate Skin** *($45 for 1.7 ounces)* contains mostly water, several thickeners, slip agent, water-binding agent, plant oil, several more thickeners, silicone, and preservatives. Nothing in here is even vaguely nutritional, and the gimmicky ingredients, yeast and DNA, are at the end of the list.

☹ **Claircilane Whitening Formula Hydro Whitening Creme for All Types** *($75 for 1.7 ounces)* doesn't contain hydroquinone or kojic acid, which means it can't lighten skin.

☹ **Claircilane Hydro Whitening Masque for All Skins** *($55 for 1.7 ounces)* is similar to the one above and the same comments apply.

☹ **Claircilane Hydro Whitening Serum for All Skins** *($100 for 1 ounce)* is similar to the one above and the same comments apply.

☺ **$$$ After Sun Creme for Face** *($30 for 1.7 ounce)* is just a good standard moisturizer for dry skin. It contains mostly water, thickeners, silicone, plant oils, water-binding agents, and preservatives.

☹ **After Sun Moisture Balm** *($25 for 4.2 ounces)* contains too much alcohol to be recommended.

☹ **B21 Sol-Energic Serum Soleil Visage Energizing System Before and After Sun** *($120 for 1 ounce)* is supposed to encourage protection from the sun while you tan, which is not humanly possible, and completely disingenuous.

☺ **$$$ Creme Solaire Total Block Sun Cream For the Face 30+ UVA 11** *($30 for 1.7 ounces)* is a very good in-part titanium dioxide– and zinc oxide–based sunscreen for someone with dry skin.

☺ **$$$ Creme Solaire Vulnerable Points Sun Cream 30 Ultra Protection** *($19.50 for 1.7 ounces)* is similar to the one above, and the same review applies.

☹ **Self-Tanning Moisture Balm SPF 4** *($25 for 4.2 ounces)* not only has a terrible SPF, this product doesn't contain avobenzone, zinc oxide, or titanium dioxide, and is absolutely not recommended.

☺ **$$$ B21 Bio-Energic Hydro-Energizing Masque for All Skins** *($55 for 1.7 ounces)* contains mostly water, thickeners, slip agent, silicone, plant oil, water-binding agents, and preservatives. There are lots of ingredients in here that would be problematic for someone with oily or combination skin, though it can be a good mask for dry skin.

☹ **Normalane Balancing Mask for Mixed and Oily Skins** *($35 for 1.7 ounces)* is a standard clay mask with some thickeners and water-binding agents. Some of these thickeners can be problematic for someone with oily skin.

☹ **Treatment Blue Mask for Combination and Oily Skins** *($26.50 for 2.5 ounces)* is a standard clay mask with several thickening agents that can cause breakouts.

☺ **$$$ Treatment Rose Mask for Dry and Very Dry Skins** *($26.50 for 2.5 ounces)* is a Vaseline-based clay mask with lanolin, mineral oil, and thickeners. I'm concerned about the menthol in here, which can be irritating for all skin types, but the other ingredients are fairly emollient for dry skin.

☹ **Progressive Tanning Cream SPF 6 for Fair Skin** *($20 for 4.2 ounces)* encourages tanning, even with its low SPF, so this product is like a cancer specialist offering you cigarettes. It is just an unethical thing for a skin-care line selling all sorts of antiwrinkle creams to do.

☹ **Safe Tanning Cream SPF 10 Maximum Protection for Sensitive Skin** *($20 for 4.2 ounces)* has an SPF 10, which is hardly maximum protection, and while this one does contain zinc oxide as part of the sunscreen protection, with so many good SPF 15s on the market why bother with it?

☺ **$$$ Safe Tanning Cream SPF 18 Ultra Sun Protection for Delicate Skin** *($20 for 4.2 ounces)* is a good in-part zinc oxide sunscreen with a great SPF number. However the notion that this one is for delicate skin doesn't prove out; it is just a good moisturizing base for normal to dry skin.

☺ **$$$ Vulnerable Skin Sun Cream 25 Ultra Protection for Children & Fragile Skin** *($25 for 4.2 ounces)* is a good in-part zinc oxide sunscreen with a great SPF number. However, this product contains padimate O, a close relative of PABA, which is considered a fairly irritating sunscreen ingredient.

Orlane Makeup

☹ **FOUNDATION:** **B21 Teint Absolu Foundation** *($50)* contains spleen extract, which is supposed to explain its price tag. It does have a good soft texture, but it also has an extremely poor selection of six colors. **These colors are OK:** Perle and Dore. **The other colors are too peach, ash, or pink for many skin tones.**

☺ **$$$ Satilane** *($35)* is a matte foundation with a great light finish, and **all of the colors are great**, although there are only five to choose from.

☹ **Creme to Powder Foundation** *($40)* is a standard cream-to-powder foundation that goes on very sheer and comes in six colors. It would be an option if the colors were more neutral. **These colors should be avoided:** Extra Rose and Extra Dore, which can turn peach, and Extra Blanc, which is extra-white and looks ghostly.

☹ **CONCEALER:** **Conceal Creme** *($18)* is an OK concealer that comes in two colors. Clair is good for light to medium skin tones, but Tres Clair is too pink for most skin types.

☹ POWDER: Velvet Pressed Powder *($32)* is not all that velvety, and all the colors have shine. What a waste—to put shine in a product that is meant to eliminate shine!

☺ Translucent Powder *($35)* is a talc-based powder with a small amount of plant oil. It has a silky texture and all three of the shades available are excellent. There are two bronzer shades, Soleil Cuiver and Soleil Clair; both are shiny, and I do not recommend them.

☺ $$$ BLUSH: Velvet Blusher *($35)* is not what I would call velvety, but it does have a soft texture. Most of the colors have some amount of shine. **These colors are OK:** Quest, Rose d'ete, Rouge d'ete, Vendanges, and Muscat.

☹ EYESHADOW: Velvet Eyeshadow *($30)* comes in duo, trio, and quad sets, and all are shiny.

☺ $$$ EYE AND BROW SHAPER: The Eye and Brow Pencils *($20)* are the same standard German-made pencils found in every line from Almay to Chanel.

☺ $$$ LIPSTICK AND LIP PENCIL: Orlane's small selection of Lipsticks *($20)* comes in two types, one that is matte and one that is creamy, bordering on greasy. The handful of Lip Pencils *($16.50)* are the same standard German-made pencils found in every line from Almay to Chanel.

☺ $$$ MASCARA: Special Effect Mascara *($22.50)* goes on well and doesn't smear or smudge, but for $22.50 it should be a great mascara, and it isn't.

Oxy Balance (Skin Care Only)

In the lineup of acne products at the drugstore, Oxy Balance actually has some of the best choices, at least when it comes to good topical disinfectants in the form of benzoyl peroxide. Be careful, you still have to pick and choose in order to avoid some irritating and drying mistakes, but there are some good topical disinfectants in this line to consider. To find where Oxy Balance is distributed, call (800) 245-1040.

☹ Oxy Balance Facial Cleansing Bar Antibacterial Soap with Triclosan *($1.99 for 3.25 ounces)* is a detergent-based bar cleanser that contains several ingredients that could clog pores, including tallow. Triclosan is an OK disinfectant, but its effectiveness is just rinsed down the drain.

☹ Oxy Balance Facial Cleansing Wash Salicylic Acid Acne Medication *($4.77 for 8 ounces)* is a water-soluble, detergent-based cleanser, which would be just fine except this one adds salicylic acid, and that should not get splashed into eyes, and its effectiveness would just be washed down the drain.

☹ Oxy Balance Maximum Medicated Face Wash *($4.77 for 8 ounces)* is a water-soluble, detergent-based cleanser, which would be just fine except this one adds 10% benzoyl peroxide, and that should not get splashed into eyes, and its effectiveness would just be washed down the drain.

☺ **Oxy Balance Deep Action Night Formula** *($4.52 for 4 ounces)* is a very good 2.5% benzoyl peroxide gel with no additional irritants. Now this is the way to deal with blemish-prone skin.

☺ **Oxy Balance Emergency Spot Treatment Sensitive Skin Formula** *($4.52 for 1 ounce)* is incorrectly named (because you can't spot-treat acne); however, this is a very good 5% benzoyl peroxide disinfectant with no other irritants added. But you would always want to start with the lower concentration of benzoyl peroxide, and if you found that not to be as effective as you were wanting then you would try this one.

☺ **Oxy Balance Emergency Spot Treatment Invisible Formula** *($4.52 for 1 ounce)* is similar to the one above except in a 10% strength. This is an option if the lower strengths of benzoyl peroxide, 2.5% and 5%, have not proven to be effective. The next step beyond this formula would be a topical antibiotic prescription you would get from a dermatologist.

☹ **Oxy Balance Emergency Spot Treatment Cover Up Formula** *($4.66 for 1 ounce)* is similar to the one above, except this one is tinted; unfortunately the color leaves much to be desired.

☹ **Oxy Balance Deep Pore Cleanser Liquid Acne Medication with Salicylic Acid** *($2.61 for 4 ounces)* would be a good BHA product except that it contains menthol and alcohol, which are way too irritating for any skin type.

☹ **Oxy Balance Deep Pore Cleansing Pads, Acne Medication with Salicylic Acid** *($4.77 for 90 pads)* is similar to the one above and the same review applies.

☹ **Oxy Balance Gentle Deep Pore Cleansing Pads Acne Medication with Salicylic Acid** *($4.77 for 90 pads)* is similar to the one above and the same warning applies.

☹ **Oxy Balance Maximum Deep Pore Cleansing Pads, Acne Medication with Salicylic Acid** *($4.77 for 90 pads)* is similar to the one above, and the same warning applies.

Pan Oxyl (Skin Care Only)

These two acne products are found at drugstores but are best left on the shelf. For more information, call (800) 327-3858.

☹ **Pan Oxyl Bar Benzoyl Peroxide 5% Regular Strength** *($5.11 for 4 ounces)* is a detergent-based bar cleanser that adds 5% benzoyl peroxide to the mix. The ingredients that keep bar cleansers in their bar form can clog pores, and benzoyl peroxide is wasted in a cleanser because it would just be washed down the drain.

☹ **Pan Oxyl Bar Benzoyl Peroxide 10%, Maximum Strength** *($5.53 for 4 ounces)* is similar to the one above, only this one has 10% benzoyl peroxide.

Parthena (Skin Care Only)

I may be the only person in the world who dreams of the day when all women will change channels every time an infomercial comes on the air. Of course, that is sheer fantasy on my part. The charisma of the salesperson/celebrity/doctor, the stunning before-and-afters, and the heartfelt testimonials always drive viewers to buy.

Objective information is never part of the sales pitch anywhere in the cosmetics industry, and this is painfully so in the empire of infomercials. For as long as I have been researching and monitoring the cosmetics industry, I have wondered how many sensational beauty claims television can display (from Victoria Principal, Ethocyn, Hydron, Forever Spring, Adrien Arpel, Marilyn Miglin, Mon Amie, H+, Murad, Dr. Mary Lupo, ProActiv, and on and on) before women will start yawning (or laughing) about miracle skin-care products and skin-care regimes, and keep their money in their pockets. Or is it sadly true that women have an insatiable appetite for being misled by every slickly positioned sales pitch? It keeps me on my toes, but it wastes the consumer's time and money.

Parthena is clearly aimed at the burgeoning needs of baby boomers—"the forgotten woman," as their brochure states, though forgotten is the hardly the case for women over 40. Given the 1,700 anti-aging products that were launched last year, the over-40 woman is not only remembered, she is relentlessly pursued and reminded constantly that she is aging and that there are miracles to help her get over that plight!

Another incongruous statement in the Parthena brochure is that the creators of this line "began to notice a trend in department stores, clients no longer wanted expensive, complicated, and time consuming regimes, that in our opinion, just did not deliver the results they promised." Uncomplicated! There are over 12 antiwrinkle products in this line, plus the routine includes separate products for day versus night, a kit for the face and another for the eyes, and not a sunscreen anywhere to be found. Inexpensive? Not from this line. Their Longevity Restorative Fluid is $59 for 1 ounce and the Rapid Skin Exfoliator Kit is $69.95 for 2 ounces! Maybe in comparison to Guerlain or Orlane this stuff is inexpensive, but not from any other perspective, and definitely not given what you are getting.

If a woman between the ages of 40 and 55 is beginning to experience pre-, peri-, or postmenopausal symptoms such as hot flashes, changes in skin texture, or vaginal dryness, she would find it hard to ignore the infomercial for Parthena skin-care products. One of the products, a toner in a spray bottle, is recommended for use in cooling down a hot flash. If you've experienced or seen a friend go through one of these "warm moments," you know it takes a lot more than a spray of "toner" to cool down a hot flash. From what I've seen, it would take a complete dip in ice water to do the trick. Besides, who wants to add more dampness to a face or body already dripping in sweat?

Part of Parthena's pitch is that some of their products contain plant hormones, in this case, wild yam extract. You have to process food in a very specific and controlled way in order to extract the progesterone or estrogen and get it into a product (or pill) intact. The likelihood of that being the case in a cosmetic is at best a long shot. Besides, the wild yam extract can be anything, but is probably just wild yam juice, processed and preserved to be mixed into the cream, without any kind of hormone content whatsoever. There is no established research demonstrating that rubbing wild yams on the skin can provide any of the dietary plant hormone benefit.

The other hook for these products is a long list of AHA products. Only one per face is necessary, as there is only so much skin you can remove. If you want more information on Parthena products, call (800) 660-0666.

☹ **All in One Cleanser, Toner & Exfoliant** *($21 for 8 ounces)* is a detergent-based cleanser that also contains scrub particles and 8% AHA. I never recommend AHAs in cleansers because the effectiveness of the AHA is washed away before it has a chance to exfoliate the skin, and the AHA can potentially irritate the eyes. I suspect this cleanser may not pose much of a problem in that regard because it seems to have a high pH (an AHA has little effect at a pH higher than 4). Given that you wouldn't want to get this near the eyes or mouth (as the directions very nicely explain), you would need another cleanser to remove eye makeup. Parthena claims the essential oils in this cleanser prevent stripping of the skin's acid mantle. That's not true in the least. Essential oils are more fragrance than anything else and are not related to pH balancing, besides, essential oils tend to be skin sensitizers and irritants that can hurt the surface of the skin, not balance it. Between this product, the line's Exfoliation System, and the two moisturizers with AHA, you're likely to experience exfoliation overkill. This product also contains grapefruit, clove, and loofah pieces; all together this just adds up to irritation.

☹ **Echinacea and Camphor Antibacterial Wash** *($19.50 for 8 ounces)* contains camphor, a skin irritant that can hurt skin and the burn eyes if you accidentally splash this in the wrong direction.

☹ **Sense & Sensibility Milk Orchid Cleanser** *($19.50 for 8 ounces)* is basically cold cream with AHAs. You have to wipe off your makeup with a tissue or washcloth to get it off. Wiping pulls at the skin, which can sag it, but this is far more gentle than the product above. The pH of this cleanser isn't low enough for it to work as an exfoliant.

☺ $$$ **Cool Off Moisture Magnet Mist** *($7.50 for 2 ounces)* is mostly water, yam extract, slip agent, witch hazel, water-binding agents, vitamin C, and preservatives. This is basically just a toner, and the witch hazel could be an irritant, but the amount of any of the ingredients other than the water is at best negligible.

☺ $$$ **Rapid Skin Exfoliation System for Skin, Eyes, and Lips** *($69.95 for* *three 2-ounce bottles plus a skin lightener)* is a three-part system (much like Elizabeth Arden's Alpha Ceramide) that starts you off with a 5% AHA concentration for two to three weeks, then a 10% concentration for two to three weeks, and finally a 15% concentration for another two to three weeks. You then rotate back to the 5% concentration and start all over again. Building up to gradually higher concentrations of AHAs is an interesting concept. The logic for this approach is to slowly increase exfoliation so your skin has a chance to get used to the potential irritation. However, I completely disagree that the goal with AHAs is increased superexfoliation. If anything, increased exfoliation with high concentrations of AHAs is very risky for the skin. I have explained this repeatedly in my books and newsletter. I would never encourage concentrations over 10% (in a base of pH 3.5 to 4.5). Too much irritation runs a risk of skin damage. And how much exfoliation does the skin need? It doesn't erase one more wrinkle except through swelling, and that can cause problems. For these products though, this whole discussion is moot, because the first two bottles have a pH of 5 and so they can't exfoliate the skin; the other one has a pH of 4, but I suspect the concentration isn't as high as they claim.

The above Rapid Skin exfoliation Kit also includes **On Target Skin Lightening Cream with Sunscreen.** This skin lightener does contain a good amount of hydroquinone as well as kojic acid and anti-irritants, but the sunscreen is minimal and has no UVA protection. While this lightening product can lighten, the amount you get is shockingly small given how much and how often you would need to use it to get any benefit.

☹ **All In One Improvement Cream** *($37.50 for 6 ounces)* is an interesting mixture of AHA and sunscreen for a distressing price. Again, who needs this many AHA products? The pH is too high for this to be an effective exfoliant and the sunscreen doesn't use avobenzone, titanium dioxide, or zinc oxide, so it is ineffective for UVA protection.

☺ **$$$ Anhydrous Extreme** *($24.95 for 4 ounces)* contains mostly silicone, plant extract, thickeners, plant oil, slip agent, vitamin E, water-binding agents, and preservatives. This contains a lot of silicone, which feels like silk on the skin, as anyone who uses the new hair laminates already knows. I bet this would feel great on dry skin. To find out, a much cheaper and easier approach would be to purchase one of the hair laminate products, such as St. Ives Hair Repair No Frizz Serum. This is mostly pure silicone, but you can apply a mere drop over or under the moisturizer you are already using. Every time I use St. Ives Hair Repair on my hair, I also rub it over my legs and arms and then apply moisturizer. It does feel great.

☺ **$$$ Longevity Daily Line Smoothing Fluid** *($24.50 for 1 ounce)* uses an interesting formula that will probably show up in a lot of cosmetic lotions and potions. It contains wild yam extract, a plant progesterone, but there is no way to know what is actually in this cream. How reliable is the extract? If this cream did somehow work to provide plant progesterone to the body through the skin, given the risks associated with the body's progesterone level, you could be randomly altering your hormone balance in a way you don't want to do. Aside from the yam extract, Longevity contains mostly water, slip agent, aloe, several thickeners, water-binding agents, silicone, vitamins, and preservatives. This would be a good moisturizer for someone with normal to dry skin, but don't believe for one second that it will replace the need for medically prescribed estrogen replacement therapy.

☺ $$$ **Longevity Resource Cream** *($37.50 for 4 ounces)* is similar to the one above only in cream form.

☹ **Stress Line Reducing Cream** *($16 for 0.5 ounce)* is another AHA product. It's supposed to contain sunscreen, but it neither contains UVA protection or states the SPF.

☺ $$$ **Eye Power Lift** *($19.95 for 2 ounces)* is just a lightweight moisturizer for normal to dry skin; it won't lift skin anywhere.

☹ **Hydro-Enzymatic Line Digesting Mask** *($24.99 for 4 ounces)* is a great name for a product that is nothing more than a standard plasticizing mask that digests little more than your money! It contains mostly witch hazel, alcohol, and some enzymes. You already know about witch hazel and alcohol being irritants, and enzymes are a poor way to exfoliate the skin.

☹ **Liquid Oil Blotting Matte Spray** *($19.50 for 8 ounces)* contains witch hazel, camphor, and eucalyptus, all serious skin irritants that can hurt skin.

☺ $$$ **Metamorphosis** *($37.50 for four ampoules, total of 1 ounce)* is more wild yam with a host of other gimmicks like bio-engineered placenta extract (meaning fake placenta), collagen, shark cartilage powder, and a host of vitamins. None of this will change anything, but this is a good lightweight moisturizer for normal to slightly dry skin. It is supposed to be worn under the All-In-One Cream, which clearly isn't so complete or you wouldn't need this stuff underneath.

☹ **Sulfur and Mint Vacuum Mask** *($16 for 4 ounces)* has a name that speaks for itself. Mint (menthol) is a skin irritant that, combined with sulfur, can cause more problems than it can help.

Paula's Choice (Skin Care Only)

By now many of you are aware that I created my own skin-care line called, aptly, Paula's Choice. Some of you may find that shocking, while others, about 20,000 of you as this book went to press, thought I had formulated a great, inexpensive line of skin-care products. It's not that I haven't had returns—not everyone's skin can tolerate everything—but for the most part it has been a successful venture.

For those of you not familiar with my work, you may just be wondering why I decided to create a line of skin-care products at all. Isn't that like Ralph Nader designing and selling cars? Good question (except, personally, I wish Ralph would come out with a reliable group of insurance policies).

Believe me when I say I did not undertake this endeavor without much consideration. Actually it is where I started more than 20 years ago when I owned my own cosmetics stores that included my own skin-care line. If anything, it has been a full circle, except now I know far more than I did back then! Basically, after 20 years of analyzing and reviewing hundreds of cosmetics lines and thousands upon thousands of skin-care and makeup products, it seemed like a natural extension of my work. As you already know, I have been continually frustrated by the endless array of products making claims that are either untrue or misleading. And even when I find products that meet my criteria for performance, they often fall short in other ways. For example, many products I otherwise like contain fragrance (a major cause of skin irritation), coloring agents, problematic preservatives, irritating or sensitizing plant extracts, are tested on animals, have (for AHAs and BHA) the wrong pH or concentration to be effective, or, more often than not, are just absurdly overpriced.

Paula's Choice is a line of skin-care products that meet my criteria when it comes to skin-care products. None of my products contain coloring agents, fragrance (including masking fragrances), or any of the irritating ingredients I've been warning about for years, and they aren't tested on animals. I make no exaggerated claims and, better yet, these products are inexpensive—every product is under $14, and they come in generous-size containers.

I've always said I want to stop the cosmetics industry from bamboozling and misleading women; that is why I continue to write books and newsletters on cosmetics. Offering a line of inexpensive products that do what they say they will do feels like an extension of that work, and not in the least a conflict.

I worked diligently for two years with a major cosmetic manufacturer to establish my criteria for the ingredients, the formulations, and the way the products are supposed to work. After the basic requirements were established, more than half a dozen versions were created before I accepted the final prototypes. Then, back in January 1996, I sent out 110 sets of the products, along with a detailed survey, to women who subscribe to my newsletter, *Cosmetics Counter Update*. Fifty-five women received skin-care products for normal to oily/combination skin, and 55 received products for normal to dry skin types. All 110 women returned their completed surveys. The results? About 80 percent of the women said they really liked the products they received and were quite pleased with the way they worked, about 10 percent had concerns about two of the products, but thought the other three were great, and about 10 percent didn't like the products at all or had allergic reactions to them. Eight women commented that they would prefer products with fragrance. However, since I feel strongly that fragrance can cause problems for the skin, I will not be adding any.

A few women were concerned that I would be abandoning my cosmetics and hair-care research, as well as my objectivity, for cosmetics sales. This is not my intent. I truly believe that offering women inexpensive, high-quality skin-care products that live up to my expectations is a service that should not get in the way of my judgment. However, all of you will be the best judges of whether I indeed remain objective. I believe my reviews speak for themselves. Clearly there are lots and lots of products I recommend that aren't mine.

I am committed to maintaining my standards. There will always be great products for me to recommend, and terrible overpriced products for me to caution you about. My products are one option from what my research indicates are many reliable and effective products: nothing more, nothing less.

I debated at length about how to review my products. After all, this is an area where it is the hardest for me to be impartial. I attempted as best I could to review them as if they weren't my own, and decided to just give it a go, trying to be as impartial as I could possibly be. Basically, this section is just a way to give you a better understanding of my products. I did decide to leave them unrated (without faces), because I couldn't possibly be that impartial! Paula's Choice products are available by calling (800) 831-4088 or (206) 444-1622. You can also order through my Web page at *http://www.cosmeticscop.com.*

One Step Face Cleanser for Normal to Oily/Combination Skin *($9.95 for 8 ounces)* is a standard detergent cleanser that takes off all the makeup, including eye makeup, without irritating or drying the skin.

One Step Face Cleanser for Normal to Dry Skin *($9.95 for 8 ounces)* is a standard detergent cleanser that takes off all the makeup, including eye makeup, without irritating or drying the skin. It contains some glycerin to soften and soothe skin.

Final Touch Toner for Normal to Oily/Combination Skin *($8.95 for 8 ounces)* is a nonirritating toner that contains mostly water-binding agents, slip agent, soothing agent, and preservatives. It should leave a clean, soothing feeling on the skin.

Final Touch Toner for Normal to Dry Skin *($8.95 for 8 ounces)* is a nonirritating toner that contains mostly water-binding agents, slip agent, soothing agent, and preservatives. It should leave a clean, soothing feeling on the skin.

8% Alpha Hydroxy Acid Solution *($10.95 for 4 ounces)* is an 8% gel/serum-type AHA liquid with a pH of 3.5. It also contains an anti-irritant, water-binding agents, and preservatives. It can be mixed with other moisturizers or used under sunscreens. It is an effective exfoliating product for the entire face and body.

Essential Moisturizing Sunscreen SPF 15 *($10.95 for 6 ounces)* is a partly titanium dioxide–based sunscreen that contains thickeners, plant oil, vitamins (antioxidants), and preservatives. This would be a good emollient moisturizer for someone with dry skin.

Essential Non-Greasy Sunscreen SPF 15 *($10.95 for 6 ounces)* is an avobenzone-based sunscreen in a lightweight lotion form. It is irritant-free and leaves a matte finish on the skin.

Completely Non-Greasy Moisturizing Lotion *($10.95 for 4 ounces)* contains mostly water, thickener, plant oil, more thickeners, water-binding agents, vitamin E, anti-irritant, and preservatives. This would be a good lightweight moisturizer for someone with normal to oily skin. It can and should be used around the eye area if that area needs moisturizer.

Completely Emollient Moisturizer *($10.95 for 4 ounces)* contains mostly water, plant oils, vitamin E, thickeners, water-binding agents, vitamins, soothing agent, and preservatives. This would be a good emollient moisturizer for someone with normal to dry skin. It can and should be used around the eye area if that area needs moisturizer.

Extra Emollient Moisturizer for Extra Dry Skin *($10.95 for 4 ounces)* is formulated so it can also be used around the eyes. It is best for someone with dry to very dry skin. It is very emollient but soothing. It contains anti-irritants and extra water-binding agents.

Remarkable Skin Lightening Lotion for All Skin Types *($12.95 for 4 ounces)* is an interesting way to improve the appearance of sun-damaged skin, brown spots, or ashen-colored skin. It contains a combination of kojic acid, glycolic acid, and 1% hydroquinone in a lightweight moisturizing base. This product can be used on the face, hands, arms, legs, or neck, and is best for someone with normal to dry skin.

Blemish/Acne Fighting Solution for All Skin Types *($12.95 for 6 ounces)* is a 2.5% benzoyl peroxide solution in a lightweight base. It also contains anti-irritants. For years, I have been recommending 3% hydrogen peroxide to disinfect blemishes, and that is a good option for some, but for others 2.5% benzoyl peroxide lotion or gel is the next step.

1% Beta Hydroxy Acid Solution *($12.95 for 4 ounces)* is designed to gently exfoliate the skin and unclog pores without feeling greasy or dry. There are no waxy ingredients to clog pores or make skin feel layered with too many products, and it includes special anti-irritants help soothe the skin. This is best for someone with blemishes and blackheads.

All Day Cover Moisturizing Sunscreen SPF 30+ with Antioxidants Waterproof *($11.95 for 6 ounces)* is similar to my Essential Moisturizing Sunscreen SPF 15. I put slightly more antioxidants in this one, more SPF protection (it's still part titanium dioxide), and made it waterproof.

All Day Cover Non-Greasy Sunscreen SPF 30+ with Antioxidants Waterproof *($11.95 for 6 ounces)* is similar to my Essential Nongreasy Sunscreen SPF 15. I put slightly more antioxidants in this one, more SPF protection (it's still part avobenzone), and made it waterproof.

Total Protection Lip Care SPF 15 *($7.95 for 0.5 ounce)* is a very good emollient balm, but that isn't so unusual. What is special about this product is that it has an in-part titanium dioxide base. That helps with sun protection and prevents dry lips.

Exfoliating Lip Treatment *($8.95 for 0.5 ounce)* is a unique way to get dry skin off your lips without irritation. You use a tiny amount and rub it into your lips, and you keep rubbing until the excess skin starts to flake off. Simply brush off what remains, and then apply the Total Protection Lip Care SPF 15 above or another emollient lip balm. You will never have dry, chapped lips again if you do this regularly!

Oil-Absorbing Facial Mask Oily/Combination Skin *($8.95 for 6 ounces)* absorbs excess oil from the surface of the skin and from within the pore without irritation or dryness. There are no clays to dehydrate skin or waxy ingredients to clog pores. This mask is best for someone with oily or blemish-prone skin.

philosophy

philosophy has come up with an intriguing twist on the same old cosmetic theme. In some ways it is the most amazing marketing campaign I've ever seen. It has a quality of upscale department-store élan, with a touch of Zen, family values, and a heavy dose of twentysomething attitude thrown into the mix. It's hard to tell if you are shopping a cosmetics line or looking for a new religious experience. In many ways this is the least cosmetics-oriented line I've ever seen. That's not to say philosophy isn't in the business of selling cosmetics, because that is exactly what they do, and with expensive price tags to boot (who says a philosophical point of view has to be inexpensive, although that happens to be my philosophy), and some pretty typical cosmetic claims about wrinkles and healing skin.

philosophy's philosophy is to capture the attention of women in all age ranges, but chiefly those between 18 and 30, as evidenced by the large number of acne products as opposed to wrinkle creams. That alone is unique when everyone else is going after the 40-and-over crowd, which is petrified about getting older. Younger women who are not yet fighting off the unwanted advance of time seem to want more from life than just beauty. They also want meaning and fun. philosophy meets that need with a brochure that looks like a volume of poetry, not a sales catalog. The only graphics are a series of photographs, circa 1950 and up, of children, parents, and grandparents, on outings or enjoying life. No glamour shots to be found anywhere. Unbelievable.

Inside, philosophy retails everything from books to perfume as well as skin care and hair care. One book, *Philosophy of Love,* is described as "a must-read, early-20th-century reproduction, a secret jewel from the literary world that examines the dynamics of love" by Eleanor Glyn, price $18. Or you can read *Reality*, described as "the discovery and reality of being a woman as seen by flowers," story by Grace and illustrations by Grammi (they are two members of the family that owns the company), price $12.

When it comes to retailing perfume, there is nothing subtle about their philosophy concerning what kind of fragrance a woman needs: **falling in love** *($60 for 4 milliliters)* is supposedly a synthetic human pheromone. That's the stuff humans and animals secrete that creates the instant attraction called chemistry, except this time you put it on artificially, which kind of negates the concept of "natural chemistry," but we're talking marketing here, not facts. Falling in love (the product) is sold as the precursor to really falling in love. The brochure waxes lyric: "Love . . . definitely one of life's greatest mysteries. What makes us fall in love? Can we affect the outcome? Perhaps we can now." Obviously even the company isn't sure, but for $60 they know a lot of women will be curious to try.

Skin care is philosophy's real raison d'être, and their line is more entertaining than anything else. The company preaches about cause and effect, offers the product they say you need to create the effect, and gives it a fetching name. It's hard to not be curious about something named "hope and a prayer" (philosophy likes to use lowercase letters for product names, much like the BeneFit line of products).

The "philosophy" statements that appear on each and every product are another fascinating aspect of the way this line is marketed. Their sunscreen with SPF 15 is called the naked truth, and the label reads "philosophy: if withholding the truth is an act of love, then is telling the truth only an act of courage?" Wow. Heavy. What that has to do with sunscreen is anyone's guess, but it makes for thought-provoking reading. The eyeshadows are romantically called windows of the soul. The rest of the label reads "philosophy: to know the true story of the soul, look deeply into the eyes," presumably past the eyeshadow. (I added that last part.) I've never seen products with such engaging copy.

Most of the basic information in the philosophy brochure is actually quite good, such as advice about weight loss, sun care, exercise, relaxation, and basic facts about skin aging. But there's also a fair share of nonsense about vitamins and botanicals being the beneficial ingredients in their products. On a less whimsical note, some extremely misleading information is tossed around, and that is not a philosophy I care for. The brochure recommends that you determine how sensitive your skin is by whether or not you tan. If your skin always burns, they claim, you know you have sensitive skin; if you usually tan, you can use most products. That isn't the least bit accurate. What about women of color? Don't they have sensitive skin sometimes? Sensitive skin has little to do with a woman's ability to tolerate sun exposure.

This line will be getting a lot of attention in the fashion magazines for a while and it will be strong and hard to ignore. Although there are definitely some very good products in this line, many are overpriced for what you get. For more information on philosophy products call (888) 2-NEW-AGE (doesn't that phone number just figure?).

philosophy skin care

☹ **on a clear day cleanser** *($14 for 4 ounces)* is a very strong detergent-based cleanser that uses sodium lauryl sulfate as the cleansing agent. That's strong stuff in this concentration, and can cause allergic reactions and irritate the skin.

☹ **real purity cleanser** *($15 for 6 ounces)* is almost identical to the product above, and the same review applies.

☺ **wiped out two-in-one cleanser/moisturizer** *($15 for 4 ounces)* contains mostly water, several thickeners, silicone, more thickeners, detergent cleansing agent, plant extracts, and preservatives. This isn't a very effective cleanser, but it can be OK for someone with dry skin who doesn't wear very much makeup.

☹ **deeply superficial enzyme scrub** *($18 for 2 ounces)* is a cornmeal-based scrub that also contains papaya and pineapple, which can cause irritation.

☺ **$$$ under your skin, face and body scrub** *($18 for 4 ounces)* is a gel-based scrub that uses synthetic particles as the abrasive. It does work, but boy is this stuff ordinary.

☺ **$$$ quick change** *($12 for 4 ounces)* is a standard detergent-based eye-makeup remover that works well, but wiping off makeup is always a problem for the skin.

☺ **$$$ dark shadows eye brightener** *($25 for 0.5 ounce)* is just water, silicones, slip agents, plant oil, thickeners, vitamin K, and preservatives. Vitamin K can't brighten anything, but this is a good lightweight moisturizer for someone with slightly dry skin.

☺ **$$$ eye believe** *($25 for 0.5 ounce)* contains mostly water, thickener, water-binding agents, thickener, more water-binding agents, vitamin E, thickener, beta carotene, anti-irritant, and preservatives. This is a good moisturizer for dry skin, with antioxidants if you are interested, though not very much of them.

☹ **hope in a bottle oil-free moisturizer normal to oily skin** *($30 for 2 ounces)*. With the new research about BHA being a good exfoliant for blemish-prone skin, I was excited about this product. Sadly, the ingredients have changed, the BHA is gone, and now there are avocado oil and other thickening agents that can leave the face greasy and shiny. How disappointing.

☹ **hope in a jar moisturizer for normal to dry skin** *($30 for 2 ounces)* is about a 6% AHA in a moisturizing base, except that the pH isn't low enough for it to exfoliate the skin.

☺ **$$$ hope and a prayer topical vitamin C** *($45 for 1 ounce)* is philosophy's attempt to keep abreast of the vitamin C craze. The gimmick here is that you mix this product up every time you use it; the kit comes with a bottle of vitamin C powder and a bottle of silicone-based liquid. Of course you're supposed to believe this concoction keeps the vitamin C fresh, but that doesn't answer the question about why that's necessary (there are plenty of stable forms of vitamin C), and why in the devil vitamin C is such an integral, one-of-a-kind ingredient. It isn't; it's just the most overhyped around, with vitamin A running close behind.

☺ **$$$ the present oil-free moisturizer sensitive skin** *($20 for 2 ounces)* is just thickeners and silicone, and that's nice for normal to slightly dry skin, but really really basic. The lavender oil in here doesn't make this the best for sensitive skin types.

☺ **$$$ thin skin** *($24 for 2 ounces)* is a good emollient moisturizer for someone with dry skin, but there is nothing special about this moisturizer regardless of how thick or thin your skin is.

☺ **$$$ between the lines topical vitamin A** *($20 for 0.5 ounce)* contains mostly water, glycerin, plasticizer, vitamin A, plant oil, water-binding agents, and preservatives. This is a good lightweight moisturizer that is supposed to go under a more emollient moisturizer. The vitamin A won't help lines in any way, but it sounds good.

☹ **the damage is done glycolic acid cream** *($24 for 2 ounces)* is a about a 6% AHA product, but it doesn't have a low enough pH to work as an exfoliant.

☺ **the healthy tan self tanning gel** *($16 for 4 ounces)* is a standard self-tanner that uses the same ingredient every other self-tanner does to turn the skin brown.

☺ **the naked truth non-chemical sunscreen SPF 15 tinted moisturizer in light, medium, and dark shades** *($16 for 4 ounces)* is a titanium dioxide–based sunscreen that also contains mostly water, silicones, thickeners, and preservatives. It's fairly basic stuff, but good for sun protection. The colors aren't for everyone but they blend to almost nothing.

☹ **shelter moisturizing lotion sunblock for the face SPF 15** *($16 for 2 ounces)* doesn't contain avobenzone, zinc oxide, or titanium dioxide, and is not recommended.

☹ **shelter spray gel sunblock for the body SPF 15** *($16 for 4 ounces)* doesn't contain avobenzone, zinc oxide, or titanium dioxide, and is not recommended.

☹ **a pigment of your imagination** *($20 for 1 ounce)* contains mostly alcohol, hydroquinone, kojic acid, glycerin, and thickeners. This product contains two reliable skin lightening agents, but the alcohol can be irritating and not just in your imagination.

☺ **$$$ when lightening strikes** *($45 for 4 ounces)* is a good hydroquinone-based skin-lightening product.

☹ **exit strategy facial cream for skin that burns** *($12 for 1 ounce)* contains mostly water, aloe, plant extract, clay, thickeners, sulfur, camphor, more thickeners, and preservatives. Several of the thickeners in this product can cause breakouts, and that's not great. The sulfur in here can be a disinfectant, but a very irritating one, and camphor is just plain irritating.

☹ **forest gunk detox facial mask** *($18 for 2 ounces)* contains several irritating plant oils, including pine and orange.

☺ $$$ **never let them see you shine oil absorbing serum** *($12 for 1 ounce)* is nothing more than milk of magnesia, except it's a lot more expensive. This product contains mostly water, slip agent, magnesium, and preservatives. They must have read my book.

☹ **out of control blemish gel for skin that tans** *($18 for 1 ounce)* is mostly alcohol with some AHA and BHA. The alcohol is unnecessarily drying and irritating for all skin types.

☹ **rescue mission deep cleansing mask** *($16 for 1 ounce)* is a clay mask that contains eucalyptus and orange oil, which are too irritating for all skin types.

☺ $$$ **stuck in the mud** *($18 for 2 ounces)* is a good basic clay mask that also contains a tiny bit of charcoal. There is no evidence that charcoal has any positive (or negative) effect on the skin.

☺ $$$ **kiss me lip balm** *($8 for 0.5 ounce)* is little more than Vaseline and lanolin in lipstick form. It's fine for dry lips.

☹ **the great awakening** *($25 for 1 ounce of gel and 2 ounces of foam)* might better be called a rude awakening. It's supposed to be a two-part facial: the gel is a cleanser to prepare the skin, and the foam is meant to bring oxygen to the skin. How does it do that? Easy: with hydrogen peroxide. Yes, the good old 3% hydrogen peroxide you buy at the drugstore in a brown bottle for 89 cents. But even if this were a good way to deliver oxygen to the skin (and it isn't), hydrogen peroxide deteriorates almost immediately on exposure to air and sunlight, which means the extra oxygen would be gone after you first opened it. Charging $25 for hydrogen peroxide and a teensy bit of basic cleanser is a rude awakening.

☹ **the big skinny, cellulite cream for legs, arms, and tummy** *($18 for 6 ounces)* is a mix of plant oils, thickeners, and a tiny bit of coffee, and if you believe that can affect fat, I have a bridge in Brooklyn I'd love to sell you.

philosophy makeup

☺ $$$ <u>FOUNDATION:</u> philosophy's **our foundation** *($25)* comes in a gorgeous but limited group of colors; there is nothing here for women with darker skin tones. The texture is quite smooth and moist, which makes it best for someone with normal to dry skin, and it provides light to medium coverage.

☺ $$$ <u>BLUSH:</u> philosophy has had a politically correct name change for their blushes. Originally called "he makes me blush" they are now called **you make me blush** *($15)*. Regardless, this is a very nice, but small, group of soft matte blushes. Avoid the colors called infatuation, vision, sun bronze, and attract, which are all rather shiny, unless shine is what makes you blush these days.

☺ $$$ <u>EYESHADOW:</u> This one wins the best name contest. **windows of the soul** *($14)* are great matte eyeshadows with a handful of shiny options in subtle neutral shades. These would be better without any shine, but here it's so minute that you can easily overlook it.

☺ $$$ <u>LIPSTICK AND LIP PENCIL:</u> These are definitely not the line's strong point. The **coloring crayons** *($12.50)* are a small collection of typical lip and eye pencils. **word of mouth** *($14)* is a small but good selection of lip colors in three styles: an excellent soft **Matte** creamy finish; sheer with **SPF 15** (but not with UVA protection); and a **Creme** that is more glossy than creamy.

☹ $$$ <u>BRUSHES:</u> There are more interesting and reasonably priced brushes than the ones offered from this line. The **Blending Brush** *($18)* is a strange shape, the **Crease Brush** *($18)* is too floppy to control color placement, the **Eye Liner Brush** *($18)* has a square, thin edge, which is one way to line the eye, but not my favorite for control (it can be too thick to control a small line), the **Lip Brush** *($16)* is too sparse, the **Powder Brush** *($25)* is too big for most faces to control placement of the powder and not get it in your eyes, and the **Brow Brush** *($10)* is painfully scratchy. The **Blush Brush** *($25)* and **Eye Shadow Brush** *($18)* were quite nice but not really worth the money.

☺ $$$ <u>SPECIALTY PRODUCTS:</u> **the coloring book** *($160)* is a great group of ten eyeshadows, four blushes, five lip colors, two liner pencils and a decent set of makeup brushes in one convenient kit. Convenient only if you don't have to pack the whole thing in your makeup bag. **custom coloring book** *($180)* is the same thing as the one above, only you choose which colors you want. Of course I feel there are far less expensive ways to put together the same array, but this is definitely one-stop shopping.

☹ $$$ **the pocket book** *($45)* is a small, tri-fold wallet of products including one blush, one eyeshadow, four small lipsticks, and a small, almost unusable, tiny brush set. There are better and more reasonable ways to put together a usable makeup bag.

pHisoDerm (Skin Care Only)

For more information about pHisoDerm call (800) 745-2429.

☹ **Daily Cleanser and Conditioner, Sensitive Skin Formula, Normal to Dry Skin Formula,** and **Normal to Oily Skin Formula** *($7.93 for 14 ounces)* are both standard detergent-based cleansers with mineral oil. The mineral oil can leave skin feeling greasy, and makes rinsing difficult. This isn't the best way to gently clean skin, but if you have dry skin it can be an option.

☺ **Gentle Skin Cleanser for Baby** *($5.41 for 8 ounces)* is similar to the ones above, and has nothing in it that is more appropriate for children or babies, but it is an option for cleaning skin if leaving a residue behind is something you don't mind.

☹ **Skin Cleanser and Conditioner Regular Formula Unscented** *($7.93 for 14 ounces)* is a detergent-based cleanser that includes petrolatum and mineral oil; talk about a greasy residue.

☹ **Sensitive Skin Cleansing Bar** *($1.99 for 3.3 ounces)* is a standard tallow-based bar cleanser that includes petrolatum and lanolin. Tallow and lanolin are both known skin sensitizers, and make the name for this product completely inappropriate.

☹ **Phisopuff** *($3.18)* is a round puff of scrubbing material that can be too irritating and abrasive for all skin types.

Physicians Formula

Logically, you would assume that all of the Physicians Formula products are formulated by physicians. Wrong. According to David Lozano, vice president of marketing and research for the company, the chemists at Physicians Formula are neither doctors nor dermatologists. They are just chemists, like the ones working for every other cosmetics line. So why the name Physicians Formula, besides the fact that it sounds very professional?

In 1937, Dr. Frank Crandell, an allergist, created Physicians Formula's first product, called Le Velvet, for his wife, who had photosensitive skin, hence the name Physicians Formula. (An allergist *is* a physician, after all.) Does today's Le Velvet even remotely resemble the original product that Dr. Crandell invented 56 years ago? Well, Physicians Formula claims that it still emulates Dr. Crandell, striving to create hypoallergenic, noncomedogenic products. But given the new ingredients on the market, I would be shocked if the original formula is still in use, or that any one would want it to be.

There aren't really any doctors at Physician's Formula, and no physicians sell or endorse it either. The line brags that there are a lot of potentially irritating ingredients they don't use that other lines do. As great as that sounds, some of the products in this line do contain ingredients that can pose serious irritation and skin sensitivity problems, including alcohol, sodium lauryl sulfate, camphor, and menthol, among others. Despite the nonsensical name and bogus identity, Physicians Formula does have some products in all categories that I can recommend as great buys and that are great for the skin. For more information about Physicians Formula call (800) 227-0333.

Physicians Formula Skin Care

☺ **Oil-Control Deep Pore Cleansing Gel for Normal to Oily Skin** *($6.95 for 8 ounces)* is a standard detergent-based, water-soluble cleanser that can be drying for some skin types.

☹ **Oil-Control Facial Bar for Normal to Oily Skin** *($3.50 for 3.5 ounces)* contains several ingredients that can clog pores and irritate skin.

☹ **Oil Free Eye Makeup Remover Pads for Normal to Oily Skin** *($4.75 for 60 pads)* is a detergent-based makeup remover, but it also contains witch hazel, which can be a skin irritant, especially in the area around and over the eyes.

☹ **Oil-Control Conditioning Skin Toner for Normal to Oily Skin** *($6.95 for 8 ounces)* is an alcohol-based toner that also contains camphor and menthol. This is extremely drying and irritating for all skin types.

☹ **Oil-Control Oil-Free Moisturizer for Normal to Oily Skin** *($8.50 for 4 ounces)* contains mostly water, thickeners, glycerin, soothing agent, clay, more thickeners, and preservatives. I can't imagine why the company thinks thickening agents with clay and a little bit of magnesium are oil-controlling. The thickening agents in here can clog pores and make the skin feel oily.

☹ **Oil-Control Shine Away for Normal to Oily Skin** *($6.95 for 1 ounce)* contains polyacrylamide as the second ingredient. Polyacrylamide creates a thin, plastic-like film on the skin (which can feel smooth), but it is also a potential skin irritant. The package claims that this product is clinically proven to instantly help regulate oil production and keep skin shine-free. Water is the first ingredient; others include several wax-like thickeners and two other plasticizing agents that have a smaller potential for causing skin irritation. A lot of new products contain these plasticizing ingredients (which are normally found in hair spray) because they set the skin in place and let little else in or out. That may initially benefit the appearance of the skin somewhat, but I doubt there is any long-term benefit, particularly in the case of this product, since the waxes and the plasticizing agents can clog pores.

☹ **Shine Away Acne Control Primer for Normal to Oily Skin** *($6.95 for 1 ounce)* is similar to the product above, only with the addition of salicylic acid. The BHA would be a good addition, but this product has too high a pH for it to be an effective exfoliant.

☹ **Deep Cleaning Face Mask for Normal to Oily Skin** *($5.95 for 2.75 ounces)* is a standard clay mask that contains mostly water, witch hazel, clay, alcohol, and glycerin. The clay is drying, and the alcohol and witch hazel will only make things worse. This mask won't deep-clean, but it can deeply irritate the skin.

☺ **Oil Free Nourishing Eye Gel for Normal to Oily Skin** *($5.95 for 0.5 ounce)* contains mostly water, plant extract, caffeine, slip agent, more plant extract, water-binding agent, and preservatives. This is a good lightweight moisturizer for slightly dry skin. There is no literature demonstrating caffeine's effect on the eye, so don't expect it to nourish or wake anything up.

☹ **Gentle Cleansing Lotion for Normal to Dry Skin** *($7.25 for 8 ounces)* is a standard mineral oil–based wipe-off cleanser that contains plant oil and petrolatum. It is like cold cream and so has all the problems associated with wiping off makeup.

☹ **Gentle Cleansing Facial Bar for Normal to Dry Skin** *($3.75 for 3.5 ounces)* is a detergent-based cleansing bar that can be drying for most skin types. It does contain tiny quantities of plant oil and water-binding agents, but that won't take care of the dryness caused by the other ingredients.

☹ **Eye Makeup Remover Lotion for Normal to Dry Skin** *($4.50 for 2 ounces)* is just mineral oil, some thickeners, and petrolatum. This is just very greasy stuff, and wiping off makeup is a problem for the skin.

☺ **Vital Lash Oil Free Eye Makeup Remover for Normal to Oily Skin** *($4.50 for 2 ounces)* is a standard detergent-based makeup remover. It is oil-free, but it is still meant to be wiped off.

☹ **Pore-Refining Skin Freshener for Normal to Dry Skin** *($6.95 for 8 ounces)* is an alcohol-based toner that also contains a little glycerin. It is extremely drying and irritating for all skin types.

☺ **Extra Rich Rehydrating Moisturizer for Normal to Dry Skin** *($8.50 for 4 ounces)* contains mostly water, thickener, mineral oil, more thickeners, and preservatives. It isn't as rich or as interesting as many of the other moisturizers in this group, but it is a good, ordinary moisturizer for someone with dry skin. It's poorly named, considering the mediocre ingredient list.

☺ **Elastin Collagen Moisture Lotion for Normal to Dry Skin** *($8.50 for 4 ounces)* contains mostly water, thickener, plant oil, more thickener, water-binding agents, more thickeners, mineral oil, more water-binding agents, more thickeners, and preservatives. This very emollient moisturizer would be good for dry skin. It contains elastin and collagen, but they are just water-binding agents, nothing more.

☹ **Enriched Cleansing Concentrate for Dry to Very Dry Skin** *($5.95 for 4 ounces)* is a standard mineral oil–based wipe-off cleanser that contains plant oil and petrolatum. It is like cold cream and so has all the problems associated with wiping off makeup.

☹ **Gentle Cleansing Cream for Dry to Very Dry Skin** *($5.95 for 4 ounces)* is similar to the Enriched Cleansing Concentrate above, and the same review applies.

☺ **Gentle Refreshing Toner for Dry to Very Dry Skin** *($6.95 for 8 ounces)* is a good nonirritating toner that contains mostly water, glycerin, plant extracts, water-binding agents, and preservatives.

☺ **Collagen Cream Concentrate for Dry to Very Dry Skin** *($8.95 for 2 ounces)* contains mostly water, plant oil, several thickeners, water-binding agents, silicone, more thickeners, more water-binding agent, and preservatives. This is a good emollient moisturizer for dry skin.

☺ **Intensive Therapy Moisture Cream for Dry to Very Dry Skin** *($8 for 2 ounces)* is just water, glycerin, Vaseline, thickeners, and silicone oil. It would be good for dry skin, but it is exceptionally ordinary.

☺ **Nourishing Night Cream for Dry to Very Dry Skin** *($5.95 for 1 ounce)* contains mostly plant oil, water, more plant oil, petrolatum, thickener, mineral oil, more thickeners, and preservatives. This is an extremely emollient, almost greasy moisturizer for someone with very, very dry skin.

☺ **Emollient Oil for Dry to Very Dry Skin** *($5.25 for 2 ounces)* contains plant oils, petrolatum, slip agents, and fragrance. This is a good, very emollient oil, but no more so than a pure oil from your pantry.

☹ **Beauty Buffers Exfoliating Scrub All Skin Types** *($5.95 for 2 ounces)* is a standard detergent-based, water-soluble scrub that uses synthetic particles as the scrub agent. This can exfoliate the skin, but the number of thickening agents here makes it problematic for oily skin, though it can be good for someone with normal to slightly dry skin.

☹ **Eye Makeup Remover Pads for All Skin Types** *($4.75 for 60 pads)* is just a mineral oil–based eye-makeup remover that can leave a greasy film on the skin.

☺ **Luxury Eye Cream All Skin Types** *($5.95 for 0.5 ounce)* contains mostly water, thickeners, petrolatum, plant oils, more thickeners, mineral oil, more plant oil, and preservatives. This is a very good emollient moisturizer for someone with dry skin, not for all skin types as the name implies.

☺ **Deep Moisture Cream Normal to Dry** *($6.89 for 4 ounces)* contains mostly water, thickeners, mineral oil, glycerin, petrolatum, plant oil, and preservatives. This is a good, though very standard moisturizer for someone with very dry skin.

☺ **Enriched Dry Skin Concentrate for Dry to Very Dry Skin** *($4.79 for 4 ounces)* contains mostly water, thickeners, plant oils, vitamins, and preservatives. It would be good for very dry skin.

☹ **Self Defense Protective Moisturizing Lotion with SPF 15 for Normal to Dry Skin** *($6.95 for 2 ounces)* doesn't contain avobenzone, titanium dioxide, or zinc oxide, and is not recommended.

☹ **Self Defense Protective Moisturizing Lotion with Sunscreen with SPF 15 for Normal to Oily Skin** *($6.95 for 2 ounces)* doesn't contain avobenzone, titanium dioxide, or zinc oxide, and is not recommended.

☹ **Self Defense Color Corrective Moisturizing Lotion with Sunscreen SPF 15 for All Skin Types** *($6.95 for 2 ounces)* doesn't contain avobenzone, titanium dioxide, or zinc oxide, and is not recommended. I won't even get into the strange color shades this product comes in.

☹ **Sun Shield Oil Free Formula SPF 20 for Normal to Oily Skin** *($7.25 for 4 ounces)* doesn't contain avobenzone, titanium dioxide, or zinc oxide, and is not recommended.

☹ **Sun Shield Moisture Formula SPF 20 for Normal to Dry Skin** *($7.25 for 4 ounces)* doesn't contain avobenzone, titanium dioxide, or zinc oxide, and is not recommended.

☹ **Sun Shield For Faces Formula SPF 20 for All Skin Types** *($7.25 for 2 ounces)* doesn't contain avobenzone, titanium dioxide, or zinc oxide, and is not recommended.

☹ **Sun Shield Sport Non-Stick Formula Dry Lotion Sunscreen, SPF 15** *($7.50 for 5 ounces)* doesn't contain avobenzone, titanium dioxide, or zinc oxide, and is not recommended.

☺ **Sun Shield Sensitive Skin Formula Chemical Free Sunscreen SPF 25** *($8.50 for 4 ounces)* is indeed a pure titanium dioxide–based sunscreen in a moisturizing base. Finally a great sunscreen in this lineup! It can leave a white film on the skin, but it provides excellent protection!

☺ **Sun Shield For Faces Sensitive Skin Formula SPF 15 for All Skin Types** *($8 for 2 ounces)* is similar to the one above, only in a much less moisturizing formula. This would be better for someone with normal to slightly dry skin.

☹ **Sun Shield Sunless Tanning Lotion, SPF 20, for All Skin Types** *($7.50 for 4 ounces)* contains dihydroxyacetone, which would be great, but it doesn't contain avobenzone, titanium dioxide, or zinc oxide, and for an SPF that's essential.

☹ **Sun Shield Lip Care SPF 15** *($1.95 for 0.15 ounce)* doesn't contain avobenzone, titanium dioxide, or zinc oxide, and is not recommended.

☺ **Vital Defense Sun Stick For Faces SPF 30 for All Skin Types** *($6.95 for 0.55 ounce)* is an in-part titanium dioxide–based sunscreen in a fairly standard, almost matte base.

☹ **Vital Defense Moisture Concentrate with SPF 15 for Dry to Very Dry Skin** *($8.50 for 2 ounces)* doesn't contain avobenzone, titanium dioxide, or zinc oxide, and is not recommended.

☹ **Vital Defense Moisture Cream SPF 15** *($8.25 for 2 ounces)* doesn't contain avobenzone, titanium dioxide, or zinc oxide, and is not recommended.

☺ **Vital Defense Oil Free Lotion with SPF 15 for Normal to Oily Skin** *($8 for 6 ounces)* is similar to the Self Defense Lotion for Normal to Oily Skin, and the same review applies.

☹ **Vital Defense Tinted Moisturizer SPF 15 in Light, Medium, and Dark** *($8.25 for 2 ounces)* doesn't contain avobenzone, titanium dioxide, or zinc oxide, and is not recommended.

☹ **Vital Defense Lip Treatment SPF 15** *($3.50 for 0.15 ounce)* doesn't contain avobenzone, titanium dioxide, or zinc oxide and is not recommended.

Physicians Formula Makeup

☺ <u>FOUNDATION:</u> **Le Velvet Film Makeup SPF 15** *($7.45)* is a compact foundation that goes on surprisingly moist and creamy and can blend out fairly sheer. Also, it contains a good titanium dioxide–based sunscreen and the SPF is great. What a shame there are no testers for this product and that some of the colors are iffy, because this would be a definite option for someone with dry skin. But the colors are too difficult to judge through the container, and the likelihood of going home with the wrong color is high.

☹ **Le Velvet Liquid Makeup SPF 15** *($5.95)* is marketed as having a light-weight finish. Nothing could be further from the truth. This makeup goes on heavy and thick, it is difficult to blend into a natural-looking appearance, and most of the six colors have a slight peach tone. It does have a great SPF and contains part titanium dioxide, but I would try this one only if you are interested in a medium to heavy finish (and then be sure the color matches in daylight).

☺ **Le Velvet Powder Finish with Nonchemical SPF 15** *($7.25)* is a very good cream-to-powder foundation that has a smooth, even finish and feels like you have nothing on your face. It also has some great colors for light to medium skin tones, as well as a nonchemical SPF of 15. This is definitely worth checking out, but it does take guesswork, because no testers are available; in three attempts, I still got the wrong color for my skin tone.

☺ **Sun Shield Liquid Makeup with SPF 15** *($5.25)* is a good option for someone with normal to dry skin, but there are no testers. It has a soft, smooth texture and more reliable colors than the other two liquid foundations, but it is risky to buy a foundation without trying it on first.

☹ **Oil Control Matte Makeup** *($5.25)* won't control oil, but it is oil-free. Despite the lack of oil, though, it does not have a completely matte finish and can feel heavy and thick. **Most of the shades are too peach or pink.**

☹ **Sheer Moisture Light Diffusing Makeup** *($5.25)* has a smooth, moist finish, and the phrase "light-diffusing" refers to the sparkle in the makeup. It may make the skin reflect light, but if you think that will change the way a wrinkle looks, you're mistaken; it actually makes wrinkles look worse.

☹ **Every Wear Minimal Makeup SPF 15** *($5.95)* is definitely a light, minimal foundation that has a great SPF (it contains titanium dioxide), but the colors have strong peach tones and can turn orange on the skin.

☺ **Refill Sponges** *($2.50)* for the Le Velvet foundation work well with any foundation. I prefer the round, thin shape to the thick wedge sponges you normally find at cosmetics counters and drugstores.

☻ <u>CONCEALER:</u> **Gentle Cover Concealer Stick** *($4.75)* comes in several shades, including unusable shades of yellow, green, and a peachy shade of beige. The yellow and green won't correct skin tone, they just leave a strange hue on the skin that interacts poorly with foundation. Plus, the texture is too heavy and tends to crease into the lines around the eyes. I never recommend green or blue concealers. **Gentle Cover Cream Concealer** *($4.75)* creases easily into the lines around the eyes, and the colors have the same problem as the stick version. **Neutralizer Color Corrective Primer** *($4.95)* comes in Mauve, Yellow, and Green. The texture is very greasy and thick, it can feel tacky under foundation, and it doesn't camouflage or correct skin tone. **Powder Finish Concealing Stick** *($3.99)* has the same color problems as the other "correcting" products in this line, except that the texture is grainy and it tends to cake.

☹ <u>POWDER:</u> **Translucent Loose Powder** *($5.95)* is a talc-based powder with a dry, powdery finish and a great deal of shine in a container that is very inconvenient to use.

☺ **Shine Away Neutral Oil Control Pressed Powder** *($5.95)* is a very dry, though smooth finish talc powder. The colors are great and this is definitely an option for dusting down shine as the day goes by.

☺ **Powder Palette Multi-Colored Pressed Powder** *($8.95)* is a prismatic arrangement of neutral-toned face powders that all come off as the same color and show up as one fairly sheer color on the face, which is as it should be. The color array is attractive to look at but doesn't have any effect on application or performance. The translucent version of this product is a good, standard talc-based powder for lighter skin tones only, and the only one of the color selections I recommend. It also comes in shades of yellow or green, supposedly to counteract redness. It won't; it just leaves a hint of green and yellow on the face. These all have a tad bit of shine and so are not appropriate for someone with oily or combination skin.

☺ <u>BLUSH:</u> **Matte Blush** *($5.95)* is a great find. I wouldn't call these blushes silky, but they do go on smooth and are totally matte. Only one word of warning: Most of these colors are very muted, bordering on dull. Check them out only if you are looking for a very natural tawny blush color. **Blush Palette Multi-Colored Blusher** or **Bronzer** *($8.95)* is a collage of separate blush colors that end up as a unified blush color on your cheeks. The five shades are nice, and the texture is smooth and even, though they all have some amount of shine. You just have to get past or into the gimmick to appreciate it. Women are spending a lot of money on products by Guerlain and Givenchy that are similar (if not identical) to these two.

☺ <u>EYESHADOW:</u> The **Matte Collection Singles** *($2.95)*, **Duos** *($4.25)*, and **Quad Eyeshadow** *($5.25)* have a wonderful collection of matte eyeshadows. I would suggest the Matte quad shades are a combination of some of the best neutral eyeshadows around. They go on beautifully and blend easily.

☹ **Eyebrightener Multi-Colored Eyelighter** *($5.94)* is definitely eye-catching. But this variegated display of colors ends up placing a sweep of intense silvery shine on the eyelid. If you're looking for shine, this has plenty, and it does go on smooth and even, but who needs silvery eyeshadow?

☺ <u>EYE AND BROW SHAPER:</u> **Eyeliner Palette Multi-Colored Cake Liner** *($10.20)* is a great version of a traditional cake eyeliner that you use with a wet brush to create a line. It goes on beautifully and smoothly. Aside from the great application, the gimmick with this product are the four shades of black, dark brown, tan, and white that let you create all kinds of layering lined effects. If you like a definite line this is a great option to try! Hint: it takes less water than you think to bring up the color. To much water and this stuff runs and is hard to control. **Eye Definer Automatic Eye Pencil** *($4.95)* is a twist-up eye pencil that is greasier than most, which means it can smear or smudge easily. **FineLine Brow Pencil** *($3.95)* is similar to the Eye Definer, only with a slightly drier texture.

☹ **Gentlewear Eye Pencils** *($4.75)* are fat, which makes them hard to sharpen and hard to use (it's hard to control the thickness of the line). Also, most of them are shiny and extremely creamy, which means they smear easily. These are also packaged so that you can't see the color. The matte versions are an option, but you couldn't tell which ones weren't shiny from the packaging. **Eye Brightener Liner** *($4.75)* comes in a pearlescent white and metallic shiny black. I'm sure this can create an intense evening look but Why? would be the question I'd ask.

☺ <u>LIPSTICK AND LIP PENCIL:</u> **Total Perfection Lipstick** *($4.50)* is almost too creamy; it isn't supposed to feather into the lines around the lips, but it does; still, for a more glossy lipstick it's just fine. **Bare Radiance Protective Lip Shine SPF 15** *($4.49)* is a good in-part titanium dioxide lip gloss. **Lip Defining Automatic Pencil** *($3.99)* is a very good twist-up pencil that has a smooth, dry texture.

☹ **Beyond Moisture with SPF 8** *($4.95)* is a good glossy lipstick with a poor SPF. **Vital Defense Lip Treatment** *($3.50)* and **Gloss Guard Protective Shine** *($3.95)* are petrolatum-based emollient lip glosses with an SPF of 15, but neither has UVA protection.

☹ <u>MASCARA:</u> **Length-Plus Mascara** *($4.50)* and **Full Lash Mascara** *($4.50)* don't build much length or thickness, and they tend to smear. **Plentiful Length-Plus Lengthening Mascara** *($3.72)* and **Plentiful Full Lash Thickening Mascara** *($3.72)* neither lengthen nor thicken. Furthermore, by midday they smear and smudge all over the place.

☹ **Month 2 Month Mascara** *($4.95)* and **Plentiful Thickening Mascara** *($4.95)* are both a waste of time and energy. Neither builds much, if any, length or thickness. Month 2 Month sometimes comes packaged as two mascaras rather than only one, and is supposed to provide a "freshness system." You note the date when you start one of the tubes and after a month you dispose of it and start the next one. The two ophthalmologists I spoke to said they had never heard of mascara going bad in a month. They both recommended discarding mascara after three to four months, but thought one month seemed excessive. I agree. **AquaWear Mascara** *($4.95)* builds some length but no thickness, and what is really disappointing is that isn't water-proof in the least.

Pond's (Skin Care Only)

Pond's spent over $36 million to advertise its line of AHA products, called Age Defying Complex, so it has likely caught your attention by now. Six-page ads in major fashion magazines and several sultry television commercials are the company's way of letting you know it has seriously joined the AHA competition. The ads carry on about tests showing that Pond's AHA products improved the skin of women who used them over a six-month period. Of course, the ads don't mention whether any other AHA products were tested or what other products the women were using be-forehand. They probably figured that most women wouldn't want to be bothered with such details. The ads don't really give you any information you can use to make a decision. Having said all that, and even though I consider the ads to be totally bogus, I do happen to think that Pond's has created two very good AHA moisturizers, and one of its water-soluble cleansers is terrific. Sadly, the other Pond's products are far less interesting and desirable. For more information about Pond's, call (800) 743-8640.

☺ **Cleansing Lotion & Moisturizer in One for Normal to Dry Skin** *($4.39 for 4 ounces)* is a water-soluble cleanser that doesn't remove makeup all that well without the help of a washcloth, though it can be good when you aren't wearing makeup, or for someone with dry skin.

☹ **Clear Cold Cream With Alpha Nutrium** *($4.50 for 4 ounces)*, is a clear, thick version of regular opaque, white cold cream. Neither rinses off; they need to be wiped off, which pulls at the skin and in time can cause it to sag. It can also leave a greasy residue on the skin. This one does contain a tiny amount of glycolic acid but not enough to do anything for the skin.

☹ **Cold Cream Deep Cleanser** *($5.49 for 6.1 ounces)* is a classic cold cream, greasy and thick.

☺ **Foaming Cleanser & Toner in One, for Normal to Oily Skin** *($4.39 for 4* *ounces)* is a good water-soluble cleanser that can take off all your eye makeup without causing irritation. It may be drying for some skin types.

☹ **Fresh Start Daily Wash With Alpha Nutrium** *($5.99 for 5 ounces)* is supposed to "awaken and energize your skin." If you don't mind some irritation, that's just what this exfoliating cleanser with little red scrubbing particles will do. This is a standard, very drying, detergent-based water-soluble cleanser that contains a tiny amount of glycolic acid that has no effect on skin. The glycolic acid can irritate the skin, particularly the eyelids, especially after it's been abraded by a scrub.

☹ **Lemon Cold Cream Deep Cleanser** *($4.39 for 3.5 ounces)* is mostly mineral oil and wax; that's pretty much cold cream with a lemon fragrance, and it's a greasy mess when you wipe it off.

☹ **Self-Foaming Facial Cleanser With Alpha Nutrium** *($6.99 for 4 ounces)* definitely foams, and, as the box says, you've never seen anything like it. I haven't, at least not in a facial cleanser. It is reminiscent of a man's shaving foam. I have to admit I found the self-foaming part rather fun and unique, but the novelty wore off the second I asked myself the basic questions pertaining to any facial cleanser. Unfortunately, while this product cleans well, the foam was difficult to spread, and it can dry out the skin. The detergent cleansing agent, sodium lauryl sulfate, is one of the most drying and potentially irritating ones around.

☹ **Water Rinseable Cold Cream** *($4.39 for 5.5 ounces)* is not at all water-soluble. The main ingredients are water, mineral oil, and beeswax. If anything, the cleanser leaves an oily film on the skin.

☹ **Clarifying Astringent** *($4.39 for 7 ounces)* is a standard alcohol-based toner that also contains witch hazel, menthol, and eucalyptus, all of which can seriously irritate the skin.

☺ **Age Defying Complex With Alpha Nutrium** *($10.99 for 2 ounces)* and **Age Defying Complex for Delicate Skin** *($11.59 for 2 ounces)* are both very good AHA products. Although the two creams are labeled differently (one for delicate skin and the other presumably for all skin types), they are practically identical except for the amount of AHAs: the Delicate Skin formula contains 4% AHAs; the other, 8%. These are rather impressive, reasonably priced AHA products for normal to dry skin. You can start at a weaker strength and then move to a higher-percentage product when you see how your skin reacts.

☺ **Age Defying Lotion With Alpha Nutrium** *($10.99 for 3 ounces)* and **Age Defying Lotion for Delicate Skin With Alpha Nutrium** *($12.49 for 3 ounces)* are similar to the products above, only in lotion form, and the same review applies. They contain 8% and 4% AHAs, respectively.

☺ **Age Defying Eye Cream** *($10.99 for 0.5 ounce)* contains about 3% glycolic acid in a very lightweight, standard moisturizing base, with vitamins and silicone.

☺ **Dry Skin Cream, Extra Rich Skin Cream** *($4.39 for 3.9 ounces)* is a standard mineral oil– and petrolatum–based moisturizer with thickeners and preservatives. It would be good for dry skin, but its ingredients are very ordinary and boring.

☺ **Nourishing Moisturizer Cream** *($5.99 for 2 ounces)* can't nourish the skin and it definitely isn't oil-free, but it is a good moisturizer for normal to dry skin. It contains mostly water, glycerin, silicones, thickeners, vitamins (antioxidants), water-binding agents, and preservatives.

☺ **Nourishing Moisturizer Lotion** *($5.99 for 4 ounces)* is similar to the product above, and the same review applies.

☺ **Nourishing Moisture Lotion with SPF 15** *($5.99 for 2.5 ounces)* won't nourish anyone's skin, but it does contain a good in-part titanium dioxide–based SPF 15 in a lightweight moisturizing base that contains several thickeners, silicone, vitamins, water-binding agents, and preservatives. This would be a very good sunscreen with antioxidants for someone with dry skin.

☺ **Overnight Nourishing Complex Cream** *($6.29 for 2 ounces)* contains mostly water, silicone oil (it obviously isn't oil-free), thickeners, slip agent, more thickeners, vitamins A and E, water-binding agents, fragrance, and preservatives. This is a good emollient moisturizer for dry skin, but the vitamins can't nourish the skin; they are just good antioxidants. One of the thickening agents high up on the ingredient list is isopropyl myristate, which can cause breakouts.

☹ **Prevent and Correct Cream Age Defying System with Alpha Nutrium SPF 8** *($16.99 for two products, totaling 2.5 ounces)* is simply a repackaging of the Age Defying Complex AHA cream and a sunscreen. The sunscreen part is called Prevent, and its SPF is 8, which is isn't great, and it also doesn't contain avobenzone, zinc oxide, or titanium dioxide and is not recommended. You can buy a good SPF 15 sunscreen for a lot less and buy the Age Defying Complex individually for less, and get more of both.

☹ **Prevent and Correct Lotion Age Defying System with Alpha Nutrium SPF 8** *($14.99 for 4.25 ounces)* is identical to the one above, only in lotion form.

☺ **Revitalizing Eye Capsules With Nutrium, Delicate Eye Area** *($10.99 for 0.13 ounce)* are capsules that contain silicones, slip agents, vitamins, and water-binding agents. If you want a lightweight silky moisturizer for slightly dry skin, this one is great, though overpriced.

☹ **Revitalizing Eye Gel with Vitamin E** *($5.99 for 0.5 ounce)* contains mostly water, witch hazel, slip agent, vitamin E, plant extracts, and preservatives. Witch hazel is a possible skin irritant and a problem in a product meant to be used near the delicate skin around the eyes.

☺ **Skin Smoothing Capsules with Nutrium** *($10.99 for 26 capsules)* contains mostly silicones, plant oil, thickener, vitamins, and water-binding agents. The results won't be dramatic, but this is certainly a good product for someone with slightly dry skin.

Prescriptives

Let's see: Estee Lauder owns Clinique, Prescriptives, and Origins. Estee Lauder introduced Day Wear SPF 15, then Clinique introduces Weather Everything SPF 15, and then Prescriptives launches Any Wear SPF 15. See a pattern? Here's another example: Estee Lauder brings out Diminish Retinol Treatment and then Prescriptives launches Retinol LSW. Lauder creates Nutritious and shortly afterward Origins has its look-alike version called Night-a-Mins. This happens with almost every imaginable product among these high-end department-store lines. Does anyone else notice a blatant similarity? I wonder how the salespeople handle the question, "why should I buy yours, what makes yours better than, say, that one at the Clinique counter or the Origins counter, or this counter, the Prescriptives counter?" But then, it's hard to imagine consumers challenging much of anything going on at cosmetic counters anywhere in the world.

What comes to mind when you hear the name of the Prescriptives skin-care product line called Prescriptives Px? A physician's prescription, maybe? Even some of the packaging has a medical or clinical appearance. What a great marketing concept. Of course, there is nothing medical, clinical, unique, or even particularly interesting about this new group of products, other than the marketing strategy. There are six Prescriptives Px products, each one supposedly necessary to solve a specific skin problem. The brochure poses a question and then answers it with a product, but the one question it doesn't include is why the prices are so absurdly high.

Prescriptives prides itself on having a wide range of colors that are appropriate for almost every skin color. For this, the line wins high marks. Prescriptives also has an outstanding selection of matte eyeshadows and blushes, neutral-colored foundations, and a handsome array of lip colors for every skin tone you can think of. And it's also one of the few department-store cosmetics lines that is almost entirely fragrance-free.

The major problem you may have with Prescriptives is that selecting a product is somewhat complicated. The counter personnel I interviewed had varying amounts of training, and this line requires training—you're better off talking to someone who has been with the line for a while. (Actually, that's true of almost all lines, but it's especially true of this one.)

Prescriptives' counter displays are incredibly well organized, and many of the colors are terrific. It is the job of the salesperson to color-type your skin and to indicate which foundations and which principal color group you should wear. Prescriptives' foundations are grouped in the same color categories used for the entire line: Yellow-Orange, Red-Orange, Red, and Blue-Red. A specific foundation shade is chosen for you by a process the company calls "color printing," which has since been picked up by many other cosmetics lines, including Lancome and Borghese.

Potential matches from the four foundation color groups are drawn in a line on your cheek with the Makeup #1 foundation and allowed to dry. The one that seems to disappear into your skin indicates the foundation color group that is best for you. Within that color group, there is a range of shades from light to dark.

What are the drawbacks of color printing? Some of the foundation colors that are "accepted" by your skin may look too pink or orange in the sunlight, so no matter how scientific color printing sounds, be sure to check the foundation in the daylight to assure true compatibility. As one Prescriptives salesperson told me, "Almost everyone is Yellow/Orange [which isn't orange at all; these shades are all neutral]—there really are no Blue/Red, Red, or Red/Orange people," and she's right. There aren't. When it comes to foundation, it is the exception to the rule that anyone should be wearing any of those color groups. Another hitch is that once you know what your principal color group is, you are told that you can wear certain colors in all the other groups for a more natural, dramatic, or intensified look. That's not a concept that everyone would agree with, particularly me, but it's great for selling more products. In spite of this sales tenet, I like the line's color selections. There are beautiful colors here, particularly for women of color and women with very light, white skin; you just have to be careful about finding them.

Unique to Prescriptives are their Custom Blended foundations. While this was a passing fad for many other lines, Prescriptives still allows the salesperson to create a specially blended foundation color that can be adjusted as many times as necessary until the color is exactly the way you want it. For more information about Prescriptives, call (212) 572-4400.

Prescriptives Skin Care

☺ **$$$ All Clean Gentle Lotion** *($18.50 for 6.7 ounces)* contains an exceptionally long list of thickening agents, plant oil, some plant extracts, and preservatives. It can be OK for someone with normal to dry skin, but it can't take off makeup without the aid of a washcloth.

☺ **$$$ All Clean Soothing Cream Cleanser** *($18.50 for 6 ounces)* contains mostly water, slip agent, plant oil, thickeners, water-binding agents, more thickeners, and preservatives. It is best removed by being wiped off with a washcloth, and it can leave a greasy film on the face.

☹ **All Clean Sparkling Clean Gel** *($18.50 for 4 ounces)* is a standard detergent-based, water-soluble cleanser that uses a very strong detergent cleansing agent. It also contains small amounts of lemon oil and spearmint oil, which can irritate or burn the eye area.

☺ **$$$ Eye Makeup Remover** *($15 for 4 ounces)* is a standard eye-makeup remover that contains mostly water, slip agents, detergent cleanser, more slip agent, and preservatives. It will take off makeup, but I don't recommend wiping off makeup, especially around the eye area.

☺ **$$$ Px Purifying Scrub** *($18.50 for 3.6 ounces)* is really more of a standard clay mask (which is one of the uses the company recommends) than a scrub. It also contains menthol, which can be a skin irritant.

☺ **$$$ Px Comfort Lotion** *($30 for 1.7 ounces)* contains mostly water, slip agent, several thickeners, water-binding agents, anti-irritant, vitamins, silicones, and preservatives. This would be a very good moisturizer for someone with dry skin.

☺ **$$$ Px Comfort Cream 24 Hour Care for Sensitive Skin** *($37.50 for 1.7 ounces)* is a good moisturizer for someone with dry skin. It contains mostly water, silicone, standard water-binding agent, plant oil, several thickeners, plant extracts, more thickeners, plant protein, marine extract, and preservatives. Plant extracts always pose potential problems for someone with sensitive skin. Marine extract and plant protein may sound like interesting water-binding agents, but even if they were superior for the skin (which they aren't), there isn't enough of either to make a difference.

☺ **$$$ Px Eye Specialist Visible Action Gel** *($32.50 for 0.5 ounce)* may make the lines around your eyes look temporarily diminished, but it can also irritate your skin. It contains mostly silicones and a film former. The gel looks convincing when you first put it on, but if you have dry skin you will still need a moisturizer because this product is not all that emollient.

☺ **$$$ Px Flight Cream** *($28 for 1.7 ounces)* is supposed to help skin when it's subjected to the rigors of flying conditions. It is a good standard moisturizer for dry skin, but nothing more. It contains mostly water, silicone, thickeners, plant extracts, plant oil, more thickeners, vitamin E, several more thickeners, and preservatives. It also contains balm mint, which can be a skin irritant.

☺ **$$$ Px Insulation Anti-Oxidant Vitamin Cream with SPF 15** *($40 for 1.7 ounces)* is one overpriced sunscreen but it does in part contain titanium dioxide as one of the active ingredients and is in a moisturizing base. It contains mostly water, silicone, slip agent, several thickeners, vitamins, water-binding agents, anti-irritant, and preservatives.

☺ **$$$ Px Uplift Active Firming Cream** *($45 for 1 ounce)* is a lightweight cream with the proclaimed virtue of actively firming the skin, instantly and for the long term. Wow! That's a lot to accomplish for some pretty standard cosmetic ingredients. Uplift contains mostly water, silicones (they show up everywhere these days), thickeners, slip agent, anti-irritant, water-binding agent, more thickeners, plant extracts, vitamin E, plasticizer (hair spray–like ingredient), and preservatives. Despite the claims about firming and long-term moisturization, you are

Prescriptives   579

The Reviews P.

supposed to wear it in conjunction with Prescriptives Line Preventor 3 or All You Need Action Moisturizer, and that still leaves you without sun protection. Uplift isn't all that uplifting, but it is a good lightweight moisturizer for someone with normal to slightly dry skin.

☺ **$$$ Px Uplift Firming Eye Cream** *($35 for 0.5 ounce)* is similar to the one above, and the same review applies.

☹ **Px Blemish Specialist Fast Acting Lotion, Spot Treatment for Acne** *($17 for 1 ounce)* is just another alcohol– and salicylic acid–based blemish product. It contains some glycerin and a soothing agent, but that won't counteract the irritation from the alcohol.

☹ **$$$ Immediate Matte Skin Conditioning Tonic** *($18.50 for 6.7 ounces)* and **Immediate Glow Skin Conditioning Tonic** *($18.50 for 6.7 ounces)* are two toners from Prescriptives that left me wondering what is so immediate about them. Immediate Matte is mostly alcohol and peppermint. That can be immediately drying and irritating. The Skin Conditioning Tonic contains mostly water, slip agent, mild detergent cleansing agents, a tiny amount of lactic acid (not enough to be an exfoliant), and some menthol and orange extract. Menthol can give the skin a glow, but it's also an irritant; other than that, it's just an ordinary toner.

☹ **Skin Balancer No Fragrance, Alcohol-Free** *($16.50 for 6 ounces)* contains mostly slip agents and Epsom salts, with some detergent cleansing agent and balm mint. Balm mint can be an irritant.

☺ **$$$ All You Need Action Moisturizer for Normal to Dry Skin** *($32.50 for 1.7 ounces)* contains mostly water, silicone, slip agent, several thickeners, water-binding agents, vitamin E, plant extracts, and preservatives. It doesn't have an SPF rating, so it isn't all you need for daytime. It would be fine as a nighttime moisturizer for someone with normal to somewhat dry skin, but it's nothing exceptional. This is Prescriptives' attempt at an AHA product, but it contains fruit extract, which isn't the same thing as a true AHA, and even if it were there isn't enough in the product for it to work as an exfoliant.

☺ **$$$ All You Need Action Moisturizer for Dry Skin** *($32.50 for 1.2 ounces)* is similar to the moisturizer above, and the same basic review applies.

☺ **$$$ All You Need Action Moisturizer Oil-Free** *($32.50 for 1.2 ounces)* is similar to the moisturizer above, give or take a few plant extracts and thickeners, and the same review applies.

☺ **$$$ Line Preventor 3** *($45 for 1 ounce)* won't prevent lines, although it is a good moisturizer for dry skin. It contains mostly water, slip agents, thickeners, silicone, water-binding agents, plant extracts, antioxidant, vitamin E, more thickeners, plant oil, more water-binding agents, and preservatives. There is a sunscreen in this product, but it provides only minimal protection from sun damage. There are also antioxidants, but they won't prevent lines.

☺ **$$$ Retinol LSW** *($50 for 1 ounce)* makes claims about retinol being a "poor man's" Retin-A or Renova—LSW stands for lines, spots, and wrinkles—though at almost $50 for 1 ounce this isn't about being poor. Even if retinol were an acceptable but second-rate alternative to Retin-A, why would you want to spend all this money on a product that performs only second or third best? Please keep in mind before you run out to join the retinol (the technical name for vitamin A) parade that vitamin C was the antiwrinkle flavor of the month only a short while ago. Still, you can easily give retinol a try with Neutrogena Healthy Skin Anti-Wrinkle Cream with Retinol *($10.89 for 1.4 ounces)* or Avon Anew Retinol Recovery Complex P.M. Treatment *($18 for 1 ounce)*.

☺ **$$$ Any Wear SPF 15** *($19.50 for 1 ounce)* is a very good sunscreen for someone with dry skin, mainly because it is part titanium dioxide.

Prescriptives Makeup

☹ <u>FOUNDATION:</u> **Virtual Skin with SPF 10** *($30)* isn't "virtual" skin as the name implies, it goes on like foundation. It does provide good sheer-to-medium coverage and would work best for someone with normal to slightly oily or dry skin. The SPF does not include any UVA protection, so you can't count on it for good sun protection.

☺ **$$$ Photochrome Compact Makeup SPF 15** *($35)* is supposed to have light-adjusting pigments that minimize the appearance of lines. Estee Lauder's Lucidity was supposed to do the same thing, and I see no more evidence of that with this cream-to-powder makeup than I did with Lucidity. But you can test this out for yourself if you want to check out my review. Photochrome does happen to be a very good, titanium dioxide–based foundation with a smooth, even, though somewhat dry, finish that is best for normal to slightly oily or slightly dry skin. Almost all the colors are excellent; **the only one to avoid** is Warm Toffee.

☺ **$$$ Makeup** *($30)* is a great foundation that is best for someone with normal to dry skin. **These colors are excellent:** Extra Light Cool, Extra Light Warm, Soft Ecru, Soft Cream, Soft Vellum, Soft Ivory, Soft Bisque, Soft Sepia, Soft Redwood, Soft Rosewood, Soft Pecan, Macassar, Nutria, Espresso, and Soft Gold. **These colors can turn peach, pink, orange, or ash:** Soft Pale, Soft Peach, Soft Fawn, Soft Taupe, Soft Blush, Soft Rose, Soft Mahogany, Soft Mocha, Soft Antelope, Soft Beige, Soft Ginger, Soft Amber, Caramel, Sable, Soft Petal, Soft Cameo, Soft Camellia, Soft Alabaster, Soft Rose, and Soft Porcelain.

☺ **$$$ 100% Oil-Free with SPF15** *($30)* is a wonderful matte foundation with a dry, nonshiny finish, but unfortunately the SPF does not contain titanium dioxide, zinc oxide, or avobenzone, and it is therefore not recommended as a sunscreen. **These colors are excellent:** Fresh Extra Light Warm, Fresh Extra Light Cool, Fresh Ecru, Fresh Cream, Fresh Vellum, Fresh Ivory, Fresh Bisque, Fresh Antelope,

Fresh Nutria, Fresh Peach, Fresh Taupe, Fresh Fawn, Fresh Sable, Fresh Sepia, Fresh Redwood, Fresh Porcelain, and Fresh Pecan. **These colors may turn peach, pink, orange, or ash:** Fresh Gold, Fresh Beige, Fresh Ginger, Fresh Pale, Fresh Amber, Fresh Caramel, Fresh Espresso, Fresh Petal, Fresh Mahogany, Fresh Alabaster, Fresh Rose, Fresh Rosewood, Fresh Mocha, Fresh Macassar, Fresh Cameo, Fresh Blush, and Fresh Rose.

☺ $$$ **Custom Blended Foundation Oil Free** *($55)* has a beautifully natural, smooth matte finish, but would only be best for someone with normal to slightly dry skin. **Custom Blended Foundation Moisturizing Formula** *($55),* which is mineral oil–based, has a dewy, moist finish, clearly best for very dry skin. Both are great alternatives to matching existing foundation colors to your skin. Be patient and don't rush the process, and be sure you find a salesperson who has been doing this technique for a while. This may just be the best match in a foundation you've ever found.

☺ $$$ **Prescriptives Matchstick Foundation SPF 15 (Titanium Dioxide–Based SPF)** *($35)* has a soft and powdery finish, with no moist or greasy after-feel. It claims to be oil-free (OK, it contains silicone, which can have a slick finish, but it does have waxy thickening agents that can be a problem for blemish-prone or oily skin). Though this foundation feels matte when you first put it on, it doesn't hold up well during the day if you have oily to combination skin. A word of warning: though the nonchemical sunscreen is impressive, the sheer powdery finish makes me skeptical of how well the sunscreen actually covers the skin and therefore how well it protects, so be cautious. Prescriptives Matchstick Foundation comes in 11 colors that are also quite nice. **These are the only colors to avoid:** Cool Shell, Warm Vellum, Warm Ivory, and Cool Desert, which can all be too peach or too pink for most skin tones.

☹ **CONCEALER:** **Virtual Skin Concealer** *($16)* comes in eight shades and almost all of them are excellent. It goes on smooth and doesn't crease. The only color that may be a problem is Cool Light, which can be too pink for some skin tones. **Custom Blended Concealer** *($10)* is only available if you get the Custom Blended Foundation. It does tend to crease and the colors are dependent on the salesperson's skill.

☺ $$$ **POWDER:** **All Skins Pressed Powder** *($22.50)* has an impressive array of six colors for a wide range of skin tones. The texture is light and slightly on the dry side, which is great for most skin types. **All Skins Loose Powder** *($24.50)* has a great range of colors and a soft, smooth finish. The label boasts that this powder is talc-free, but since there is nothing wrong with talc, the comment is meaningless. (There is concern that those in the talc industry are at risk for lung cancer from inhaling talc but that is vastly different from the amounts used by women in face powders.)

☺ $$$ **BLUSH:** **Powder Cheekcolor** *($14.50)* comes in beautiful shades and most have no visible shine, although some of the colors tend to go on quite sheer.

The browner tones—Sandalwood, Cherrywood, Tulipwood, and Rosewood—are superb contour colors. **All Skins Face Colors Refillable** *(blush tins $14.50 each, compact $5)* is a two-in-one blush container. What a great concept. You can pick a contour and a blush color, or two different blush colors, or a blush and a pressed powder of your choice. One caution: Most of the colors have a slight amount of shine, although not enough to be a problem. **These colors are intensely shiny and should be avoided:** Peach, Mocha, Bronze, Rose, Rosewood, Cocoa, and Orchid.

☺ **EYESHADOW:** There are some great matte colors in this line. **The Trio Eyeshadow** *($30)* compact colors includes three thin strips of matte shades. **Pick 2** *(color tins $11 each, compact $4.50)* is an eyeshadow compact that allows you to insert your own choice of two colors. Great idea, and many of the colors (and there are a lot of colors) are matte and excellent.

☺ $$$ **EYE AND BROW SHAPER:** The huge selection called **Eye Coloring Pencil** *($13)* come in good colors and have a smooth, slightly dry texture. **Automatic Eye Pencil** *($15)* is a twist-up version of the regular pencil and is very standard. **Skinny Dip Eyeliner** *($16)* is a standard liquid liner that goes on in a severe line. It only has two color options, but at least these two don't chip.

☹ **Soft Lining Pencil** *($14.50)* offers two colors in one pencil—Bronze/Cocoa, Slate/Pewter, or Navy/Jet. The texture is soft, but that translates to greasy and smeary instead of soft in appearance. I won't even get into the shine and the color selection. **1,2,3, Eye Pencil** *($16)* is supposed to be a three-in-one product; eyeliner, eyeshadow, and brow color. It comes up short in all departments. It is really too greasy for either the brows or as an eyeliner, and there are just lots better ways to apply eyeshadow. **Brow Shaping Pencils** *($13.50)* have an incredibly dry texture and are hard to apply.

☺ $$$ **LIPSTICK AND LIP PENCIL:** **Lavish Lipstick** *($16)* is a lavishly greasy, standard lipstick in a large, attractive range of colors. The salespeople carry on about a gel-type formulation. It sounds more impressive than this lipstick ends up being. **Soft Suede Lipstick** *($16)* has a more matte, creamy finish then the Lavish. **Lip Gloss** *($12.50)* is a standard gloss that will apply a good sweep of thick wet color to the lips. **Lip Coloring Pencil** *($13)* comes in a large array of colors and has a great texture, but is not unusual as far as pencils go, and you do have to worry about sharpening it. **Matte Lip Crayon** *($15)* is a fat pencil with a soft texture that you can use as a lipstick. It isn't all that matte and requires sharpening. But it can be a fun way to apply lip color and create a lip line at the same time.

☹ **Bi-Color Lip Pencil** *($12)* is a two-sides pencil, with one side being the texture of a lip pencil and the other side a lipstick. As convenient as this sounds, sharpening is a problem. Other than that, it can be a fun product, but I wouldn't take it too seriously. Neither of these will be around too long either.

☺ <u>MASCARA:</u> **Intensified Mascara** *($15)* and **Dramatic Mascara** *($15)*, while not terrible, are completely lackluster and ordinary, and despite the different names they perform the same. Don't expect any dramatic or noticeable lengthening or thickening from either. They don't smear or clump, which is nice, so if you don't want thicker or longer lashes, these may be an option.

☺ $$$ <u>BRUSHES:</u> Prescriptives has a handsome collection of brushes. The bristles are satiny soft and some of the shapes are quite workable, while others are not for everyone. The only ones to avoid are the **Powder Brush** *($32.50)*, which is too big for most faces, making it hard to control placement of the powder, and the **Buff** *($30)* which has a flat top and isn't really worth it or easy to use.

Prestige Cosmetics (Makeup Only)

Prestige, a new cosmetics line showcasing only color, has been getting more shelf space at drugstores and small beauty-supply boutiques lately. Not only are the prices absurdly low, but many of the products are surprisingly good, and some are excellent. Unfortunately, the variety of products stocked isn't the same from store to store, so you may not find all the products reviewed below. For more information about Prestige, call (800) 722-7488.

☹ <u>CONCEALER:</u> **Extreme Cover Concealer Creme** *($4.51)* comes in a small pot and is supposed to provide heavier coverage, but it doesn't have enough staying power to do that, at least not any more than any other concealer. It also has a tendency to slip into lines if you don't set it with a powder, which doesn't look great in the under-eye area. **Everyday Cover Concealer** *($2.99)* is a standard lipstick-style concealer. Its coverage is almost identical to the Extreme Cover, and it has the same problems. However, if you don't have lines around the eyes, these are decent concealers in good skin-tone shades.

☺ <u>POWDER:</u> **Pressed Powders** *($4.51)* are talc-based, have a great dry, silky texture, and come in six good neutral shades.

☺ <u>BLUSH:</u> **Soft Finish Blush** *($3.15)* comes in an extremely pretty assortment of colors that have a soft, smooth texture and application. These are quite similar to M.A.C.'s shades, and are impressively matte.

☺ <u>EYESHADOW:</u> **Shadows Accents** *($3.19)* are a bit tricky, because the mattes and pearls are hard to differentiate. Choose carefully, because the matte shades are silky and, for the most part, very nice.

☹ **Eye Accent Shadow Pencils** *($3.95)* are too greasy and hard to sharpen and most all of them are shiny.

☺ <u>EYE AND BROW SHAPER:</u> **Eye Pencils** *($2.89)* are standard pencils that have a good, soft, but dry texture and come in every color imaginable. **Waterproof Eye Pencils** *($4.19)* go on fairly creamy but stay on well. They aren't any more waterproof than any other pencil. **Waterproof Mechanical Eye Pencils** *($4.19)* are a nonsharpening version of the one above (which needs sharpening).

☺   LIPSTICK AND LIP PENCIL: The **Lipsticks** *($2.95)* have mediocre staying power and the shades are hidden under color caps that inaccurately represent what you're getting.

☺   **Lasting Lip Color** *($3.89)* is a very nice, soft, matte-finish lipstick. It doesn't stay any better than other lipsticks but it does provide good, soft, matte coverage that doesn't bleed. **Lasting Lipstick Crayon** *($4.49)* has no lasting ability whatsoever, it's just a fat pencil that can be applied like lipstick. This one has a fairly glossy finish. **Lip Pencils** *($2.89)*, like the Eye Pencils, come in a huge assortment of colors and are standard but good. **Waterproof Lipstick Pencils** *($4.19)* are identical to the Eye Pencil version. They go on fairly creamy but stay on well. They aren't any more waterproof than any other pencil. **Waterproof Mechanical Lip Pencils** *($4.19)* are a nonsharpening version of the one above (which needs sharpening). **Aromatherapy Lip Gloss** *($2.89)* are pots of standard lip gloss with fairly intense fragrance that not everyone will find all that aromatic. **Vitamin Enriched Lip Gloss** *($3.89)* is a standard tube gloss with a very slick finish. The standard tube **Lip Glosses** *($3.75)* are fine if you are interested in glosses.

☺   MASCARA: **Long Lash Mascara** and **Conditioning Mascara** *($3.89)* both build poorly and don't make the lashes very thick or long. These don't clump or smear, so they can be good if you don't want much action from a mascara.

☺   BRUSHES: Prestige has a small but good assortment of **Makeup Brushes** *($2 to $8)*. They are soft and relatively firm, with good flexibility.

Principal Secret

I've come down hard on Victoria Principal's products in the past and I admit that isn't entirely fair and I apologize. In my own defense, I imagine my snide remarks are a result of my frustration in dealing with the belief and faith people put into celebrities. In the '70s it was Bob Hope selling motor oil, and today it's Judith Light selling acne products, but the method's the same, and I still don't get why these people (with nothing more than great agents who have garnered them a lucrative endorsement contract) are perceived by the public as having instantaneous expertise. Is there something about acting talent or being beautiful that is equal to wisdom, science, and genuineness? I guess it there must be, because celebrities endorsing products is big business the world over. It is simply amazing to me that Victoria Principal can convince women that they can have great skin like she does by using her skin-care routine. In fact, Victoria Principal's infomercial is one of the most successful ever. But I should stick with the facts and not get bogged down by the phenomena of marketing and advertising spectacles and the public's unwavering acceptance of it all.

Victoria Principal's skin-care products were formulated and manufactured by Aida Thibiant, a Beverly Hills aesthetician who has run a successful skin-care boutique and cosmetic manufacturing business there for years. Because the Guthy Renker Corporation that markets and distributes the line felt they no longer needed Thibiant to establish Principal's credentials, they severed ties with her in 1995. That isn't good or bad, it just means it isn't Principal's own skin-care genius behind these products.

This is a line with deals, or at least that's what they appear to be on the surface; deep down, these are just expensive products. You can get the Gentle Deep Cleanser (6 ounces), Eye Relief (0.5 ounce), Time Release Moisture (2 ounces) for $59.85. Or a seven-piece kit called Total Skin Care that includes Gentle Deep Cleanser (6 ounces), Eye Relief (0.5 ounce), Time Release Moisture (2 ounces), Gentle Exfoliating scrub (4 ounces), Invisible Toning Mask (2 ounces), Intensive Serum with AHAs (0.5 ounce), and AHA Booster Complex (1 ounce) for $109.95. Then there is a grouping of makeup products also arranged in varying kits. The makeup and skin care just ends up being incredibly overpriced for what you get.

I should mention that several of these products aren't bad, and a few are actually quite nice, specifically for someone with normal to dry skin. (Someone with oily, sensitive, or blemished skin could have problems with this skin-care routine.) A nice feature is that none of these products are tested on animals. But my opinion about prices hasn't changed. And no one needs six to ten different products to take care of her face and body. Did I forget to mention that the claims are exaggerated?

In the following reviews, all prices listed are retail. If you decide to use these products, joining the club is a good idea, because you will need to reorder frequently; most of the products come only in 0.25- to 4-ounce sizes. Four ounces of any cleanser won't last more than a month. For more information about Principal Secret products call (800) 545-5595.

Principal Secret Skin Care

☺ **$$$ Gentle Deep Cleanser** *($22 for 6 ounces)* is a standard detergent-based, water-soluble cleanser. It cleans well but contains two ingredients that can be a problem for the eyes, and it can be drying for some skin types.

☺ **Gentle Exfoliating Scrub** *($20 for 4 ounces)* contains too many irritating ingredients to be called gentle, including polyacrylamide and salicylic acid.

☺ **$$$ AHA Booster Complex** *($45 for 1 ounce)* contains mostly water, thickeners, slip agent, glycolic acid, several more thickeners, silicone, more thickeners, plant extracts, anti-irritant, and preservatives. The handful of exotic-sounding ingredients at the very end of the ingredient list means they're almost nonexistent. However, this is a good, though absurdly overpriced, 3% to 4% AHA product. It would be good for someone with sensitive skin, but it is almost indistinguishable from Pond's Age Defying Cream for Sensitive Skin, which costs one-fourth as much.

☺ **$$$ Intensive Serum with AHAs** *($45 for 0.5 ounce)* contains mostly water, plant extracts, anti-irritant, aloe, slip agents, water-binding agents, thickeners, and preservatives. There is nothing intense about this product except the price. The plant extracts are not AHA ingredients that can exfoliate the skin.

☺ **$$$ Extra Nurturing Cream** *($40 for 2 ounces)* is a good moisturizer for dry skin; it contains mostly water, thickeners, plant oil, silicone, more thickeners, water-binding agents, more thickeners, and preservatives.

☺ **$$$ Eye Relief** *($30 for 0.5 ounce)* is a light gel with a light feel. It isn't very emollient, but it does include good water-binding ingredients. It contains mostly water, film former, slip agent, water-binding agent, plant extract, more water-binding agents, and preservatives. It would be good for someone with normal to combination skin. The label claims that it can prevent the formation of wrinkles, which is completely untrue.

☹ **Oil-Control Hydrator with SPF 8** *($38 for 2 ounces)* has an SPF of 8, and with so many good SPF 15s around why even think about this one, which also doesn't contain avobenzone, zinc oxide, or titanium dioxide, and is not recommended.

☹ **Time Release Moisture with SPF 8** *($35 for 2 ounces)* has the same review as the one above.

☹ **$$$ Time Release Tinted Moisture** *($35 for 2 ounces)* has the same review as the one above.

☺ **$$$ Sun Block SPF 20** *($17 for 4 ounces)* is a part titanium dioxide–based sunscreen in a lightweight moisturizing base. It would be good for someone with normal to slightly dry skin.

☹ **Sun Secret Self-Tanning System** *($21 for Sunless Tanner and Tan Accelerator)* uses the same active ingredient to turn the skin brown as all self-tanners do, namely dihydroxyacetone, although the Tan Accelerator is a burn. The notion of selling a product to encourage tanning is unethical and offensive for any skin-care line.

☹ **Blemish Buster Mask** *($25 for 2 ounces)* contains cornstarch, which can cause breakouts, as the third ingredient, as well as several other ingredients that can clog pores. It also contains menthol and eucalyptus, which are unnecessary skin irritants.

☹ **Blemish Buster Solution** *($20 for 0.5 ounce)* is just alcohol, sulfur, and zinc. It can irritate the skin and, like many other, much less expensive acne products with the same ingredients, it won't get rid of acne. Sulfur can be a disinfectant, but there are far gentler ones to try besides this, and the price is ludicrous.

☺ **$$$ Invisible Toning Masque** *($23 for 2 ounces)* is a moisturizing mask that won't tone anything. It contains mostly water, thickeners, egg yolk, plant oil, film former, water-binding ingredients, and preservatives. It closely resembles the Extra

Nurturing Cream. It seems unnecessary since so many of the other products contain the exact same ingredients.

☹ **Liptensive Lip Balm with SPF 15** *($10 for 0.16 ounce)* doesn't contain avobenzone, zinc oxide, or titanium dioxide, and is not recommended.

Color Principal Makeup

☺ **$$$ Blush Duo** *($22)* comes in an attractive black case with two shades of blush, one matte and the other shiny. They have a silky soft feel and go on even and smooth, but so do lots of other blushes for far less money and without the shine.

☺ **$$$ Eye Shadow Quad** *($29)* is a set of four eyeshadow colors that are surprisingly matte and have a soft, even application. I actually like the application, and the four shades are coordinated nicely, but $29 for such tiny amounts! These aren't *that* nice.

☺ **$$$ Defining Eye Liner** *($10)* is just a standard two-sided eye pencil with a smooth, slightly creamy finish.

☺ **$$$ Lipstick** *($15)* has a creamy, slightly glossy finish. These work as well as any. **Defining Lip Liner** *($10)* is a standard two-sided lip liner. The colors are fine and the application creamy but not greasy.

☺ **$$$ Double Duty Mascara** *($19)* is a very overpriced mascara. It does build a good deal of thickness and length, but it tends to clump, and the mascara tube gets incredibly gunky and gooey. The mascaras come two-sided; one has a black shade on one end and brown at the other. The other has black mascara at both ends. The two sides and different wand shapes don't improve the application.

ProActiv (Skin Care Only)

ProActiv is a group of four products aimed at those with breakouts. It was created and endorsed by two dermatologists, Dr. Katie Rodan and Dr. Kathy Fields, who market these products via infomercial. While I don't doubt these two doctors' dermatologic expertise, I still find some of their products lacking and the prices a bit steep, unless of course you join their club. In order to get your first order at the discount price, which would include the four products listed in my review below for $39.95 plus shipping, you need to agree to automatic shipments of the same four products for $39.95 plus shipping every two months. If you want to pick and choose which products work best for you the price goes up considerably. My constant reminder to all of you trying to take good care of your skin is to pick and choose carefully. For more information call (800) 950-4695.

☺ **Renewing Cleanser** *($16 for 4 ounces)* contains mostly 2.5% benzoyl peroxide, detergent cleansing agents, thickeners, silicone, and preservatives. Though benzoyl peroxide is an effective disinfectant for breakouts, putting it in a cleanser doesn't make much sense. You risk getting the disinfectant in the eyes and the effectiveness of the benzoyl peroxide is rinsed down the drain.

☺ **Revitalizing Toner** (*$16 for 4 ounces*) contains mostly water, glycolic acid, slip agents, plant extract, witch hazel, thickener, water-binding agents, and preservatives. This is a potentially good AHA liquid. However, when it comes to most kinds of breakouts, new research indicates a BHA (salicylic acid) is the best way to exfoliate within the pore.

☺ **Repairing Lotion** (*$22.95 for 2 ounces*) contains 2.5% benzoyl peroxide, water, slip agents, soothing agent, and preservatives. This is a fine benzoyl peroxide product, but it doesn't repair anything in the skin; it only disinfects. There is nothing special or unique about this benzoyl peroxide lotion; you can find several products just like it in the acne section of your local drugstore.

☹ **Daily Oil Control** (*$18 for 1.7 ounces*) contains mostly alcohol and a form of aluminum starch found in deodorants. There are better ways to deal with oil than this irritating combination.

☹ **Mask** (*$20 for 2.5 ounces*) contains at least 6% pure sulfur. Sulfur can be a good, mild antibacterial agent, but it is also a pretty good skin irritant.

PropapH (Skin Care Only)

I remember this line of acne products from when I was a kid, and they haven't changed since way back then. They are just as irritating and problematic for skin today as they were in the '70s! The company's phone number is (800) 645-4664.

☹ **PropaPh Foaming Face Wash Acne Medication and Moisturizer** (*$2.99 for 8 ounces*) is a detergent-based water-soluble cleanser, but this one contains menthol, which is too irritating, and salicylic acid, which is wasted in a cleanser.

☹ **PropapH Astringent and Cleanser Acne Medication and Moisturizer Maximum Strength** (*$3.79 for 10 ounces*) contains salicylic acid, which would have made this a nice product if it didn't also contain menthol, peppermint, and alcohol. This is a burn for the skin, causing more problems than it could ever hope to help.

☹ **PropapH Astringent Cleanser Acne Medication and Moisturizer Maximum Strength** (*$3.79 for 10 ounces*) is similar to the one above, and the same review applies.

☹ **PropapH Astringent Cleanser Acne Medication and Moisturizer Normal to Sensitive Skin** (*$4.21 for 12 ounces*) is similar to the one above, and the same review applies.

☹ **PropaPh Overnight Pore Clarifier Acne Treatment and Moisturizer** (*$3.79 for 2 ounces*) doesn't contain unnecessary irritants, but the pH of this part salicylic acid–, part AHA–based product (and it's not a great mix of these, I should mention), isn't low enough for it to be an effective exfoliant.

☹ **PropaPh Peel-Off Acne Mask Acne Treatment and Moisturizer** *($4.21 for 2.66 ounces)* is similar to the one above only in mask form, and it contains alcohol.

Purpose (Skin Care Only)

Prior to 1987, Johnson & Johnson was better known for baby care than for skin care. That has changed. Johnson & Johnson has become better known for their controversial foray into the world of serious wrinkle treatment with Retin-A and Renova. These two products represent over $200 million a year in revenue. Leaving no stone unturned, Johnson & Johnson has made great strides convincing physicians that a prescription for Retin-A and Renova should be accompanied by the Purpose line of products. Your face could easily live without most of the Purpose products, although the Dual Purpose Sunscreen is a consideration for daily sun protection. For more information about Purpose products call (800) 526-3967.

☹ **Gentle Cleansing Bar** *($3.17 for 6 ounces)* is just a standard bar cleanser that contains tallow and a strong detergent cleansing agent with a little glycerin added, but that won't counteract the drying effect of the soap. Also, the tallow can cause breakouts.

☺ **Gentle Cleansing Wash** *($4.95 for 6 ounces)* is a standard, detergent-based, water-soluble cleanser that can be drying for some skin types. However, it may be good for someone with oily skin.

☹ **Alpha Hydroxy Moisture Lotion with SPF 15** *($10.05 for 4 ounces)* and **Alpha Hydroxy Moisture Cream with SPF 15** *($9.84 for 2 ounces)* contain about 8% glycolic acid in a pH of about 3 to 4. That makes it a decent AHA product for someone with normal to dry skin. Now if only the SPF contained avobenzone, titanium dioxide, or zinc oxide, you would have a decent two-in-one AHA with a reliable SPF. Alas, it doesn't, so although this one comes close, it's still miles away from the real thing.

☺ **Dry Skin Cream** *($5.61 for 3 ounces)* is a very standard but good moisturizer for someone with dry skin. It contains mostly water, petrolatum, slip agents, thickeners, plant oil, more thickeners, mineral oil, and preservatives.

☺ **Dual Treatment Moisturizer with SPF 15 Protection** *($7.89 for 4 ounces)* is a good sunscreen for someone with normal to slightly dry skin or slighly oily skin. It is partly nonchemical and also contains water, glycerin, several thickeners, silicone, more thickeners, and preservatives.

Rachel Perry (Skin Care Only)

Health food stores have been selling Rachel Perry products for years. This is one of the original "natural" cosmetics lines, and it is now also available at some large drugstore chains. Rachel Perry products contain many, if not more, of the same natural-sounding ingredients included in more highbrow natural-product lines such as Aveda, Clarins, and Origins. For the consumer on a budget who is interested in the ballyhoo surrounding botanical skin-care products, this line could satisfy that curiosity without hurting the pocketbook. But watch out for your skin, there are skin irritants and allergens lurking in these products. For more information about Rachel Perry products call (800) 966-8888.

☹ **Citrus-Aloe Cleanser and Face Wash, for Normal to Dry Skin** *($10.50 for 4 ounces)* contains plant water, thickeners, plant oil, more thickeners, silicone, more oils, and preservatives. The oils make this more of a wipe-off product than a face wash. It can leave a greasy residue on the skin.

☹ **Tangerine Dream Foaming Facial Cleanser with Alpha-Hydroxy Acids for All Skin Types** *($10.50 for 6 ounces)* is a standard detergent-based, water-soluble cleanser that contains about 3% AHAs. AHAs are wasted in a cleanser because their effectiveness is rinsed down the drain. They are also a problem if you get this kind of concentration in your eyes. Plus, several of the plant extracts can be skin irritants.

☹ **Peach & Papaya Gentle Facial Scrub** *($10.50 for 2 ounces)* contains menthol, lemon peel, balm mint, and several other potentially irritating ingredients. Even papaya does nothing for the skin except cause irritation. Ouch!

☺ **Sea Kelp-Herbal Facial Scrub** *($10.50 for 2.5 ounces)* contains mostly water, cornmeal, glycerin, slip agent, rye flour, thickener, almond meal, sea salt, plant extracts, and preservatives. This is a pretty thick mess to use as a scrub. It would be cheaper and better for the skin to use plain cornmeal or sea salt all by itself.

☹ **Lemon Mint Astringent, for Normal to Oily Skin** *($9.50 for 8 ounces)* contains mostly plant water, AHAs, water-binding agents, peppermint, soothing agent, slip agents, and preservatives. This toner has more than its share of irritating ingredients, including mint, lemongrass, peppermint, and witch hazel.

☹ **Perfectly Clear Herbal Antiseptic, for Oily or Acne Prone Skin** *($10.50 for 8 ounces)* is mostly alcohol with a host of even more irritating ingredients, including camphor, eucalyptus oil, menthol, peppermint oil, and clove oil. This product is a skin rash waiting to happen.

☺ **Violet Rose Skin Toner** *($9.50 for 8 ounces)* contains mostly plant water, water-binding agents, soothing agent, and preservatives. It would be a good irritant-free toner for most skin types.

☺ **$$$ Visible Transition 10% Alpha-Hydroxy Serum** *($27.50 for 1.1 ounces)* is a good concentration of AHAs, but the pH is too high for it to be effective as an exfoliant.

☺ **Bee Pollen-Jojoba Maximum Moisture Cream** *($12.50 for 2 ounces)* contains mostly plant water (with a teeny amount of bee pollen), plant oils, thickeners, silicone, vitamins, water-binding agent, fragrance, and preservatives. This is a good emollient moisturizer for dry skin.

☺ **Calendula-Cucumber Oil Free Moisturizer with Sunscreen** *($13.50 for 4 ounces)* contains mostly plant water, slip agent, thickeners, silicone, water-binding agents, more thickeners, and preservatives. This isn't oil-free, and the amount of sunscreen is minimal; even the label says it isn't a sunblock, so why put it in at all?

☺ **Elastin and Collagen Firming Treatment** *($14.50 for 2 ounces)* contains mostly plant water, witch hazel extract, water-binding agents (collagen and elastin), more thickeners, more water-binding agent, and preservatives. The collagen and elastin won't firm anything, but the witch hazel can cause irritation.

☺ **Ginseng and Collagen Wrinkle Treatment** *($14.50 for 2 ounces)* contains plant water, safflower oil, several thickeners, collagen, vitamins, and preservatives. The vitamins are way down on the list, but they can provide some antioxidant benefit. This would be a good moisturizer for dry skin, but it won't change wrinkles.

☺ **Hi Potency "E" Special Treatment Line Control** *($14.50 for 2 ounces)* contains mostly water, vitamin E (16,000 I.U.), thickeners, plant oils, vitamins A and D, royal bee jelly, and preservatives. Vitamins are good antioxidants, and this one has a lot of them, though no one knows how much it takes one way or the other. This stuff also won't control lines, but it is a very good moisturizer for dry skin. The royal bee jelly is barely present here, which is fine, because it serves no purpose for the skin anyway.

☺ **$$$ Immediately Visible Eye Renewal Gel-Cream with Liposomes** *($22.50 for 0.5 ounce)* contains mostly plant water, glycerin, bee pollen extract, plant oil, vitamin A, antioxidant, water-binding agents, more antioxidant, silicone, thickeners, and preservatives. Forget the bee pollen; what's interesting about this product are the antioxidants and water-binding agents.

☺ **Lecithin-Aloe Moisture Retention Cream for Normal-Combination Skin** *($12.50 for 2 ounces)* the amount of oil in this product isn't good for combination skin and the amount of sunscreen is minimal, even the copy says it isn't a sun block (so why put it in at all?), plus it contains menthol which is a skin irritant.

☺ **Clay and Ginseng Texturizing Mask** *($10.50 for 2 ounces)* contains mostly plant water, clay (supposedly French clay, but clay is clay no matter what country it's from), talc, more clay, thickeners, vitamin E, RNA, plant oil, and preservatives. This is a standard clay mask, and several of the plant extracts may be too irritating, particularly combined with the drying effect of the clay. The RNA won't affect your skin cells, but it sounds impressive.

☺ **Lip Lover** *($2.53 for 0.2 ounce)* is a good emollient and even tasty group of lip balms in a host of flavors.

Ralph Lauren Polo Sport (Skin Care Only)

I wasn't going to include men's skin care in this book, mainly because men don't buy my book and I didn't want to include lines women would otherwise find a waste of their time. I just couldn't pass up reviewing the Polo Sport line of Men's Skin Care products for one basic reason: these products are really terrible! The masculine packaging is the best thing this line has going for it. I shudder to think of the red, irritated skin men are having to deal with from using this line, without knowing there were more gentle, far less irritating products available. If you see these jars on your significant other's counter, give him this review to read; it could save his face. For more information about Ralph Lauren products call (800) 631-7358.

☹ **Face and Body Soap** *($15 for 5.3 ounces)* is a standard bar of lard and lye. That can dry and irritate the skin and clog pores.

☹ **Scrub Face Wash** *($12.50 for 2.5 ounces)* is a standard detergent-based scrub that uses synthetic particles as the abrasive. That would be OK, but this product also contains eucalyptus, peppermint, grapefruit, and menthol. The only thing I can think of is, Ouch!

☹ **Lotion Sports Moisturizer** *($12.50 for 4.2 ounces)* contains mostly water, silicone, thickeners, film former, and preservatives. This could have been a decent though incredibly ordinary moisturizer, but for some inane, skin-irritating reason, this product also contains eucalyptus, mandarin, peppermint, and grapefruit.

☹ **After Shave** *($38 for 4.2 ounces)* contains fragrance and alcohol. Put this on the skin after a shave and you will be assured of having red dots and rashes most of the year.

☹ **Shave Comfort Gel** *($12.50 for 5.3 ounces)* would have been comforting except this product contains eucalyptus, mandarin, peppermint, and grapefruit. That isn't comforting, that's distressing.

☹ **Shave Fitness Skin Protecting Foam** *($12.50 for 5.3 ounces)* does foam, but the review for the Gel above applies here too.

☺ **Water Basics Post Shave Relief Balm** *($25 for 4.2 ounces)* is just a good emollient moisturizer with too much fragrance, but given the list of irritating ingredients in all the shave products, I imagine this balm would feel nice.

☹ **Face Fitness AHA Moisture Formula, SPF 8** *($25 for 4.2 ounces)* has an SPF 8; that's bad enough, but this product also doesn't contain avobenzone, zinc oxide, or titanium dioxide, and is not recommended.

☹ **Oil-Free Self-Tanning Spray SPF 8** *($15 for 3.5 ounces)* has the same review as the one above.

☹ **Sun Stick SPF 15** *($10 for 0.26 ounce)* has the same review as the one above.

☹ **Weatherproof Sun Block SPF 15** *($15 for 3.4 ounces)* has the same review as the one above.

☹ **Waterproof Sun Lotion SPF 8** *($15 for 3.4 ounces)* is a part titanium dioxide–based sunscreen, but the SPF 8 just doesn't cut it when so many other lines have great SPF 15s.

☹ **Weatherproof Sun Block SPF 8** *($15 for 3.4 ounces)* has the same review as the one above.

Rejuveness (Skin Care Only)

You may have noticed ads in fashion magazines for a product called Rejuveness claiming that it can magically heal scars. ☺ **Rejuveness** *($39.50 to $295, depending on the size ordered)*, and other products like it, are nothing more than pliable sheets of silicone, quite similar to the silicone used in so many skin- and hair-care products because of its texture and water-binding properties. It is not clear how these sheets of silicone work. They may increase the amount of water in the scar, and continuous rehydration of scars may soften the tissue, making it more elastic and pliable, thus encouraging natural skin-cell production and the flattening process. But work they do, and rather successfully (although I use the word successfully with caution).

Silicone sheets appear to be most effective for hypertrophic or keloidal scarring. As wonderful as this sounds, and close to wonderful it is, there are disadvantages. Users purchase one relatively inexpensive sheet of silicone that is worn over and over again. You need to keep the sheet clean, which requires some amount of care and maintenance time. You have to wear these sheets of silicone over the scar for prolonged periods of time, which means that you might not want to wear one on your face or other exposed parts of your body, at least not during the day. Also, the silicone sheet can stick to the skin (wearing camisoles or T-shirts can help), and skin reactions such as rashes or irritation can occur.

Even more difficult and uncomfortable is that you have to wear the covering for long periods—for hours at a time, over a span of at least two to nine months—in order to see a difference. But patience pays off: the longer you wear it, the more likely it is that the scar will dissipate to some extent. Of course, these sheets work best over new scars, but they also can make a difference with old ones. Even acne scarring— thick raised scars, not pits—can be reduced if the scars have been around for less than 16 years. As wonderful and hopeful as this all sounds, be aware that the word reduce can be a suspect term. Do not give these a try if you are hoping for extraordinary results, of the kind the advertising implies. Dr. Loren Engrav, associate director and chief of plastic surgery for the University of Washington burn unit at Harborview Medical Center, Seattle, explains that the "silicone strips are standard treatment for helping dissipate scars, and though the results may be good, they are absolutely not a miracle."

Some women buy the sheets to use over stretch marks, but there is no clinical evidence that this product will have any effect on them whatsoever, and the Rejuveness company will not guarantee their product for this use. These sheets use a flattening process, not a raising process, which would be required for stretch marks. Rejuveness, at (800) 588-7455 in the United States, and (800) 361-0778 in Canada, isn't for everyone, but if you are willing to be persistent, it is absolutely worth a try.

Renee Guinot (Skin Care Only)

What's in a name? If it's French, usually a high price tag and the promise of "European" skin care. Of course, in Europe the women praise American know-how when it comes to skin care—but I guess the grass is always greener in someone else's lawn. As it turns out, French products are no different from American products. All the gimmicky plant extracts and vitamins, standard thickening agents, basic detergent cleansing agents, preservatives, slip agents, emollients, lightweight silicone moisturizing gels, and problematic ingredients are virtually identical, but the claims have a French accent.

Renee Guinot is a long-established salon/spa line of skin-care products with a reputation for being an elegant, elite, serious, and intricately designed way to take care of skin. The price tag definitely makes them elite, and the packaging can be described as elegant, but in terms of formulation these products are rather ho-hum, with some downright inferior formulations. Many of them seem old-fashioned and in desperate need of an overhaul.

Despite the extravagant-sounding product names, this line seems unusually over-priced for what you get, and in need of revamping. I could go on at length about the claims, ranging from "remodels your silhouette" to "blackheads disappear," "trans-forms the appearance of oily skin," "diffuses the water needed to keep skin moist all day," and (this one's my favorite) "dynamizes the complexion, smoothing away signs of fatigue." It would take a book to do justice to this kind of obtuse profundity. That's not to say there aren't some good products mixed in here, but they just can't do what the claims lead you to believe. Renee Guinot's name turns out to be the most impressive part of this skin-care line, which means its elite, serious image is just that: image. Renee Guinot's customer service number is (800) 748-5825.

☒ **Gel Surnettoyant Peaux Grasses Super Cleansing Gel Oily Skin, Rinse with Water** (*$16.50 for 6.7 ounces*) is a standard detergent-based cleanser with a handful of plant extracts. For some reason the formulators decided to throw in some sulfur, which can irritate the skin and the eyes. Sulfur can be a disinfectant for blemishes, but it's rinsed down the drain in a cleanser.

☒ **Lait Demaquillant Hydra-Douceur Hydra Soft Cleansing Milk Dry and**

Sensitive Skin *($19.50 for 6.7 ounces)* is a standard mineral oil–based wipe-off cleanser that can leave a greasy film on the skin.

☹ **Lait Demaquillant Parfait Perfect Cleansing Milk Face and Eyes All Skin Types** *($19.50 for 6.7 ounces)* is similar to the product above, but this one contains lanolin, and can be even more greasy.

☹ **Purifiant Biologique, Deep Cleansing Cream All Skin Types Rinse with Water** *($35 for 5 ounces)* is similar to the two products above, and the same review applies.

☺ **$$$ Purifiant Biologique Gentle Wash and Cleansing Cream All Skin Types** *($26.50 for 5 ounces)* is a more emollient rinse-off cleanser that contains several waxy thickening ingredients that could be a problem for oily or combination skin types. This can be an option for someone with dry skin.

☹ **Refreshing Cleansing Milk with Flower Extracts for All Skin Types** *($19.50 for 6.7 ounces)* is a standard mineral oil–based wipe-off cleanser. There are several ingredients that would not make someone with oily or combination skin very happy, and who needs an expensive cold cream?

☹ **Lotion Yeux, Eye Makeup Remover Lotion Anti-Irritation, Soothes, Softens** *($19.50 for 0.5 ounce)* contains mostly water, slip agent, thickener, silicone, plant extracts, fragrance, and preservatives. This is a very simple silicone-based wipe-off cleanser. It shouldn't ever be necessary to wipe off eye makeup.

☹ **Lotion Seche, Clarifying Lotion Oily Skin Purifies and Matifies** *($27 for 6.7 ounces)* contains mostly water, plant extracts, slip agents, sulfur, preservatives, and fragrance. Sulfur can disinfect, but it can also be an irritant. It is an option for oily skin, but one I don't recommend, because there are far less irritating ways to treat breakouts.

☺ **$$$ Lotion Tonique Hydra-Douceur Hydra Soft Toning Lotion Dry and Sensitive Skin, Alcohol-Free** *($19.50 for 6.7 ounces)* is simply water, slip agent, plant extracts, glycerin, preservatives, and fragrance. This is a lot of money for something that's mostly water and glycerin; it is a standard irritant-free toner, if you aren't sensitive to the fragrance in here.

☺ **$$$ Lotion Tonique Rafraichissant Fresh Toning Lotion All Skin Types Alcohol-Free** *($19.50 for 6.7 ounces)* is similar to the product above, but with rose water (which is glycerin and rose fragrance). The same basic review applies.

☹ **$$$ Refreshing Toning Lotion with Flower Extracts for All Skin Types** *($19.50 for 6.7 ounces)* is mainly just rose water, slip agents, preservatives, and silicone. This is a fairly do-nothing toner that isn't bad for skin, it just doesn't do anything.

☺ **$$$ Base Hydratante, Continue Day Long Moisturizer with Essential Oils, Dry/Dehydrated Skin** *($34.50 for 1.7 ounces)* contains mostly water, thickener, slip agent, more thickeners, acrylate, shea butter, plant oil, water-binding agent, fragrance, vitamin E, preservatives, and fragrant oils. This would be a good moisturizer for someone with dry skin, but the essential oils are a minute part of the formula and they are primarily fragrance additives, not emollients for the skin.

☺ $$$ **Creme Fermete 777, Restructurant Firming Night Cream 777, with Cell Vitalizers, Slackened Skin** *($38.50 for 1.7 ounces)* contains mostly water, thickeners, slip agent, lanolin, water-binding agents, plant extract, fragrance, and preservatives. This rather standard moisturizer has a small amount of collagen and something called serum protein, which supposedly will help support your skin; they can't, but they are good moisturizing agents.

☹ **Gommage Douceur, Gentle Exfoliating Cream, for a Renewed Complexion, All Skin Types, Even Sensitive** *($36 for 1.7 ounces)* contains mostly water, clay, petrolatum, thickeners, mineral oil, silicones, acrylates, plant oils, fragrance, and preservatives. With all the greasy ingredients in here, this is hardly good for any skin type. This scrub can leave an oily residue on the skin that can inhibit, not help, exfoliation.

☺ $$$ **Hydrallergic, Day/Night Desensitizing Care, Ultra-Sensitive Skin** *($40 for 1.6 ounces)* is accompanied by claims about taking care of ultra-sensitive skin. That is pushing things when the product contains fragrance, polystyrene (a strong hair-spray ingredient), and vitamin E. All of these are potential irritants. Other than that, this is a good but ordinary moisturizer for someone with dry skin, though it is not recommended for daytime use because it lacks a sunscreen.

☺ $$$ **Hydrazone Moisturizing Face Cream, Dry Skin** *($67 for 1.6 ounces)* contains mostly water, plant oil, mineral oil, thickeners, shea butter, more thickeners, more plant oil, silicone, plant extract, water-binding agent, preservatives, and fragrance. This is a very good, but extremely overpriced, standard moisturizer for someone with dry skin.

☺ $$$ **Liftosome, Day/Night Cream, All Skin Types** *($72 for 1.6 ounces)* contains mostly water, slip agent, thickeners, shea butter, silicone, more thickeners, water-binding agents, plant oil, more thickeners, preservatives, and fragrance. Without a sunscreen, this moisturizer is acceptable for use only at night, but it is a very good moisturizer for someone with dry skin. Several thickening agents in here make it problematic for other skin types.

☺ $$$ **LongueVie Cellulaire, Vital Face Care, Day/Night Cream, Triple Action Formula** *($67 for 1.6 ounces)* contains mostly water, several thickeners, plant oil, more thickeners, silicone, more thickeners, preservatives, fragrance, and a long list of water-binding agents. The extensive list of water-binding agents in this product would have been interesting, but they are present in such minuscule amounts they don't really add up to much. This is still a good moisturizer for someone with dry skin, but only at night, because there is no sunscreen.

☺ $$$ Surgenerant Profond, Skin Revitalizing Concentrate, Day/Night *($85 for 1 ounce)* contains mostly water, silicone, thickener, slip agents, more thickeners, more silicone, preservatives, and fragrance. This is a good lightweight moisturizer for someone with normal to dry skin, but without a sunscreen it would be appropriate only at night.

☺ $$$ Surtenseur Cou, Firming Neck Serum Cream, Tightening, Anti-Wrinkle *($40 for 1 ounce)* contains mostly water, water-binding agent, thickeners, shea butter, silicone, slip agent, more thickeners, egg white, preservative, and fragrance. Egg white doesn't tighten skin, but this is a good basic moisturizer for someone with dry skin.

☹ Teint Hydratant, Tinted Moisturizing Cream, All Dehydrated Skin *($32 for 1.7 ounces)* contains mostly water, thickeners, shea butter, water-binding agents, glycerin, silicones, more thickeners, plant oil, silica, preservatives, and fragrance. Without a sunscreen, a tinted moisturizer doesn't make much sense for daytime. This product is not recommended.

☺ $$$ Anti-Fatigue Yeux, Gel Crystal Anti-Fatigue Gel for the Eyes, Heavy Eyelids, Shadows, Bags *($28 for 0.5 ounce)* contains mostly water, glycerin, slip agent, plant extracts, thickener, preservatives, and fragrance. Absolutely nothing in this product will have any effect on shadows, bags, or heavy eyelids. This is little more than a lightweight gel with some ordinary moisturizing agents.

☺ $$$ Anti-Rides Yeux, Cream for the Eyes, Wrinkles, Crow's Feet *($34 for 0.5 ounce)* contains mostly water, thickeners, slip agent, shea butter, silicone, more thickeners, plant oil, water-binding agent, and preservatives. This is a good moisturizer for someone with dry skin, but it can't take care of wrinkles any more than the one above can take of sagging skin!

☹ Base Protectrice Anti-Rides, Anti-Wrinkle Day Long Protection, with Cell Vitalizers, Devitalized Skin *($34 for 1.7 ounces)* contains mostly water, slip agents, several thickeners, preservatives, water-binding agents, fragrance, and egg white. This unbelievably ordinary, do-nothing product isn't even a good basic moisturizer. It is mostly waxy thickening agents and some token amounts of collagen and elastin. This product is not recommended.

☹ Creme Anti-Irritation 600A, Soothing Repair Treatment 600A, with Natural Active Ingredients, Irritated Skin *($30 for 1.7 ounces)* contains both cornstarch and lavender oil, which can be problematic for sensitive skin. Cornstarch can be an irritant, and lavender oil can be a photosensitizer.

☺ $$$ Creme Anti-Rides 888, Regenerate, Anti-Wrinkle Night Cream 888, with Cell Vitalizers, Devitalized Skin *($48.50 for 1.7 ounces)* contains mostly water, petrolatum, thickeners, water-binding agents, slip agent, plant extracts, preservatives, and fragrance. This is a very good basic moisturizer for someone with dry skin.

☹ **Creme Anti-Rougeurs 109, Diffuse Redness Treatment 109, with Natural Active Ingredients, Blotchy, Sensitive Skin** *($34 for 1.7 ounces)* contains nothing that makes it appropriate for someone with sensitive or blotchy skin. It contains water, slip agent, thickeners, silicone, plant extract, preservatives, and fragrance.

☹ **Creme Normalisant Matifiant, Matte Finish Normalizer, with Plant Extracts, Oily Skin with Blemish Problems** *($27 for 1.7 ounces)* contains mostly water, thickeners, slip agents, more thickeners, silicone, preservatives, plant extracts, salicylic acid, soothing agent, and fragrance. Several thickening agents in this product are known for clogging pores. This product is not recommended.

☹ **Gel Regulateur Intensif, Oil-Free Normalizing Gel, One Month Treatment with Plant Extracts, Oily Skin with Blemish Problems** *($34.50 for 1.6 ounces)* contains mostly water, water-binding agents, acrylates, thickeners, more acrylates, witch hazel, plant extracts, camphor, and fragrance. Nothing in here can reduce oil or stop blemishes. If anything, several ingredients in here can clog pores and irritate the skin.

☺ **$$$ Masque Anti-Rides Defatigant, Instant Relaxing Anti-Wrinkle Mask with Cell Vitalizers, Devitalized Skin** *($31 for 1.7 ounces)* contains mostly water, mineral oil, thickeners, glycerin, more thickeners, shea butter, water-binding agents, plant extract, soothing agent, preservatives, and fragrance. This would be a good mask for someone with dry skin, but the price is outrageous for a standard, mineral oil–based product.

☹ **Masque Dermique Purifant, Instant Purifying Mask, with Plant Extracts, Oily Skin with Blemish Problems** *($24.50 for 1.7 ounces)* contains mostly water, thickener, clay, glycerin, more thickener, balm mint, preservatives, and camphor. Clay can absorb oil, but the mint and camphor in here can irritate skin, and that's not a great trade-off.

☹ **Masque Essential Dynamisant, Instant Radiance Mask, with Essential Oils, All Types of Dehydration** *($28 for 1.7 ounces)* contains mostly petrolatum, water, lanolin, mineral oil, thickeners, plant oils, camphor, menthol, and preservatives. This is one greasy mask. It would be great for someone with dry skin, but why menthol and camphor are in here is a complete mystery: they can irritate the skin.

☹ **Masque Yeux, Instant Eye Mask, Swollen Eye Lids, Shadows, Wrinkles** *($31 for 1 ounce)* contains mostly water, slip agent, witch hazel, plant extract, egg white, and fragrance. This is a lot of money for water and egg white. Surely you have something better to do with your money!

☹ **Correcteur Traitant, Spot Treatment Concealer, with Plant Extracts** *($16 for 0.4 ounce)* contains mostly water, thickener, clay, more thickeners, preservatives, plant extracts, salicylic acid, and camphor. Several thickening agents in here are well-known for causing breakouts. Salicylic acid may be helpful, but not with camphor and not in this kind of formulation, at least not for someone trying to deal with breakouts.

Renew (Skin Care Only)

In regard to the skin-care line Renew, which advertises in small newspapers throughout the United States and Canada without providing a referring phone number (I have not been able to locate one either), I received the following letter from a reader of my newsletter:

Dear Paula,

I am 46 years old and recently came to the conclusion that there must be something better out there for my skin. About a month ago I came across a full-page advertisement in our local newspaper for Renew Skin Care Formula. I have been using their products for several months and am not sure if they are doing anything for my skin or if they are worth the money. I would appreciate if you would evaluate the products and give me your opinion. Thanks again for all you do, Paula.

Eileen, Colorado Springs, Colorado

My response was as follows:

Dear Eileen,

Renew Skin Care Formula products are nothing more than a poor assortment of AHA products with a cleanser and a poor version of a vitamin C liquid. These "amazing new face-lift-in-a-jar" products you've been using since July clearly are not so amazing or you would not be wondering if they work and writing me. Amazing products should perform amazingly, don't you think? I wonder how many women have been duped by this ad, with a smiling Terri Welles telling you to expect unbelievable results. I've seen it in almost every local newspaper all over the United States and Canada. What a sad, expensive mistake for many women. Not only are these products a waste of money, but they are unnecessarily expensive, poorly formulated (at least when it comes to the AHA and vitamin C products), and the line does not include a sunscreen, so women are left with no way to really stop wrinkling and take good care of their skin. All this from some "famous" plastic surgeon. I would hate to be this doctor's patient. What dermatologist or plastic surgeon would encourage all this nonsense without discussing Retin-A, Renova, well-formulated AHA products, or sunscreen?

Here's what Eileen's hard-earned money *($65 for six products totaling 7 ounces)* bought her:

☹ **$$$ Glycolic Facial Shampoo** *(2 ounces)* is a standard detergent-based water-soluble cleanser, except the cleansing agent is extremely drying for most skin types. Plus, it contains citrus oils, which can irritate the skin and eyes. It also contains a small amount of glycolic acid, but its effectiveness is washed down the drain.

☹ $$$ **Fruity Skin Tonic** *(2 ounces)* is a glycolic acid–based toner, but this product has the wrong pH to be an effective exfoliant, and the citrus ingredients in here provide no benefit but can definitely irritate the skin.

☹ $$$ **Oil-Free Moisture Gel** *(2 ounces)* could have been a good lightweight AHA product in a light moisturizing base, but the pH isn't adequate for exfoliating the skin.

☺ $$$ **Topical Vitamin C** *(0.25 ounce)* is just what the name says, but it isn't that different from Avon's product Anew Formula C Treatment Capsules. Vitamin C won't save skin or change it, and if you are interested there are far less expensive versions than this one.

☺ $$$ **Wrinkle Cream with Topical C and AHAs** *(0.25 ounce)* contains mostly water, film former, thickeners, water-binding agents, lactic acid, egg white, and preservatives. The amount of AHA in this product isn't even 2%, which makes it a moisturizing ingredient, not an exfoliant. The vitamin C, though in a different form than that used in the product above, is also unstable and has no proven effect on the skin; and about the egg white I have no comment.

☺ $$$ **Vitamin Enriched Natural Moisture Factor** *(0.5 ounce)* contains mostly water-binding agent, thickeners, vitamins, and silicone oil. This would be a good moisturizer for someone with normal to dry skin, but that's about it.

Revlon

I reported in the past that Revlon improved its bottom line by becoming a public stock. Revlon models Naomi Campbell, Cindy Crawford, and Elle Macpherson made a personal appearance on the floor of the New York Stock Exchange the day of the initial public offering. You can imagine the commotion that ensued! Revlon has maintained their profitability with two remarkably successful product lines: first, the Age Defying products, and then ColorStay. The ColorStay and Age Defying lines serve two distinct age groups, the former being the 35-and-under crowd and the latter those over 35, and they serve them well, with some excellent options. The first ColorStay product was ColorStay Lipstick (which was really a clone of LipSexxxy by Ultima II, a company owned by Revlon). It was advertised as the first lipstick that wouldn't kiss off. Well, it does kiss off if it's a really good kiss, but if it's your average little friendly peck on the cheek, then it pretty much stays on your lips with no telltale imprint. This single product spawned a new generation of lipsticks with a consistency that is ultra-matte and dry.

To attract the young teen and twentysomething crowd, Revlon is one of the few drugstore lines with a color line to compete with Hard Candy and Urban Decay at the department store. Street Wear is Revlon's line of extreme color nail polishes, lip glosses, and face shine. They are reasonably priced (under $5) and if you are in the market for lime green nail polish, intense shine face powder, or yellow lip gloss, it beats the $15 price tags for these items at the department store and the quality in the Revlon products is as good if not better.

Revlon's standard lines—Eterna '27', Natural Collagen Complex, and Moon Drops—are still around and have some great products to consider, while Revlon Results, a quasi-AHA line, has been put out to pasture. For more information about Revlon call (800) 4-REVLON.

Revlon Skin Care

☹ **Moon Drops Extra Gentle Cleansing Cream Water-Rinseable for Sensitive/Delicate** *($5.99 for 4 ounces)* is a standard mineral oil–based wipe-off cleanser that can leave a greasy film on the skin. This isn't water rinseable in the least.

☹ **Moon Drops Replenishing Cleansing Lotion Water Rinseable for Normal to Dry** *($5.99 for 8 ounces)* is similar to the one above and the same review applies.

☺ **30 Second Eye Makeup Remover** *($4.99 for 2 ounces)* is a standard detergent-based wipe-off cleanser. It will take off eye makeup, but why wipe and pull at the eyes if you don't have to?

☺ **ColorStay Makeup Remover Pads** *($5.47 for 80 pads)* is a standard detergent-based makeup remover that definitely will help you (and you will need help) to get the ColorStay products off.

☺ **Waterproof Eye Makeup Remover** *($4.99 for 0.8 ounce)* is a greasy mess. It contains mostly petrolatum, mineral oil, thickeners, and preservatives. It will take off waterproof eye makeup, but that's the problem with wearing waterproof makeup.

☺ **Moon Drops Softening Toner Normal to Dry** *($5.99 for 8 ounces)* is a good irritant-free toner that contains mostly water, slip agents, vitamins, water-binding agents, and preservatives.

☹ **Age Defying Performance Skin Care Face Cream, SPF 15** *($12.61 for 1.75 ounces)* and **Age Defying Performance Skin Care Oil-Free Face Lotion, SPF 15** *($12.61 for 1.7 ounces)* are both average moisturizers but poor sunscreens; neither contains avobenzone, titanium dioxide, or zinc oxide, and therefore neither is recommended.

☺ **Eterna '27' All Day Moisture Lotion** *($11.99 for 2 ounces)* is a very emollient, good moisturizer for dry skin. It contains mostly water, slip agent, thickener, plant oil, more thickeners, silicone, water-binding agents, more thickeners, more water-binding agents, and preservatives.

The Reviews R

☺ **Eterna '27' All Day Moisture Cream** *($11.99 for 1 ounce)* is very similar to the lotion above, but with more thickeners and mineral oil. It would be good for dry skin.

☹ **Eterna '27' with Exclusive Progenitin** *($15.69 for 2 ounces)* is going to sound strange, but remember, I'm only describing this product, I didn't formulate it. The active ingredient is called pregnenolone acetate. It is derived from the urine of pregnant women, and is considered an anti-inflammatory agent. Therefore, this moisturizer is actually a very mild topical cortisone-type cream. In my opinion, unless your dry skin is a result of slight dermatitis, this cream is unnecessary because cortisone can eventually break down the skin.

☹ **Moon Drops Nourishing Moisture Lotion SPF 6 Normal to Dry** *($6.93 for 4 ounces)* with its SPF 6 is bad enough, but this product also doesn't contain avobenzone, zinc oxide, or titanium dioxide, and is not recommended.

☹ **Moon Drops Soothing Moisture Cream SPF 6 Extra Moist for Sensitive/ Delicate Skin** *($5.99 for 4 ounces)* is similar to the one above, and the same review as above applies.

☹ **Natural Collagen Complex Protective Moisture Cream with SPF 6** *($8.92 for 3 ounces)* is similar to the one above, and the same review as above applies.

☹ **Natural Collagen Complex Protective Moisture Lotion SPF 6 with Vitamin E** *($8.92 for 3 ounces)* is similar to the product above, and the same review applies.

☹ **Natural Collagen Complex Protective Eye Cream with SPF 4** *($7.99 for 0.5 ounce)* is a nonchemical sunscreen that would be good for someone with normal to dry skin, but SPF 4—this is a joke, right?

☹ **Pure Radiance Self Tanner for Face SPF 8 Light to Medium** *($5.33 for 2 ounces)* with its SPF 8 isn't worth the trouble when there are so many good SPF 15s out there, plus this one doesn't contain avobenzone, zinc oxide, or titanium dioxide, and is not recommended.

☹ **Pure Radiance Self Tanner for Face SPF 8, Medium to Deep** *($5.33 for 2 ounces)* is similar to the one above, and the same review applies.

☹ **Pure Radiance Tinted Face Creme SPF 8 Light to Medium** *($5.33 for 2 ounces)* has the same review as the one above.

☹ **Pure Radiance Tinted Face Creme SPF 8 Medium to Deep** *($5.33 for 2 ounces)* has the same review as the one above.

Revlon Makeup

FOUNDATION: Revlon provides testers for some of its new foundations, which makes it more likely that you'll be able to find the right color.

☺ **Age Defying Makeup with SPF 10** *($9.34)* is best for someone with normal to somewhat dry skin, and provides light to almost medium coverage. The nonchemical (titanium dioxide–based) SPF 10 is good, though SPF 15 would be better. The color selection and texture are both quite good.

☺ **Age Defying Extra Cover Creme Makeup with SPF 12** *($9.34)* comes in colors that are all surprisingly excellent, the texture is very smooth and emollient, and the titanium dioxide–based SPF 12 is a nice touch. For someone with normal to dry skin, this is a definite option if testers are available, and they often are.

☹ **Age Defying Smoothing Powder** *($6.69)* comes in nine shades of which only two look like skin tone, the rest are two peach or pink to recommend.

☺ **ColorStay Makeup SPF 6** *($9.34)* is beyond matte, beyond no shine, and far beyond the claim of "It won't come off on him." It won't come off even when you want it to. This is one of the most stubborn makeups I've ever seen. Get it on right the first time, because once it dries, it won't budge. I didn't notice in the daylight that I had a bit too much foundation above my mouth and a little streaking on my nose. All the blending in the world, even with my oily skin, wouldn't smooth it out. It was there to stay. If you get even the slightest wrong color it can look like a chalky mask. Removing it at night takes some effort, including several attempts with your cleanser and a washcloth. ColorStay Foundation is appropriate only for someone with truly oily skin and a deft hand at blending. The SPF is not one you can rely on; though the SPF is titanium dioxide–based, the SPF 6 is too low a number. Nevertheless, the colors are superior, except for the lightest shade, Ivory, which can be too pink; the rest are stunning neutral shades, in a range of 12 colors. There are no shades for very light or very deep to dark skin tones, which is a serious limitation, but the medium skin tones have a wide selection.

☺ **ColorStay Lite Makeup SPF 15** *($9.69)*. Kudos to Revlon for responding quickly to a major complaint about their ColorStay foundation. The Lite version is an excellent matte foundation with a wonderful nonchemical (titanium dioxide) SPF. If you have oily skin, this is a must-try foundation! All the colors are excellent— there's not one in the bunch you need to avoid—and the color range is fairly extensive! One complaint: The container for the foundation is a terrible design. It stands on its head, which isn't helpful for this very liquid foundation. The only way to put it down is on its side, and then it tends to run out. Not good.

☺ **New Complexion One-Step Makeup SPF 15** *($8.78)*. This cream-to-powder foundation is virtually identical with Clinique's City Base Compact Foundation. I simply could not tell the difference in a side-by-side face test of the two products. They felt, looked, applied, and wore the same. Revlon offers more colors than City Base, and the shades are, for the most part, fairly neutral, but the range of tones is strange. The selection of lighter shades is extremely limited, and the darker shades tend to be a bit too coppery. If you have a more medium skin tone, you're in luck; all the comments about Clinique City Base Foundation apply to Revlon's New Complexion Makeup (that means that if you have normal to slightly dry skin this is a great option, but it can be too greasy for someone with oily skin). **Avoid** Natural Beige, Cool Beige, Warm Beige, and Sun Beige.

☺ **New Complexion Even Out Make Up Oil-free SPF 20** *($10.69)* is a mixed bag and I'm not sure whether to recommend it or tell you to wait until Revlon gets the kinks out. This foundation is trying to be a little bit of everything and it comes up far too short in some areas yet way ahead in others. The sunscreen is excellent and one of the better combinations for dry skin on the market, using both zinc oxide and titanium oxide! Still, the color selection is 50/50; half of the shades are really too peach, pink, or ash to be suitable on most skin tones and the other half are a strange jumble and, to say the least, quite limited. The consistency is rather light and moist, which would be great for a sheer finish if you have dry skin. Yet, this product contains salicylic acid (BHA) which is a waste in a foundation. Not everyone should be using a BHA all over their face, or using it every day. But not to worry, the pH of this product is too high for it to be effective as an exfoliant. All in all there are more problems with this foundation than positive points, and I wouldn't use it over Revlon's New Complexion One-Step Makeup SPF 15 reviewed above. If you do consider this product, the only shades that look like skin are Sand Beige, Caramel, and Natural Tan.

☹ **New Complexion Makeup for Normal to Dry with SPF 4** *($8.75)* has been improved. In the past, all the shades for this foundation were too pink, orange, peach, or rose. However, Revlon has recently added new colors that are much more neutral and impressive. Still, there are never any testers, and SPF 4 is too low to provide reliable protection.

☺ <u>CONCEALER:</u> **New Complexion Concealer** *($6.75)* comes in three shades: Light, Medium, and Deep. This lightweight concealer leaves a sheer residue that covers beautifully. It is one of the better concealers I have tested. **ColorStay Concealer** *($7.29)* ranks up there with the best of them. It absolutely doesn't crease, stays well, isn't as heavy or thick as the ColorStay foundation, and comes in four very good neutral colors. It tends to be better for someone who needs more coverage rather than less, and it can be a problem if you want to hide instead of accentuate the lines under the eyes, but it does take good care of dark circles all day long.

☺ **New Complexion Oil-Free Concealer** *($6.29)* is a very good matte concealer with a dry, smooth finish. It blends on evenly and doesn't crease into lines, which should make it worth checking out. Unfortunately, several of the colors are very strange, ranging from a very drab yellow shade to brownish peach. Check this one closely in daylight to be sure the color doesn't look strange around your eyes.

☹ **New Complexion Correct & Conceal Blemish Stick** *($8.59)* contains 1% BHA, which isn't the best in a makeup product, but again, not to worry: the pH of this product is over 5, and that means it has no exfoliation properties, which means it is completely wasted in here. While that isn't problematic for skin, it isn't helpful either. What is damaging to the skin is the menthol in this concealer, which is unnecessarily irritating and completely purposeless for the skin. I won't even get into the strange assortment of colors this product has.

☹ **Age Defying Concealer with Nonchemical SPF 12** *($6.59)* comes in a a just passable range of colors, but it creases into the lines around the eyes as the day goes by, and that helps accentuate wrinkles, not diminish them. The titanium dioxide–based SPF 12 is nice but the application leaves much to be desired.

☹ **POWDER: Love Pat Pressed Powder** *($8.34)* colors are too pink or peach for most skin tones.

☺ **ColorStay Powder** *($9.34)* is virtually identical to the Almay Amazing Lasting Powder reviewed at the beginning of this book. My review for the Revlon version is better. The application is similar to most cream-to-powder foundations, but this one then dries into place and doesn't budge. If you have any dry skin or lines and the powder slips into them it will make them look more pronounced and there is no way to smooth over this. For a cream-to-powder foundation this is an option, but it's really best for someone with normal to oily skin.

☹ **New Complexion Powder Oil-Control Normal to Oily Skin** *($6.59)* is a standard talc-based powder with a great color selection. It does blend on smooth and soft, but nothing about this product will control oil in the least and most of the colors are too peach or pink to recommend.

☺ **Age Defying Pressed Loose Powder** *($9.34)* is a puzzle. Pressed loose powder is a contradiction in terms, isn't it? This product is just a lightweight pressed powder that goes on rather sheer but slightly chalky. It has a silky texture, and the colors are OK.

☺ **Street Wear All Over Face Shine** *($4.99)* is, as the name indicates, a face highlighter with sparkle. It goes on sheer and the shine is tenacious. If you want all-over shine this is as good as any.

☺ **BLUSH: Age Defying Cheek Color** *($9.34)* is a cream blush with a slight powdery finish, no matter what Revlon calls it. Cream blushes are hard to blend and don't hold up all that well during the day. Powder blushes rest on top of the skin, while cream blushes merge into it; that's the nature of creams. Unless you have flawless skin, they tend to accentuate every dent and imperfection. If you have perfect, even skin, you may like this blush—it does have a great texture—but if not, you're likely to have the same problems I did, plus all the colors are slightly shiny. **ColorStay Cheek Color** *($8.56)* is virtually identical to Almay's Amazing Lasting Cheek Color and the same review applies.

☺ **Naturally Glamorous Blush-On** *($8.03)* has a great color selection and a smooth application. Most of the colors are excellent (I've been wearing Toast of New York for years as a blush and/or contour color).

☺ **EYESHADOW:** The **Custom Eyes Single Eyeshadows** *($3.10)* will work for anyone who wants a soft, natural-looking eye design. Be careful—not all of the colors are matte, and many have quite a bit of shine. The only ones I recommend are the matte shades, and they are nicely, and accurately, labeled as matte.

☹ **Overtime Eyeshadows** *($5.69)* come in sets of two or four colors, respectively, that are either too shiny, or in strange combinations.

☹ **Age Defying Eye Color** *($6.59)* is a cream eyeshadow that dries to a powder finish, but before it can do that, it seeps into the lines around the eyes and emphasizes every wrinkle. In any case, cream eyeshadows are just hard to work with; they're awkward to blend with the applicator they come with, and even harder to blend with your fingers. They're supposed to blend out softer than powders, but I don't find that to be true. Also, cream eyeshadows crease faster than powders, and it's hard to blend other colors over them to build any kind of interesting, blended eye design.

☹ **ColorStay Eyecolor** *($5.48)* comes in a tube, which is not my favorite way of applying shadow. Blendability is essential, and that isn't easy with such a dry, immovable eye color. These colors are all about as stubborn as they come: The shadow "grabs" before you can blend it. Subsequent applications are impossible, and once the color "sets" efforts to blend result in clumps and eyeshadow fingerprints. The only positive point is that they can make it through the day when others may long since have smeared and disappeared.

☺ **EYE AND BROW SHAPER:** **Time Liner Eye Pencil** *($4.99)* is a great standard pencil with a smooth creamy application. **Jetliner Intense** *($4.84)* is a liquid eyeliner with a soft, pen-shaped tip. It applies a very dramatic, intense line. **Fine Line Natural Brow Pencil** *($5.99)* is an ultra-thin pencil with a twist-up applicator. It also takes refills. It can easily stroke on thinner lines than other pens for a more natural-looking brow.

☺ **ColorStay Brow Color** *($6.94)* is a two-sided product: one side is a mascara-like wand with color to stroke on a brow, and the other is a pencil. In some ways this is the best of both worlds. If you're a woman who uses a pencil but also likes applying a brow thickener to make your brows look denser and keep them in line, it's all right here. The brow gel is a great product that goes on easily and stays very well. The pencil is just a pencil, nothing special, and it doesn't stay any better than most pencils. Still, the two-in one gimmick is appealing. **ColorStay EyeLiner** *($5.48)* is a standard, twist-up eyeliner with a creamy application that then dries to an almost immoveable finish. That staying power is nice, but it doesn't hold up well over moisturizers or moisturizing foundations and concealers.

☺ **StreetWear Jumbo All Over Pencil** *($3.99)* and **StreetWear Slim All Over Pencil** *($3.99)* are standard two-sided pencils that have a creamy finish. One side is shiny and the other matte, in an interesting group of colors. They work, but this is about preference in terms of color choice not application.

☹ **Revlon ColorStay Liquid Liner** *($6.30)* has a strange, hard applicator that scratches at the eye as you apply it. Why Revlon couldn't make this a brush is beyond me. It does stay well, as the name implies, but getting it on in the first place isn't easy. **SoftStroke PowderLiner** *($6.94)* does have a slight powdery finish but all the shades are slightly shiny and the color tends to pill and chip when blended.

☺ <u>LIPSTICK AND LIP PENCIL:</u> Most of the **Moon Drops Moisture Creme** *($6.20)* and **Super Lustrous Creme or Shine** *($6.20)* lipsticks have great colors and smooth, creamy, not glossy, textures. **Moon Drops Color Lock Anti-Feathering Lip Base** *($6.20)* really does keep lipstick from bleeding—what a find! **MoistureStay Lipcolor** *($7.99)* is moist and creamy, not glossy, and relatively matte, a nice combination for someone who wanted to like the original ColorStay but found it too lip-crackingly dry. **Time Liner Lip Pencil** *($4.93)* comes in a nice variety of colors and has a good soft texture. **ColorStay Lip Liner** *($4.89)* is undeniably tenacious and less greasy than most.

☺ **StreetWear Lip Gloss** *($3.99)* is a standard lip gloss with an angle; the colors offered include green, brown-black, blue, purple, and a few other less than traditional shades. These work as well as any lip gloss; it's only the color that differentiates this group of products. **New Complexion Condition & Color Lipstick** *($5.39)* lets Revlon join the trend of pencil lip products. One side is slightly more glossy than the other in this two-side application of color, but both provide a nice creamy texture. Sharpening is tricky but obviously essential and, from my perspective not worth the trouble. Still, it can be a convenient way to apply color.

☺ **Line & Shine** *($7.64)* is a two-in-one combination that appears to give you more for your money. What you really end up with are tiny amounts of each. Line & Shine comes with a decent but standard lip gloss at one end and a nice soft lip pencil at the other. It does seem minimally more convenient than packing two regular-size products, so maybe it's an option for your purse, nice and compact, but why bother with the extra product?

☺ **ColorStay Lipstick** *($4.95)* from Revlon has been revamped, and they did a pretty good job of making it slightly, and I mean *slightly*, less ultra-matte. That reduced the chipping/peeling problem (the lipstick tended to come off in chunks or rolled off in clumps, not nearly as pretty as Cindy Crawford made it seem in the commercials), but it still peels off from the inside of the lip out, not exactly a pretty picture.

☹ **ColorStay Lip Tint SPF 15** *($7.95)* isn't anywhere near as drying as the original ColorStay Lipstick, but the sunscreen component lacks ingredients that will protect your lips from UVA rays.

☺ <u>MASCARA:</u> **Lengthwise Mascara** *($5.48)* is excellent, and I strongly recommend it. **Lashful Mascara** *($5.48)* is another very good mascara that goes on well and really makes it through the entire day. **Lashful Mascara Curvaceous** *($5.48)* is identical in application to the regular Lashful only with a curved brush. This one is about preference, though I find the curved brush more difficult to use and it doesn't improve application in the least.

☺ **StreetWear Mascara** *($3.99)* is an assortment of uniquely colored mascaras ranging from blue to green. When you have these kinds of mascara colors, does application really matter?

☹ **ColorStay Lashcolor** *($5.99)* goes on quickly and definitely lengthens, but it tends to clump.

☹ <u>BRUSHES:</u> Revlon has several brushes in good shapes and sizes, but the **Blush Brush** *($6.50)* and **Eyeshadow Brush** *($4.25)* have oversized handles that are cumbersome and hard to carry in a makeup bag for touch-ups during the day. Also, the bristles are too soft to apply the color evenly.

ROC (Skin Care Only/Canada Only)

ROC prides itself on gentle, sensitive skin care. It would have been nice if they had been that way when I tried to contact them for information. Nevertheless, this line does contain far fewer irritating ingredients than most cosmetics lines do. There are a handful of exceptions, but for the most part these simple formulations are distinctive for their concern in preventing skin irritation or skin sensitivity. The product line as a whole is definitely a consideration for sensitive or dry-skin types, though if you have oily or blemish-prone skin there really aren't any options or solutions among these products. For more information about ROC in Canada call (519) 836-6500; in the US call (800) 526-3967. All prices are in Canadian dollars.

☹ **Cleanser and Refresher for Face and Eyes 2 In 1** *($16 for 200 ml)* is a standard wipe-off makeup remover. Wiping off makeup is not recommended because pulling at the skin can encourage sagging.

☹ **Cleansing Milk Pure and Balancing, Normal to Combination Skin** *($14.50 for 200 ml)* contains isopropyl myristate, an ingredient known for blocking pores. This product is not recommended.

☹ **Cleansing Milk Pure and Soothing, Dry Skin** *($14.50 for 200 ml)* contains lanolin oil, which is a known skin sensitizer, and that's a little surprising; however it is also exceptionally emollient if you aren't allergic to it. Nevertheless, this is a cleanser and needs to be wiped off, and it can leave a greasy film on the skin, while pulling at the skin can encourage sagging.

☺ **Rinse-off Facial Cleanser** *($14.50 for 125 ml)* is a good standard detergent-based cleanser that isn't the best at removing makeup but can be good for normal to dry skin.

☺ **Eye Makeup Remover Lotion** *($14.50 for 125 ml)* is a standard detergent-based wipe-off cleanser. Wiping off makeup isn't the best idea, especially around the eyes, because pulling can encourage sagging.

☺ **Gentle Exfoliating Cream** *($14 for 50 ml)* is a mineral oil–based scrub that uses synthetic scrub particles. This one can leave a greasy film on the skin.

☹ **Skin Toner Refreshing and Balancing, Normal to Combination Skin** *($14.50 for 200 ml)* contains alcohol as the second ingredient; it is a skin irritant and not recommended for any skin type.

☺ **Skin Toner Refreshing and Soothing, Dry Skin** *($14.50 for 200 ml)* is a good, detergent-based, irritant-free toner. It does help clean the skin but it isn't very moisturizing.

☺ **Amino Moisturizing Cream, Dry Skin** *($20.50 for 50 ml)* is a very good, extremely emollient moisturizer for dry skin that includes water, plant oil, mineral oil, thickeners, lanolin oil, more thickeners, water-binding agent, and preservatives.

☹ **Hydra+ Effet Reservoir Enriched Texture** *($23.50 for 40 ml)* contains mostly water, thickeners, silicone, and preservatives. This is a very unimpressive, useless moisturizer for normal to slightly dry skin.

☹ **Hydra+ Effet Reservoir Light Texture** *($23.50 for 40 ml)* is similar to the one above, and the same comments apply.

☺ **Hydra+ Mat, For Combination Skins** *($23.50 for 40 ml)* contains mostly water, thickeners, glycerin, film former, and preservatives. This isn't all that matte or moisturizing. It can be an OK lightweight moisturizer for someone with normal to slightly dry skin.

☹ **Hydra+ Teint Tinted Moisturizing Cream: Clair, Hale, Dore** *($23.50 for 40 ml)* comes in colors that are too peach for most all skin tones.

☺ **Melibiose Anti-Aging Action Enriched Texture** *($30 for 40 ml)* contains melibiose, a dissacharide (sugar) that is a good water-binding agent; it doesn't change wrinkles anymore than other sugars found in cosmetics such as glucose and fructose do. This is a good emollient moisturizer for dry skin but that's about it.

☺ **Melibiose Anti-Ageing Action Light Texture** *($30 for 40 ml)* is similar to the one above, and the same comments apply.

☺ **Melibiose Anti-Ageing Action Eye Contour** *($23 for 15 ml)* uses the sugar melibiose along with retinyl palmitate; neither can affect wrinkles or aging, but this is a good lightweight moisturizer for normal to slightly dry skin.

☺ **Moisturizing Cream, Normal to Combination Skin** *($20.50 for 50 ml)* contains mostly water, plant oil, thickeners, lanolin oil, water-binding agent, and preservatives. This is a good emollient moisturizer for someone with extremely dry skin, but the ingredients are completely inappropriate and terrible for someone with combination skin.

☺ **Revitalizing Night Cream** *($28.75 for 40 ml)* contains mostly water, thickeners, plant oil, glycerin, water-binding agents, and preservatives. This is a very good moisturizer for someone with dry skin.

☺ **Hydra+ Masque Moisturizing Mask** *($19.50 for 40 ml)* contains mostly water, thickeners, witch hazel, more thickeners, clay, and preservatives. The clay can be drying and the witch hazel irritating, but as a mask that's on briefly it can be OK for someone with normal to dry skin.

☺ **Retinol Actif Pur Eye and Lip Contour** *($28.75 for 15 ml)* contains only a negligible amount of retinol, so even if that could make a difference in the skin, it can't: there isn't enough of it to count. Other than that, this is a good, ordinary moisturizer for normal to slightly dry skin.

☺ **Retinol Actif Pur Moisturizing Anti-Wrinkle Day Cream** *($32.75 for 30 ml)* is similar to the one above only with more emollient, and is better suited to dry skin. But without a reliable SPF and UVA protection, this product is useless for daytime and can't fight wrinkles in the least.

☺ **Retinol Actif Pur Night Treatment Cream** *($35.75 for 30 ml)* is a good emollient moisturizer for dry skin, and the same comments about retinol above apply here as well.

☺ **Retinol Actif Pur Radiance Anti-Wrinkle Mask** *($32 for 40 ml)* contains only a negligible amount of retinol, so even if that could make a difference in the skin, it can't: there isn't enough of it to count. This is just glycerin and thickeners, boring but OK and hardly worth the trouble.

☹ **Soothing Eye Gel** *($19 for 15 ml)* contains sodium borate and witch hazel, and both of those are skin irritants, particularly the sodium borate. This product is not recommended.

☹ **Lipo-Moisturizing Treatment, Very Dry Skin** *($28 for 50 ml)* contains mostly water, thickeners, silicone, vitamins, and preservatives. There are several ingredients in here that are completely inappropriate for dry skin, including talc and silica.

☺ **Lipo Vitamin Treatment, Very Dry Skin** *($24 for 50 ml)* contains mostly water, thickeners, silicone, water-binding agent, anti-irritant, vitamin, and preservatives. This isn't the best for very dry skin but it is a good ordinary moisturizer for normal to slightly dry skin.

☺ **Lip Protector** *($7.25 for 3 grams)* is a good basic petrolatum-based lip balm. It's good but ordinary.

R Pro (Makeup Only)

Revlon has a small line of makeup products it distributes through beauty-supply houses that are open to the public. It is a surprising group of products that has some solid strengths and some strange weaknesses. The strong points are an excellent group of matte blushes and eyeshadows, a very good group of brushes, and an attractive selection of lipsticks, glosses, and pencils. Weak points include a lack of testers at most outlets, which makes choosing a foundation fairly impossible, no concealer, a poor mascara, and pressed powders packaged in a way that hides the color. There are definitely products to check out, but I would call first to make sure you find a store that offers testers before you make a special trip out to shop this line. For more information about R Pro, call (800) 4-Revlon.

☹ <u>FOUNDATION:</u> There were no testers for the R Pro foundations at any of the stores I called that carried the line. The **Liquid Foundation** *($8.99)* is a very good, lightweight, sheer foundation with a great range of colors. **Concealer & Makeup** *($8.99)* is a stick foundation that has a sheer, smooth finish that can work well for drier skin types. As a concealer it works OK, but it does tend to slip into the lines around the eyes. Sadly, the packaging for this product doesn't even let you see the color.

☹ <u>POWDER:</u> **Pressed Powder** *($7.99)* and **Loose Powder** *($7.99)* come in an attractive range of colors and have a soft, smooth finish. Unfortunately, the packaging is such that you can't see the color, so unless you find a store with testers you would have no idea whether or not the shade you were buying matched your skin tone.

☺ <u>BLUSH:</u> Simply named, **Blush** *($5.99)* comes in a superior range of matte, neutral shades. The application is smooth and soft, without any streaking or flaking.

☺ <u>EYESHADOW:</u> **Eyeshadow Single** *($3.49)* comes in a superior range of matte, neutral shades. The application is smooth and even, without streaking or flaking.

☹ **Eyeshadow Trio** *($4.99)* comes in attractive groups of mostly neutral combinations, but all of these combos are shiny, and the application is not nearly as smooth or even as the Eyeshadow Singles from this line.

☺ <u>EYE AND BROW SHAPER:</u> **Eye and Brow Pencil** *($5.99)* are very standard but good pencils in a nice range of colors. It would be better if these were twist-ups, but they are just fine as pencils go. **Liquid Eyeliner** *($5.99)* is about as standard a liquid eyeliner as they come. With a pen-tip applicator, this one works just fine for a dramatic, defined line.

☺ <u>LIPSTICK AND LIP PENCIL:</u> The lipsticks for R Pro come in three types. **Shimmer** *($5.99)* has a glossy finish; **Creme** *($5.99)* has a good, creamy, opaque application; and **Matte** *($5.99)*, which isn't all that matte but does have good opaque coverage. **Lip Pencil** *($5.99)* is a very standard but very good lip pencil in a nice range of colors. It would be better if it were a twist-up, but these are just fine as pencils go.

☹ <u>**MASCARA:**</u> R Pro's **Mascara** *($5.99)* isn't terrible, just unimpressive, plus it tends to clump and takes forever to build any length or definition. Well, maybe it is terrible.

☺ <u>**BRUSHES:**</u> Brushes are a strong point for this group of makeup products. The assortment has some great options, from the **Blush Brush** *($8.99)* to a clever **Retractable Blush Brush** *($8.99)* and **Eyeshadow Brushes** *($4.99 to $5.99)*. The only ones to be cautious of are the **Face Brush** *($8.99)*, which is just huge and hard to adjust and control for different areas of the face, and the **Lipstick Brush** *($6.99)* which has an unnecessarily long, cumbersome handle.

St. Ives (Skin Care Only)

For more information about St. Ives products, call (818) 709-5500.

☺ **Alpha Hydroxy Facial Renewal Cleanser** *($3.34 for 12 ounces)* contains minimal AHAs in a pH that is too high to make them effective, so you don't have to worry about that part. This is a mineral oil–based cleanser with several thickeners. It's just cold cream with some plant extracts.

☹ **Alpine Mint Antibacterial Facial Cleansing Gel** *($3.34 for 12 ounces)* does contain a disinfectant, but it also contains peppermint, which is too irritating for any skin type.

☺ **pH-Neutral Extra Gentle Facial Cleansing Liquid** *($3.34 for 12 ounces)* is a standard detergent-based water-soluble cleanser with some plant extracts thrown in. It isn't all that gentle but it can be good for someone with normal to oily skin.

☹ **Swiss Formula Peaches and Cream Extra Moisturizing Facial Beauty Wash** *($3.34 for 12 ounces)* is similar to the product above, except this one also contains a small amount of plant oils, which can help decrease the dryness caused by the detergent cleansing agents. It also contains mint and peppermint, which can burn the skin and eyes!

☹ **Soothing Aloe Medicated Cleansing Cream** *($3.47 for 12 ounces)* is supposed to fight blemishes with a BHA, but it contains so many greasy, pore-clogging ingredients that seems ludicrous. Why would anyone trying to deal with breakouts want to put mineral oil, safflower oil, or petrolatum on their skin? What were the people formulating this product thinking?

☺ **Swiss Formula Facial Cleanser and Makeup Remover** *($2.32 for 7.5 ounces)* is a fairly standard mineral oil–based, cold cream–type cleanser that contains more greasy ingredients than you can imagine, including lanolin oil and plant oil! This is not water-soluble in the least, and it can leave a greasy residue on the skin.

☹ **Vanilla & Honey Moisture Rich Face & Body Wash In One** *($3.34 for 12 ounces)* is just shampoo with some plant extracts. The lime can irritate the eyes and skin.

☹ **Medicated Apricot Scrub with Soothing Elder Flower** *($2.32 for 6 ounces)* is supposed to fight blemishes with a BHA, but it contains so many greasy, pore-clogging ingredients it seems ludicrous. Why would any one trying to deal with breakouts want to put lanolin oil on their skin?

☹ **Swiss Formula Apricot Scrub with Soothing Elder Flower** *($2.32 for 6 ounces)* is a cornmeal scrub that uses sodium lauryl sulfate, which is a strong skin irritant and can also be drying, as its main detergent cleansing agent.

☹ **Alpha Hydroxy Facial Renewal Treatment Cream** *($2.32 for 6 ounces)* contains AHA and BHA, but not in a low enough pH for it to work as an exfoliant.

☺ **Swiss Formula Alpha-Hydroxy Moisturizing Facial Renewal Lotion** *($3.47 for 12 ounces)* is similar to the one above, and the same review applies.

☹ **Aloe Vera Protective Facial Moisturizer SPF 4** *($2.32 for 6 ounces)* fails with its useless SPF and because it doesn't contain any UVA protection.

☺ **Extra Relief Collagen Elastin Dry Skin Lotion** *($3.19 for 18 ounces)* is a very good, though standard, moisturizer for dry skin. It contains mostly mineral oil, glycerin, thickeners, Vaseline, silicones, water-binding agents, vitamins, and preservatives.

☺ **Swiss Formula Antibacterial Collagen Elastin Antiseptic Dry Skin Lotion** *($3.19 for 18 ounces)* is a moisturizer that does include a disinfectant, but don't count on this fighting germs for very long unless you keep on reapplying it.

☺ **Swiss Formula Collagen Elastin Essential Moisturizer** *($3.47 for 12 ounces)* is a very good moisturizer for someone with dry skin. It contains mostly water, mineral oil, slip agents, thickeners, water-binding agents, plant oil, plant extracts, thickeners, silicone, and preservatives.

☺ **Swiss Formula Instant Relief Collagen Elastin Dry Skin Lotion** *($3.19 for 18 ounces)* is similar to the moisturizer above, and the same review applies.

☺ **Swiss Formula Peaches and Cream Moisturizing Beauty Lotion** *($2.32 for 6 ounces)* is similar to the moisturizer above, but even more emollient.

☹ **Alpha Hydroxy Exfoliating Peel-Off Masque** *($2.32 for 6 ounces)* is an alcohol-based mask which is too irritating for all skin types.

☺ **Swiss Formula Firming Masque with Pure Mineral Clay** *($2.29 for 6.7 ounces)* is a standard clay mask and little else.

☺ **Swiss Formula Sunflower & Silk Moisture Lotion with Antioxidant Vitamins A&C** *($3.19 for 18 ounces)* is just mineral oil, thickeners, and plant extracts with a few vitamins added. It is a good though very standard moisturizer for dry skin.

☺ **Swiss Formula Swiss Vanilla Cream Lotion with Soothing Milk Protein** *($3.19 for 18 ounces)* is similar to the one above, and the same review applies.

Sea Breeze (Skin Care Only)

Like so many lines aimed at those struggling with breakouts, Sea Breeze adds the most absurd combination of irritating, skin-damaging ingredients to its products. I suspect all these companies think consumers who have acne-prone skin want a cool tingling feel from their acne products. While that may or may not be true, the truth is that cool and tingling means irritating and skin damaging, and that these ingredients are bad for all skin types, especially someone with acne. After all, what color is acne? Red. And what color do these irritating ingredients make the skin? Redder. That's not smart, that's painful. Irritation also reduces the skin's ability to fight infection, and that too would cause more breakouts. The phone number for Sea Breeze is (800) 831-2684.

☹ **Sea Breeze Exfoliating Facial Scrub** *($3.78 for 3.5 ounces)* would have been an OK synthetic scrub, but they just had to add camphor to it so it would irritate the skin.

☹ **Sea Breeze Whipped Facial Cleanser** *($4.99 for 6 ounces)* is similar to the scrub above; they added camphor for no reason other than irritation.

☹ **Sea Breeze Facial Cleansing Bar, for Normal to Oily Skin** *($2.99 for 3.25 ounces)* is a standard tallow-based bar cleanser. The tallow can clog pores, which just doesn't make sense in a product for oily skin.

☺ **Sea Breeze Foaming Face Wash for Normal to Oily Skin** *($3.78 for 6 ounces)* is a detergent-based, water-soluble cleanser that can be more drying than most, but it would be an option for someone with oily skin.

☺ **Sea Breeze Foaming Face Wash for Sensitive Skin** *($3.78 for 6 ounces)* is similar to the one above, only definitely less drying. This would be an option for someone with normal to oily skin.

☹ **Sea Breeze Astringent for Oily Skin** *($3.78 for 10 ounces)* is the product for you if you want red, irritated skin; it contains a great list of toxic ingredients, including alcohol, camphor, clove, eucalyptus, and peppermint.

☹ **Sea Breeze Astringent for Sensitive Skin** *($3.78 for 10 ounces)* is similar to the one above, which makes this product's label for sensitive skin inexcusable.

☹ **Sea Breeze Astringent Original Formula** *($4.99 for 16 ounces)* is similar to the one above, and the same review applies.

☹ **Sea Breeze Breezers Astringent Facial Towelettes** *($4.19 for 24 towelettes)* is similar to the one above, and the same review applies.

Selleca Solution (Skin Care Only)

Celebrities are believed no matter what they are endorsing. All it takes is celebrity status to convince consumers that something is worth buying, which is clearly the situation with Selleca Solution products. The first major problem with this small line of products is the glaring lack of a sunscreen. The second issue is the limited range of products, with no differentiation between skin types. There is really only one narrow skin type represented here, namely normal to somewhat dry skin. The last problem is that these products are especially standard, boring formulas in very small quantities for way too much money.

What you are supposed to believe about these products, besides that they make Connie look great, is that sea algae extract works wonders. Even if algae could have some benefit for skin (it can't, but let's just say it can), there isn't enough in here to even notice. Don't get me wrong: These aren't bad products, just a waste of time and energy for the consumer—but lots of consumers won't know that.

Please note that the first price is retail and the second is the club members' price (but this isn't a club worth joining, because either way the products are truly overpriced). For more information about Selleca Solution, call (800) 365-1974.

☺ $$$ **Soothing Cleanser with Chamomile** *($28, $19.50 for 6 ounces)* is a standard detergent-based cleanser that would be almost identical to Cetaphil Gentle Skin Cleanser except that this one contains fragrant oils, including rose, clove, and sandalwood oil, that can cause allergic reactions and skin sensitivities. By the way, Cetaphil retails at about $10 for 16 ounces and you don't have to join a club.

☺ $$$ **Gentle Eye Makeup Remover** *($25, $17.50 for 4 ounces)* is a good, standard eye-makeup remover that contains mostly water, fairly gentle detergent cleansing agents, slip agent, plant extracts, and preservatives. Effective, but incredibly overpriced.

☺ $$$ **Daily Difference Moisturizer** *($42, $29.50 for 2 ounces)* lacks sunscreen. Without sunscreen, the only difference this moisturizer can make is to cause more wrinkles by leaving the skin unprotected from the sun. At night it would be a good but very standard moisturizer for normal to dry skin. It contains mostly water, thickeners, slip agent, silicone, water-binding agents, plant extracts, and preservatives. There is a tiny amount of algae in here, but don't count on seaweed being a cure for wrinkles.

☺ $$$ **Firming Eye Gel** *($35, $24.50 for 0.5 ounce)* contains mostly water, thickeners, algae extract, and preservatives. This is a very lightweight, almost do-nothing gel moisturizer. It can be OK for very slightly dry skin, but for the most part you're buying some gel thickening agents and a teeny bit of algae.

☺ $$$ **Hydrating Eye Cream** *($38, $26.50 for 0.5 ounce)* is a good emollient moisturizer for dry skin that contains mostly water, thickeners, plant oils, and preservatives. Why this basic formula needs to be so pricey is a complete mystery.

☺ $$$ **Nighttime Miracle Cream** *($47, $32.50 for 1.7 ounces)*. Calling this a miracle is a piece of fiction that makes *Star Trek* look like fact. This cream for normal to dry skin contains mostly water, thickeners, water-binding agents, Vaseline, algae extract, fragrance (several that can be skin irritants), silicone, and preservatives.

☺ $$$ **Quick Lift Facial Firming Gel** *($55, $38.50 for 0.5 ounce)* is virtually identical to the Firming Eye Gel. The redundancy and change in price is bizarre. Did they think no one would notice?

☺ $$$ **Essential Moisture Body Lotion** *($35, $19.50 for 6 ounces)* contains mostly water, thickeners, silicone, fragrance, plant oil, and preservatives. This doesn't even come close to improving on moisturizers like Lubriderm and the price difference is one not to ignore.

Dr. Semel (Skin Care Only)

While there are lots of "famous" dermatologists and plastic surgeons with their own skin-care lines, Dr. George Semel is the first one to be selling his products at Nordstrom (call 800-7-BEAUTY for more information). Despite the prestige outlet for Semel's products, I'm at a loss as to how I should approach the intolerable, offensive claims Dr. Semel is making for his very expensive, very overpriced, silicone-based products.

For me, the most shocking claims concern DNA repair. DNA repair from some ordinary vitamins and moisturizing ingredients? Please! And it is amazing how many different ingredients you're supposed to believe are capable of helping your DNA, because many of Dr. Semel's products, with different ingredients, make that claim.

Perhaps the most unprincipled product in the lot is Aspire After Sun, which, according to the company's brochure, is supposed to "enhance melanin activity already started by prior sun or tanning bed exposure. Apply after tanning." Is this doctor endorsing getting a tan? Using a tanning bed? Encouraging melanin production? I think I'm going to be sick.

☺ $$$ **Collagen Stimulator** *($85 for 1 ounce)* contains mostly water, thickeners, water-binding agents, silicone, slip agents, preservatives, plant oil, vitamins, and preservatives. This absurdly expensive cosmetic formulation is as standard as they come, though it could be a good lightweight moisturizer for someone with normal to dry skin.

☺ $$$ **DNA Repair Aspire** *($45 for 2 ounces)* contains mostly water, plant oil, enzyme extracts, water-binding agents, silicone, thickeners, vitamins, and preservatives. Enzymes are unstable in cosmetic formulations, and I've seen no evidence that they help DNA repair. Other than that, this absurdly expensive product could be a good lightweight moisturizer for someone with normal to dry skin.

☺ $$$ **Triple Moisture** *($45 for 1 ounce)* contains mostly water, thickener, silicone, plant oil, slip agents, water-binding agent, and preservatives. It is just a good moisturizer for someone with dry skin.

☺ $$$ **UVA/UVB SPF 19** *($50 for 4 ounces)* is a partly titanium dioxide–based sunscreen that also contains water, water-binding agents, thickeners, silicone, and preservatives. This is an extremely overpriced sunscreen, but it does contain titanium dioxide, so the claim about UVA protection is valid.

☺ **$$$ Licorice Lightning DNA Repair—UVA/UVB SPF 19** *($50 for 4 ounces)* is a partly titanium dioxide–based sunscreen that also contains thickeners, silicone, water-binding agents, plant enzyme, licorice, more thickeners, and preservatives. The sunscreen can prevent further sun damage to the skin, which can allow DNA to repair itself, but so can lots of other well-formulated sunscreens.

☺ **$$$ Tightener** *($45 for 1 ounce)* contains mostly water, thickener, silicone, plant oil, slip agent, water-binding agent, and preservatives. What can I say? It's a good moisturizer for normal to dry skin, but will it tighten the skin? Nah.

☹ **After Sun Tanning Enhancer** *($50 for 4 ounces)* contains mostly water, plant oil, plant enzymes, silicones, thickeners, and preservatives. This product encourages tanning and is one of the most objectionable skin-care products I've seen in quite some time.

☺ **$$$ Easy Peel** *($45 for 0.5 ounce)* contains mostly water, lactic acid, salicylic acid, water-binding agent, thickeners, plant oil, silicone, slip agents, and preservatives. It is actually a decent lightweight skin exfoliant, with a good AHA and BHA concentration in a pH 3 base. But other good products of this nature are available for much less money, and I do not recommend BHA for sun-damaged skin; it is more effective for clogged pores or breakouts.

Serious Skin Care (Skin Care Only)

Serious Skin Care has changed a lot since it first launched as a line featuring a small group of acne products. Their successful infomercial has created lots of extensions to the line, and the simple three or four step routine has become complicated and more of a problem than I thought it was originally. It's not that there aren't some good products in this line, because there are, it's just that several of these are fairly serious when it comes to irritation and others can clog pores. There are products to consider, so just be sure to choose carefully. And this isn't an inexpensive line! I think the prices are steep for what you get. For more information about Serious Skin Care, call (800) 540-8662.

☹ **Glycolic Cleanser** *($18 for 4 ounces)* is a standard detergent-based cleanser that contains about 5% to 6% glycolic acid. In a moisturizer or gel that would be fine, but in a cleanser the chances of getting it in the eyes are pretty good and a problem. The instructions suggest leaving this product on the face for two to five minutes, which is certainly one way for the glycolic acid to have more effect instead of being washed away down the drain. Of course, that also means leaving the detergent cleansing agents on the skin for two to five minutes, and running a strong risk of irritation or skin sensitivity.

☹ **Mother of Pearl Soap** *($16.50 for four bars)* is a standard tallow-based bar cleanser that contains emollients, which can be a problem for lots of skin types. There is mother of pearl in here, but it is rinsed down the drain, so even if it had some purpose other than shine, it would be eliminated when you were done washing.

☹ **Sulfur Soap** *($16.95 for four bars)* is almost identical to the soap above except that it contains sulfur. If you are considering trying sulfur for disinfecting it would be better not to have it in a cleanser where the effectiveness would be rinsed down the drain.

☹ **Tea Tree Oil Soap Bar** *($16.95 for four bars)* is a fairly standard detergent-based bar cleanser. It contains the tiniest amount of tea tree oil, which isn't going to help acne, and the cleansing agents can be drying, while the ingredients that keep the bar in its bar form can clog pores.

☺ **$$$ Eye Sweep** *($15 for 2 ounces)* is a standard, detergent-based gel makeup remover. It will do the job, but this is exceedingly pricey for a very ordinary product.

☹ **Serious Buff Polish** *($19.95 for 4 ounces)* is a standard detergent-based cleanser with walnut shells and a tiny bit of AHAs. It will work as a scrub, but not nearly as well as Cetaphil Gentle Skin Cleanser and baking soda mixed together. This product also contains several potentially irritating ingredients that can hurt skin, including lemon oil, citrus oil, and balm mint oil.

☹ **Toner** *($14.95 for 4 ounces)* is an irritating mix of alcohol and eucalyptus. The AHA is good but the other ingredients can hurt skin.

☺ **$$$ Glycolic Renewal Gel** *($20 for 4 ounces)* is a good gel/liquid 8% AHA product. I question bombarding the skin with all of these potentially irritating products at once, but by itself this is a good option for someone with normal to oily/combination skin.

☺ **$$$ 1 Million IU Vitamin A Cream** *($26.50 for 2 ounces)* contains 1 million international units (I.U.) of vitamin A. I realize 1 million is an impressive number, and vitamin A sounds like it can help acne. Lots of women know there are several forms of prescription-only vitamin A products recommended for treating breakouts. Retin-A (tretinoin), Differin (adapelene), and Accutane (isotretinoin, an oral drug for acne) are all related to vitamin A. But being related doesn't mean they work the same. Moldy bread is related to penicillin, but you wouldn't consider eating moldy bread for an infection. Currently, there is minimal to no real information about the effect vitamin A has topically (on the skin). I have searched and searched, and while there are a few small studies indicating it can be a good moisturizer adjunct, it is not more so than other antioxidants like vitamin E. Hanging your hopes on vitamins sounds healthy, but there is no evidence that they can make a difference, and there may be some serious concerns about the risks associated with them, depending on how much is used.

☺ **$$$ A Force Vitamin A Serum** *($25 for 1 ounce)* is a serum version of the above; see my comments there for this. This one is an option for normal to oily skin as a lightweight moisturizer.

☺ **$$$ Mega Mins** *($28 for 1 ounce)* has the same comment as the serum above.

☺ **$$$ Emu & Aloe Soothing Cream** *($24.50 for 2 ounces)* is a good moisturizer for dry skin. Too bad about the poor emu and the poor consumer who is being sold the notion that this is the best oil on earth; it isn't, though it is a good moisturizing agent just like any other oil, though I do prefer plant-derived oils.

☺ **$$$ Eye Help** *($19.95 for 0.05 ounce)* is mostly silicone oil and film former; it can feel quite soothing on dry skin.

☺ **$$$ Super Hydrate** *($19.95 for 4 ounces)* contains mostly plant water, glycerin, slip agent, aloe, plant extract, water-binding agents, thickener, and preservative. This is a good lightweight gel/serum that would be quite soothing after all these incredibly irritating products on the face. It is more of a toner than a moisturizer, though.

☹ **Serious Shade Sun Block, SPF 15** *($16.50 for 4 ounces)* doesn't contain avobenzone, zinc oxide, or titanium dioxide, and is not recommended.

☹ **Acne Treatment Pads** *($19.95 for 45 pads)* contain a lot of alcohol, which can hurt skin and negate the effectiveness of the BHA in this product.

☺ **$$$ Clarifying Treatment with 2% Salicylic Acid** *($19.95 for 4 ounces)* is just that: 2% salicylic acid in a liquid base of water, glycerin, and slip agent. While I am not fond of high concentrations of BHA, this is a good version because of its lightweight base. If you want to try a salicylic acid exfoliant for acne, this is one to check out.

☺ **$$$ Clearz–It with 5% Benzoyl Peroxide** *($19.95 for 4 ounces)* is, as the name implies, 5% benzoyl peroxide in a liquid base of water, glycerin, and slip agent. It is just fine, although 5% benzoyl peroxide is a little strong to start with, particularly when used with all these other irritating products. I would suggest starting off with a more gentle 2.5% benzoyl peroxide product and seeing if that works, though 5% can be a great option for many with stubborn acne.

☹ **Dry-Lo** *($24.95 for 1 ounce)* contains several irritating ingredients that can hurt the skin's healing process, including alcohol and camphor.

☺ **$$$ Fading Fluid** *($22.50 for 2 ounces)* is an OK hydroquinone-based skin-lightening product, but it also contains sodium sulfite and sodium bisulfite, which are both potential skin irritants.

☹ **Lipo-Fix** *($19.95 for 0.23 ounce)* contains witch hazel, grapefruit oil, lavender oil, and orange oil, which won't fix anything but can cause irritation and dryness.

☺ **$$$ Phase Out** *($19.95 for 0.5 ounce)* is supposed to be "specifically for the problem of dark circles underneath the eyes," yet there is nothing in here unique or special for dark circles. It contains mostly water, standard thickeners, vitamins, water-binding agents, and preservatives. There is vitamin K in here, but that has no effect on dark circles.

☺ **$$$ Pure E** *($24 for 4 ounces)* includes an amount of vitamin E that is hardly worth mentioning, but it is in here. This very standard moisturizer for dry skin contains mostly water, silicone, thickeners, vitamins, fragrance, and preservatives.

☺ **$$$ Skin Relief** *($24.50 for 2 ounces)* is an emollient hydrocortisone product, which is helpful for irritation, but this is no different than Lanacort or Cortaid at the drugstore for a fraction of this price. Plus, you would never use a cortisone cream on a regular basis because it can break down the skin's collagen and cause breakouts.

☹ **$$$ Triple Acting Glycolic Mask** *($12 for 2.5 ounces)* contains mostly water, clays, plant extracts, thickeners, glycolic acid, lactic acid, thickeners, water-binding agents, and preservatives. If your skin survives this mask in addition to all the other products, it must be as tough as nails. You just don't need multiple AHA products, a BHA product, disinfectants, and drying masks. If you choose a few of these products your skin may do well, but if you use all of them I just can't imagine anything but red, irritated skin.

☹ **$$$ Unplugged** *($22 for 2 ounces)* contains mostly water, slip agent, water-binding agent, preservatives, and an ingredient called isolutrol, which is supposed to be effective in unclogging pores. This product is the only one in the line that contains the ingredient isolutrol. I have been unable to find and the company has not provided independent research indicating what isolutrol does for the skin. The only information I've been able to find is from the company selling the ingredient, and that is hardly independent and there is no supporting documentation to be had.

☹ **$$$ Zero Shine** *($14.95 for 0.05 ounce)* is merely powder with silicone. That wouldn't be bad, but it is hardly special; the problem is that it contains eucalyptus oil, which can be a skin irritant.

☺ **$$$ Mini Facial Peel Program** *($28 for six towelettes)* is a good AHA product that would work well for exfoliation, especially for someone with oily skin, but how much exfoliation can one face take? The price is overkill, and the number of exfoliating products in this line is overkill too.

Shaklee (Skin Care Only)

Shaklee has introduced a new line of skin-care products called Enfuselle. Their claims about this product portray it as nothing less than outstanding. Patented formulations and substantial research about to be published from two independent labs are the basis of their primary marketing push.

The brochure says, "In collaboration with physicians from the Dermatology Division of the Scripps Clinic and Research Foundation, Enfuselle products have been clinically tested at the independent laboratories of the California Skin Research Institute for safety and performance." The results quoted are "154% increase in skin elasticity and firmness in 4 weeks, 88% reduction of in the appearance of fine lines in 2 weeks, 104% reduction in the appearance of facial wrinkles in 8 weeks." While that all sounds wondrous, it doesn't tell you anything. Without knowing something about the subjects' skin, age, what their skin-care routine was before they entered the test, or what product or products these were tested against, these numbers can be true for thousands and thousands of moisturizers the world over. This is what moisturizers do!

As a matter of fact, the brochure says as much: "The results of the Enfuselle clinical tests dramatically reflect the difference between one side of the face being untreated and exposed to changing climatic conditions, and the other side of the face being treated with Enfuselle under the same climatic conditions." That's all true. If the skin is dry, and you leave one side of the face without any moisturizer, it's going to look wrinkly and dehydrated. So much for scientific research. One more point: the actual studies were not made available to me, so I can't tell anything about how they were done or what they were trying to prove. However, I am familiar with one of the so-called independent labs that performed the "research," and it is not in the least independent. It is a claims substantiation lab used by most of the cosmetics industry to get data that looks like a scientific study. The protocols they use allow the cosmetics company to always get the results they want. I've repeatedly seen this sort of work done at "skin research" labs.

Shaklee is very proud of the antioxidants used in their products, and that seems to be the reality behind the brouhaha. Antioxidants are theoretically good for skin, and most skin-care products contain them; however, there is no research anywhere proving that they can affect or stop aging or change one wrinkle on your face.

As it turns out, nothing in these products makes them unique in any way, and several have serious problems that you need to be aware of. Several of the products contain potentially irritating ingredients that are just bad for skin and completely unnecessary. Further, for all the patented ingredients and "serious scientific" research that is supposed to be supporting the claims, whoever these scientists are, they don't have any information about UVA sun protection, because none of the sun products contain avobenzone, zinc oxide, or titanium dioxide. The line also glaringly lacks any BHA or AHA products, exfoliants that are helpful for many different skin types. Plus there are no disinfectants for breakouts. Shaklee needs to go back to the drawing board with this line. For more information about Shaklee, call (800) 848-2532.

☹ **Enfuselle Gentle Action Cleansing Bar** *($15.25 for 4.5 ounces)* is a standard bar cleanser that can be drying to the skin, and the ingredients that keep the bar in its bar form can clog pores.

☺ **$$$ Enfuselle Hydrating Cleansing Lotion** *($16.50 for 6 ounces)* is a standard wipe-off creamy cleanser that can leave a slight film behind on the skin. Wiping off makeup is always a problem for skin because pulling can help cause sagging.

☺ **$$$ Enfuselle Purifying Cleansing Gel** *($16.50 for 6 ounces)* is a good detergent-based water-soluble cleanser for most skin types. There are a handful of antioxidants in this formula, just as in most of the Enfuselle products, but even if these could somehow be effective in fighting wrinkles, they would simply be rinsed down the drain.

☺ **$$$ Enfuselle Eye Makeup Remover** *($9.15 for 2 ounces)* is an extremely standard detergent-based eye-makeup remover. It can work, but why bother wiping off makeup if the cleansers above could do the job?

☹ **Enfuselle Refining Polisher** *($16.50 for 2.5 ounces)* contains menthol and alcohol, which are too irritating for all skin types, particularly in a product that is supposed to be an exfoliant.

☹ **Enfuselle Hydrating Toner** *($12.75 for 6 ounces)* contains both witch hazel and menthol, which makes it too irritating for all skin types.

☹ **Enfuselle Purifying Toner** *($12.75 for 6 ounces)* is almost identical to the one above, and the same comments apply.

☺ **$$$ Balancing Moisturizer** *($19.95 for 2 ounces)* contains mostly water, silicone, thickeners, vitamins, more thickeners, preservatives, and fragrance. This does contain good antioxidants, but so do lots of other skin-care products. This is a good moisturizer for normal to dry skin but it won't change a wrinkle.

☺ **$$$ Enfuselle Eye Treatment** *($19.95 for 0.5 ounce)* is similar to the one above, and the same comments apply.

☺ **$$$ Enfuselle Hydrating Moisturizer** *($19.95 for 1.7 ounces)* is similar to the ones above, and the same comments apply.

☹ **Enfuselle Time Repair A.M. SPF 15** *($45 for 2 ounces)* doesn't contain avobenzone, titanium dioxide, or zinc oxide, and is not recommended.

☹ **Enfuselle For Body, SPF 15** *($16.50 for 4 ounces)* doesn't contain avobenzone, titanium dioxide, or zinc oxide, and is not recommended.

☹ **Enfuselle For Body SPF 30** *($16.50 for 4 ounces)* doesn't contain avobenzone, titanium dioxide, or zinc oxide, and is not recommended.

☺ **$$$ Enfuselle Calming Complex** *($45 for 2 ounces)* contains mostly water, water-binding agents, slip agents, alcohol, thickeners, and preservatives. If it weren't for the alcohol, this would be a good lightweight moisturizer for normal to slightly dry skin.

☺ **$$$ Enfuselle C+E Repair P.M.** *($45 for 1 ounce)* contains mostly silicone and vitamins. Silicones leave a nice silky feel on the skin, but that's about it. If you're looking for a vitamin C product this one isn't it (though you shouldn't be looking for a vitamin C product, but I've already discussed that at length in the introduction and in my other books). The vitamin C in here is ascorbic acid, and is not considered the best version of vitamin C to use.

☺ **$$$ Enfuselle Infusing Mineral Masque** *($16.50 for 2.5 ounces)* is a standard clay mask with a tiny about of BHA; however, the pH is too high for it to work as an exfoliant. It also contains menthol, which is a completely unnecessary skin irritant.

Shiseido

Shiseido is the largest cosmetics company in Japan. They have a strong footing here in the United States, and several other Japanese cosmetics lines would love to chip away at their popularity. So far none has come close to knocking Shiseido off its pedestal. In terms of product selections, I was surprised to find that very few of Shiseido's skin-care and makeup products had changed since I last reviewed the line two years ago. The makeup line is rather limited, although some products are excellent, especially the foundations and lipsticks. One drawback to the Shiseido experience is their displays, which are attractive but inaccessible.

In contrast, the skin-care line is huge. There are several skin-care divisions, yet despite these categories, the various cleansers, moisturizers, and toners aren't really all that different. Beware of the products in the oily skin group: they are confusing and poorly formulated. Imagine moisturizers with pore-clogging ingredients and Vaseline for someone with oily skin, or toners and cleansers with seriously irritating ingredients. Even more frustrating is the Vital Perfection line, which is supposed to be for oily skin with a dehydrated surface; maybe if you didn't use the line's irritating toners and drying cleansers you wouldn't have a dehydrated surface!

Perhaps most distressing is that Shiseido is one of the few cosmetics lines that has a group of products for "Tanning In The Sun." These products are showcased as helping someone get tan. I guess this way Shiseido can sell more antiwrinkle products. Isn't that sort of like a lung cancer specialist handing out cigarettes? For more information on Shiseido products, call (800) 354-2160.

Shiseido Skin Care

☺ **$$$ Benefiance Creamy Cleansing Emulsion** *($27 for 6.7 ounces)* is a standard mineral oil–based wipe-off cleanser that can leave a greasy residue on the skin.

☹ **$$$ Benefiance Creamy Cleansing Foam** *($27 for 4.4 ounces)* is a very standard, detergent-based, water-soluble cleanser that can be drying for most skin types and doesn't clean makeup off all that well.

☺ **$$$ Benefiance Balancing Softener** *($34 for 5 ounces)* is good irritant-free toner that contains mostly water, glycerin, several slip agents, and preservatives. There are some water-binding agents at the very end of the ingredient list, which makes them completely irrelevant.

☹ **Benefiance Enriched Balancing Softener** *($34 for 5 ounces)* is similar to the product above, except that it contains alcohol, which can irritate and dry the skin.

☹ **Benefiance Daytime Protective Emulsion SPF 8** *($35 for 2.5 ounces)*, besides being a lowly SPF 8, doesn't contain avobenzone, zinc oxide, or titanium dioxide, and is not recommended.

The Reviews S

☹ **Benefiance Energizing Essence** *($47 for 1 ounce)* is an alcohol-based serum and is not recommended.

☹ **Benefiance Neck Firming Cream** *($40 for 1.8 ounces)*. What makes this special for the neck is a mystery. However, what isn't a mystery is that this cream contains alcohol, menthol, and witch hazel, which are irritating and drying for every part of the body.

☺ $$$ **Benefiance Revitalizing Cream** *($40 for 1.3 ounces)* contains mostly water, plant oil, glycerin, petrolatum, thickeners, silicone, water-binding agents, more thickeners, and preservatives. There is trivial amount of vitamin E at the end of the ingredient list. This is a good but standard moisturizer for someone with normal to dry skin.

☹ **Benefiance Daytime Protective Cream SPF 8** *($35 for 1.4 ounces)*, besides being a lowly SPF 8, doesn't contain avobenzone, zinc oxide, or titanium dioxide, and is not recommended.

☺ $$$ **Benefiance Revitalizing Emulsion** *($40 for 2.5 ounces)* is similar to the Revitalizing Cream above, and the same review applies.

☺ $$$ **Benefiance Revitalizing Eye Cream** *($40 for 0.51 ounce)* contains mostly water, plant oil, mineral oil, petrolatum, slip agent, water-binding agent, more thickeners, and preservatives. This is a good but ordinary emollient moisturizer for dry skin.

☺ $$$ **Benefiance Firming Massage Mask** *($37 for 1.9 ounces)* contains mostly water, glycerin, slip agents, thickener, silicone, water-binding agent, plant oil, fragrance, and preservatives. This is a good, but very ordinary, moisturizer; calling it firming is a gross exaggeration.

☹ **Pureness Cleansing Foam Oil-Control** *($15 for 3.7 ounces)* contains potassium stearate, a highly irritating cleansing agent, and other irritating foaming agents. This is one is not recommended.

☹ **Pureness Cleansing Gel** *($15 for 5.4 ounces)* is a standard detergent-based, water-soluble cleanser that uses sodium lauryl sulfate, which is extremely drying and irritating for most skin types, as the cleansing agent.

☺ $$$ **Pureness Cleansing Water** *($15 for 5 ounces)* is an irritant-free toner that can be good for someone with normal to oily skin.

☺ $$$ **Pureness Exfoliating Treatment Gel** *($18 for 3.6 ounces)* uses synthetic scrub particles as the exfoliant in a fairly gentle water-soluble base. It can be a good scrub for most skin types.

☹ **Pureness Balancing Lotion Oil Control** *($18 for 6.7 ounces)* is an alcohol-based toner that won't balance anything, but it will irritate the skin. It also contains a small amount of sodium phenolsulfonate, which can be a skin irritant and cause breakouts.

☹ **Pureness Balancing Lotion Oil-Control** *($18 for 6.7 ounces)* is an alcohol-based toner that also contains clays, sulfur, and salicylic acid. It won't control oil, but it can be drying and irritating for most skin types.

☹ **Pureness Moisturizing Emulsion** *($20 for 1.6 ounces)* is part of the Pureness line of products, and is supposed to be ideal for getting rid of breakouts, yet this product contains several ingredients that are notorious for clogging pores!

☹ **Pureness Moisturizing Cream** *($20 for 1.3 ounces)* is similar to the Emulsion above, and the same review applies.

☹ **Pureness Moisturizing Gel Oil-Free** *($20 for 1.6 ounces)* contains too many irritating and drying ingredients, including alcohol, sodium phenolsulfonate, and a small amount of salicylic acid, to make it worthwhile for any skin type.

☺ $$$ **Pureness Blemish Control Cream** *($15 for 0.53 ounce)* contains mostly sulfur, water, clay, talc, and alcohol. Sulfur is a disinfectant, but also a skin irritant. This is not the best way to control breakouts.

☺ $$$ **Pureness Hydro Purifying Masque, Peel-Off** *($18 for 2.7 ounces)* is basically plastic and alcohol. It dries on the face like a film and then peels off. That can make the face feel smooth, but it won't purify anything; also, the alcohol and plastic can be drying and irritating for some skin types.

☺ $$$ **Pureness Oil-Blotting Paper** *($10 for 100 sheets)* is just what the name implies. You press these small sheets over your face to help absorb oil during the day. The sheets are coated with a light layer of clay that can absorb oil. It's an option, but plain old powder and permanent-wave endpapers do essentially the same thing.

☺ $$$ **Vital Perfection Cleansing Cream** *($22 for 3.9 ounces)* is a standard mineral oil–based cold cream that must be wiped off the face, and can leave a greasy film on the skin.

☺ $$$ **Vital Perfection Cleansing Foam** *($22 for 4.5 ounces)* is almost identical to the Benefiance Creamy Cleansing Foam above, and the same review applies.

☺ $$$ **Vital Perfection Advanced Makeup Cleansing Gel** *($23 for 4.2 ounces)* is a mineral oil–based eye-makeup remover with detergent cleansing agents. It works, but it shouldn't be necessary.

☺ $$$ **Vital Perfection Balancing Softener** *($30 for 5 ounces)* is a good irritant-free toner that contains mostly water, slip agents, glycerin, water-binding agents, and preservatives. It would be good for someone with normal to dry skin.

☹ **Vital Protection Soothing Lotion** *($27 for 5 ounces)* isn't in the least soothing; it contains menthol which can be a skin irritant.

☹ **Vital Perfection T-Zone Balancing Toner** *($25 for 2.5 ounces)* is similar to the Pureness Balancing Lotion above, meaning too much alcohol, and the same review applies.

☹ **Vital Perfection Daytime Protection Moisturizer SPF 8** *($30 for 1.4 ounces)* is a disappointing SPF, though it does contain in part titanium dioxide, but with so many great SPF 15s available, why bother with this?

☺ $$$ **Vital Perfection Moisture Active Cream** *($32 for 1.3 ounces)* is a good emollient moisturizer for dry skin. Vital Perfection is a line of products meant for someone with oily skin and a dry surface; I suspect if the cleansing products in this group weren't so drying, you wouldn't have a dry surface! Even more to the point is, why would someone with any amount of oil want to put Vaseline on their skin? There are other ways to treat a dry skin surface than adding oil to it.

☺ $$$ **Vital Perfection Moisture Active Emulsion** *($32 for 2.3 ounces)* is similar to the cream above, and the same review applies.

☺ $$$ **Vital Perfection Moisture Active Lotion** *($32 for 2.3 ounces)* is a more lightweight version of the emulsion above. The alcohol it uses to lessen the emolliency can be a slight problem for some skin types but someone with oily skin should not be applying the other ingredients to their face.

☺ $$$ **Vital Perfection Daily Eye Primer** *($30 for 0.5 ounce)* contains mostly water, slip agents, glycerin, mineral oil, thickeners, plant oil, more thickeners, and preservatives. This is a good moisturizer for normal to dry skin, but it's incredibly ordinary.

☺ $$$ **Vital Perfection Hydro-Intensive Mask** *($28 for 1.4 ounces)* contains mostly water, glycerin, slip agents, alcohol, thickeners, plant oil, more thickeners, and preservatives. This very ordinary mask can be drying for some skin types, plus the oils in here can be problematic for oily skin types.

☹ **Vital Perfection Rinse-Off Clarifying Mask** *($25 for 3 ounces)* is basically just clay and alcohol. It can be drying and irritating for most skin types.

☺ $$$ **Vital Perfection Protective Lip Conditioner SPF 4** *($20 for 0.14 ounce)* doesn't have much of a sunscreen, so there isn't much else to say about this otherwise very emollient lip balm that doesn't contain any UVA protection.

☺ $$$ **Bio-Performance Advanced Super Revitalizer Cream** *($60 for 1.7 ounces)* contains mostly water, glycerin, silicones, thickener, slip agent, more thickeners, more silicone, petrolatum, and preservatives. This is a very standard but good moisturizer for someone with dry skin. But silicone and petrolatum for $60 is a burn!

☹ **Bio-Performance Advanced Super Revitalizer Whitening Formula** *($60 for 1.7 ounces)* contains none of the ingredients known to lighten skin, such as hydroquinone or kojic acid.

☺ $$$ **Bio-Performance Synchro Serum** *($75 for 0.03 ounce of Powder and 0.5 ounce of Essence)* is incredibly overpriced. You're supposed to combine the contents of the two vials in this package. The Powder contains a thickener, several water-binding agents, and preservatives. The Essence contains water, slip agents, alcohol, more slip agents, and preservatives. Mixed together, these two compounds do make an OK moisturizer, but nothing more, and the alcohol can be drying.

☺ $$$ **Revitalizing Cream** *($125 for 1.4 ounces)* is hopelessly ordinary, and the price is unspeakable. It contains mostly water, plant oil, petrolatum, slip agent, mineral oil, thickener, water-binding agent, more thickeners, more water-binding agent, preservative, fragrance, and more preservative. There are minute amounts of placenta extract and vitamin E, but they come well after the preservatives and are meaningless in both amount and what they can do for the skin.

☹ **Self-Tanning Moisturizing Gel** *($18 for 5 ounces)* contains too much alcohol and can be drying to the skin.

☹ **Sun Block Lip Treatment, SPF 15** *($15 for 1 ounce)* doesn't contain avobenzone, titanium dioxide, or zinc oxide, and is not recommended.

☺ $$$ **Gentle Sun Block Cream SPF 22** *($20 for 3.8 ounces)* is a very good pure titanium dioxide–based sunscreen in a slightly moisturizing base. It would be best for someone with normal to dry skin.

☺ $$$ **Sun Block Face Cream SPF 35** *($22 for 1.7 ounces)* is a very good in part titanium dioxide–based sunscreen for someone with dry skin.

☹ **Sun Block Stick SPF 35** *($18 for 0.31 ounce)* is a very good in-part titanium dioxide–based sunscreen with a small amount of tint for someone with dry skin. Unfortunately, with the amount you get this product wouldn't last you a week, and you need more protection than that.

☹ **Sun Protection Emulsion SPF 8 Waterproof** *($16 for 5 ounces)* has a low SPF 8, doesn't contain avobenzone, zinc oxide, or titanium dioxide, and is not recommended.

☹ **Translucent Sun Block Stick SPF 30** *($20 for 0.31 ounce)* is a good in-part titanium dioxide–based sunscreen, but the amount you get in this product is so tiny as to be useless for any amount of sun protection. Given the amount necessary to assure sun protection this product wouldn't last more than a week or two.

☺ $$$ **Ultra Light Sun Block Lotion SPF 30** *($25 for 3.3 ounces)* is a very good in-part titanium dioxide–based sunscreen in a slightly moisturizing base. It would be best for someone with normal to dry skin.

☺ $$$ **B.H.-24-Day/Night Essence** *($65 for two 0.5-ounce containers)* consists of two very small bottles, each containing a liquid that is supposed to be worn under your regular moisturizer. The Day Essence contains mostly water, slip agents, alcohol, thickeners, water-binding agents, a useless amount of sunscreen, vitamin E, and preservatives. The Night Essence has essentially the same formulation minus the sunscreen. The alcohol in both liquids is an irritant. Basically, this is an overpriced toner, and if the moisturizer you are using is good, you shouldn't need a second undercoat. If you have dry skin, you shouldn't be using a moisturizer with alcohol.

Shiseido Makeup

☺ **$$$** <u>FOUNDATION</u>: **Stick Foundation** *($29)* is for dry skin only because it tends to go on fairly greasy; after blending, though, it can be surprisingly sheer, and it does feel great on dry skin. These colors are excellent: I2, I4, B2, B4, B6, and G1. These colors are too orange or pink for most skin tones: P2, P4, P6, and C1 (this last one is a green primer color for the skin, something I never recommend because it places a strange tone on the skin that can interact poorly with a foundation turning, it an unnatural color).

☺ **$$$ Fluid Foundation** *($29)* has a great consistency and blends easily on the skin. These colors are excellent: Natural Light Ivory, Natural Fair Ivory, Natural Light Beige, Natural Fair Beige, Natural Fair Pink (almost too pink), Natural Warm Beige, Natural Deep Beige, and Warm Bronze. These colors should be avoided: Natural Light Pink (no one is this pink) and Natural Deep Pink.

☺ **$$$ Creme Powder Compact Foundation** *($35)* looks like a cream but has a silky light finish, which is nice, but all the shades have some amount of shine and the color range leans toward the pink and peach side and won't work for everyone.

☺ **$$$ Dual Compact Powdery Foundation** *($30)* is basically a talc– and mineral oil–based pressed powder that can be used wet or dry (though wet can go on streaky and smeary). It comes in an excellent assortment of sheer colors, and you can wear it as a foundation although it is more a pressed powder than anything else.

☺ **$$$ Liquid Compact Foundation SPF 15** *($35)* isn't liquid at all, but rather a very dry finish, cream-to-powder foundation. If you've been disappointed by a lot of cream-to-powder foundations because they ended up being more creamy than matte, take a closer look at this one. It has an attractive group of neutral colors with a only a few must-avoid shades (they include O8, B2, and B8); you'll find these three either two ash (meaning green) or peach for most skin tones. By the way, the SPF 15 is pure titanium dioxide and that's great!

☹ **Shiseido PreMakeup Cream SPF 8** *($24.50 for 1.4 ounces)* is really just a good moisturizer for someone with normal to dry skin, despite the claims that it will hold makeup and fill in lines. The demonstration on the lines on my hand was not the least bit convincing. Even the salesperson commented that it didn't look like it was working the way she was taught by the line representative who trained her. Although this SPF 8 cream does contain titanium dioxide, the SPF still leaves something to be desired.

☺ **$$$ Shiseido Vital Perfection Tinted Moisturizer SPF 10** *($26)* is a titanium dioxide–based sunscreen that comes in four prime shades for light to medium skin tones. Although it contains mineral oil it also contains a small amount of talc, so it has a slightly matte finish.

☺ **$$$ Sun Block Compact SPF 32** *($25 for 0.42 ounce)* is a very good in-part titanium dioxide–based sunscreen for someone with dry skin. This foundation isn't bad, but this amount wouldn't last you a week, and you need more protection than that.

☹ **CONCEALER: Concealer for Circles** *($18)* comes in only two shades; 01 is too peach for most skin tones, and 02 is too gold for most skin tones. I wish the colors were better, because the texture of this product is smooth and it blends well. **Concealer for Lines** *($18)* is a standard pencil that comes in two light shades; one is rather peach and the other pink. They don't hide lines in the least, they just look like a very different color from the foundation, and they can easily crease.

☺ **$$$ POWDER: Natural Pressed Powder** *($23)* is a standard talc-based powder that goes on very sheer and soft, and the colors are great.

☺ **$$$ BLUSH: Singles** *($28)* and **Tri-Effect Blush** *($28)* are available in a small number of colors, and they blend on smoothly and evenly. The Tri-Effect is just three blush colors in a row that mix together on the brush to create one color. It looks more clever in the compact than it does on the face. **All of the colors are beautiful.**

☺ **$$$ EYESHADOW: Single** *($21)*, **Duos** *($21)*, and **Tri-Effect Eye Shadow** *($23)* are available in a limited number of acceptable colors. **These colors are excellent:** Bronze Gold, Soft Brown, Grey Brown, Lemonade, and Melon Matches. **These colors are extremely shiny or too blue or green:** Soft Gold, Blue for Beginners, Roseate, Tortoise Shells, Moss, Teddy Brown, Cinders, Anthracites, Purple Quartz, Raspberry on Fire, Steely Blues, Clove/Violet, Red Madness, Desert Hues, Ultra Violet, and Bronze Copper.

☹ **$$$ EYE AND BROW SHAPER:** The **Eye Liner Pencil** *($13)* and **Eye Brow Pencil** *($11)* both have a good soft texture and come in an attractive array of muted colors; however, the brow pencils go on heavier than most and need to be blended carefully. **Eyebrow Shapeliner** *($20)* is a brow gel that goes on just fine, but the only shade is slightly taupe, and how many eyebrows can that match? **Shadow Liner** *($25)* is a trio of eyeshadow colors—black, brown, or navy—that can be used wet or dry. This is just very expensive matte powder.

☺ **Eyebrow Shadow Liner** *($23)* is simply two eyeshadows in a single compact. It's the best way to apply brow color, but the packaging is strange. One set of colors is Light Brown and Chestnut, the other Black and Dark Brown. Since your brow color is one or the other but not both, you are buying an extra color you will probably never use. **Pen Liner** *($23)* is a felt-tip style liquid liner. The color goes on evenly and dries matte, but there is only one shade, sort of a black brown. **Liquid Liner** *($23)* is a traditional liner in a tube that you apply with a tiny eyeliner brush. It too comes in only one shade, black, and it can easily chip.

☺ <u>LIPSTICK AND LIP PENCIL:</u> **Advanced Performance Lipstick** *($16)* has a wonderful creamy texture with a semi-matte finish that is really quite nice. **Advanced Performance Lip Gloss** *($15)* is a traditional lip gloss that comes in lipstick form; it's nothing special, but it is a good gloss. **Matte Variations Lipstick** *($14.50)* has a good creamy, opaque finish, but it isn't all that matte. The **Lip Liner Pencil** *($13)* has a very good dry texture and comes in a lovely array of colors.

☹ **$$$ Staying Power Lipstick** *($18.50)* is supposed to stay on so well that it even comes with its own **Staying Power Lipstick Remover** *($13 for 1.6 ounces)*. Nice try, Shiseido. It's a decent imitation of ColorStay, but the real thing is better. Also, Staying Power Lipstick comes in only a handful of colors, while ColorStay has a wide range to choose from. The special remover is actually not all that special, and the lipstick comes off all by itself or after wiping with a tissue, just like any other lipstick.

☹ <u>MASCARA:</u> **Advanced Performance Mascara** *($18)* and **Mascara Fiber Blended** *($18)* are just OK but not great, and the fiber mascara can flake and get in the eyes.

☺ **$$$ Shiseido Waterproof Mascara** *($18)* is a good mascara. It goes on fairly quickly and easily without any clumps, makes lashes long and thick, and stays on under water.

Shu Uemura

Shu Uemura is a makeup artist who started his skin-care line back in 1968. His Tokyo-based line has been available in the United States for the past ten years. It isn't well known, but it gets attention in fashion magazines and is sold at Barneys in New York and Los Angeles, Nordstrom in San Francisco, and at the Shu Uemura boutique in Los Angeles. The line has an exclusive yet simple flair. The products are plainly packaged and the descriptions are straightforward and refreshingly uncomplicated. Unfortunately, I can't say the same for the prices.

Shu Uemura's literature claims that "recent environmental conditions for our skin have taken a turn for the worse, due to the aggravating air pollution, the increase of social stresses, and the recent trends in foods and lifestyle. . . . [The products are] composed effectively to promote the skin's natural metabolism without giving more nourishing materials than it needs."

None of these products can provide nourishment for the skin, nor can they counteract the effects of pollution or stress, because we don't know what those effects are. More to the point, none of these products contains anything new or different, just the same old standard stuff, and without a sunscreen. (So much for preventing environmental damage.) Several of the products contain DNA. We all know putting DNA on the skin, or even taking DNA pills, can't affect our own DNA, right? If it could, you would be risking cancer and all kinds of possible mutations. It is just a gimmick—nothing more, nothing less.

Where Uemura does excel is in eyeshadows, blushes, and brushes. The colors aren't much to look at, but the textures are some of the most exquisite around. It is worth the trouble to check out the application of these shades just to see how creamy, smooth, and evenly they cover. And don't forget to check out this vast collection of brushes. Some of the prices are just absurd, but it is one of the most extensive collections of brush sizes being sold anywhere. For more information about Shu Uemura, call (800) 743-8205 or (310) 652-6230.

Shu Uemura Skin Care

☹ **Cleansing Beauty Oil Balancer** *($40 for 8.4 ounces)* contains mostly mineral oil, plant oils, thickeners, detergent, preservatives, and vitamin E. This is a lot of money for mineral oil and corn oil. It will cut through makeup as you wipe it off, but you could just use pure mineral oil mixed with a little corn oil from your kitchen cabinet. It is supposed to be washed off, but it can leave a greasy film on the skin.

☹ **Cleansing Beauty Oil Fresher** *($40 for 8.4 ounces)* is almost identical to the product above, and the same review applies.

☹ **Cleansing Oil Foam** *($15 for 1.9 ounces)* is almost identical to the ones above and the same review applies.

☺ **$$$ Cleansing Water** *($25 for 8.4 ounces)* is a detergent-based gel cleanser that would be good for most skin types, but it can be on the drying side.

☺ **$$$ Gommage Extra Gentle Facial Peeling Cream** *($38 for 2.3 ounces)* contains mostly water, talc, slip agent, clay, polyethylene (synthetic scrub particles), mineral oil, plant oils, and preservatives. It will exfoliate the skin, but it can also leave a greasy film. The talc and clay can cause dryness and irritation, so I would be skeptical of the term "gentle."

☺ **$$$ Moisture Lotion** *($35 for 8.4 ounces)* contains mostly water, slip agents, water-binding agents, thickeners, vitamins, preservatives, and fragrance. This is a good lightweight moisturizer for normal to dry skin.

☺ **$$$ Moisture Fluid** *($40 for 1.6 ounces)* is similar to the one above, and the same review applies.

☺ **$$$ Refreshing Lotion** *($35 for 8.4 ounces)* isn't all that refreshing, but it is a good lightweight moisturizer for slightly dry skin, similar to the one above.

☺ **$$$ Absolute Cream** *($40 for 1.05 ounces)* is mostly, water, slip agents, thickeners, plant oils, water-binding agents, silicone, vitamins, preservatives, and fragrance. This is a good moisturizer for dry skin.

☺ **$$$ Eye Care Jell** *($27 for 0.7 ounce)* contains mostly water, thickener, water-binding agents, plant oils, thickeners, and preservatives. This light-textured gel would be a fairly emollient moisturizer for someone with normal to dry skin.

☺ $$$ **Aid Oil** *($39 for 0.8 ounce)* contains mostly mineral oil, thickeners, plant oils, fragrance, and preservatives. This is indeed oily and would be very good for dry skin, but for the money and what you get, you would be better off mixing some safflower oil and mineral oil on your own.

☺ $$$ **Balancing Mask** *($33 for 2.2 ounces)* is supposed to be ideal for oily skin, but the thickening agents and plant oils in here would be a problem, leaving the face more oily and risking clogging pores. It could be good for someone with dry skin.

☹ **Mask Moisturizer** *($39 for 2.3 ounces)* contains mostly water, mineral oil, talc, water-binding agents, plant oils, clay, thickeners, and preservatives. This is a lot to pay for mostly mineral oil, talc, and clay. It isn't all that moisturizing either; the effect of the oils is negated by the presence of the talc and clay.

☺ $$$ **Principe 21 Bio-Energizing Concentrate** *($60 for 1 ounce)* is supposed to contain revolutionary ingredients to increase cell production (the cosmetic industry has more revolutionary ingredients than the world of medicine). It just contains emollients and water-binding agents that make it a really overpriced good moisturizer for dry skin.

☺ $$$ **Utowa Beaute Douce Eye Pads** *($33 for 12 packets)* is one of the Utowa products that are supposed to "act in harmony with the biorhythms of your skin" as well as replace lost elasticity and deliver a range of other skin wishes. The ingredients don't live up to those claims in the least. This lightweight moisturizer is soaked on eye pads. That feels good but it doesn't do anything other than moisturize.

☹ **Utowa Beaute Douce Moisture Mask** *($66 for eight packets)* contains too much alcohol to be recommended for any skin type.

☹ **Utowa Day/Night Double Concentrate** *($125 for 1 ounce each of the Day Concentrate and Night Concentrate)* includes no sunscreen, and without that there is little reason to bother with the Day part, plus the Day part contains alcohol as the third ingredient which makes it too drying for all skin types. The Night Concentrate has the same problem.

☹ **Cicica Water** *($9.50 for 1.7 ounces)* is, despite the claims, just nitrogen and slip agents. Nitrogen is a gas, not bad for the water, but a do-nothing for your skin, because it would just be released into the atmosphere.

Shu Uemura Makeup

FOUNDATION: There are eight foundation types in this line, and all but two have an exceptionally narrow range of colors. Trying to find your shade among four or five selections is a joke. Consolidation would be a good idea for this line, or increasing the color options.

☺ **$$$ Foundation Fluide S SPF 8** *($26)* is a titanium dioxide–based sunscreen, but the SPF would be far better if it were a higher number. This one does go on sheer and smooth and the colors are quite good, but there are only four of them. Avoid #130.

☺ **$$$ Foundation Fluid N SPF 8** *($26)* is a liquid foundation with an even, soft finish. The SPF is titanium dioxide–based, but the number is disappointing. The color range is large and quite good, and the texture is one of the better options in this line for normal to dry skin. **The colors to avoid are:** #185, #325, #375, #584, #754, and #775.

☹ **$$$ UV Powder Foundation** *($30)* comes with a brochure that claims this product contains titanium dioxide–based SPF 26, but that is not reflected on the product or its ingredient listing. Without ingredient disclosure, I am very skeptical that this product lives up to the claim, especially since there are no powders with SPF ratings (because powders cling so unevenly). That's a shame, because this smooth, sheer, finish powder has great colors.

☹ **$$$ UV Cream Foundation** *($30)* is supposed to be a titanium dioxide–based SPF 31 foundation, but unfortunately the ingredients listed on the box don't support this. It has a smooth, fairly greasy cream-to-powder finish and a small range of colors that are all excellent. It would be best for someone with normal to dry skin.

☹ **Make-Up Cake** *($22)* is a very thick, heavy, mineral oil–based foundation that isn't the best unless you want opaque, noticeable coverage.

☹ **$$$ Nobara Cream Foundation** *($19.50)* is a cream-to-powder foundation with a matte powder finish. Unfortunately the powder finish doesn't hold up; the waxes and oil in here show through fairly fast, so it's only appropriate for normal to dry skin.

☹ **CONCEALER: Cover Crayon** *($18)* is a two-sided pencil concealer. Both pencils and all four shades are too peach or pink for most all skin tones. **Base Control** *($26)* is a group of color correctors in a mineral-oil base that go on extremely sheer but add a strange color to the skin and don't help correct color problems. Isn't that what foundation is for? This just adds another layer to the skin, and if you have any other skin type than dry this is going to feel greasy.

☺ **$$$ POWDER: Face Powder** *($25)* is a standard talc-based loose powder with a soft, dry finish. Most of the colors are excellent, but avoid peach, purple, pink 100, 200, and 300, and pink 5.

☹ **Compact Powder** *($30)* has a smooth finish but strange colors. The one called One Colorless works, but the rest don't look like skin color.

☺ $$$ <u>BLUSH:</u> **Glow On** *($18)* has an ultra-sheer, soft finish. There are a huge range of colors to choose from, and some excellent matte shades. The shiny ones are clearly identified.

☺ $$$ <u>EYESHADOW:</u> **Pressed Eyeshadows** *($15)* have the most silky-smooth texture you have ever felt, and they go on beautifully, without streaking or flaking. Most powders this smooth have a difficult time clinging evenly, but not these. I wish the color choices were better; they are mostly a strange assortment of pastels. Still, that texture makes a closer look worthwhile.

☺ $$$ <u>EYE AND BROW SHAPER:</u> The price for these ordinary pencils is just beyond belief, I had to check the prices twice just to be sure I wasn't seeing things. The pencils are decent, but the prices are completely indecent. **Retractable Eyeliner** *($28)* and **Retractable Eyebrow Pencil** *($37)* are standard twist-up pencils with a smooth application. **Eyebrow Pencil** *($15)* is a very standard pencil that goes on almost the same as the retractable.

☻ $$$ **Kajal Eye Liner** *($13)* comes in two shades and is a fairly greasy pencil. **Hard Formula Eyebrow Pencil** *($20)* is just that, hard to get on. It does have a more dry appearance on the brow.

☻ $$$ <u>LIPSTICK AND LIP PENCIL:</u> **Lip Rouge** *($15)* has three types of finishes: Sheer, which isn't all that sheer but does have a good creamy, slightly glossy finish; Matte, which is fairly creamy and not really all that matte; and Neutral, which is a standard cream-finish lip color. Be careful, lots of these colors are shiny.

☺ $$$ **Powder Lipstick** *($27)* is Shu Uemura's version of Revlon's ColorStay Lipstick and it has lots in common with it. This one has a dry finish, and like the new version of ColorStay, doesn't feel powdery; it also tends not to flake or chip like some ultra-matte lipsticks can. Why you would want to spend $27 on this one instead of the $4.95 for ColorStay is hard for me to fathom. **Lip Gloss** *($20)* is a group of standard, incredibly overpriced pot glosses that have a slightly sticky texture. **Pencil Lipliner** *($15)* and **Retractable Lipliner** *($28)* are almost identical. Both are very standard lip pencils with smooth applications, but the one you don't have to sharpen is by far easier to use.

☺ $$$ <u>BRUSHES:</u> *($9 to $260).* There is an amazing selection of **brushes** in the Shu Uemura lineup, with dozens to choose from. If you want to see what a really skinny eyeliner brush looks like, this line gives you several to select from, and in varying lengths. (I should mention that M.A.C., Lancome, and Make Up For Ever also offer versions of this type of eyeliner brush, which is the type I recommend using.) Their prices are just as astounding as their range of eyeshadow brushes. There is no reason to spend over $15 on any makeup brush. Despite the claims about exotic hair sources, a brush doesn't have to be sable or badger to work. Fortunately, the line has many reasonably priced brushes too.

Signature Club A (see Adrien Arpel)

Sisley (Skin Care Only)

What a shame you just can't wear the boxes and containers of the skin-care products you buy, because more often than not the packaging has more value than the stuff inside. I get sticker shock every time I see a product priced over $20 for nothing more than standard cosmetic ingredients, but when I see a product for more than $200 I can barely breathe. I want to yell at the top of my lungs, "This is absurd; there is nothing in here worth this amount of money."

I often wonder what it would be like to be a fly on the wall at a meeting of Sisley marketing executives when they sit down to establish the prices for their products. I imagine it must go something like this: "Let's see, this product is really similar to a drugstore moisturizer that costs $9 for 6 ounces, but if we package it in an elegant gray and white box, put it in a matching jar with a shiny black cap, play up the European know-how angle with French words on the label, and stick in some exotic-sounding plant extracts and oils, we can probably charge $145 for 2 ounces. Women love that kind of foolishness. We can tell them it heals the skin naturally and all that kind of rot. Let's also tell them the products are really concentrated and they will last a year." Even if that isn't what they are really saying behind closed doors, it comes through loud and clear on the product label and in the brochures.

Perhaps I'm just in one of my moods. For some reason I've received a barrage of requests to review this line over the past few months, so you can imagine my dismay when I discovered Sisley is almost embarrassingly ordinary yet outrageously and insultingly overpriced. What is most distressing to me is that women would even wonder if these products are worth the expense. Sigh!

Forgive my frustration. It is completely valid to ask me about any cosmetic, and I will always do my best to let you know if it can live up to its claims or if it is worth the price. In Sisley's case, besides some plant extracts, which I feel strongly are more of a problem than a help, there is nothing in these products you can't find at the drugstore from lines such as Nivea, Pond's, Eucerin, and L'Oreal; actually, those lines and more have far better and more interesting products than this one does. That truly sums it up, so before I find myself ranting and raving, let's look at Sisley's offerings. For more information about Sisley products, call (800) 753-1362.

☹ **Botanical Cleansing Milk with Hawthorn for Dry/Sensitive Skin** *($65 for 8.4 ounces)* is a lotion version of cold cream. This wipe-off cleanser can leave a greasy film on the skin.

☹ **Botanical Cleansing Milk with Sage for Combination/Oily Skin** *($65* *for 8.4 ounces)* is similar to the product above, only with sage, and the same review applies.

☹ **Botanical Soapless Cleanser for All Skin Types** *($55 for 4 ounces)* is indeed soapless, but it does contain several very drying and potentially irritating standard detergent cleansing agents, including sodium lauryl sulfate as the first ingredient!

☹ **Buff and Wash Botanical Facial Gel for Daily Use** *($74 for 3.5 ounces)* contains standard synthetic scrub particles in a base of thickeners. It also contains lemon, and that can be a skin irritant. Baking soda and Cetaphil Gentle Skin Cleanser would be far better for the skin as a scrub than this any day.

☹ **Botanical Gentle Facial Buffing Cream, for All Skin Types** *($60 for 1.3 ounces)* is just wax, clay, and synthetic scrub particles. This is very drying and not appropriate for most skin types. See my comments for the one above.

☺ **$$$ Botanical Eye and Lip Special Cleansing Lotion** *($65 for 4.2 ounces)* is a standard detergent-based makeup remover, and when I say standard I mean very standard!

☹ **Botanical Floral Spray Mist** *($61 for 4.2 ounces)* is just water, witch hazel and preservatives, for the most absurd amount of money I've ever seen. Witch hazel is a skin irritant, as is the orange water in here.

☹ **Botanical Floral Toning Lotion for Dry/Sensitive Skin** *($60 for 8.4 ounces)* is similar to the Mist above, and the same review applies.

☹ **Botanical Grapefruit Toning Lotion, for Combination/Oily Skin** *($61 for 8.4 ounces)* contains alcohol and grapefruit, which are useless for oily skin. These two ingredients can leave skin feeling irritated, dry, and red.

☹ **Botanical Lotion with Tropical Resins for Combination/Oily Skin** *($56 for 4.2 ounces)* contains too much alcohol to be recommended for any skin type. The tropical resins are just standard plant extracts.

☺ **$$$ Hydra-Flash with B-Hydroxyacid and Natural Plant Extracts for All Skin Types** *($160 for 2.1 ounces)* is just an extremely overpriced, standard moisturizer. There's really nothing else to say.

☹ **Botanical Day Cream with Lily for Normal to Oily Skin** *($115 for 1.6 ounces)* has isopropyl myristate as its second ingredient, and the fifth is mineral oil. Why anyone with oily skin would want to spend this kind of money on ingredients known to make oily skin worse is anyone's guess.

☹ **Botanical Fluid Compound with Tropical Resins, for Combination/Oily Skin** *($127 for 1.7 ounces)* contains even more oil than the one above.

☺ **$$$ Botanical Intensive Day Cream** *($220 for 1.7 ounces)* isn't even remotely intensive, and as a day cream it is actually a problem, because it has no sunscreen. It contains mostly water, thickener, plant extracts, mineral oil, more thickeners, water-binding agent, more thickeners, and preservatives. There are some plant extracts at the very end of the ingredient list, which makes them nonexistent at best. If you can get over the price—wait, there is no reason to get over this price.

☺ **$$$ Botanical Intensive Night Cream for All Skin Types** *($248 for 1.6 ounces)* contains mostly petrolatum, water, thickeners, plant oils, mineral oil, more thickeners, preservatives, and plant extracts. I don't have any good words for this overpriced standard moisturizer.

☺ **$$$ Botanical Moisturizer with Cucumber** *($115 for 1.5 ounces)* is a standard mineral oil–based moisturizer with nothing else of any consequence.

☺ **$$$ Botanical Night Complex for All Skin Types** *($237 for 1 ounce)* contains mostly water, several thickeners, plant extracts, more thickeners, preservatives, and plant oils. This isn't all that botanical—most of the plant stuff is at the end of the ingredient list—but even if it were that wouldn't make it better for the skin. This is a really average moisturizer that would be OK for someone with normal to dry skin.

☺ **$$$ Botanical Night Cream for Dry/Sensitive Skin** *($137 for 1.5 ounces)* is a Vaseline-based moisturizer with thickeners, plant oil, and minimal water-binding agents. It contains arnica, a plant extract that can be irritating for most skin types, but especially for sensitive skin.

☺ **$$$ Botanical Night Cream with Collagen and Woodmallow** *($137 for 1.6 ounces)* is a mineral oil– and lanolin–based moisturizer. It would be good for dry skin, but the price is what's painful for this 50-cent formula.

☺ **$$$ Botanical Protective Day Cream for Dry/Sensitive Skin** *($115 for 1.6 ounces)* is similar to the one above, and the same review applies.

☺ **$$$ Botanical Restorative Facial Cream with Shea Butter for Day and Night** *($137 for 1.6 ounces)* is similar to the one above and the same review applies.

☺ **$$$ Botanical Super Night Cream** *($205 for 1 ounce)* contains mostly water, mineral oil, thickeners, plant oil, more thickeners, plant extracts, and preservatives. This is a good emollient moisturizer for someone with dry skin, but calling it super is a stretch. The only thing super about this is the price.

☺ **$$$ Botanical Tensor Immediate Lift** *($143 for 1.05 ounces)* contains mostly water, plant extracts, slip agents, witch hazel, thickeners, plant oils (fragrance) and preservatives. These plants won't lift your skin anywhere. The irritation from the witch hazel can tighten skin, but that isn't good for the skin in the long run.

☺ **$$$ Botanical Throat Cream** *($127 for 1.5 ounces)* is a mineral oil–based moisturizer with thickeners and plant extracts.

☺ **$$$ Botanical Tinted Moisturizer for All Skin Types** *($78 for 1.4 ounces)* has a tint that isn't for everyone.

☺ **$$$ Ecological Compound Day and Night for All Skin Types** *($176 for 4.2 ounces)* is a mineral oil–based moisturizer with just thickening agents, fragrance, preservatives, and plant extracts. Someone at Sisley has to be laughing at the women willing to spend money on wax and mineral oil.

☺ **$$$ Botanical Self Tanning Lotion Medium** *($93 for 3.5 ounces)*, like all self-tanners, uses dihydroxyacetone to turn the skin brown, but unlike other self-tanners this one is the most expensive one I've reviewed and the most ordinary for the money.

☹ **Botanical Facial Mask, with Tropical Resins for Combination/Oily Skins** *($71 for 1.5 ounces)* is a clay mask that contains several ingredients that would be a problem for someone with oily skin.

☺ **$$$ Botanical Purifying and Hydrating Green Mask for All Skin Types** *($88 for 1.4 ounces)* is just wax, clay, and mineral oil, with some plant extracts, all for the inane price of $88.

☺ **$$$ Botanical Toning and Hydrating Pink Mask for All Skin Types** *($88 for 1.4 ounces)* is similar to the one above, and the same comments apply.

☺ **$$$ Botanical Eye and Lip Contour Complex** *($137 for 0.5 ounce)* contains mostly water, thickeners, plant oil, slip agents, fragrance, preservatives, and plant extracts. What a waste of money for an ordinary moisturizer.

Smash Box

How Smash Box got launched is a question worth asking, because there is nothing remotely exciting about the products and they are ridiculously overpriced. The mascara is terrible, the pencils are extremely standard, the eyeshadows are almost all shiny, and the blush is almost too soft to show depth on darker skin tones. That's a lot of negatives, which means Smash Box is not all that smashing after all. This line pales in comparison to the other designer lines such as Laura Mercier, Bobbi Brown, M.A.C., Stila, or even Trish McEvoy (a line I also find wanting in many respects). So what gives?

Most of this line's raison d'être is in its name and in the heritage of the company's creators. Smash Box is aimed directly at the twenty- to thirtysomething crowd. It is very Generation X to come at beauty through the back door, to make cosmetics about something other than beauty. (The Urban Decay or Hard Candy lines come to mind.) Moreover, the creators of this line have built-in celebrity status: Davis and Dean Factor are great-grandsons of the late makeup master Max Factor.

Of course, the story of these great-grandkids makes up only an inconsequential portion of what you need to know. The most significant element is whether you want to spend your money on clever marketing and some captivating names, or on really great products. This line seems to be hoping for the former. If Max Factor knew what his descendants had created, he would assuredly be turning over in his grave. For more information about Smash Box, call (310) 558-1490.

Smash Box Skin Care

The two skin-care products here seem to have been a complete afterthought, and the line would be better off without them. ☺ $$$ **Cleanser** *($26 for 3.5 ounces)* is a standard detergent-based face wash that cleans well, but can be somewhat drying for some skin types. It is best for someone with normal to oily skin. ☺ $$$ **Moisturizer** *($28 for 3.5 ounces)* contains mostly water, thickeners, glycerin, more thickeners, soothing agent, plant extracts, vitamins, preservatives, and fragrance. This is about as ordinary as a moisturizer can get. It isn't even worth mentioning, but I couldn't exactly pretend it doesn't exist. You should.

Smash Box Makeup

☺ $$$ <u>FOUNDATION:</u> Smash Box's main strengths are its foundations. **Anti-Shine Foundation** *($32)* is an intriguing product. It is mostly water and magnesium (sort of like milk of magnesia, the stuff I recommend using as a facial mask for oily skin because magnesium absorbs oil so well) with color. It goes on extremely matte and dry and has very good staying power. It also doesn't blend on heavy like Revlon ColorStay; the texture is more like Lancome MaquiControle, only lighter in weight. The major flaw is the lack of color choice. This foundation comes in only four shades, and they are a strange group of colors. I don't know whose skin tones these will fit, but they *are* neutral, so if you have oily skin that happens to match one of these shades, it is a definite option.

☺ $$$ **Liquid Foundation** *($28)* is a water-based foundation that contains a small amount of oil, making it best for someone with normal to dry skin. It blends on evenly, with a silky-soft finish. The colors are all wonderful, although Mocha could turn ashy on some skin tones.

☺ $$$ **Stick Foundation** *($28)* blends out very sheer and soft, but it takes some patience to get it to do that. It is more like a cream-to-powder foundation than a traditional stick foundation. If you have any dry patches on your face, this will make them more noticeable. The colors for the most part are excellent. **The only colors to avoid** are Ivory (can be slightly pink), Mocha, and Warm Bronze. Beige, Warm Beige, Camel, Natural, Sand, Honey, Suntan, and Mahogany are great neutral shades.

☺ $$$ <u>CONCEALER:</u> **Concealer Stick** *($16)* comes in two shades: Light and Medium. It blends on easily but tends to crease.

☺ $$$ <u>POWDER:</u> **Pressed Powder** *($24)* is a fairly standard powder with a lovely texture and a smooth finish. Only three of the six shades are worth considering: Hot Chocolate, Ivory, and Light are beautifully neutral, but Clay, Translucent, and Bone are too peach or pink to recommend. **Loose Powder** *($28)* is a good loose

The Reviews S

powder with a very smooth, translucent application. Color choice is more reliable here than in the pressed powders.

☺ $$$ <u>BLUSH:</u> **Blush Compact** *($24)* comes in six beautiful shades (one is iridescent for some reason, but it's easily avoided). The only potential problem with this small group of colors is that they blend on almost too soft, which is fine for lighter skin tones or for those who want a more natural look, but they don't deliver for darker skin tones or for those who want more color.

☹ $$$ <u>EYE SHADOW:</u> **Eye Shadow Duo** *($24)* must have been designed by someone who has been in a deep sleep for the past five years. All of the eyeshadows come packaged in sets of two (most other "designer" lines provide single shades, allowing consumers to decide which colors to combine), and in most of these duos either one or both colors are shiny! The only matte colors in the bunch are Fleetwood/ Chocolate and Sarah/Brooke. They are both fine, but talk about a limited selection! This one is pathetic.

☹ $$$ **Cream Eye Shadow** *($18)* is for women who want a cream eyeshadow. Why anyone would want it is another story altogether. As is true for most cream eyeshadows, this one tends to crease and is hard to blend evenly across the eye. Of the four shades available, two are matte and the other two are shiny.

☺ $$$ <u>EYE AND BROW PENCIL:</u> The large selection of **Eye** and **Brow Pencils** *($12)* is impressive. They have a drier texture than most, which makes them a little harder to apply, but they also have less chance of smearing than others.

☺ $$$ <u>LIPSTICK AND LIP PENCIL:</u> There is only one type of **Lipstick** *($14)* in this line, and although the color range is very attractive, the lipstick is rather greasy and many of the shades are shiny. **Lip Gloss** *($12)* is just, well, lip gloss; what more can I say? The **Lip Pencils** *($12)* come in an extensive range of colors, but they go on rather dry, which may not be for everyone.

☹ <u>MASCARA:</u> How inferior can you get? This **Mascara** *($16)* is a clumpy, thick, smeary mess. I rarely return the cosmetics I buy, even when they don't live up to their claims. Given what I do for a living, I don't want to alienate the sales-people I deal with any more than I already do, but this one absolutely deserved to be returned.

☹ $$$ <u>BRUSHES:</u> The small assortment of brushes range in price from $19 to $62. The only one of interest in this group is the **Eye Liner Brush** *($19)*, which is one of the better ones of this type around. It is thin enough to use for both the upper and lower eye, so you can make the line as thin or thick as you like. It can be used with almost any eyeshadow, wet or dry. The other brushes are undistinguished—either too soft, too large (the handle on the lipstick brush is almost 8 inches long), or with limited application (the fan brush is good for something, but I've never been sure what or why).

Sothys Paris (Skin Care Only)

It would take an entire book to deal with all of the exaggerated claims attributed to Sothys's exceedingly ordinary, overly hyped products. Sothys has the same élan and prestige that are associated with other high-end French lines, and, from my perspective, this line relies on prestige and has very little to offer in product content. As is typical with many cosmetics lines that don't yet know about the insidious risk of sun damage, Sothys's daily skin-care routine recommendations do not include a reliable SPF. Dozens of moisturizers later and not one SPF means your face is just asking for wrinkles, and for this you are asked to spend hundreds of dollars on taking care of your skin. There are many other areas where Sothys falls short. The blemish products either contain useless irritants or pore-clogging ingredients, but no disinfectant or effective exfoliant; the cleansers use cleansing agents known for their irritation or are little more than expensive cold creams; and the AHA products are poorly formulated and completely ineffective for exfoliation. There are great moisturizers, lots of them, but, for the money they are fairly basic.

Sothys does an outstanding job of making their products sound remarkable and scientifically sound. For example the Desquacreme Deep Pore Cleanser is supposed "to increase the complexion's receptiveness by unclogging and desincrustating the follicular ostium as well as eliminating dead cells." As impressive as that sounds, though I have no idea how skin becomes "receptive," this simply says it exfoliates skin in the pore and on the surface of skin. Then the copy carries on to say "due to its high content of poamino acid salts, Desquacreme improves and regulates sebaceous secretions." While there are amino acids in this cleanser, they can't regulate oil production in any way shape or form; these are water-binding agents, and that's it. What the copy doesn't mention is that Desquacreme contains sodium lauryl sulfate as the main cleansing agent, which is a serious skin sensitizer and potential irritant and not recommended for any skin type. I guess they decided to leave that part out. I wish I had space to explain to you why the claims for these products are so bogus, but there just isn't room. Suffice it to say there are far better less-expensive products to choose from. Though if you think selecting expensive products is the only way you can take care of your skin, this isn't the best expensive line to shop. For more information about Sothys call (800) 325-0503.

☹ **Desquacreme Deep Pore Cleanser** *($29 for 6.7 ounces)* contains sodium lauryl sulfate as the main cleansing agent, which is a skin sensitizer, potential irritant, and not recommended for any skin type.

☹ **Purifying Cleanser for Oily/Problem Skin** *($26 for 6.7 ounces)* is similar to the one above and the same comments apply; plus, this one contains camphor, an unnecessary skin irritant.

☹ **Nettoyant du Matin Morning Cleanser Face Wash** *($28 for 4.2 ounces)* is a standard detergent-based cleanser that uses some of the more irritating cleansing agents. This product does contain emollient and plant oil, which is confusing. While the cleansing agents dry out the skin the emollients grease it back up?

☹ **Lait Demaquillant Comfort Soothing Skin Cleanser, Avocado Extract, for Sensitive Skins** *($26 for 6.7 ounces)* is just plant oil and thickeners, which makes it a wipe-off cleanser. Wiping off makeup tugs at the skin and encourages sagging.

☺ **$$$ Lait Demaquillant Douceur Softening Skin Cleanser, Aloe Vera Gel, for Dry Skin** *($26 for 6.7 ounces)* contains the tiniest amount of aloe imaginable. Other than that, this is mostly water, thickeners, and a detergent cleansing agent, extremely standard, but OK for someone with dry skin.

☹ **Lait Demaquillant Satine Normalizing Skin Cleanser, Grapefruit Extract, for Normal or Combination Skin** *($26 for 6.7 ounces)* includes grapefruit, a skin irritant that serves no purpose for any skin type, plus several ingredients that would be problematic for someone with combination skin, including coconut oil, acetylated lanolin, and sorbitan palmitate.

☹ **Peau Seche Skin Cleanser for Dry Dehydrated Skins** *($26 for 6.7 ounces)* is mostly water, slip agent, a tiny amount of vitamins, and an even tinier amount of collagen. This is a strange wipe-off cleanser for dry skin.

☹ **Purifying Beauty Milk, Camphor Extract, for Oily Skin with Blemish Problems** *($26 for 6.7 ounces)* contains camphor, a significant skin irritant.

☺ **$$$ Eye Make-Up Remover Gel, Special Waterproof** *($24 for 1.7 ounces)* is a standard detergent-based eye-makeup remover and will work as well as any.

☺ **$$$ Lotion Demaquillante Pour Les Yeux, Eye Make-Up Removing Lotion, Sage Extract, for All Skin Types** *($25 for 6.7 ounces)* contains mostly thickeners and plant oil. It is as standard a wipe-off makeup remover as you can get.

☹ **Peau Normal Normalizing Lotion, Hypericum Extract, for Normal or Combination Skin** *($24 for 6.7 ounces)* contains mostly witch hazel, and that won't normalize anything though it will cause irritation.

☹ **Peau Grasse Purifying Lotion, Rosemary Extract, for Oily Skin with Blemish Problems** *($26 for 6.7 ounces)* contains camphor, which is a skin irritant and doesn't help skin in the least. This product also contains film former as the main ingredient and that can clog pores.

☹ **Soothing Skin Lotion, with Allantoin Extract, for Sensitive Skin** *($26 for 6.7 ounces)* contains the tiniest amount of allantoin (0.3%), which is indeed a standard anti-irritant; the other ingredients are water, film former, and water-binding agents. This tends to have sticky feel on the face, though it shouldn't be irritating to the skin.

☹ **Alpha Serum 3% AHAs** *($32 for 1.7 ounce)* is honest about the amount of AHA it contains, but in this quantity it isn't effective as an exfoliant.

☺ **Time Interceptor Mask with AHA, 3% AHAs** *($32 for 1.7 ounces)* is nothing more than a good, ordinary moisturizer for dry skin. It's nice Sothys told us how much AHA this product of theirs contains, but I guess they didn't know that it takes at least 5% to begin exfoliation on the skin. The quantity here is not a terrible problem for the skin, it's just that at 3% these AHAs are just moisturizing ingredients, that's all.

☺ **Noctuelle with AHA, Universal Night Creme 8% AHAs** *($60 for 1.7 ounces)* has a better amount of AHAs (8%) than the one above, but the pH of this product is too high for it to work as an exfoliant. At this price you should have an AHA product that works to exfoliate.

☺ **Time Interceptor Alpha-Serum Intensive Care with AHA** *($67 for 1 ounce)* contains less than 2% AHA, which makes it ineffective as an exfoliant; other than that it is just an ordinary, very overpriced moisturizer for dry skin.

☺ **Active Creme, Nourishing Creme for Oily Skin with Blemish Problems** *($39 for 1.7 ounces)* is mostly waxy thickening agents and plant extracts, none of which are helpful for oily or blemish-prone skin. If anything, this product can clog pores.

☺ $$$ **Active PhytoContour Anti-Wrinkles, Anti-Circles Eye Serum** *($47 for 0.5 ounce)* is an ordinary, emollient moisturizer for dry skin and contains mostly water, slip agent, plant oil, thickeners, silicone, film former, water-binding agents, and preservatives.

☺ **Bio-Relaxing Eye Contour Gel** *($31 for 0.5 ounce)* contains mostly water, plant extracts, water-binding agent, witch hazel, silicone, thickeners, and preservatives. This ordinary, lightweight moisturizer can irritate the skin due to the amount of witch hazel present.

☺ $$$ **Cream for All Skin Types, for Fragile Capillaries** *($31 for 1.7 ounces)* contains aorta extract, which I assume is supposed to imply that if you put heart tissue on your skin it will affect your blood flow. How inane! This is just a good, ordinary moisturizer with plant oil and thickeners.

☺ **Creme de Jour, Day Creme for Couperose Skin** *($38 for 1.7 ounces)* is only suitable for use at night as an ordinary moisturizer, since it is without sunscreen.

☺ **Creme de Jour, Day Creme for Dry Skin** *($35 for 1.7 ounces)* is only suitable for use at night as an ordinary moisturizer, since it is without sunscreen.

☺ **Creme de Jour, Day Creme for Normal or Combination Skins** *($35 for 1.7 ounces)* has as its second ingredient isopropyl palmitate, which, along with the acetylated lanolin in this creme, is known for clogging pores. This product is not recommended for combination skin.

☺ **Creme de Jour, Day Creme for Sensitive Skin** *($39 for 1.7 ounces)* is only suitable for use at night as an ordinary moisturizer, since it is without sunscreen.

☹ **Creme de Jour, Day Creme to Firm Normal to Dry Skins** *($39 for 1.7 ounces)* is only suitable for use at night as an ordinary moisturizer, since it is without sunscreen.

☹ **Creme de Jour, Day Creme to Oxygenate All Skin Types** *($39 for 1.7 ounces),* because it is without sunscreen is an ordinary moisturizer only suitable for use at night, plus there isn't enough oxygen in this product to oxygenate one skin cell.

☹ **Creme Special, Day Creme for Dry or Couperose Skin** *($41 for 1.7 ounces)* is an exceptionally ordinary moisturizer and is only suitable for use at night since it is without sunscreen.

☹ **Creme Ultra Protectrice, Day Creme to Control Climatic Influences on the Skin** *($47 for 1.7 ounces)* is an ordinary moisturizer only suitable for use at night since it is without sunscreen.

☺ $$$ **Creme de Nuit, Night Creme for Dry Skins** *($39 for 1.7 ounces)* is a good standard moisturizer for dry skin that contains mostly water, plant oil, thickeners, vitamins, water-binding agents, and preservatives.

☺ $$$ **Creme de Nuit, Night Creme for Normal or Combination Skins** *($39 for 1.7 ounces)* contains several ingredients that can be a problem for combination skin types, including plant oil and acetylated lanolin, but for dry skin it's fine.

☺ $$$ **Creme de Nuit, Night Creme for Sensitive Skins** *($39 for 1.7 ounces)* is a repetitive version of thickeners, plant oil, and water-binding agents, and preservatives. There is nothing in here special for sensitive skin, but it is good for dry skin.

☺ $$$ **Creme de Nuit, Night Creme to Firm Normal to Dry Skins** *($39 for 1.7 ounces)* is similar to the one above, and the same comments apply.

☺ $$$ **Creme de Nuit, Night Creme to Oxygenate All Skin Types** *($39 for 1.7 ounces)* doesn't contain enough oxygen to oxygenate one skin cell, but it can be a good moisturizer for dry skin.

☺ $$$ **Hydrobase Light Moisture Base** *($33 for 1.7 ounces)* is a very standard moisturizer of water, slip agent, thickeners, and preservatives. There is about 1% lactic acid in this product, but that's not enough for it to be effective as anything but a water-binding agent.

☺ $$$ **Immuniscience Cream for Sensitive Skin** *($36 for 1.7 ounces)* is a very good moisturizer for dry skin that contains mostly water, plant oils, thickeners, shea butter, silicone, water-binding agents, and preservatives.

☺ $$$ **Immuniscience Fluid for Ultra-Sensitive Skin** *($36 for 1.7 ounces)* is similar to the one above, but it won't do anything about redness.

☹ $$$ **Intenspheres 2, Two Phase Firming Complex** *($77 for 0.5 ounce of each)* is a standard gel and standard moisturizer for an absurd amount of money. These contain ingredients fairly similar to many of the formulations found in all of these products; why the tiny size and higher price is sheer marketing fantasy.

☺ **$$$ Moisturizing Intensive Care Liposomes Hydrogel** *($62 for 1.7 ounces)* is a good, though extremely standard, moisturizer for dry skin. It's just water, thickeners and plant oil.

☺ **$$$ Perfection Creme, Time Interceptor Line** *($67 for 1 ounce)* claims an all-natural formula. But how do they explain the presence of caprylic/capric triglyceride, propylene glycol, and triethanolamine? What a joke: this is a standard moisturizer that would be good for someone with normal to dry skin.

☺ **$$$ Placentyl Cell Renewal Cream, with Vegetable Protein** *($37 for 1.7 ounces)* is a very ordinary moisturizer of water and thickeners. There is no reason to consider this product.

☺ **$$$ Repairing Serum, Regulating Intensive Care** *($50 for 1 ounce)* contains alcohol as the second ingredient, which inhibits the skin's repair process, it doesn't help skin of any skin type.

☺ **$$$ Retinol-15 Night Cream, Time Interceptor Line** *($48 for 1 ounce)* is a good moisturizer for dry skin and that's about it. There is no evidence that retinol can do anything for lines or behave in any way like the active ingredient in Retin-A or Renova.

☺ **$$$ Retinol-30** *($48 for 1 ounce)* is similar to the product above and the same review applies.

☹ **Serum Clarte, Clearness Serum, Fragile Capillaries Line** *($50 for 1 ounce)* is mostly water, slip agent, arnica (a skin irritant), castor oil, salt, fragrance, and preservative. I can't think of why you would need this for skin, and arnica can only make skin red and worsen the presence of capillaries.

☺ **$$$ Serum Nourissant, Nourishing Serum for Dry Skins** *($50 for 1 ounce)* is a good emollient moisturizer of plant oil, thickeners, silicone, and water-binding agents, and while it won't feed the skin it is very good for dry skin.

☹ **Serum Vivifiant, Vitality Serum for Normal or Combination Skins** *($50 for 1 ounce)* is just slip agent, witch hazel, and a tiny amount of water-binding agents. This is a crazy amount of money for ingredients that don't add up to a few pennies!

☹ **Active Sun Spray, SPF 4** *($25 for 5.1 ounces)* has an embarrassingly low SPF number that would encourage someone to seriously hurt their skin.

☹ **Hydrating Tanning Lotion, SPF 8** *($25 for 5.1 ounces)* has a low SPF number. With so many good SPF 15s on the market, why bother with an SPF 8?

☺ **$$$ Self-Tanning Emulsion** *($20 for 4.2 ounces)* is a standard self-tanner that uses dihydroxyacetone to tan the skin. This one works as well as any.

☹ **Self-Tanning Lotion, SPF 4** *($25 for 4.2 ounces)* has an embarrassingly low SPF number that would encourage someone to seriously hurt their skin.

☹ **Sun Tanning Oil, SPF 2** *($16 for 6.7 ounces)* has an embarrassingly low SPF number that would encourage someone to seriously hurt their skin. Products with this level of SPF should be illegal!

☹ **Total Sun Block, Complete Block, SPF 16** *($20 for 2.5 ounces)* doesn't contain avobenzone, zinc oxide, or titanium dioxide, and is not recommended.

☹ **Waterproof Sun Cream, SPF 9** *($18 for 2.5 ounces)* has a low SPF number. With so many good SPFs on the market, why bother with a 9?

☹ **Waterproof Sun Gel, SPF 6** *($18 for 2.5 ounces)* has an embarrassingly low SPF number that would encourage someone to seriously hurt their skin.

☹ **Beauty Mask, Diffused Redness Line for Delicate and Fragile Skins** *($31 for 1.7 ounces)* is a standard clay mask with plant oil, but it also contains arnica, a skin irritant, fairly high up on the ingredient listing, which isn't best for red or fragile skin.

☺ **$$$ Beauty Mask for Normal to Combination Skin** *($31 for 1.7 ounces)* contains plant oil, which isn't the best for combination skin; other than that, it is just a good, standard clay mask for normal to dry skin.

☹ **Beauty Mask for Sensitive Skin** *($30 for 1.7 ounces)* is similar to the one above, only this one contains witch hazel and arnica, which aren't good for sensitive skin in the least. Other than that, it is just a very ordinary clay mask for normal to dry skin.

☹ **Clarifying Mask, Mask for Oily/Acne Skins** *($29 for 1.7 ounces)* contains several ingredients that are a problem for oily skin, including zinc oxide, caprylic/capric triglyceride, and mineral oil.

☹ **Matt Creme, for Oily Skin with Blemish Problems** *($35 for 1.7 ounces)* contains lanolin wax and mineral oil, absolutely a terrible problem for oily, blemish-prone skin.

Stila (Makeup Only)

Stila is a line of cosmetics designed by makeup artist Jeanine Lobell. Like many of the other makeup artist–designed lines, this one has its share of matte eyeshadows and blushes, great yellow-to-neutral–based foundations, matte concealers, and great brushes. It is a relatively small line with few color choices and no foundation options for darker skin tones, but the colors that are here are excellent. This line is growing and it has some intriguing options. It isn't anything to run out and buy, but if you are near a counter there are some items worth checking out. For more information on Stila, call (323) 913-9325 or (800) 883-0400.

☺ **$$$ FOUNDATION:** There are two types of foundation here: **Oil Free Liquid Makeup** *($30)*, which blends on very sheer and light, and **Complete Coverage** *($40)*, which is extremely emollient and provides even, medium coverage. Both are actually quite impressive, with a beautiful range of foundation colors. If you want to check out really neutral foundation colors, this line is one of the better options you'll find.

☺ **$$$ CONCEALER:** For some reason this line offers two concealers. **Face Concealer** *($16)* comes in seven shades and is slightly more matte than the **Eye**

Concealer *($16)* that has only three shades. Both tend to be on the thick side and don't blend on all that easily. The colors are beautifully neutral enough, but the texture isn't for everyone. Test this one for yourself, because for most it will crease. Nevertheless, for extra coverage on the face, the reason to consider the Face Concealer is that it's one of the few that has enough color choices to go with most foundation colors in this line so it won't show up on the face as a strange color over a blemish or reddened areas.

☺ $$$ <u>POWDER:</u> The **Loose Powder** *($27)* has a soft, smooth texture that is on the dry side. It is a standard talc-based powder with excellent colors. The container is hard to use without making a mess; it comes in an aluminum, salt-shaker type container. **Pressed Powder** *($32)* while pricey and incredibly standard (it's just talc and aluminum starch) has good colors and a great feel.

☺ $$$ <u>EYESHADOW AND BLUSH:</u> The **Eyeshadows** *($15)* and **Blushes** *($15)* have some great matte, neutral colors and are virtually indistinguishable from many of the other "designer lines" from M.A.C. to philosophy, or from M Professional at the drugstore, for that matter.

☹ $$$ **Eye Rouge** *($13)* is a group of intensely shiny eyeshadows. These are up to you, you already know how I feel.

☺ $$$ <u>LIPSTICK AND LIP PENCIL:</u> The small selection of lipstick colors is available in **Creams** *($16)*, which are more glossy than creamy, and **Mattes** *($16)*, which are more creamy than matte. Both have a good amount of stain that helps keep the color on the lips. **Lip Gloss** *($16)* comes in a squeeze tube and provides a very wet, moist finish; it has very good staying power. **Pencil** *($14)* for the eyes and lips are standard only in application; unlike other pencils, the pencil part is made of recycled paper.

☹ $$$ **Lip Rouge** *($26)* claims to be a '90s magic marker for the lips. I wouldn't call it indelible, but it has some staying power, just not what you would expect for the money. What is also a disappointment is that there are only two color choices, if you can even call that a choice.

☹ <u>MASCARA:</u> Stila's **Mascara** *($16)* is a glumpy mess that takes forever to build any length or definition, and then it still disappoints.

☺ $$$ <u>BRUSHES:</u> This line offers a large, extremely usable group of brushes. These are some of the best selections of **Brushes** *($14 to $53)* around (best of all is M.A.C.).

☺ $$$ <u>SPECIALTY PRODUCTS:</u> **All Over Shimmer** *($28)* is an intensely shiny, liquid cream that dries to a powder finish. It does have a smooth sheer finish, but why are we drowning in a sea of shine nowadays! **Nail Shimmer** *($13)* is just shiny nail polish, nothing more, but it does match the All Over Shimmer, which can make for an alluring evening look.

Stridex (Skin Care Only)

Although I can't think of a reason why, but just in case, for more information on Stridex products call (800) 761-1078.

☹ **Stridex Antibacterial Cleansing Bar with Triclosan Maximum Strength** *($1.99 for 3.5 ounces)* is a confusing product because one of the main ingredients is acetylated lanolin alcohol which can clog pores. Plus the detergent cleansing agents in this product are fairly strong and drying.

☹ **Stridex Clear Antibacterial Face Wash Maximum Strength** *($4.93 for 8 ounces)* contains a small amount of disinfectant, but mostly this is just a detergent-based cleanser that doesn't clean the face all that well.

☹ **Stridex Dual Textured Super Size Pads Maximum Strength** *($3.44 for 32 pads)* has alcohol and menthol added; for this BHA product, that becomes too irritating to even think of using.

☹ **Stridex Maximum Strength Pads** *($3.44 for 55 pads)* is similar to the one above, and the same review applies.

☹ **Stridex Invisible Clear Gel Maximum Strength** *($4.93 for 1 ounce)* doesn't contain much alcohol, so it may be an option for someone wanting an effective BHA product, but be careful.

☹ **Stridex Pads for Sensitive Skin with Aloe Acne Medication with Salicylic Acid** *($3.44 for 55 pads)* is a puzzle: how a company can rationalize calling a product with menthol and 28% alcohol content good for sensitive skin is beyond me.

☹ **Stridex Regular Strength Pads** *($2.99 for 55 pads)* contains menthol and alcohol and is way too irritating for all skin types.

☹ **Stridex Super Scrub Pads, Oil Fighting Formula** *($3.44 for 55 pads)* is similar to the one above, only it contains even more alcohol.

Suave (Skin Care Only)

More often than not, I'm a big fan of inexpensive skin-care and makeup products. If the same thing exists for less money, unless you can't live without the image and packaging, there is no reason to spend extra cash. I was hoping that concept would hold up for the Suave line of skin-care products, but, alas, it doesn't. What a shame, because the prices for these products are killer. Two of the cleansers are an option for some durable skin types, but you have to get past the bad taste they leave in your mouth and the slight irritation over the eyes; the moisturizers are dated, pointless formulations; and there is no sunscreen. For more information about Suave, call (312) 661-0222.

☺ **Balancing Facial Cleansing Gel** *($2.75 for 8 ounces)* is supposed to gently clean and maintain the skin's moisture balance. It does clean, but it doesn't maintain any moisture balance. This standard, detergent-based cleanser is pretty drying for some skin types.

☺ **Foaming Face Wash** *($2.75 for 8 ounces)* is similar to the Cleansing Gel but slightly more drying.

☹ **Greaseless Medicated Cleansing Cream** *($1.99 for 10 ounces)* includes enough irritating ingredients to cause problems for almost anyone's face. It contains, in part, clove oil, camphor, phenol (I didn't think anyone was using phenol anymore), eucalyptus oil, and menthol. This product is absolutely not recommended. Suave must think medicated and irritating are synonymous.

☹ **Water Rinseable Cold Cream** *($1.99 for 4 ounces)* is a standard wipe-off cold cream made with mineral oil and wax. If you don't have clogged pores before using this product, you probably will after; the second ingredient is isopropyl palmitate.

☹ **Exfoliating Peach Facial Scrub** *($1.99 for 12 ounces)* is a strange mixture of talc, thickeners, walnut shells, detergent cleanser, and plant oils. Several of the plant oils, especially lemon oil, can be irritating, and the talc feels tacky on the skin. Despite the low, low price, there are much better ways to exfoliate the skin than this.

☹ **Clarifying Facial Astringent** *($1.93 for 10 ounces)* is mainly water and alcohol, plus a touch of menthol. Ouch!

☹ **Age Defense Renewing Cream, 8% Alpha Hydroxy Complex** *($3.47 for 4 ounces)* contains mostly water, glycolic acid, thickeners, silicone, soothing agent, and preservatives, and is not the right pH to be an effective exfoliant.

☺ **Replenishing Moisture Cream** *($3.47 for 2 ounces)* contains mostly water, glycerin, thickeners, silicone, and preservatives. This isn't a bad moisturizer, just an incredibly boring, ordinary one.

☺ **Replenishing Moisture Lotion** *($3.47 for 4 ounces)* is similar to the Moisture Cream, but with fewer thickening agents.

☺ **Replenishing Moisture Lotion for Sensitive Skin** *($3.47 for 4 ounces)* is an OK but fairly ordinary moisturizer for someone with normal to slightly dry skin. It contains mostly water, glycerin, thickeners, and preservatives. Nothing about this product makes it preferred for sensitive skin.

Sudden Youth (Skin Care Only)

If you flipped the book open to check out this line first, you need to read the section on skin care; it will remind you that you can't buy youth from the cosmetics industry, despite this product's enticing name. Sure, the before-and-after pictures are enough to make believers out of many women. But as a professional makeup artist, I know how to create that kind of effect. If you look closely, you'll see that the lighting, facial position, backdrop, and makeup in each "before" photograph are different from those in the "after" photograph. Sudden Youth would like you to believe that its products created the difference in the way these women look, but that is not the whole truth. Also, when you look at the ingredient lists, you'll find that these products are remarkably ordinary. The ingredients are not unique or sufficiently different from those in other face lift–type products or moisturizers to warrant the hoopla. For your information, the company's telephone number is (800) 542-5537.

☺ **$$$ Deep Pore Cleanser** *($22.50 for 8 ounces)* is a standard wipe-off cleanser that contains nothing more than thickeners, mineral oil, plant oil, more thickeners, and preservatives. It can leave a greasy residue, and wiping off makeup can encourage skin to sag.

☺ **$$$ Pearlized Facial Wash** *($22.50 for 8 ounces)* is a standard detergent-based, water-soluble cleanser that can be good for some skin types. It contains several plant oils, which can leave a greasy residue.

☹ **Facial Wash** *($15.75; $40.75 for Pro-Size)* is a standard detergent-based, water-soluble cleanser. The main detergent cleansing agent is TEA-lauryl sulfate, which can be drying and irritating on the skin. Also in this cleanser are plant oils, which can help soften the dryness, but why use such an irritating cleansing agent in the first place?

☹ **Alfalfa-Cleansing Bar** *($8.95)* is a standard bar cleanser made of fats and lye (sodium hydroxide). This can be very drying and irritating for the skin.

☹ **Oat-Cleansing Bar** *($8.95)* is almost identical to the cleansing bar above, and the same review applies.

☹ **Honey-Cleansing Bar** *($8.95)* is almost identical to the Alfalfa-Cleansing Bar above, and the same review applies.

☹ **Celery-Cleansing Bar** *($8.95)* is almost identical to the Alfalfa-Cleansing Bar above, and the same review applies.

☺ **Eye Make-up Remover Gel** *($14.75 for 1 ounce)* is a standard wipe-off makeup remover. It can indeed remove eye makeup, but repeatedly pulling at the eye area can cause the skin to sag.

☹ **Skin Freshener** *($16.50 for 8 ounces)* is a very standard detergent-based toner that also contains witch hazel and arnica, both of which can be skin irritants.

☹ **Facial Lift Gel** *($13.95 for 1 ounce)* is nothing more than aloe, water, thickener, and preservatives. It is meant to be mixed with **Facial Lift Powder** *($26.95 for 1 ounce)*, which is nothing more than cornstarch and egg white. There are some plant extracts and water-binding agents listed after the preservatives, which means they are not present in any significant amount. If you're thinking that this expensive little mixture is little more than what you could whip up in your kitchen, you're right. Cornstarch and egg white for $40—how depressing. By the way, cornstarch can be a skin irritant and cause breakouts.

☺ $$$ **Essential Beauty Oils** *($15.95 for 1 ounce)* is, as the name implies, a blend of plant oils. You could easily, and for far less money, mix up something like this from items in your kitchen cabinet and get the same benefits for dry skin.

☺ $$$ **Moisture Lotion** *($15.75 for 8 ounces)* contains mostly aloe, water, mineral oil, thickeners, slip agent, plant oils, more thickeners, water-binding agent, and preservatives. It is a good emollient moisturizer for someone with dry skin.

☺ $$$ **Sleeping Beauty Cream** *($24.95 for 2 ounces)* contains mostly aloe, water, slip agent, thickener, plant oils, and preservatives. This is a good emollient moisturizer for dry skin, but it's incredibly ordinary for the price. There are some vitamins, more plant oils, and collagen at the end of the ingredient list, which in larger quantities could have made this product more interesting, but there aren't enough of them in this cream to have any benefit for your skin.

☺ $$$ **Elastin Elegance** *($42.50 for 2 ounces)* contains mostly water, water-binding agent, slip agent, plant oils, thickeners, a tiny amount of AHAs, and preservatives. This is a good but ordinary moisturizer for someone with dry skin. It does contain collagen, but that can't affect the collagen in your skin.

☹ **Mint Julep** *($26 for 4 ounces)* is mostly aloe, alcohol, film former, thickeners, plant oil, soothing agent, plant extracts, and preservatives. This is supposed to be a pick-me-up for the face, but the alcohol can dry out the skin and cause irritation.

☺ $$$ **Eye Cream** *($24.95)* contains mostly aloe, petrolatum, plant oil, thickeners, water-binding agents, and preservatives. This is a very good emollient moisturizer for someone with dry skin.

☺ $$$ **Miracle Moisture Masque** *($32 for 4 ounces)* contains mostly water, aloe, slip agent, water-binding agents, thickeners, plasticizer, and preservatives. This is an OK mask if you're not allergic to the plasticizer.

TheraCel (Skin Care Only)

On many occasions readers provide product reviews that echo mine exactly or almost exactly. Even when they disagree, readers provide insights that I always appreciate. In the case of TheraCel, I heard from two readers who had completely different experiences. Here are their comments. For more information about TheraCel, call (800)943-5844.

Dear Paula,

I am 32 years old and have very fair skin. I do everything I can possibly do to keep my skin in good shape. I have read many informative books (including yours) on such maintenance. Through your books, I have grown somewhat savvy about being taken by the beauty industry and I use your books as a personal guide before trying new products. On occasion, however, I must admit that I have let myself be lured into the seductive promises of the infomercial. Those darn before-and-after pictures get me every time. Such is the case with the TheraCel infomercial.

I'm sure you have seen (and cringed when you saw) Shelley Hack in Paris with this "breakthrough product." I watched her and TheraCel's creator, Ardiss Boyd, and they both seemed so down-to-earth and honest that I was sold.

When I got the products in the mail, an instructional video came along. I watched it and did exactly what it said to do. The kit contained a bar of soap, a night moisturizer, a day moisturizer, and these vials of "serum." You are supposed to wash your face with this soap until it is "squeaky clean." This right away made me a little nervous, but I trusted it was a good product so I did as it instructed. As you may suspect, my skin felt very tight and dried out. The next step was to apply one third of the serum vial onto my face in even, light strokes, and keep my face still for ten minutes. This should have tipped me off that something was faulty with a product that is supposed to moisturize your skin and does not allow you to move it. Reluctantly, I applied this watery fluid in the instructed fashion and waited. As it dried during those ten minutes, it felt as though there was a light solution of water and egg whites tightening my face. When it was completely dry, I curiously touched my face and it felt like there was a piece of cellophane over it.

Now that my skin was thoroughly dried out, and artificially tightened, the next step was the day moisturizer. I hoped, at this point, that this product would somehow make this whole experience reach some kind of balance and undo all the bad effects that it had already done to my skin, so I applied this watery "moisturizer." My skin continued to feel tight, but I had spent all of this money and I really wanted it to work so I gave it a week, hoping for a positive change.

During this time, I did not see any positive results with my skin, let alone the "instant results" that the infomercial had so generously promised. In fact, my skin got very dry and flaky, the lines I was hoping to get rid of around my eyes looked more defined, and a rash developed under my chin and around my eyes. Needless to say, the product got shipped back and the company credited my account. A few days after that, a company representative called my house to see how I was "enjoying" the product. I politely told her about my experiences and was not surprised when she confided in me that many people she had talked to had some similar statements. I didn't feel quite so naive upon realizing that there were quite a few trusting souls who saw that same infomercial and bought it; however, my heart goes out to them, knowing they had comparable unpleasant experiences with this line, and I hope they sent the products back as well.

I don't know if you were going to review this product for your newsletter, but I thought you might be interested in my experiences with it. I feel that if you do review this line, you will find similar discoveries and will be able to warn your readers about this, in my opinion, bogus product line. This is the last time I ever try a new product until you have reviewed it first. Keep up the good work, Paula!

Theracelled Out, via e-mail

And now for another reader's comments:

Dear Paula,

Thank you for considering evaluating the skin-care line TheraCel. I do not work for TheraCel. I just recently bought the product (from their infomercial) and am interested in your opinion.

I have found the product really does reduce lines after only ten minutes! The Advanced Procellular Formula is the key to it. I am 38 years old and the results were quite dramatic. The delicate skin under my eyes was turned into perfect baby skin!

There are three products you get in the initial starter kit: night serum, moisturizer, and the stuff that gives the miraculous (no joking) results, the Advanced Procellular Formula (vials).

The only problems are:

1. The product is drying to my slightly oily skin type.
2. The products are too expensive for the average person. Ninety-nine dollars for a 30-day supply of the Advanced Procellular Formula vials alone is a bit much!
3. Deep lines on the throat are not affected (even though the product directs the user to apply only to the face).
4. The night serum and moisturizer do little to moisturize.

I also wonder where they get the placental protein and embryo extract from. (Could it be from aborted humans, or is it just chicken eggs?) What on earth is emu oil? Maybe you could develop a similar product and work out the kinks in this version.

Renee, Boise, Idaho

To Theracelled Out, Renee, and all my readers: My review of the TheraCel products reflects both Renee's and Theracelled Out's experiences, at least in terms of the products' overall performance. However, I find the notion of "miracle" skin-care products or *any* anti-aging skin-care routine that doesn't include an effective sunscreen to be unethical and harmful! I also found TheraCel's ingredient list to be most likely incomplete. There is no way these products can perform and feel the way they do—that is, the plastic layer on the skin and the watery mess of the serums—and contain what the label says, not to mention the lack of any preservatives. The only product that seems to have an accurate ingredient list is the bar soap. **Emu Cleansing Bar** *($8.33 for a 2-ounce bar)* is a standard tallow-based bar with detergent cleansing agents and a tiny amount of emu oil (an emu is a bird native to New Zealand). Emu oil has no miraculous properties to help skin.

In regard to the improvement Renee had with the Advanced Procellular Formula, there will always be women who experience success with this kind of product. The improvement may be a result of the extremely lightweight nature of the products as well as the film-forming ingredients. Hair spray–like ingredients can make skin look smoother, but they also leave the face feeling sticky and dry, as both women experienced. About the placental and embryo stuff, the company says it is from animals, but they weren't sure which ones.

☹ **Emu Cleansing Bar** *($49.95 for six 2-ounce bars)* is a standard tallow-based bar with detergent cleansing agents and a tiny amount of emu oil (an emu is a bird native to New Zealand). Emu oil has no miraculous properties to help skin.

☺ $$$ **Advanced Procellular Moisturizer** *($49.95 for 2 ounces)* is accompanied by an ingredient list that is probably incomplete. Aloe can be considered a soothing agent, and beta glucan is a decent antioxidant, but they can't keep water in the skin or provide any emolliency. This product also won't generate cell production, as the name seems to promise. As a toner this could be a viable option, but not to keep moisture in the skin.

☺ $$$ **Emu Promoist** *($39.95 for 2 ounces)* is identical to the moisturizer above except this one has emu oil. Again, I doubt the ingredient list is complete, but in any case this is a lot of money for some bird oil, vitamin A, and aloe. This would be a good toner for someone with normal to dry skin, but not a good moisturizer by itself.

☹ $$$ **Advanced Procellular Formula** *($99.95 for ten 0.07-ounce vials)* has an ingredient list that is personally offensive to me. It reads as follows: serum protein, placental protein, embryo extract, hydrolyzed collagen. While protein and collagen can be good water-binding agents, animal placentas and embryos seem inappropriate and unnecessary given the excellent plant sources available for these ingredients. This product also leaves a tacky, stiff feeling on the skin, like that caused by a film-forming ingredient, which leads me to believe the list isn't accurate.

☺ $$$ **Advanced Procellular Night Serum** *($49.95 for 2 ounces)* is just aloe, betaglucan, and a marine source of elastin. Again, I doubt this list is complete; if it is, spoilage would be a major issue. This $50 product would last for only a week or two, even in your refrigerator. If you have normal to slightly dry skin, this could be a good toner, but that's about it.

☺ **$$$ Emu Oil** *($120 for 4 ounces; $200 for 8 ounces)* is pure emu oil. Women believed for a while that mink oil was the answer for wrinkles, so why not emu oil?

T. Le Clerc (Makeup Only)

Whatever the hype surrounding this sparse but inflated cosmetics line, I can assure you there is nothing here to warrant the $45 price tags. In fact, these are just standard talc-based powders with a little rice starch and zinc. Rice starch doesn't add anything special to the formula and can actually cause problems for those with sensitive skin or a tendency toward breakouts. It's not that these are bad powders; in fact, quite the contrary is true. These are excellent powders, with a dry, soft, silky feel. But that describes dozens of other pressed and loose powders that range in price from $5 to $30. There just is no extra value or quality for the cost.

Both the pressed and loose powders come in 15 shades each. The colors are fine. **The only colors to avoid** are Banane (which is too ashy, not yellow as you might think), Soleil (which is shiny), and Orchide (which is lavender, for some reason).

Tova (Skin Care Only)

This is the line that made Oscar-winner Ernest Borgnine look like a new man—at least that's what the ads claimed years ago when Tova Borgnine was first selling her small group of skin-care products via ads in newspapers (lately she's been on QVC). The pitch by an attractive Beverly Hills woman who shared her beauty secrets with her famous husband and then with the American public had a following. Is Tova the answer for skin-care ills and can we all look as good as Ernest, or, more hopefully, Tova?

I have to admit to being intrigued by all these products piled on my desk—not necessarily by their quality, but by the very nature of cosmetic marketing. The essence of these skin-care products is presumably an ingredient called cactine 1. This ingredient is extracted from cactus plants supposedly once developed by the Aztecs. Because of its cactus origin, cactine is supposed to help skin do what these desert plants can do, namely protect itself against water loss. Interesting concept, but there is no supportive evidence for this, and botany experts say cacti can go without water for many different reasons, not just because of one ingredient. Anecdotally, I've never seen a cactus plant or an Aztec with skin I've envied. A closer look at Tova reveals ingredients that are more standard than anything else. What is decidedly not standard are the prices ($19 to $40), which lean toward the higher end of the cosmetic spectrum.

I get the feeling the popularity of this line has mostly to do with the moisturizing products designed for women with dry skin (along with some amount of celebrity élan). These are very emollient products with good absorption, not fancy or state-of-the-art, but good and reliable. If you have dry skin or if you buy their theory on cactine, some of these may be worth checking out. Avoid buying sets of these products (one of the skin-care groupings sells for $166), because you are more than likely to end up with products that are a total waste of money and not great for your skin. For more information about Tova's products, call (800) 852-9999.

☺ $$$ **Cactine Skin Renewal Cleanser** *($22 for 6.7 ounces)* is a detergent-based cleanser with some oils and thickener agents known for clogging pores. This can leave a greasy film on the skin. It contains some AHA, but too small a quantity to be effective as an exfoliant. And in a cleanser they would be useless anyway because their effectiveness would be washed away.

☺ $$$ **Cactine Eye Makeup Remover** *($29 for 6.7 ounces)* is a standard detergent-based, incredibly ordinary eye-makeup remover. It will take off eye makeup but no better than hundreds of other products priced far more reasonably.

☺ $$$ **Cactine Cream Scrub** *($24.50 for 3.2 ounces)* is almost identical to the Renewal Cleanser above except for the addition of synthetic plastic scrub particles. The same problems apply for this product.

☹ **Cactine Skin Refresher** *($20 for 6.7 ounces)* contains mostly water, witch hazel, slip agent, and fragrant plant oils. The witch hazel is too irritating for all skin types, and the fragrant oils can be sensitizing.

☹ **Cactine Skin Toner** *($18 for 6.73 ounces)* is almost identical to the Skin Refresher above, except this one contains alcohol, which is even worse for the skin.

☺ $$$ **Cactine CelRenual** *($41 for 1 ounce)* contains mostly film former, water, water-binding agents, and preservatives. This is a very overpriced but very good moisturizer for someone with normal to slightly dry skin.

☺ $$$ **Cactine EyeRenual Treatment** *($31 for 0.5 ounce)* is similar to the one above and the same review applies.

☺ $$$ **Cactine Emollient** *($23.50 for 1 ounce)* is a Vaseline-based moisturizer that also contains plant oil, lanolin, and waxes. This is a very greasy, very thick moisturizer that would be very good for someone with exceedingly dry skin.

☺ $$$ **Cactine Eye Lift** *($28 for 0.5 ounce)* contains mostly water, aloe, water-binding agents, plant extracts, vitamins, salicylic acid (BHA), and preservatives. This product won't lift anything. The pH of this product isn't enough for the salicylic acid to work well as an exfoliant, and I would question using a BHA in an eye product.

☺ $$$ **Cactine Moisture Milk** *($19.50 for 3.38 ounces)* contains mostly water, slip agent, vitamin E, thickeners, and preservatives. This is a good though standard moisturizer for normal to slightly dry skin.

☺ $$$ **Cactine Moisture Rich Cream** *($26.50 for 1 ounce)* contains mostly water, thickeners, water-binding agent, plant oil, and preservatives. This is a good ordinary moisturizer for someone with dry skin.

☺ $$$ **Cactine Skin Renual Cream** *($31 for 1.7 ounces)* is supposed to be an

AHA product, but it contains neither enough AHA or the right pH for it to be an effective exfoliant.

☺ **Fragrance Free Block, SPF 30** *($18.50 for 4 ounces)* contains neither avobenzone, titanium dioxide, nor zinc oxide, and is not recommended.

☹ **Cactine Masque** *($29.50 for 4 ounces)* contains primarily witch hazel and rice starch, which are both potential skin irritants. This product is not recommended.

☺ **$$$ Cactine Moisture Masque** *($29.50 for 4 ounces)* is mostly thickeners, plant oils, and water-binding agents. While that might be good for dry skin, it is no different than other moisturizers in this line.

☺ **$$$ Cactine Lip Renual Masque and Lip Renual Serum** *($21.50 for both 1 ounce of the Masque and 0.25 ounce of the Serum)* is mostly wax that can rub off dry skin, but the witch hazel and rice starch can be irritating. The serum is mostly film former and water-binding agents. That can make the lips feel tight and slightly smoother, and hold lipstick in place, but it can also eventually cause dryness because there are no emollients in the product.

Trish McEvoy

It isn't easy to put together a new cosmetics line that incorporates both skin-care and makeup products. Creating a reliable skin-care regime that works for many different skin types is a daunting task in itself, but add to that the requirements of a makeup line—foundations, concealers, blushes, eyeshadows, lipsticks, lip liners, brushes, eyeliners, and powders—and you can literally drown in a sea of products. Very few people develop the whole ball of wax all at once; instead, they often start with skin care and slowly add makeup, or vice versa.

New York makeup artist Trish McEvoy couldn't wait. Instead, she (or whoever worked with her) created an entire line all at once, with a broad variety of products. The displays are completely user friendly but with no names of products or colors you're in the dark as to exactly what you are using. The large brush selection is impressive, but the blush and powder brushes have a stiff, hard texture and the prices are high for what you get. Given the line's six foundations, all women should be able to find a suitable shade or product, but that isn't really the case. There are two cream-to-powder foundations (one is oil-free) but neither has a suitable SPF, which makes these pale in comparison to Clinique's, Prescriptives', or Revlon's. There are some good color matches to be found but there are also far too many peach and pink shades mixed in.

McEvoy is clearly competing with her neighbors at the department store, such as M.A.C., Bobbi Brown, Stila, Nars, Lorac (Carol Shaw), and Laura Mercier. For the money you would be wise to check out M.A.C. first; their prices and colors are far better—McEvoy's eyeshadows are $16 each; M.A.C.'s are $10.

You might expect expensive skin-care products to have something distinct or individual that you wouldn't necessarily find in similar products. I rarely, if ever, find that the so-called "special" ingredients often found in more expensive cosmetics live up to the claims made about them, but at least their presence shows that the formulator put some energy and research into the products or tried to come up with a unique combination of ingredients.

What do I consider unique? A mixture of interesting water-binding agents such as hyaluronic acid with sodium PCA, perhaps; or an AHA product with a unique anti-irritant ingredient such as green tea; or, although I'm loath to say it, even a bizarre concoction of plants—these would all be more distinctive than the standard stuff in Pond's or Nivea. Not that Pond's or Nivea are bad, but while I expect the standard good stuff in the less-expensive products, I hope for more from the expensive stuff—something special that partially justifies the higher cost. Besides, these "special" ingredients and "unique" formulas provide a challenge when I do my research.

Not this line, though. Most of the skin-care products go beyond ordinary to downright boring. On one hand, I was thrilled to see a department-store line that didn't include an obnoxious list of plants or sea extracts, but on the other I was disappointed to find such standard formulations with such unreasonable price tags.

One very unique aspect of the McEvoy line is her Face Planner. It's worth a visit to the counter just to check this one out. For more information about Trish McEvoy, call (800) 431-4306.

Trish McEvoy Skin Care

☹ **Astringent Cleansing Bar** *($20 for 3.7 ounces)* uses sodium tallowate (lard) as the primary ingredient. Tallow can cause eczema and blackheads. I wouldn't recommend this for any skin type, and definitely not for someone with problem skin. It also contains mud, mineral oil, and glycerin. The mud can feel heavy on the skin, and the mineral oil isn't great for someone with oily skin.

☺ **$$$ Essential Cleanser** *($37 for 8 ounces)* is a standard detergent-based, water-soluble cleanser that can be drying for some skin types. The price for this cleanser is completely unwarranted. There are dozens of other cleansers equal to if not far better than this one.

☹ **Essential Wash** *($37 for 8 ounces)* uses sodium C14-16 olefin sulfonate as the main detergent cleansing ingredient, and that makes this cleanser potentially irritating and drying for all skin types. There are far more gentle ways to effectively clean the skin for far less money.

☺ **$$$ Gentle Cleansing Lotion** *($37 for 5 ounces)* may indeed be gentle for some skin types, but it could wreak havoc if you tend to break out, are prone to bumps under the skin, or have blackheads. The second ingredient is isopropyl myristate, notorious for clogging pores. Other than that, this is an OK water-soluble makeup remover.

☹ **Glycolic Wash** *($37 for 8 ounces)* can be very drying, and you shouldn't wash your face with a product that contains glycolic acid, because you may inadvertently get it in your eyes. Anyway, one glycolic acid product is enough for any face, and it is best to use one that stays on the skin. In a cleanser, some of the acid may be rinsed off, making for an uneven application.

☹ **Moisture Retaining Bar** *($20 for 3.7 ounces)* is almost identical to the bar above, minus the mud. It can be extremely drying, and it has the same potential to cause eczema and blackheads.

☹ **Eye Makeup Remover** *($15 for 2 ounces)* would be a fine eye-makeup remover if it didn't contain PVP, a film former, rather high on the ingredient list. It can definitely be a problem around the eyes and leave a sticky feel on the skin.

☺ $$$ **Waterproof Mascara Remover** *($15 for 2 ounces)* is mostly silicone with a few additional slip agents. It will work, but this is very expensive for silicone.

☺ $$$ **Dry Skin Normalizer, Extra-Rich Improvement Cream** *($40 for 1 ounce)* contains mostly petrolatum, water, thickener, mineral oil, plant oil, more thickeners, lanolin oil, and preservatives. This is little more than Vaseline with a bunch of oils. For this kind of money, they should at least throw in some interesting water-binding agents. It is indeed a good moisturizer for someone with dry skin, just shockingly expensive for what you get.

☺ $$$ **Enriched Moisturizer** *($37 for 2 ounces)* is almost a joke, at least at this price. All this very expensive product contains is water, mineral oil, thickener, lanolin, vitamins A and D, and preservatives. It is definitely a very rich emollient moisturizer for someone with dry skin, but there are cheaper versions of products like this.

☺ $$$ **Extra-Light Moisturizer** *($37 for 2 ounces)* is similar to the moisturizer above, minus the silicone. It isn't all that light, but it would be a good moisturizer for someone with normal to slightly dry skin.

☺ $$$ **Glycolic Face Cream** *($37 for 1 ounce)* contains mostly water, water-binding agents, thickeners, glycolic acid, several more thickeners, and preservatives. This is about a 4% AHA concentration, which is just fine for someone with sensitive skin. There are much cheaper AHA products on the market; nothing about this one makes it worth the expense.

☺ $$$ **Glycolic Lotion** *($37 for 2 ounces)* has a very simple ingredient list of water, glycolic acid, two thickeners, and preservatives. This would be a very good (but overpriced) 8% AHA product for someone with oily skin.

☺ $$$ **Light Moisturizer** *($37 for 2 ounces)* contains mostly water, slip agent, thickeners, silicone, more thickeners, water-binding agents, film former, vitamins E and A, and preservative. The vitamins are at the end of the ingredient list, meaning they are practically nonexistent. This is as ordinary a moisturizer as you can find, but that doesn't mean it's bad. It would be a good moisturizer for someone with normal to slightly dry skin; it's just not worth the exorbitant price tag.

☺ $$$ **Line Refiner** *($25 for 0.18 ounce)* contains mostly water, a long list of thickening agents, emollient, silicone, water-binding agents, plant oils, plant extracts, and preservatives. This won't change a line on your face, but it is a good moisturizer for someone with dry skin.

☺ $$$ **Moisture Gel (Oil-Free)** *($19 for 1 ounce)* is a silicone-based light-weight moisturizer that is more boring than it is helpful. The silicone can feel good on skin, but it would be better if this product contained some interesting water-binding agents or soothing ingredients than what is in here.

☺ $$$ **Oil-Controlling Gel** *($19 for 1 ounce)* is similar in some ways to plain milk of magnesia. It contains merely water, a form of magnesium, slip agent, preservative, and dye. It will work to absorb oil, but so will milk of magnesia for far less.

☺ $$$ **Protective Shield Moisturizer SPF 15** *($37 for 2 ounces)* is similar to the Light Moisturizer above, but with SPF 15. SPF 15 provides the same protection no matter what price tag is attached to it, and you can find it much more cheaply elsewhere.

☺ $$$ **Natural Sunscreen SPF 17 Waterproof** *($19 for 5 ounces)* is a very good titanium dioxide–based sunscreen for normal to dry skin.

☹ **Sunscreen Spray SPF 15** *($18 for 4.5 ounces)* doesn't contain avobenzone, zinc oxide, or titanium dioxide, and is not recommended.

☹ **Waterproof Sunscreen, SPF 30 (Oil-Free)** *($18 for 5 ounces)* doesn't contain avobenzone, zinc oxide, or titanium dioxide, and is not recommended.

☺ $$$ **Soothing Exfoliating Mask, Normalizing Mask for All Skin Types** *($30 for 2 ounces)* contains mostly water, clays, glycerin, thickener, and preservatives. This is a very standard clay mask, and if you want clay with no other irritants, you've found the right mask. I wouldn't call clay soothing, however; it can be drying.

Trish McEvoy Makeup

☺ $$$ <u>FOUNDATION:</u> **Natural Tint Foundation Oil-Free** *($35)* goes on evenly and smoothly, and quite sheer. Most of the colors are good, with only a handful to really avoid. For the money, this is just an ordinary foundation with nothing really to highlight. **Avoid** C1, C2, C4, N6, and W6.

☺ $$$ **Cream Powder Makeup** *($40)* is just what it says—a creamy-feeling makeup that spreads smoothly and sheer and then leaves a soft, powdery finish. It can be OK for dry skin types, but could be a problem for someone who tends to break out. It contains plenty of wax (including carnauba), and the second ingredient is isopropyl myristate, which can clog pores. Most of the colors are very good but these colors should be avoided: C2, C3, C6, W4, W5, W6, and N4.

☺ $$$ Cream Powder Makeup Oil-Free SPF 8 *($40)* may not contain oil but it contains plenty of waxes that can be a problem for someone with oily or blemish-prone skin. Also, the SPF does not have UVA proteciton. It does have a soft, powdery, smooth finish and can work well for someone with normal to slightly oily or slightly dry skin. Most of the colors are very good but these colors should be avoided: C2, C3, C6, W5, W6, and N4.

☺ $$$ Dual Powder *($28)* is meant to provide all-over face color as an alternative to traditional foundation. This product has a dry, powdery finish though it does have a silky feel. This can be great for a regular pressed powder.

☹ CONCEALER: Protective Shield Cover-up *($23)* gives great coverage, and blends out nicely to a subtle finish, but it does tends to crease and some of the colors are poor. Avoid Light, 1C, 2E, and 2C.

☺ $$$ POWDER: Loose Powder *($20)* is talc-based, with a very silky, soft texture, but the four color choices are appropriate only for light to medium skin tones. Did someone forget that this line has foundation colors for dark to very dark skin tones? What are those women supposed to use?

☺ $$$ All Over Face Powder*($28)* is a group of rather ordinary talc-based powders.

☺ $$$ Face Shine *($28)* is a cream-to-powder that has a more greasy finish and adds the requisite trendy shine women seem to want.

☺ $$$ BLUSH: Sheer Blush *($20)* are a group of soft matte shades that go on quite sheer. The regular Blush *($20)* colors are nice but fairly ordinary, and there are a few strange or shiny colors to watch out for.

☺ $$$ The very fat Lip & Cheek Pencils *($18.50)* are soft enough to be used as lipsticks or blushes. They feel like very glossy lipsticks or very creamy blushes. The pencils are convenient if you can somehow figure out how to keep them sharpened all the time.

☺ $$$ EYESHADOW: Six types of eyeshadows might sound like overkill, but in this case you can ignore the categories and just look for the colors you like, because they are all fairly similar. The Glazes have some amount of shine; Shapers are supposed to be softer colors; Definers are intense deep colors for liner; and Enhancers are medium shades for the crease *($18 each)*. All of the colors are interchangeable and the matte ones are, of course, the best. Most of the eyeshadows, particularly the darker shades, are a bit on the "wet" side and tend to crease.

☺ $$$ Face Essentials Kit *($35)* is a compact quad group of colors with a strip for blush, eyeliner, and two eyeshadows. The way the colors are organized makes it hard to prevent the blush brush from getting into the eyeshadows, and the colors tend to flake into one another. Additionally, any time you buy sets, you rarely end up using all the colors, which makes this kind of product a waste of money. On the other hand, some of the color groupings are beautifully matte, and the color that is meant to be used as the blush can be used around the eyes, so if you find a selection that meets all your needs, this can be an essential kit for you.

☺ $$$ <u>EYE AND BROW SHAPER:</u> The **Eye Pencils** *($15)* are incredibly standard, in a very typical assortment of colors.

☺ $$$ <u>LIPSTICK AND LIP PENCIL:</u> **Sheers** *($16)* are like a gloss, with the same staying power. **Sheers with SPF 15** *($16)* are identical to the Sheers except they contain sunscreen but no UVA protection. **Lip Colors** *($16)* are creamy lipsticks with good staying power, a wonderful texture, smooth application, and a very impressive color selection. **Semi-Matte** *($16)* has a good opaque, creamy finish. **Highlights Lip Gloss** *($16)* comes in a tube applicator and offers an interesting array of colors, including red, a shiny lavender, and a shiny gold, as well as soft, pale shades of pink, mauve, and peach. These glosses go on very thick and rich, looking more wet than glossy. **Lip Essential** *($20)* is a compact of four lip colors and types. One is glossy, the others creamy, semi-matte, and sheer. It works, but I prefer a traditional lipstick tube. **Lip Pencils** *($16)* come in a nice assortment of colors, and one side of the pencil is a lip brush. It's a nice touch, but Max Factor sells almost the exact same pencil for a quarter of the price.

☹ **Matte Over** *($16)* is supposed to be used as a lipstick base to help keep lipstick on longer or as a top coat to make any cream lipstick look matte. Either way, it is a problem. Used as a base it tends to peel, and used over lipstick it is just messy.

☺ $$$ <u>MASCARA:</u> The **Mascara** *($16)* stays on wonderfully and doesn't smear or clump, it also builds decent length and some amount of thickness.

☺ $$$ <u>BRUSHES:</u> It takes good professional brushes to apply makeup well and there are definitely some options in this group. The prices range from $38 to $18 but most are overpriced and have far less pricey counterparts. Stay away from the blush and powder brushes, the texture is stiff and coarse. (I was told they were getting new ones due to this problem but as this book went to press the old ones were still there.)

☺ $$$ <u>SPECIALTY:</u> **Face Planner** *($35 to $45 for the case/$12 to $14 for the pages)* is a very clever way to assemble a makeup bag that resembles a day planner. A two-ring binder inside a pouch holds "pages" that can be filled with the color of your choice. It's pricey, but this is an intriguing assortment and exceedingly convenient, especially if you're loyal to McEvoy's color line of eyeshadows and blushes.

Tyra (Skin Care Only)

Tyra's brochure is quite extensive and long, but the primary message is that skin needs water. "Both the medical community and the cosmetic industry agree that loss of water is the leading cause of most skin problems." Their brochure also claims that "Dehydration, the natural loss of moisture during aging, is the main cause of wrinkles in the skin… As dehydration occurs, the fatty tissues lose moisture and begin to shrivel. Without the firm, plump, fatty tissues for support, the surface layers wrinkle and the skin begins to look older." None of that is accurate in any way, shape, or form. There isn't a dermatologist or plastic surgeon anywhere in the world who would say dryness causes wrinkles or acne. Dehydration causes dry skin, but few other skin problems. Sun damage is the major culprit in causing wrinkles, not dryness. Fatty tissues are not comprised of water, they are comprised of fat, and fat is not affected by water. Fat tissue doesn't shrivel with age, though it can get thinned out. More typically, the fat tissue under the skin droops and sags, and that makes the skin look full in areas where you don't want it to look full. Thankfully, you can't plump fat tissue up, or your jowls would look fuller and the lines around your mouth would too.

Tyra wants you to believe that most skin problems are somehow related to water loss, even acne. "This condition [acne] can not be improved unless the impurities in the pore are cleaned out. Bringing water into the skin will soften the plug and eventually, it will be brought to the surface and cleaned away. The more water we put into the skin, the quicker we can help eliminate this oily condition." What fiction! The oil in the pore is not water-soluble, or water-permeable. Water won't flush out a pore, it just isn't possible, you can swim for days and days, and your pores will not become unplugged.

At several points, the copy explains that Tyra products will not clog pores. Tyra needs to check their ingredient lists more closely, because their products contain ingredients that definitely could cause problems for some skin types. For more information about Tyra, call (888) 444-6242.

☹ **Phase I, Premiere Cleanser** *($15 for 8 ounces)* is a standard detergent-based cleanser. It also contains lanolin oil and jojoba oil, which can clog pores. This can leave a greasy film on the skin.

☺ **Phase II, Premiere Normalizer** *($15 for 8 ounces)* is a good but extremely standard toner that contains mostly slip agents, soothing agents, and water-binding agent. That's fine, but unimpressive.

☺ **$$$ Phase III, Premiere Moisturizer** *($36 for 4 ounces)* contains mostly water, thickeners, plant oil, more thickeners, and preservatives. It is a good moisturizer for someone with dry skin, but the price is absurd. This is so standard it's almost a joke.

☺ **$$$ Plus IV Deep Moisturizer** *($44 for 4 ounces)* contains water, plant oil, thickeners, a tiny amount of vitamins, soothing agent, more thickeners, and preservatives. It is an emollient but rather standard moisturizer. The only thing wrong with it is the price.

Ultima II

At some point, Ultima II decided to appeal more to women in their 20s than to the over-50 crowd. The products went from ultra-moisturizing to ultra-fun and clever. New names include The Nakeds and LipSexxxy, the new skin-care products are called Interactives, and the shades in the color line are all matte and neutral.

At the forefront of this shift in direction are the Interactives, a six-step grouping of products that stack (almost interlocking) on top of each other. Supposedly, the design was influenced by ergonomics, the science of accommodating the human body. As impressive as that sounds, I don't get the feeling that these products relate to the human body in any way. In fact, getting the products unhooked from each other isn't all that easy, and the wide jars encourage bacteria growth. But if storage is an issue, this line is definitely an option; the packaging concept offers an attractive solution to the dilemma of how to store cosmetics in a snug bathroom.

What about the Interactives products themselves? According to the brochure, the six products are supposed to cover three skin-care needs: "prevention, protection, and repair." Antioxidants are supposed to provide prevention; protection is tackled by an SPF of 15; and "lipid fluidizers" are supposed to repair "the lipid barrier." Of those three, the only one that really makes sense is the SPF 15. The only way antioxidants could really have an effect on the skin would be if they blocked off all air, and that means suffocation—not a great idea. That's why the theory that antioxidants can prevent free-radical damage is only a theory. Lipid fluidizers, in the form of lecithin and glycerin, are nothing more than lipid water-binding agents added to the product to replace fats (sebum or oil) that may be missing from your skin. Thousands of products contain these ingredients.

Turning to the rest of the product line, the display units are attractive, though it's tough to figure out which are The Nakeds, WonderWear, Beautiful Nutrient, or Sexxxy products. Wherever I went, I found the Ultima II sales staff less aggressive than most, which made shopping at their counters less intimidating, but being left on your own isn't the best when a makeup line is this confusing. From lipsticks to eyeshadows and blushes, some of the colors are very good and matte, but there are a lot of problems to wade through. There are over seven types of foundation! There are a wide range of lipstick shades that vary from natural to full, bold colors, but the distinctions between the different types of lipstick are unclear. For more information about Ultima II call (800) 4-Revlon.

Ultima II Skin Care

☺ **CHR Cream Cleanser** (*$18.50 for 4 ounces*) is a standard mineral oil–based cleanser that must be wiped off and that can leave a greasy film on the skin.

☺ **CHR Lotion Cleanser** *($18.50 for 6 ounces)* is similar to the cleanser above, only in lotion form, and the same review applies.

☺ **Interactives Refreshing Cleanser Normal to Dry** *($16.50 for 4.5 ounces)* is almost identical to the cleansers above, except that it is aimed at a younger consumer.

☺ **Interactives Refreshing Cleanser Normal to Oily** *($16.50 for 5 ounces)* is a standard detergent-based cleanser that uses sodium lauryl sulfate rather high up on the ingredient list, which can make this too drying for most skin types.

☺ **Eye Makeup Remover for Sensitive Eyes** *($12.50 for 3.6 ounces)* is a standard detergent-based eye-makeup remover. There are too many detergent cleansers here to make it good for sensitive skin.

☺ $$$ **Going Going Gone Makeup Remover** *($13.50 for 4 ounces)* is just an expensive cold cream. It also contains isopropyl myristate, which can cause breakouts.

☺ $$$ **Brighten Up, Tighten Up Eye Cream** *($20 for 0.5 ounce)* contains mostly water, a very long list of thickeners, glycerin, silicone, water-binding agents, plant extract, vitamins, anti-irritants, more water-binding agents, plant oil, more water-binding agents, more thickeners, and preservatives. This is a very good moisturizer for dry skin. The ingredient list is immense; if you want to try almost every water-binding agent in the book, this is the product to buy. Of course, it won't do anything a hundred other moisturizers can't do.

☺ $$$ **CHR Cream Concentrate** *($32.50 for 2 ounces)* contains mostly water, thickener, slip agent, lanolin oil, more thickener, mineral oil, plant oil, more thickeners, water-binding agents, more thickeners, and preservatives. This is a very good moisturizer for someone with exceptionally dry skin.

☺ $$$ **CHR Double Action Night Cream** *($42.50 for 2 ounces)* is similar to the one above, and the same review applies.

☺ $$$ **CHR Double Action Eye Cream** *($22.50 for 0.5 ounce)* is similar to the one above, and the same review applies.

☹ **CHR Double Action, Day Lotion with Ceramides SPF 15** *($45 for 1.7 ounces)* doesn't contain avobenzone, zinc oxide, or titanium dioxide, and is not recommended.

☺ $$$ **CHR Extraordinary Cream** *($68.50 for 1.13 ounces)* contains mostly water, plant oils, mineral oil, slip agent, thickener, lanolin, more thickeners, water-binding agents, more plant oil, more thickeners, fragrance, and preservatives. This is an overpriced, but extremely emollient, moisturizer for someone with dry skin.

☺ $$$ **CHR Extraordinary Lotion** *($68.50 for 2 ounces)* contains mostly water, thickeners, collagen, protein, water-binding agents, almond oil, rice oil, mineral oil, more thickeners, and preservatives. This is a good emollient moisturizer for dry skin, but it's very overpriced.

☺ **$$$ CHR Lotion Concentrate** *($32.50 for 3 ounces)* contains mostly water, slip agent, thickeners, water-binding agents, more thickeners, and preservatives. It would be good for dry skin, but don't expect the collagen and protein to change anything about your skin.

☺ **$$$ Interactives Balanced State Antioxidant Skin Control Hydrator** *($20 for 1.75 ounces)* contains mostly water, slip agents, thickeners, BHA, water-binding agents, vitamins, plant extracts, preservatives, and fragrance. This huge ingredient list is wrapped around salicylic acid, but the pH of this product isn't low enough for it to be an exfoliant. This is still a good emollient moisturizer for dry skin; it would not be good for any other skin type.

☺ **$$$ Interactives Booster Shot Antioxidant Firming System** *($28.50 for 1.7 ounces)* contains mostly water, glycerin, film former, thickener, several antioxidants, water-binding agents, plant extracts, more thickeners, and preservatives. Calling hair spray "firming" is stretching the truth; film formers can make the skin look smoother, but they can also irritate sensitive skin. This is an OK lightweight gel for someone with normal to slightly dry to combination skin, but it isn't a booster shot for any type of skin.

☺ **$$$ Interactives Eye Site** *($18.50 for 0.39 ounce)* contains mostly water, silicone, slip agents, thickeners, water-binding agents, vitamin, water-binding agents, vitamins, and preservatives. One of the main thickening agents is a potential skin irritant.

☹ **Interactives Line Manager Antioxidant Retexturizer SPF 15** *($20 for 1.73 ounces)* doesn't contain avobenzone, zinc oxide, or titanium dioxide, and is not recommended.

☺ **$$$ Interactives Night Cap Antioxidant Skin Smoother** *($25 for 1.72 ounces)* contains mostly water, several thickeners, water-binding agents, silicone, more thickeners, a form of acrylate (like hair spray), more water-binding agents, antioxidants, plant oil, and preservatives. This is a good moisturizer for dry skin, although one of the thickening agents can be a skin irritant.

☹ **Interactives Oil Check Antioxidant Oil-Free Hydrator with SPF 15** *($20 for 1.81 ounces)* doesn't contain avobenzone, zinc oxide, or titanium dioxide, and is not recommended.

☹ **Interactives Thirst Buster Antioxidant Hydrator with SPF 15** *($20 for 1.73 ounces)* doesn't contain avobenzone, zinc oxide, or titanium dioxide, and is not recommended.

☹ **ProCollagen Eyes with Sunscreen** *($27.50 for 0.8 ounce)* doesn't contain avobenzone, zinc oxide, or titanium dioxide and for some strange reason no SPF is indicated. Without knowing the amount of protection you're getting and with no real UVA protection, this product is absolutely not recommended.

☹ **ProCollagen Face and Throat with Sunscreen** *($40 for 2 ounces)* is similar to the one above, and the same comments apply.

☺ **$$$ Smart Move** *($25 for 1.7 ounces)* contains mostly water, water-binding agent, thickener, slip agent, more thickeners, silicone oil, plant oil, more thickener, vitamin E, soothing agent, more thickeners, and preservatives. This is a good moisturizer for someone with dry skin.

☺ **$$$ Under Makeup Moisture Cream** *($22 for 2 ounces)* is a very emollient moisturizer for very dry skin, but the second ingredient is isopropyl myristate, and the lanolin oil can cause breakouts. The cream contains mostly water, thickener, lanolin oil, slip agent, mineral oil, more thickeners, plant oils, more thickeners, fragrance, and preservatives.

☺ **$$$ Under Makeup Moisture Lotion** *($27.50 for 4 ounces)* is identical to the cream above except that it is slightly less emollient, and the same review applies.

☹ **Vital Radiance Skin Perfecting Lotion SPF 15** *($22.50 for 1.5 ounces)* and **Vital Radiance Skin Perfecting Cream SPF 15** *($22.50 for 1.5 ounces)* are supposed to be beta hydroxy acid (BHA—salicylic acid) formulations with SPF. Even if they had a low pH to make the BHA effective, the sunscreen agents don't include titanium dioxide, zinc oxide, or avobenzone to assure protection against UVA sun damage. Without those ingredients, these two aren't vital; at best they're trivial and unimportant.

Ultima II Makeup

☹ <u>FOUNDATION:</u> **Ultimate Coverage** *($18.50)* is an accurate self-description. This is thick stuff with poor colors to choose from.

☺ **Beautiful Nutrient Nourishing Makeup SPF 15** *($24)* has a great in-part titanium dioxide–based sunscreen. The foundation has a sheer, soft, lightweight coverage, which makes it great for a natural look. There are 15 shades, but almost none for darker skin tones. The only colors to watch out for are: Cream, Alabaster, Dawn, Aurora Beige, and Almond. All of these are too peach or pink for most skin tones.

☺ **Beautiful Nutrient Nourishing Compact Makeup** *($24)* is a cream-to-powder foundation that is more cream, with only a minimal powder finish. It goes on soft and even and most of the nine shades are quite nice. The only shades to watch out for are: Ginger and Almond.

☺ **Vital Radiance Sheer Makeup** *($25)* has some great colors, and there are over 15 to choose from. The drawback to this foundation is that it has shine, and lots of it. I can't imagine why sparkling during the day is supposed to be a natural fashion statement. The only colors to stay away from (that is, if you don't mind shining) are: Bone, Ginger, and Nutmeg, which are all too peach for most skin tones.

☺ **WonderWear Foundation with SPF 6 Oil-Free Makeup** *($21.50)* comes in great colors, goes on matte, and it wears and wears and wears. This is Ultima II's version of ColorStay Foundation, and they share the same problems: they dry into place quickly and then don't budge, which makes blending difficult; they are hard to get off; and if you get the foundation on your nails it will wreck your manicure. It does last all day for someone with oily skin, but this kind of wear may not be so wonderful. You also can't rely on the SPF, which is an utterly disappointing number. **These colors are too peach, pink, or ash:** 0-Neutral, 2-Neutral, 3-Neutral Cool, 6-Neutral Cool, 9-Neutral Cool, 11-Neutral, 12-Neutral Cool, Nutmeg, Mocha, and Espresso.

☺ **WonderWear Cream Makeup SPF 6** *($21.50)* has a creamy application, providing thick, opaque coverage. This is an option for heavy coverage, but the SPF 6 is dismal. Most all of the nine shades are very good, only Ginger may be too ash for most skin tones.

☹ **The Nakeds Smoothing Line Makeup with SPF 10** *($20)* won't smooth lines and the colors are for the most part too peach or ash to recommend. Only one has any potential of looking like skin tone.

☹ **Glowtion with SPF 15** *($20)* is a tinted moisturizer with SPF 15 and part titanium dioxide. It would be an OK option for a sunscreen with a hint of color, except that this product has sparkles that make the skin shine and really terrible peach shades.

☺ **CONCEALER: WonderWear Concealer** *($14.50)* has a smooth, even application that is neither too dry or greasy, and that means it is an excellent choice. There is only a small chance it will slip into the lines around the eyes. There are four shades that are all quite good, only Ivory may be slightly too pink for some skin tones.

☹ **POWDER: The Nakeds Pressed Powder** *($16.50)* is a standard talc-based powder that has a great, silky-soft texture but colors that are too pink, peach, or rose for most skin tones. **The Nakeds Loose Powder** *($21.50)* has a slight shine, which defeats the purpose of a powder. **WonderWear Pressed Powder** *($16.50)* has a great texture and better colors than The Nakeds Pressed Powder, but this one has shine too.

☹ **BLUSH: Powder Blush** *($15.50)* is a group of extremely shiny blushes, and if you don't mind the shine the colors are excellent.

☺ **$$$ WonderWear Cheek Color** *($16.50)* goes on smooth and even, and the beautiful colors only have a hint of shine that barely shows up at all. **The Nakeds Cheek Color** *($16.50)* comes in a subtle range of colors, all of which are agreeably matte. **Beautiful Nutrient Blushing Stick** *($14)* is a standard cream blush in a twist-up container. The shades are lovely and all matte. I generally don't recommend cream blush, but this one has a very smooth texture and a slightly powdery finish.

☹ <u>EYESHADOW:</u> **Eye Shimmer Quad** *($20)* is just what the name implies, and I do not recommend it. **The Nakeds Eye Color Duet** *($15.50)* comes in colors that are all shiny.

☺ **WonderWear Eye Color** *($13.50)* and **The Nakeds Eye Color Single** *($13.50)* come in a great selection of neutral matte shades that blend on evenly. Watch out for the shiny ones. **Beautiful Nutrient Cream Eye Color** *($13.50)* comes in a squeeze tube and has a sheer matte finish. All of the shades are beautiful and quite matte. The trick is blending them on, which takes a deft hand. These do create a soft look and they stay great.

☺ <u>EYE AND BROW SHAPER:</u> **EyeSexxxy Liner** *($12)* is an extremely standard pencil that comes in a twist-up applicator. **Kohl Eye Pencil** *($11)* is just another standard eye pencil that goes on smooth and creamy. **WonderWear Liquid Eye Definer** *($12)* is a liquid eyeliner that dries to a solid, though soft, matte finish.

☺ **BrowSexxxy** *($12)* is a standard pencil with a creamy finish, probably too creamy for the brows! **Brow Pencil** *($11)* is the same thing as Brow Sexxxy; it just has a different name and doesn't come in a twist-up container.

☺ <u>LIPSTICK AND LIP PENCIL:</u> **The Nakeds** *($13.50)* is a good creamy, slightly glossy lipstick with great neutral shades. **LipSexxxy** *($12.50)* is the original ultra-matte lipstick; it has a very dry, extremely matte finish. It doesn't feel like a powder, but it definitely doesn't feel like a lipstick, nor is it all that sexy; as it wears off, it tends to peel. The texture isn't for everyone, but it is an ultra-matte look. Be careful with ultra-matte lipsticks during the winter; they make chapped lips worse. **Beautiful Nutrient Lip Color** *($13.50)* is a standard creamy, somewhat glossy lipstick. It doesn't provide more moisture or benefit for your lips than any other lipstick (as if any lipstick could feed the skin!). **Lip Glossy** *($12)* is a standard lip gloss in a tube applicator. **The Lip Liner** *($11)* comes in a nice variety of colors and has a smooth texture, but is strictly standard-issue. **LipSexxxy Lip Liner** *($12)* is a standard lip pencil in a twist-up applicator that comes in a large array of colors.

☺ **Full Moisture Lip Color SPF 25** *($13.50)* has no UVA protection. It is more of a lip gloss than lipstick.

☺ <u>MASCARA:</u> **Flutters Lengthening Mascara** *($13)* is simply sensational. It builds long, thick lashes easily and quickly, without a smudge or smear to be seen all day long. **WonderWear Mascara** *($13)* builds long lashes with no clumping or smearing but it doesn't have any more staying power than other mascaras. The claim about keeping mascara on 18 hours is impressive but lots of mascaras can do that.

☺ **Beautiful Nutrient Mascara** *($13.50)* is just an OK mascara; it doesn't build much length or thickness but it does clump and smear.

Urban Decay (Makeup Only)

Please look at my comments about the cosmetic line Hard Candy in reference to my overall feelings about Urban Decay. In essence it isn't for me to comment on any cosmetics line that has shiny cranberry mascara and lime green lipstick. What am I supposed to say about black metallic nail polish, glittery peacock-blue eyeliner, or gold lamé body paint? Clearly, any one who wants to wear shiny peacock-blue eyeliner or iridescent body paint should take a very close look at this line. But I will still encourage women of all ages to think about why they get dressed in the morning and what they want from their life, and then figure out how metallic, black, sparkling nail polish fits into that plan. For more information on Urban Decay call (800) 784-URBAN.

Eyeshadows are called ☹ **Potholes** *($15)* in the Urban Decay city angst–filled marketing regulations. These are extremely overpriced eyeshadows with a handful of ordinary matte shades and a larger assortment of sparkles and iridescent ones. The texture overall leaves much to be desired, but when you're thinking glitter I'm not sure smooth application or wearability matters, maybe a choppy application is part of the look?

☺ **Nail Polish** *($11)* are standard nail polishes in completely unstandard colors. The price is about the color, not the quality. Ozone is a clear top coat that dries in three minutes, and it does a pretty good job. But it will chip in the same amount of time as any other polish and for the money doesn't work any differently than Revlon's or Maybelline's fast-drying polishes.

☺ **Lipsticks** *($12)* are iridescent to the max and have a more glossy than creamy finish. The colors are what you would expect. The same is true for the **Lip Pencils** *($12)*. These are extremely standard, with color and shine being the distinctiveness you are paying for. **Lip Gunk** *($12)* is just purple to yellow lip gloss. Very emollient and very overpriced for what you get, except for the color that is.

☺ **Liquid Liner** *($14)* comes in an intriguing range of colors, from shiny Violet to shiny Black. The color goes on smoothly but it does tend to chip, and **Eye Pencils** *($12)* are extremely standard with shine and some interesting color options.

☺ **Mascara** *($12)* is an OK mascara that builds minimal length and thickness and tends not to smear. This isn't an exciting mascara but the colors are. If you want magenta lashes, this would be one of the few places to find that option.

☺ **Body Haze Hair and Body Paint** *($18)* is a very gunky, thick spread of color that is applied in a stick over any part of the body. It can also be combed through the hair, and even comes with a tiny comb for that purpose. It applies easily and you can spread it to any coverage level, though it does tend to chip. But again, I can never tell if that's part of the "look" or not. **Body Jewelry** *($11)* speaks for itself and is a fascinating way to get dressed for an evening look, but don't overdo.

Vaseline Intensive Care and Dermasil
(Skin Care Only)

For more information about Vaseline or Dermasil products, call (800) 743-8640.

☺ **Aloe Vera Triple Action Formula** *($3.29 for 10 ounces)* contains mostly water, glycerin, thickeners, aloe, plant oils, more thickeners, vitamins, several water-binding agents, silicone, and preservatives. This is a very good emollient moisturizer for someone with dry skin.

☺ **Dermasil Dry Skin Treatment Cream** *($7.79 for 4 ounces)* is similar to the product above, except this one contains petrolatum, and the same review applies.

☺ **Dermasil Dry Skin Treatment Lotion** *($7.79 for 8 ounces)* is similar to the one above but with mineral oil, but the same review applies.

☺ **Dermatology Formula** *($2.29 for 11 ounces)* contains mostly water, petrolatum, mineral oil, glycerin, silicone, a long list of thickeners, and preservatives. This is a very emollient, but very standard, moisturizer for someone with dry skin.

☺ **Dry Skin Triple Action Formula** *($3.29 for 10 ounces)* contains mostly water, glycerin, thickeners, plant oil, vitamins, water-binding agents, a tiny amount of AHAs, silicone, and preservatives. The amount of AHAs is hardly worth mentioning; nevertheless, this is a good emollient moisturizer for someone with dry skin.

☺ **Dry Skin Triple Action Formula, with Vitamins, Lipids, Alpha Hydroxy Complex** *($3.29 for 10 ounces)* is similar to the one above, and the same review applies.

☺ **Extra Strength Formula** *($3.29 for 10 ounces)* is similar to the product above, and the same review applies.

☺ **Extra Strength Triple Action Formula with Petroleum Jelly** *($3.29 for 10 ounces)* is similar to the Dermatology Formula above, and the same review applies.

☹ **Petroleum Jelly Cream Enriched with Vitamin E** *($2.99 for 4.5 ounces)* has, as its second ingredient, aluminum starch, which can be a skin irritant and cause breakouts.

☹ **Sensitive Dry Skin Triple Action Formula** *($3.29 for 10 ounces)* contains menthol, which makes it completely unacceptable for sensitive skin.

☺ **Sensitive Skin with Natural Oatmeal** *($4 for 15 ounces)* is similar to most of the good moisturizers in this group of products, and the oatmeal doesn't add anything of interest.

☹ **UV Daily Defense Lotion for Hands & Body SPF 4 Enriched Skin-Softening Formula with Ultraviolet Screen** *($4.79 for 9 ounces)* has an SPF 4, and that's a burn; it also doesn't contain avobenzone, zinc oxide, or titanium dioxide, and is not recommended.

Vichy (Skin Care Only/Canada Only)

Vichy took a long time to give Canadians ingredient listings on their products, which up to now has prevented me from reviewing this line. That was always disappointing, because this relatively inexpensive line of skin-care products looked interesting. It turns out, finally, that there are some good, reasonably priced products in this line that would be worthwhile to check out. The areas where Vichy really falls short are in its AHA and acne products. It excels in moisturizers and sunscreens! All prices are in Canadian dollars. For more information about Vichy products, call (888) 45-VICHY.

☺ **Demaquillant Integral One-Step Cleanser for Face and Eyes** *($13.50 for 200 ml)* is a detergent-based cleanser that can be good for gently cleaning the face.

☹ **Dermatological Cleansing Bar** *($7.95 for 100 g)* is a standard detergent-based bar cleanser that can be drying, and the ingredients that keep the bar in its bar form can clog pores.

☹ **Normaderm Express Cleansing Gel, for Acne Prone Skin** *($9.99 for 150 ml)* is a standard detergent-based cleanser with a tiny amount of disinfectant and a small amount of AHA. The AHA isn't enough to exfoliate the skin and the disinfectant would be rinsed down the drain before it had much of an effect on the skin.

☹ **Normaderm Express 2-In-One Lotion, for Acne Prone Skin** *($11.99 for 150 ml)* is mostly alcohol, and that hurts all skin types.

☹ **Purete Thermale Soap-Free, Rinse Off Cleanser** *($13.50 for 50 ml)* is a standard oil-based wipe-off cleanser. Wiping off makeup can pull at the skin and cause sagging.

☹ **Purete Thermale Cleansing Milk** *($13.50 for 200 ml)* is a standard wipe-off cleanser. It can leave a greasy film behind on the skin, and wiping off makeup tugs at skin and can encourage sagging.

☹ **Demaquillant Yeux Sensibles Eye Makeup Remover for Sensitive Eyes** *($13.50 for 150 ml)* is a standard detergent-based cleanser that contains way too many cleansing agents to make this good for any eyes, much less sensitive ones.

☺ **Purete Thermale Gentle Exfoliating Gel** *($13.50 for 50 ml)* is a standard detergent-based scrub that uses synthetic scrub particles. It isn't gentle, but it can exfoliate. This also contains BHA, but the pH is too high for it to be effective as an exfoliant.

☹ **Purete Thermale Dermo Protective Toning Lotion, for Dry Skin** *($13.50 for 200 ml)* contains witch hazel, which can be a skin irritant.

☹ **Purete Thermale Dermo Protective Toning Lotion, for Normal to Combination Skin** *($13.50 for 200 ml)* contains even more witch hazel than the one above, and is not recommended.

☺ **Thermal Spa Water** *($4.88 for 50 ml)* is just water, and serves no more special purpose in any way for skin than any other water from the tap. It just evaporates and then leaves the skin drier than before.

☺ **Adaptive Skin Balancing System, for Combination Skin** *($21.50 for 40 ml)* contains mostly water, silicone, glycerin, thickeners, film former, fragrance, plant oil, water-binding agents, and preservatives. This is a good but standard moisturizer for dry skin.

☹ **Lift-Active** *($28 for 50 ml)* contains silicone, cornstarch, thickeners, shea butter, plant oil, water-binding agents, preservatives, and fragrance. The cornstarch may make the skin feel tighter but it is also drying and irritating for the skin. What a waste, because every other aspect of this product makes for a good moisturizer.

☹ **Lift Active Eyes** *($26 for 15 ml)* is similar to the one above, and the same review applies.

☹ **Lift Active Lotion** *($18.95 for 40 ml)* is almost identical to the one above; the same review applies.

☺ **Lumiactive Rejuvenating Daily Filter-Care** *($26 for 50 ml)* is a very good UVA-protecting sunscreen that contains both avobenzone and Mexoryl SX. It also contains a small amount of AHA but not enough to be effective as an exfoliant.

☺ **Lumineuse Sheer Radiance Tinted Moisturizer, Dry Skin** *($19 for 30 ml)* has a tint color that isn't the best, but this is a good emollient moisturizer for dry skin. It also contains some plant extracts that you're supposed to believe act like AHAs, but they don't.

☺ **Lumineuse Sheer Radiance Tinted Moisturizer, Normal to Combination Skin** *($19 for 30 ml)* is similar to the one above, only this product contains ingredients that can be a problem for combination skin, including several plant oils.

☺ **Nutritive 1 Balanced Nutrient Cream for Dry Skin** *($26 for 40 ml)* is a good basic moisturizer for dry skin that includes mostly water, silicone, glycerin, thickeners, plant oils, shea butter, preservatives, vitamins, and water-binding agents. It would be better if the vitamins and water-binding agents came before the preservatives, but this is still a good moisturizer.

☺ **Nutritive 2 Reinforced Nutrient Cream for Very Dry Skin** *($26 for 40 ml)* contains mostly water, mineral oil, petrolatum, waxes, emollients, preservatives, and fragrance. This is a very heavy but good moisturizer for parched skin.

☺ **Optalia Restructuring Eye Gel** *($28.50 for 15 ml)* is a good lightweight moisturizer for normal to slightly dry skin, which includes water, glycerin, water-binding agents, thickeners, vitamins, plant oil, and preservatives.

☺ **Regenium Night Renewal Cream** *($31 for 40 ml)* is an emollient moisturizer for dry skin that contains mostly water, thickeners, silicone, plant oils, petrolatum, water-binding agents, preservatives, and fragrance.

☺ **Thermal S1: Long Lasting Hydration** *($21.50 for 50 ml)* contains mostly water, silicones, glycerin, thickeners, mineral oil, petrolatum, water-binding agents, vitamins, plant oils, preservatives, and fragrance. This is a very good moisturizer for dry skin.

☺ **Thermal S2: Long Lasting Hydration for Very Dehydrated Skin** *($21.50 for 50 ml)* is similar to the one above, and the same review applies.

☺ **Thermal S2 Lotion: Long Lasting Hydration** *($21.50 for 50 ml)* is similar to the one above, and the same review applies.

☺ **Therma S Oil Free Lotion** *($21.50 for 100 ml)* is a good lightweight moisturizer for normal to slightly dry skin. It does contain cornstarch, which isn't the best because it can clog pores.

☺ **Capital Soleil Protective Gel-Cream SPF 15** *($15.50 for 120 ml)* is a very good sunscreen for normal to dry skin that contains titanium dioxide, avobenzone, and Mexoryl SX.

☹ **Capital Soleil Protective Lotion SPF 8** *($15.50 for 120 ml)* has a low SPF; with all the great SPF numbers in this line, why bother with such an unprotective number?

☺ **Capital Soleil Protective Lotion SPF 15** *($15.50 for 120 ml)* is a very good sunscreen for normal to dry skin; it contains titanium dioxide, avobenzone, and Mexoryl SX.

☺ **Capital Soleil Sunblock Cream for the Face SPF 25** *($15.50 for 50 ml)* is a very good sunscreen for normal to dry skin; it contains titanium dioxide, avobenzone, and Mexoryl SX.

☺ **Capital Soleil Sunblock Lotion SPF 25** *($15.50 for 120 ml)* is a very good sunscreen for normal to dry skin; it contains titanium dioxide, avobenzone, and Mexoryl SX.

☺ **Capital Soleil Sunblock Lotion for Children SPF 25** *($15.50 for 120 ml)* is a very good sunscreen for normal to dry skin; it contains titanium dioxide, avobenzone, and Mexoryl SX.

☺ **Capital Soleil Total Sunblock Lotion SPF 30** *($15.50 for 120 ml)* is a very good sunscreen for normal to dry skin; it contains titanium dioxide, avobenzone, and Mexoryl SX.

☺ **Capital Soleil Total Sunblock Cream SPF 45** *($15.50 for 50 ml)* is a very good sunscreen for normal to dry skin; it contains titanium dioxide, avobenzone, and Mexoryl SX.

☹ **Heliocalm Soothing and Hydrating After-Sun Milk** *($15.50 for 150 ml)* would have been a great moisturizer, but this one contains menthol, which is a skin irritant and can hurt the skin's healing process.

☺ **Heliocalm Calming Reparative Gel For Face and Body** *($15.50 for 100 ml)* is a very basic lightweight gel that contains mostly water, glycerin, silicone, film former, water-binding agent, anti-irritant, preservatives, and plant oil. This won't repair anything, but it is a good moisturizer for someone with normal to slightly dry skin.

☺ **Normaderm Express Tinted Treatment Cream, For Acne Prone Skin** *($11.99 for 30 ml)* has a tint that isn't the best color, and this product is meant to be an AHA exfoliant, except it doesn't contain enough AHA to do that.

☹ **Normaderm Express Treatment Cream, For Acne Prone Skin** *($11.99 for 30 ml)* is almost identical to the one above and the same comments apply, plus this product contains cornstarch, which can clog pores and encourage bacteria growth.

☹ **Normaderm Patch Express, For Acne Prone Skin** *($10.99 for 24)* contains a tiny amount of disinfectant and BHA. The disinfectant is OK but not the best for breakouts, and the pH isn't low enough for the BHA to be effective as an exfoliant.

☹ **Normaderm Stick Express Treatment Stick for Imperfections, For Acne Prone Skin** *($9.99 for 0.28 g)* contains lots of ingredients that would be a problem for blemish-prone skin, including castor oil, titanium dioxide, thick waxes, and aluminum chlorohydrate (that's deodorant!).

☺ **Purifying Thermal Mask** *($18 for 50 ml)* is a very standard clay mask that can be good for normal to oily skin.

☺ **Rehydrating Thermal Mask** *($18 for 50 ml)* contains mostly water, silicone, thickeners, glycerin, water-binding agents, and preservatives. The interesting ingredients in here come well after the preservatives, so this ends up being not as beneficial for skin as many of the moisturizers in this line.

Victoria Jackson

Victoria Jackson Cosmetics had one of the first cosmetics infomercials to hit the airwaves, and it has been amazingly successful. Almost everything you need to do a complete makeup application and cleansing routine is part of the ☹ **$$$ Introductory Kit** *($119.85, $234.35)*. The makeup items include a brush set (no sponge tips), four eyeshadows, two shades of foundation in one compact, a retractable lip pencil, three retractable eye or brow pencils, four shades of lip color that come in a compact, two blushers, pressed translucent powder, mascara and lash conditioner, a packet of instruction cards, an instructional videotape, and reorder forms. Whew! Each item is marked with a price that's higher than what it costs as part of the kit. For example, the foundation is marked $24.95, although you receive it for $12.95 when you get it in the kit. In fact, all the Victoria Jackson products have two prices. If you order a certain number of products, you can get the cheaper price every time. This is a cosmetics line that likes making deals.

But what about the products? Most of the makeup items are fine, although nothing special; a few don't work well at all. The few skin-care products are supposed to be suitable for all skin types. It's an interesting and unusual concept, but skin-care products for someone with oily skin cannot be the same as products for someone with extremely dry or even normal skin. This line is best for women with normal to dry skin; women with normal to oily or combination skin are not going to be happy. Still, I liked some of these products very much, and the prices (if you buy more than $20 worth of products at a time) are quite reasonable.

Once you place an order, you also start getting the product catalog. One of the "money-saving" offers includes groups of eyeshadows, eye pencils, blushes, and lipsticks divided into ☺ $$$ **Morning, Noon, and Night** *($41.95, $82.75)*.These are three different intensities of makeup (a total of 15 products) in a color family of Red, Peach, or Pink; Morning is the softest, Noon is a little deeper, and Night is the darkest. This is more makeup than anyone needs, and it also assumes that you need drastically different makeup for morning than you need for afternoon and night. There are easier ways to change morning makeup into night makeup than buying entirely different sets of makeup! And that's not all: the eyeshadows are shiny and the lip colors are greasy. The blushes and pencils are nice enough, but they are fairly pricey when purchased individually.

One other product offered in the catalog is the **Ultimate Space-Saving Makeup Kit** *($52.95)*. It looks great in the picture—all your makeup packaged in a neat little box that unfolds in an organized, orderly fashion. It is indeed small and looks convenient, but the containers are not refillable, so once one runs out, refilling it is an expensive proposition.

The makeup demonstration videotape that came with the introductory kit was good and understandable, although I didn't always agree with Ms. Jackson's application techniques. For example, she recommends applying eyeliner and brow color before the eyeshadows, but that means the eyeshadows would likely undo or mess them up. Those are minor points, though. A more annoying feature is that half of the tape is like sitting through another ad, listening to Ms. Jackson and a guest celebrity talk about how great the products are. If you've got the tape, you've already bought the products; now you want to learn how to use them. I suppose that sometimes it's hard to stop selling.

The prices listed in the reviews below are the prices for the individual products, not the lower prices you get if you order a number of products (the first price is for club members; the second is the retail price). For more information about Victoria Jackson's products call (800) V-MAKEUP.

Victoria Jackson Skin Care

☺ **Facial Cleanser and Eye Makeup Remover** *($9.25, $13.50 for 4 ounces)* is a standard detergent-based wipe-off cleanser. You are supposed to wipe off your makeup using this watery cleanser applied to a cotton ball, and then rinse off any residue. Wiping off makeup pulls at the skin and over time can cause it to sag.

☺ **Sensitive Facial Scrub** *($12.95, $19.95 for 4.7 ounces)* claims that this product is oil-free, but there are several ingredients in here that would not make someone with oily or combination skin happy. This is a group of thickeners with cornmeal as the scrub agent. You would be far better off with baking soda and some Cetaphil Gentle Skin Cleanser than with this waxy scrub.

☺ **Toning Mist** *($9.75, $14.50 for 4 ounces)* is a very good nonirritating toner that contains mostly water, aloe, water-binding agents, slip agent, and preservatives.

☺ **$$$ Eye Repair Gel** *($12.50, $19.50 for 0.5 ounce)* contains mostly water, slip agent, several water-binding agents, and preservatives. This would be a good lightweight moisturizer for the skin around the eyes.

☹ **Moisture Enhancer with Sunscreen SPF 8** *($12.75, $19.50 for 1.9 ounces)*. SPF 8 doesn't count, and this product doesn't contain avobenzone, zinc oxide, or titanium dioxide, and is not recommended.

☺ **$$$ Moisturizer** *($13.75, 20.50 for 2 ounces)* contains mostly water, thickeners, slip agents, more thickeners, water-binding agents, vitamins E and A, and preservatives. This would be a very good moisturizer for someone with dry skin.

☺ **Nourishing Skin Revitalizer** *($12.95, 19.95 for 1 ounce)* isn't all that revitalizing, but it is a good moisturizer for someone with dry skin. It contains mostly water, water-binding agents, vitamins, thickeners, anti-irritant, and preservatives.

☺ **Skin Renewal System** *($30.95, $39.95 for 0.14 ounce of Extra-Intensive Eye Cream and 1.25 ounces of Extra-Intensive Night Cream)* is somewhat unusual. The Night Cream is in the bottom half of the jar, and the Eye Cream is in the top half. Very cute. However, the ingredients in each are not all that different, so the division seems unnecessary. The Eye Cream contains mostly water, thickener, tissular extract (it's anyone's guess as to what this is, but it certainly can't change your skin tissue), plant oil, mineral oil, water-binding agents, vitamins, and preservatives. The Night Cream contains mostly water, several thickeners, water-binding agents, anti-irritant, silicone, and preservatives. Both creams are very good moisturizers for dry skin.

☹ **Firming Gel Masque** *($11.95, $17.50 for 4 ounces)* won't firm anything, and the second ingredient is a strong skin irritant. If your skin looks tighter after you take this mask off, it's due to the irritation.

☹ **Moisturizing Lip Conditioner SPF 15** *($9.95, $15.95)* doesn't contain avobenzone, zinc oxide, or titanium dioxide, and is not recommended for sun protection.

Victoria Jackson Makeup

☺ **FOUNDATION:** Victoria Jackson offers only one type of **Foundation** *($14.95, $25.95);* it comes in a single compact with two shades each for four categories of skin tones: Light, Medium, Tan, and Dark. The colors are good, though the Medium shades are a tad ashy green, the Light shade is a bit pink, and there is only one option for darker skin tones. To create the right color for your skin, you are supposed to mix the two shades together, which is fine if you know how to mix them in the right proportions. If you don't, you're likely to have trouble. The foundation is quite thick, and I would not call the application sheer, as the commercial claims. The foundation is petrolatum-based and therefore somewhat greasy. Oily or combination skins would not do well with this one.

☹ <u>CONCEALER:</u> There is no individually packed concealer in the Victoria Jackson line. The line suggests using the lighter shade of foundation in the dual-foundation compact for the under-eye area. This would be a great idea if the foundation weren't so greasy. It easily slips into the lines under the eyes, and any liner you use will probably smear.

☺ $$$ <u>POWDER:</u> **Pressed Powder** *($11.95, $17.95)* comes in four shades—Light, Medium, Tan, and Dark—and is talc-based. The colors are all fine and the texture is sheer and light.

☺ $$$ <u>BLUSH:</u> Each color-family kit (Peach, Red, and Pink) comes with a **Blush Compact** *($11.95, $20.95)* that contains two colors. One is always a pale shade of peachy pink, and the other is more vivid. The textures and colors are very good. The Red kit's blush is a nice shade of coral (which is not red, by the way); the Pink kit's blush is a soft shade of pink; and the Peach kit's blush is a brown-peach shade that is probably too brown for most skin tones.

☹ <u>EYESHADOW:</u> The **Eyeshadow Compact** *($11.95, $20.95)* is a single compact of four different colors. The combinations are excellent; unfortunately, almost all are slightly shiny.

☺ <u>EYE AND BROW SHAPER:</u> All of the **Eye Pencils** and **Brow Pencils** *($7, $10.95)* are twist-up and have a great smooth texture, a bit on the dry side. There are three eye or brow pencils in each kit—Black, Chocolate Brown, and Taupe.

☹ <u>LIPSTICK AND LIP PENCIL:</u> Each Victoria Jackson color kit includes a **Lip Compact** *($11.95, $18.95)* that contains three shades of lip cream and a lip-color powder. The colors are fine, but the lip creams are very greasy; if you have any problem with bleeding lipstick, these are not for you. The lip powder is a problem because it tends to cake on the lips and dry them out when used alone or when worn for an extended period of time. Lipsticks that come in tubes are listed on the order sheet, but there are no color swatches to assist you in making a decision. The kit includes a **Lip Pencil** *($7, $10.95)* that matches the color categories of Peach, Pink, and Red.

☺ <u>MASCARA:</u> Every introductory kit comes with **Dual Black Mascara** *($8.50,*

$13.95): one end is a clear conditioner, the other a black mascara. The mascara is good, but the conditioner consists mostly of a plastic-like substance and glycerin. It won't do much for the lashes, and I didn't notice any difference when I used it. Victoria Jackson's traditional black **Mascara** *($14.95)* is great just by itself.

☹ **BRUSHES:** Victoria Jackson includes a set of brushes in the introductory kit that are adequate but not great. A **Retractable Brush Set** *($40)* that includes a retractable blush brush and a retractable lip brush is overpriced. The **Professional Brush Set** *($18.95)* includes a lip brush, an eyebrow brush/comb, a two-sided eyeshadow brush, and a blush brush. The brush bristles are sparse and not firm enough to hold the color well. There are better brushes on the market.

Victoria's Secret Cosmetics (Makeup Only)

I admit it, I'm not a sexy lingerie fan. I've been wearing cotton briefs for as long as I can remember. I learned way back when that cotton underwear was far better for women for lots of health reasons, and ever since then I've stocked up on Calvin Klein's whenever they've gone on sale. I'm also not one for skimpy underwear in general. I hate anything that can inch up my backside. Lacy, sheer bras are attractive, but the straps tend to slip during the day and the cup just never fits right. I do own a satiny bathrobe and one satiny nightgown but that's it! I prefer my cotton T-shirt for serious sleeping. Evidently I am not a big of a fan of Victoria's Secret. I'm not even on their mailing list and believe me, I get dozens and dozens of a catalogues every month! Imagine my chagrin when I learned they had launched a new cosmetics line. What could this be about? When they introduced their fragrant body-care products and sachets, that made sense; lingerie and bathing do go hand in hand. But lipsticks and foundations?

When I walked in the store it seemed plain as day that Victoria's Secret Cosmetics (makeup products only) were about the same sleek, coy, sexuality that the rest of their merchandise is about. It was all inclined toward a woman feeling sexy and beautiful head to toe. Donning a silky teddy or lacy corset with a freshly clean face just loses something in the translation. It almost begs for full, glossed pouty lips and softly blushed cheeks. Plus, what woman can pass a cosmetics counter and not start to play, which is exactly what was taking place on several of my visits to a few Victoria's Secret stores—women were shopping for makeup and the lingerie part of the store was empty. It will be hard not to stop and try these products: the large, imposing display is easily accessible, and the sales staff eager and enthusiastic. Plus, the polished silvery containers and boxes are indeed beautiful and the names sweet and winsome. Draw Me a Line Lip Pencil and Play Around Makeup Adjuster or Hint Hint Sheer Lip Color are irresistibly cute. But cute doesn't always mean quality, and beyond the packaging there needs to be good product quality that works. It would be easy to get waylaid by the impulse buying this line (or any line for that matter) can attract, but let me encourage you to pick and choose wisely. What won't be a secret after you read my review is which products work and which ones don't. For more information about Victoria's Secret cosmetics call (800) 888-8200.

☹ **Oil-Free Cream-to-Powder Makeup SPF 10** *($19.50)* what were the creators of this foundation thinking? This oil-free product has shiny glitter, and lots of it. Isn't an oil-free makeup supposed to reduce shine, not add more to the face? Plus, the colors are just terrible, an unimpressive group of peaches and pinks! What a shame, because the application has a nice matte finish and the SPF 10 a decent nonchemical base. **Seamless Cover Moisture Rich Cream-to-Powder Makeup SPF 10** *($19.50)* also has poor colors, but, even more disappointing, it lacks any UVA protection. The texture is rather thick and creamy, which isn't bad, just heavy and hard to blend. **Play Around Oil-Free Makeup Adjustor SPF 10** *($17)* and **Play Around Moisture Rich Makeup Adjustor SPF 10** *($17)* are supposed to work with the corresponding liquid makeups (reviewed below) to help you get just the right color. The idea of custom blending a foundation is great, but having to do that every morning is time-consuming, and if you don't mix it just right, it can streak and look terribly uneven.

☹ **Liquid Lingerie Moisture Rich Makeup SPF 10** *($17.50)* has a very soft, sheer finish but the color selection is poor; of the ten shades, half are too pink, peach, or ash to recommend, plus the SPF doesn't include UVA protection.

☺ **$$$ Liquid Lingerie Oil-Free Makeup SPF 10** *($17.50)* has all the benefits the Moisture Rich version lacks, far better colors—and there are over 15 of them, and a titanium dioxide–based sunscreen (though a higher SPF would be better). The application isn't as sheer as the name implies, but you do get light to medium coverage with a dry smooth finish! This one is worth checking out if you have normal to oily skin!

☺ **$$$ Keep Your Secret Cream Concealer** *($10)* comes in a tube with four excellent shades! It does have a smooth, even finish, but it can crease, so test this one before you consider buying.

☹ **All an Illusion Skin Tone Primer** *($17.50)* is your standard group of green, peach, and lavender colored color-correctors. They don't change skin tone, they only add a strange cast to the skin and interact even more strangely with your foundation. Even if you're sold on this kind of product, this one contains isopropyl myristate (the second ingredient), which is known to cause breakouts. **Trick Stick Corrector Crayon** *($10)* has the same concept as the Primer only in pencil form, and for some reason comes in only two shades, yellow and green. **Thick Stick Concealer Crayon** *($10)* is a chubby pencil with three shades, of which two are way too peach for most all skin tones. The Light shade is just fine, but the texture is heavy and hard to blend, and it tends to easily crease into lines.

☺ $$$ **Powdered Silk Finishing Powder** *($15)* is a standard talc-based powder with a wonderful smooth silky texture. Of the eight shades #2, #5, #6, and #8 can be too rose, peach, or pink. The other four shades are excellent skin tones.

☺ $$$ **Sudden Blush Sheer Blushing Powder** *($15)* has a gorgeous silky texture, with a beautiful range of matte shades.

☹ **Dream Dust Face & Body Shimmer Powder** *($17.50)* is actually not all that shiny or iridescent and the texture is not as soft or even as that of the other powders in this line. While I'm not a fan of shiny, this product wouldn't past muster even if I did like shine.

☹ **Silky Wear Eye Colour** *($11)* is a good-looking group of very workable eyeshadow colors. Unfortunately, most of the shades are iridescent, even though the salesperson tried to convince me otherwise. The only matte shades were In the Buff, Hazelnut Cream, Java, Shell, Love at First Sight (this one is pink), and Bisque. **Party of 4 Eye Colour Quad** *($15)* is a set of four shiny shades of white, off-white, cream, and tan. For shiny this is fine, but how much shine can any one face handle?

☺ $$$ **Pencil Me in Brow Pencil** *($10)* has an exceptionally dry finish, which can make brows look less "penciled," but this one is hard to get on in the first place. All in all this is just a very standard brow pencil with a comb on one end to soften the application. **Draw Me a Line Eye Pencil** *($10)* is a standard, rather creamy finish pencil. It will definitely tend to smear along the lower lashes, though it will be easier to apply over eyeshadow. **Unruffled** *($12.50)* is a brow mascara that comes in a clear gel (like a gel hair spray) and two colors—blond and dark brown. The color choice is limited, but this one works well, though not well enough for me to give up my Borghese Brow Milano.

☺ $$$ **Stroke of Brilliance Mascara** *($12)* is a group of glittery mascaras. They don't make lashes very long or thick, but they do add a bit of silvery or purply iridescent color. I imagine there is a reason for this (everything these days is about shine), but I wouldn't recommend it. **Stroke of Brilliance Shimmery Liquid Eye Liner** *($12)* will one work as well as any if you want shiny gold or shiny black eye liner.

☹ **Brush with Greatness Thickening Mascara** *($12)* and **Exaggeration Lengthening Mascara** *($12)* both leave much to be desired. The Lengthening Mascara doesn't lengthen in the least, and the Thickening Mascara doesn't thicken, though it does work somewhat better than the Lengthening, but only somewhat. Both of these are not worth the money.

☺ $$$ **Smooth Talk Creamy Lip Colour** *($12.50)* is a huge array of lipsticks with a great color selection. The application is definitely creamy, so if you have any lines around your lips this one will bleed in an instant. **Hint Hint Sheer Lip Colour SPF 15** *($12.50)* is a small group of richly colored lipsticks with a glossy finish. Sadly, the SPF 15 doesn't have UVA protection. **Liquid Gleam Shiny Lipstick** *($11)* is a high-gloss lip gloss with sparkles that comes in a tube. **Mirror Mirror Shiny Lipgloss** *($10)* is similar to Liquid Gleam, only this one comes in a pot. **Draw Me a Line Lip Pencil** *($10)* is a large range of standard lip pencils that have a creamier application than most.

☺ $$$ **Quick Draw Lip Crayon** *($11)* is a chubby pencil that works as a lipstick, but has a very smeary, glossy application. **Matte Kisses Intense Lip Colour** *($12.50)* comes in eight rather limited strange shades. Try this on before you buy it; the colors are not the prettiest. It also isn't all that matte. You'll find this is just a good, opaque, creamy lipstick. **Mouth to Mouth Long Wear Lip Colour** *($12.50)* isn't all that long-wearing and the finish isn't all that different from the Matte Kisses lipstick. The colors for this one are also limited, and the shades too dark for lighter skin tones.

☹ **Lip Plump** *($12)* was sold at two of the Victoria's Secret stores I went to, and no wonder—the salespeople were selling it as a type of "spackle" that fills in the lips, making them smooth and perfect. It doesn't work. It's just a matte-finish concealer that sits on the surface of the lips for several minutes until it settles into the lines. **Party of 4 Lipgloss Quad** *($15)* is a group of four lip glosses ranging from black to white. It's supposed to change the color of any lipstick you own. It will indeed do that, but it also gives the lipstick a bizarre color quality.

If there is one solid area of interest for this line, it is the handful of handsome, silver-handled brushes. The feel is soft and the density great for application. The **Face Powder Brush** *($17.50)*, **Blush Brush** *($14.50)*, and the **Retractable Blush Brush** *($14.50)* are very good, as are the **Eye Colour** *($10.50)*, **Eye Colour Blender** *($10.50)*, and the **Retractable Lip Brush** *($8.50)*. The only one I question is the **Eye/Lip Definer Brush** *($8.50)*; it is really too small for the mouth and too big to use for the eyes, but if you are in need of this specific size brush (say, to smudge eyeliner), it is an option.

Wet 'n' Wild (Makeup Only)

It doesn't get any cheaper than this in the world of cosmetics. There are actually a few interesting items to consider in this small selection of products, but overall, it isn't the most exciting of the drugstore lines, and it definitely is neither wet or wild. For more information about Wet 'n' Wild call (914) 353-3000.

☹ **Oil-Free Makeup** *($1.44)* isn't the least bit oil-free, and the color selection is minimal. It tends to separate and doesn't blend well over the skin. **Matte Finish Liquid Makeup** *($1.44)* isn't all that matte, and it becomes greasy rather quickly, which isn't surprising given the lanolin and oils in the ingredient list.

☹ **Coverall Stick** *($1.99)* is extremely greasy, easily creases under the eye, and the shades are poorly suited to most skin tones.

☺ **Pressed Powder** *($2.49)* is a standard talc-based powder with a smooth, silky feel. It does have a slight bit of shine, which makes it appropriate only for someone with dry skin. This is a surprisingly nice, inexpensive powder.

☺ **Silk Finish Blush** *($1.86)* is slightly shiny, but not bad. I've complained in the past that these colors went on streaky, but no longer: the problem seems to have been fixed, and it goes on smooth and even. The color range has improved, too: there are some good soft colors here.

☺ **Eyeshadow Kit** *($1.42)* would be a possibility, because these are wonderfully smooth and soft, but the color selection is shiny and extremely limited (though what I've seen is mostly neutral). If only there were more matte colors it would be an option, and the same is true for the **Single Eyeshadows** *($1.42)*.

☺ **Liquid Lip Colour** *($1.99)* is just a good standard emollient gloss. **Lip Tricks Mood Lipstick** *($1.59)* isn't much of a trick, just one of those mood lipsticks that turn a different color on the lips. It is just a gloss with a hint of color. **MegaColors Lipstick** *(1.99)* is more of a glossy, shiny lipstick, but it's a good one for a sheer look and the texture is just fine. **MegaMatte** *($1.99)* isn't matte, but it is a very good creamy lipstick to consider with a great feel and soft finish. **Silk Finish Lipstick** *(99 cents)* is Wet 'n' Wild's standard lipstick. It is just a very sheer, shiny hint of color and it's fine for a minimal lipstick look. **Liner for Lips and Eyes** *(99 cents)* is a group of standard pencils that work as well as any in the rest of the cosmetics world. Don't be afraid of the price—go ahead and give these a try. They do need to be sharpened, which isn't my favorite, but at these prices, sharpening isn't so bad.

☹ **Protein Mascara** *($1.99)* doesn't build any length or thickness. **MegaLash Mascara** *($1.99)* is an awful sticky mess that clumps and doesn't build much length or thickness. **MegaLash Lengthening Mascara** *($1.99)* doesn't do a thing for lashes. It isn't a terrible mascara, just a waste of time and energy.

Youngblood (Makeup Only)

What a great name for a cosmetics line! Youngblood suggests all kinds of images to women in search of beauty. Aside from the trendy name, this line's claim to fame is an assortment of loose powders called ☺ **Youngblood Natural Mineral Cosmetics** *($29.95)*. These supposedly revolutionary powders are promoted as an all-in-one product—foundation, concealer, and powder. The brochure states, "You'll be amazed at how lightweight and long lasting" this powder is, plus it's "water resistant, [it] won't run, smear, or fade," it contains no "talc, fillers, perfumes, [and] dyes," and it isn't supposed to cause breakouts. The good news is that 50 percent of Youngblood's claims are valid: this is an amazing foundation that can double as concealer or loose powder. The bad news is that 50 percent of their claims are embellished and misleading, although that doesn't diminish the positives. Even better, they send out small sample packets of the powder in three or more shades, which makes this stuff incredibly easy to check out. (At least for those of you with normal to oily, combination, or normal skin. If your skin is even slightly dry this powder will cause flaking, and if your skin is very oily it can pool into the pores and look patchy.)

The brochure describes one of the ingredients, bismuth oxychloride, as a natural antiseptic that can be healing for problem skin. It can't. This earth mineral does have antiseptic properties, but it can also be a skin irritant, which doesn't make it all that healing. Also, the powder is supposed to give the skin "a translucent glow." The powder imparts a glow because it contains shiny, sparkly ingredients, including mica and iron oxides. If you have oily skin, you will not be happy with this much shine. However, these powders really do provide surprisingly even, smooth coverage; the colors are wonderfully neutral and easy to blend; they stay on incredibly well; and for most of the day they give the face a nice glow that only starts to look *too* shiny at the end of the day. Like most powder foundations, the Youngblood products did feel quite light, but they still provided completely opaque coverage and evened out most imperfections, especially when applied with a sponge instead of a brush.

One definite drawback is that at the end of the day, when you wash off the Youngblood foundation powder, you may very well find dry, flaky-looking skin all over your face (that's what happened to me). That may tone down with time or if you exfoliate your skin on a regular basis, but the bottom line is, this stuff can be drying.

A word of caution: Youngblood contains a fair amount of titanium dioxide, which explains why, as a loose powder, it can provide opaque coverage and stay in place so well. When I asked about an SPF rating, the salesperson explained that it wasn't rated ("It hasn't undergone the expensive testing required to give it an SPF number"), but, she said, "it is comparable to an SPF 15." If this company doesn't want to spend the money necessary to rate this product that's up to them, but making any statement about sun protection is disingenuous and irresponsible. If a product doesn't have an SPF rating, you can't know how much protection you are getting.

If Youngblood Natural Mineral Cosmetics piques your interest, you can call them at (888) YOUNGBLOOD.

Yves Rocher (Skin Care Only)

If you have ever tuned in to the Home Shopping Channel, you've likely encountered a pitch for Yves Rocher products. Like any other cosmetics line, Yves Rocher capitalizes on hyperbole and misleading information. Every gimmick in the book can be found in this vast assembly of products, from DNA and RNA in their A.D.N.

line (as if you would want a cosmetic to affect your genetic structure), to yeast, a cornucopia of plants (of course, plants are always the answer for everything from acne to wrinkles), and vitamins.

Yves Rocher does have its good points. The products are not tested on animals, all of them have a 100 percent money-back guarantee, there are some very good products to be found (especially moisturizers), the company often has sales of their products, and the prices aren't all that steep (although the sizes of the products are skimpy). You have to get past the extremely exaggerated claims and the really unnecessary diversity of the line to make a decision, and avoid some really bad products for acne. Stay away from the sunscreens and cleansers. If you are interested, the Yves Rocher customer service number is (800) 321-9837.

☺ **Acaciane Rinse-Off Cleanser** *($7.95 for 6.7 ounces)* is just shocking: the second ingredient in this cleanser for oily skin is Vaseline, and there are a host of other oils and thickeners that would be ludicrous for oily skin.

☺ **Acaciane Refreshing Floral Toner for Skin Prone to Oiliness** *($7.95 for 6.7 ounces)* contains alcohol and grapefruit, useless for oily skin, although they can cause redness and irritation.

☺ **Acaciane Matte Finish Skin Care Cream** *($9.95 for 1.7 ounces)* is not a good idea for someone with oily skin. Several of the thickening agents can clog pores, and though it contains clay for a matte finish to dry things up, why bother?

☺ **Acaciane Moisture Balancing Cream** *($9.95 for 1.7 ounces)* contains mineral and coconut oil, and how they are supposed to balance oily skin is anyone's guess. This is a good moisturizer for dry skin, but this line is aimed at those with oily skin.

☺ **Acaciane Replenishing Treatment** *($13.95 for 1.7 ounces)* is similar to the Cream above, and the same comments apply.

☺ **Acaciane Deep Cleansing Mask for Skin Prone to Oiliness** *($9.95 for 1.7 ounces)* is a standard clay mask with several thickening agents that can clog pores.

☺ **A.D.N. Revitalizing Resource Rinse-Off Cleansing Lotion, for Devitalized Skin** *($14 for 6.7 ounces)* is a fairly standard mineral oil–based cleanser with emollients that doesn't rinse off easily, if at all. It can leave a greasy film behind on the skin and really needs to be wiped off, and wiping at the skin can cause sagging.

☺ **A.D.N. Revitalizing Resource Refreshing Toner, Alcohol-Free, for Devitalized Skin** *($14 for 6.7 ounces)* contains mostly water, plant extracts, slip agents, detergent cleanser, water-binding agents, and preservatives. This is a very average, irritant-free toner that can be good for someone with normal to dry skin.

☺ **$$$ A.D.N. Revitalizing Resource Age Defense Eye Contour Treatment, for Wrinkles and Puffiness** *($30 for 1 ounce)* contains mostly water, plant extracts, thickener, slip agent, castor oil, water-binding agent, and preservatives. This very standard, overpriced moisturizer claims to have DNA and RNA that can somehow affect your skin; they can't, and it is insulting that the company suggests otherwise.

☺ $$$ A.D.N. **Revitalizing Resource Firming Intensive Night Cream, for Devitalized Skin** *($22 for 1.35 ounces)* contains mostly water, thickener, plant extract, corn oil, emollient, mineral oil, several thickeners, and preservatives. This is a good but extremely ordinary moisturizer for someone with normal to dry skin.

☺ $$$ A.D.N. **Revitalizing Resource Intensive Firming Serum, for Face and Throat** *($30 for 1.7 ounces)* contains mostly water, plant extract, several thickeners, water-binding agent, plant oil, emollient, more water-binding agents, and preservatives. This is a good but rather ordinary moisturizer for someone with normal to dry skin.

☹ A.D.N. **Revitalizing Resource Vital Defense Lotion, SPF 15 for Devitalized Skin** *($19 for 1.7 ounces)* doesn't contain avobenzone, zinc oxide, or titanium dioxide, and is not recommended.

☹ A.D.N. **Revitalizing Resource Vital Energizing Complex, for Devitalized Skin** *($24 for 1.35 ounces)* is supposed to contain fruit acids, a bogus name for AHAs. It doesn't contain any ingredients that can exfoliate the skin.

☺ $$$ A.D.N. **Revitalizing Resource Vital Moisture Day Cream, for Devitalized Skin** *($16 for 1.7 ounces)* contains mostly water, mineral oil, thickeners, plant oil, emollient, more thickeners, another plant oil, and preservatives. This is a good, but extremely standard, moisturizer for someone with dry skin, but because it lacks sunscreen, this "day" cream should only be used at night.

☺ $$$ A.D.N. **Revitalizing Resource Energizing Mask, for Devitalized Skin** *($16 for 1.7 ounces)* contains water, thickener, plant extract, emollient, more thickeners, water-binding agents, plant oil, silicone, preservatives, and vitamins. This is a good emollient mask for someone with dry skin.

☹ A.D.N. **Revitalizing Resource Vital Defense For Hands SPF 12** *($16 for 3.4 ounces)* doesn't contain avobenzone, zinc oxide, or titanium dioxide, and is not recommended.

☺ **Bio-Calmille Gel Cleanser** *($9.95 for 3.4 ounces)* is a standard detergent-based, water-soluble cleanser, good for most skin types. It can be drying for someone with dry to sensitive skin.

☹ **Bio-Calmille Gentle Cleansing Lotion** *($9.95 for 6.7 ounces)* is a fairly standard mineral oil–based cleanser with emollients that doesn't rinse off easily, if at all. It can leave a greasy film behind on the skin and really needs to be wiped off, and wiping at the skin can cause sagging. Any soothing benefit the Bio-Calmille products would have is reduced by the addition of fragrance in of all them.

☺ **Bio-Calmille Eye Makeup Remover Gel** *($9.95 for 3.4 ounces)* is a standard detergent-based eye-makeup remover. This one should work as well as any.

☺ **Bio-Calmille Soothing Alcohol Free Toner** *($9.95 for 6.7 ounces)* contains mostly water, slip agent, plant extracts, cleansing agent, and preservative. This is a very simple, ordinary, irritant-free toner. It would be OK for someone with normal to dry skin.

☺ **Bio-Calmille Long-Lasting Day Cream** *($11.95 for 1.7 ounces)* contains mostly water, plant oil, petrolatum, water-binding agents, thickeners, more plant oils, more thickeners, fragrance, and preservatives. Day cream without sunscreen should not be used during the day! At night this would be a good moisturizer for someone with dry skin.

☺ **Bio-Calmille Relaxing Soothing Mask** *($11.95 for 1.7 ounces)* is a standard mineral oil–based mask with thickening agents. It isn't particularly interesting, but it could be good for dry skin.

☺ **Bio-Calmille Soothing Night Cream** *($15.95 for 1.7 ounces)* contains mostly water, thickeners, slip agent, water-binding agent, silicone, thickener, plant oils, petrolatum, and preservatives. It is a good moisturizer for someone with normal to dry skin.

☹ **Bionutritive Essential Cleansing Lotion** *($9.95 for 6.7 ounces)* is a fairly standard mineral oil–based cleanser with emollients that doesn't rinse off easily, if at all. It can leave a greasy film behind on the skin.

☺ **Bionutritive Essential Toning Lotion** *($9.95 for 6.7 ounces)* contains mostly water, plant extracts, emollient, castor oil, water-binding agents, and preservatives. This is a good irritant-free toner for someone with dry skin.

☺ **Bionutritive Enrichment Day Cream** *($11.95 for 1.35 ounces)* contains mostly water, thickeners, plant oils, more thickeners, silicone, more thickeners, and preservatives. Day cream without sunscreen should not be used during the day! At night this would be a good moisturizer for someone with dry skin.

☺ **Bionutritive Nourishing Night Cream** *($17.95 for 1.35 ounces)* contains mostly water, thickener, plant oils, silicone, thickeners, slip agent, more thickeners, and preservatives. This is a good moisturizer for someone with dry skin.

☹ **Cel Defense Protective Foaming Cleanser** *($10 for 5 ounces)* is a standard detergent-based cleanser that contains sodium lauryl sulfate somewhat high up on the ingredient list. That can be a skin irritant and drying for most skin types.

☹ **Cel Defense Age-Defying Toner** *($10 for 5 ounces)* is an alcohol-based toner and absolutely not recommended.

☺ **Cel Defense Age-Defying Day Cream** *($17.50 for 1.35 ounces)* isn't much of a day cream (it has no sunscreen), but it is a very good moisturizer for very dry skin. It contains mostly water, plant oils, thickeners, silicone, fragrance, a teeny amount of AHA, vitamins, and preservatives.

☺ **Cel Defense Age-Defying Night Cream** *($19.50 for 1.35 ounces)* is similar to the one above, only more emollient.

☹ **Derma Controle Foaming Gel Cleanser** *($9.95 for 2.5 ounces)* contains a small amount of BHA (salicylic acid), which is completely wasted in a water-soluble cleanser because it would be rinsed down the drain before it could have an effect on the skin.

☹ **Derma Controle Normalizing Gel** *($11.95 for 2 ounces)* is yet another salicylic acid product, this time in a gel, along with ingredients that could possibly cause breakouts!

☹ **Derma Controle Purifying Lotion** *($9.95 for 4.2 ounces)* is an alcohol-based salicylic-acid toner. Alcohol only irritates the skin, causing dryness and redness that would be a problem for the skin in the long run.

☺ **Hydra Advance Hydrating Facial Wash for Dehydrated Skins** *($9.95 for 6.7 ounces)* is a detergent-based cleanser with mineral oil and several plant oils. The oils can definitely eliminate the dry feeling from the cleansing agent but they also leave a greasy film on the skin. This can be good for very dry skin types.

☺ **Hydra Advance Hydrating Toner, for Dehydrated Skins** *($9.95 for 6.7 ounces)* is a good irritant-free toner that contains mostly water, slip agents, water-binding agents, and preservatives.

☺ **Hydra Advance Maximum Moisture Renewal Gel for Dehydrated Skins** *($19.95 for 1.35 ounces)* contains mostly water, slip agents, film former, silicone, thickeners, water-binding agents, plant oils, fragrance, and preservatives. This can be a good moisturizer for someone with dry skin.

☺ **Hydra Advance Replenishing Moisture Base for Dehydrated Skins** *($15.95 for 1.35 ounces)* is a very emollient moisturizer for very dry skin that contains mostly water, plant oils, silicone, emollients, thickeners, water-binding agents, fragrance, and preservatives.

☹ **Hydra Advance Solaire Intensive Moisture Sun Lotion SPF 8** *($13.95 for 5 ounces)* doesn't contain avobenzone, zinc oxide, or titanium dioxide, and is not recommended.

☹ **Hydra Advance Solaire Intensive Moisture Sun Lotion SPF 15** *($15.95 for 5 ounces)* doesn't contain avobenzone, zinc oxide, or titanium dioxide, and is not recommended.

☺ **Hydra Advance Solaire Moisture Replenishing Lotion After-Sun** *($11.95 for 5 ounces)* is a very good emollient moisturizer for very dry skin. It contains mostly water, plant oils, mineral oil, thickeners, emollient, silicones, thickeners, water-binding agents, fragrance, and preservatives.

☺ **Hydra Advance Soliare Moisturizing Self-Tanning Spray** *($15.95 for 4 ounces)*, like all self-tanners, uses dihydroxyacetone to turn the skin brown; this one will work as well as any.

☺ **Hydra Advance Solaire Moisturizing Sun Block SPF 25** *($17.95 for 5 ounces)* is a good in-part titanium dioxide–based sunscreen for someone with dry skin.

☹ **Hydra Advance Solaire Self-Tanning Face Cream SPF 10** *($11.95 for 1.35 ounces)* doesn't contain avobenzone, zinc oxide, or titanium dioxide, and is not recommended.

☹ **Pro-Balance Skin-Balancing Cleanser** *($9.95 for 6.7 ounces)* is a fairly standard oil-based cleanser with emollients that doesn't rinse off easily, if at all.

☹ **Pro-Balance Toner with Botanical Self Regulator** *($9.95 for 6.7 ounces)* contains mostly water, glycerin, thickener, plant oil, and preservatives. The oil part of this product will not make someone with combination skin happy.

☺ **Pro-Balance Day Cream with Botanical Self Regulator** *($11.95 for 1.7 ounces)* contains mostly water, glycerin, thickener, plant oil, silicone, more thickeners, slip agent, and preservatives. A day cream without sunscreen should not be used during the day! At night this would be a good moisturizer for someone with normal to slightly dry skin, but the oil would not be great for oily parts of the face.

☹ **Pro-Balance Fluid** *($13.95 for 1.7 ounces)* contains mostly water, glycerin, cornstarch, plant oil, thickeners, silicone, plant oil, and preservatives. Cornstarch can cause bacteria growth, increasing breakouts as well as irritation. This product won't balance anything.

☹ **Pure Systeme Micro-Grain Gentle Cleansing Bar** *($15.95 for 4.4 ounces)* is a standard tallow- and detergent-based bar cleanser. Tallow can cause breakouts and irritate the skin.

☺ **Pure Systeme Gentle Foaming Scrub** *($15.95 for 3.4 ounces)* is a standard detergent-based scrub that uses synthetic particles as the exfoliant. It's OK, but it does contain grapefruit and menthol, which can be irritating to the skin and won't do anything to reduce oil or breakouts.

☹ **Pure Systeme Gentle Skin Clarifier** *($16.95 for 6.7 ounces)* contains mostly water and alcohol. It won't control oil and can cause dryness and irritation.

☹ **Pure Systeme Oil-Free Balancing Gel, for Oily Skin** *($19.95 for 1.7 ounces)* contains mostly water, alcohol, slip agent, silicone, thickeners, grapefruit extract, more thickeners, and preservatives. Alcohol and grapefruit extract are serious irritants, and one of the thickeners used in this gel can clog pores.

☹ **Pure Systeme Oil-Free Moisturizing Lotion** *($19.95 for 1.7 ounces)* contains mostly water, thickeners, slip agent, silicone, grapefruit extract, more thickeners, and preservatives. The grapefruit can be a skin irritant and can only hurt the skin; it provides no benefit for oily or acne-prone skin.

☺ **Pure Systeme Oil-Free Absorbent Mask** *($14.95 for 2 ounces)* is a standard clay mask that can indeed help absorb oil. It does contain grapefruit, but hopefully not enough to cause problems for the skin.

☺ **Response Nature Time Defense Radiance Defense Complex with Triple Fruit Acids** *($26 for 1 ounce)* doesn't contain AHAs and can't exfoliate the skin. This cream does contain lemon juice high up on the ingredient list, and that can be a skin irritant.

☺ **Response Nature Time Defense Radiance Renewal Fluid with Triple Fruit Acids** *($14 for 5 ounces)* is similar to the one above, and the same review applies here.

☺ **$$$ Response Nature Time Defense Eye Contour Treatment** *($19 for 0.5 ounce)* contains mostly water, slip agents, thickeners, silicone, water-binding agent, mineral oil, preservatives, and vitamins. This is a good moisturizer for dry skin.

☹ **Response Nature Time Defense Daytime Protective Cream SPF 8** *($14 for 1.35 ounces)* doesn't contain avobenzone, zinc oxide, or titanium dioxide, and is not recommended.

☹ **Response Nature Time Defense Fluid Day Cream, SPF 8** *($19 for 1.7 ounces)* doesn't contain avobenzone, zinc oxide, or titanium dioxide, and is not recommended.

☺ **Response Nature Time Defense Night Recovery Treatment** *($24 for 1.35 ounces)* is a very good emollient moisturizer for someone with dry skin. It contains mostly water, slip agents, thickeners, plant oils, emollients, water-binding agents, and vitamins. It does contain a tiny amount of vitamin A, as the name claims, but it won't help skin recover from anything.

☹ **Riche Creme Rinse-off Creme Cleanser, with 10 Botanical Oils** *($14 for 5 ounces)* is a fairly standard mineral oil–based cleanser with emollients, and it doesn't rinse off easily, if at all. It can leave a greasy film behind on the skin and really needs to be wiped off, and wiping at the skin can cause sagging.

☺ **Riche Creme Alcohol-Free Toner, with Floral and Herbal Extracts** *($14 for 6.7 ounces)* is a good irritant-free toner (if you aren't allergic to the plant extracts). It contains mostly water, glycerin, plant extracts, cleansing agent, slip agent, and preservatives.

☺ **$$$ Riche Creme Line Smoothing Serum, with Plant Extracts** *($14 for 0.3 ounce)* contains mostly water, slip agents, thickener, silicone, plant oil, more thickeners, another plant oil, and preservatives. This is a good, lightweight moisturizer.

☺ **$$$ Riche Creme Smoothing Throat Cream, with Botanical Extracts** *($24 for 1 ounce)* contains mostly water, thickener, plant oil, more thickeners, mineral oil, plant extracts, more thickeners, silicone, and preservatives. This would be a good moisturizer for dry skin anywhere on the body.

☺ **$$$ Riche Creme Wrinkle Fighting Concentrate** *($26 for 1 ounce)*, as the name implies, is a very rich moisturizer. It contains mostly plant oils, thickeners, and a tiny amount of vitamins. It won't change wrinkles but it is great for very dry skin.

☹ **$$$ Riche Creme Wrinkle Refining Complex with Triple Fruit Acids**

($26 for 1.7 ounces) contains mostly water, slip agent, thickeners, silicone, plant extracts, more thickeners, water-binding agents, several plant oils, and preservatives. This would be a good moisturizer for someone with dry skin, but it is a terrible AHA product, it neither contains enough nor the right form of AHAs to be considered an effective exfoliant.

☺ **Riche Creme Wrinkle Smoothing Day Cream, with 10 Botanical Oils** *($19 for 1.7 ounces)* contains mostly water, slip agent, thickeners, silicone, plant extracts, more thickeners, water-binding agents, several plant oils, and preservatives. This would be a good moisturizer for someone with dry skin. Of course, because it doesn't contain a sunscreen, this product should not be used during the day.

☺ $$$ **Riche Creme Wrinkle Smoothing Eye Cream, with Floral Extracts** *($24 for 0.5 ounce)* contains mostly water, slip agent, plant oil, thickeners, lanolin, more thickeners, plant extracts, another plant oil, and preservatives. This is a good moisturizer.

☺ $$$ **Riche Creme Wrinkle Smoothing Night Cream with 10 Botanical Oils** *($24 for 1.7 ounces)* does contain a lot of plant oils, lanolin, and emollients, but the first oil is mineral oil. This is a very good emollient moisturizer for someone with very dry, parched skin.

☺ **Cap Soleil Sunless Self-Tanning Cream** *($11.95 for 3.5 ounces)*, like all self-tanners, uses dihydroxyacetone to turn the skin brown. This one would work as well as any.

Yves St. Laurent

While I'm often quite opinionated about varying aspects of most cosmetics lines, I actually don't have much to say about the very blue-blooded Yves St. Laurent line of cosmetics. This upper-end cosmetics line has an air of snobbery about it that doesn't help the quality of its products in the least. In many ways this is the least impressive of all the French lines. The skin care is just OK, the foundation colors terrible, and the eyeshadows and blushes are all shiny. All of that combined with salespeople who seem to sniff at you in disdain if you look as though you don't have money to spend makes this line one to approach with an overall skeptical eye. For more information about Yves St. Laurent, call (212) 621-7300.

Yves St. Laurent Skin Care

☹ $$$ **Creme Demaquillant Douceur/Soothing Creme Cleanser** *($24 for 5 ounces)* is a standard mineral oil–based cleanser. It can leave a greasy film on the skin and requires a washcloth to really get off all the makeup, which is not very soothing.

☹ **Gel Mousse Purete/Foaming Cleansing Gel** *($24 for 5 ounces)* is a standard detergent-based, water-soluble cleanser that rinses well and takes off all the makeup.

The detergent cleansing agent can be very drying and may cause skin irritation, not to mention burn the eyes.

☺ $$$ **Lait Demaquillant Fraicheur/Instant Cleansing Milk** *($24 for 6.6 ounces)* is similar to the product above, and the same review applies.

☺ $$$ **Doux Demaquillant Pour Les Yeux/Gentle Eye Makeup and Lipstick Remover** *($22.50 for 2.5 ounces)* is a silicone-based wipe-off makeup remover. Pulling at the eye area to remove makeup causes the skin to sag and is never a good idea.

☹ **Tonique Soin Douceur/Extra-Gentle Tonic Alcohol-Free** *($24 for 6.6 ounces)* contains mostly slip agents, fragrance, film former, plant extracts, and preservatives. This is mostly fragranced water. It's about as do-nothing a skin-care product as I've ever seen.

☺ $$$ **Tonique Soin Fraicheur/Mild Clarifying Tonic** *($24 for 6.6 ounces)* is a silicone-based toner that also contains sodium phosphate, which can be a skin irritant. This isn't all that mild, and it's overpriced for what you get.

☺ $$$ **Tonique Soin Purete/Oil-Control Tonic** *($24 for 6.6 ounces)* is a standard alcohol-based toner that won't control oil, but will irritate the skin.

☺ $$$ **Creme de Nuit Revitalisante/Nighttime Revitalizer, for Combination to Dry Skin** *($55 for 1 ounce)* is almost identical to the Intensive Nighttime Revitalizer below, with a few minor differences (like no sunscreen) and a tiny amount of AHAs—only enough to be water-binding agents, not exfoliants. This is a good emollient moisturizer for dry skin, but it's nothing special.

☺ $$$ **Creme de Nuit Revitalisante Peaux Seches a Tres Seches/Intensive Nighttime Revitalizer, for Dry to Very Dry Skin** *($55 for 1 ounce)* contains mostly water, thickener, silicones, water-binding agents, more thickeners, plant oil, mineral oil, a small amount of sunscreen (which is strange in a night cream), preservatives, and fragrance. Vitamins A and E are in here, but they're too far down on the list to count. This is a good emollient moisturizer for dry skin, but it's nothing special.

☺ $$$ **Day/Night Concentrate, Concentrated Revitalizer** *($90 for two 0.5-ounce bottles)* consists of two products. The Day Concentrate contains mostly water, film former, slip agent, plant extracts, thickener, and preservatives. Several water-binding agents and vitamins are included, but they are present in such minuscule amounts that they don't benefit the skin at all. The Night Concentrate contains mostly plant oils, thickeners, water-binding agents, vitamin E, and preservatives. This is one of the most overpriced combinations of ordinary moisturizers you may encounter. They're not bad for your skin; they're just not very good.

☺ $$$ **Fruit Jeunesse/Firming Renewal Complex Glucohydroxy Acid** *($50 for 1.6 ounces)* contains mostly water, silicone, glycerin, thickener, AHAs, slip agent, more silicones, vitamin E, water-binding agent, plant oil, soothing agent, and preservatives. This is a good 4% AHA product that can be helpful for someone with dry, sensitive skin, but there are plenty of cheaper and equally good, if not better, AHA products on the market.

☺ **$$$ Hydra Fluide/Hydro-Light Day Lotion Oil-Free with SPF 15** *($35 for 1.3 ounces)* contains mostly water, slip agent, vitamin E (antioxidant), thickeners, and preservative. The long list of other ingredients following the preservative means they are barely present. This is an extremely ordinary but good basic daytime sunscreen for someone with normal to oily skin, but it's a waste of money to spend this much for something so dull.

☺ **$$$ Hydratant Absolu/Absolute Hydration** *($57 for 1 ounce)* contains mostly water, thickener, silicones, more thickener, slip agents, more thickeners, plant extract, preservative, and fragrance. There are some interesting water-binding agents at the end of the ingredient list, but that placement means they amount to little more than air. This is a good moisturizer for someone with dry skin, but it's completely standard and hardly worth the price.

☺ **$$$ Hydra Fluide/Hydro-Light Day Lotion, SPF 15** *($50 for 1.3 ounces)* contains mostly water, silicone oil, film former, glycerin, thickeners, vitamin E, more silicone, plant oil, more thickeners, mineral oil, and preservatives. There are some interesting water-binding agents at the end of the ingredient list, and that means they amount to little more than air. This is still a good sunscreen for someone with dry skin, but it's completely standard and hardly worth the price.

☺ **$$$ Precurseur Anti-Temps/Time Interceptor Fortifying Complex** *($65 for 1 ounce)* contains water, slip agent, mineral oil, water-binding agent, preservatives, and fragrance. There are some other interesting water-binding agents here, but they come well after the preservatives, which makes them worthless. This is a lot of money for mineral oil and thickeners, but the product can be good for dry skin.

☺ **$$$ Prevention + /Time Prevention Day Creme** *($65 for 1.7 ounces)* contains mostly water, thickener, silicone, a long list of other thickeners, vitamins E and C, more thickeners, and preservatives. This is a good but standard moisturizer for someone with dry skin. The vitamin C is supposed to be wonderful for the skin; it can be a good antioxidant, but that's it. This cream is one of many vitamin C products making great claims for being a fountain of youth; it isn't.

☺ **$$$ Soin Beaute Instantanee/Instant Firming Gel** *($60 for 1 ounce)* contains mostly water, slip agents, water-binding agents, thickeners, vitamins, and preservatives. This won't firm anything but it is a good lightweight moisturizer for dry skin.

☹ **$$$ Soin Contours/Firming Eye and Lip Creme** *($55 for 0.5 ounce)* is a very standard moisturizer that contains water, thickeners, mineral oil, and preservatives, and is way overpriced for this very basic moisturizer for normal to dry skin.

☺ **$$$ Soin Lissant Immediat Contour de L'oeil/Smoothing Eye Contour Gel** *($45 for 0.5 ounce)* contains mostly water, slip agent, thickener, plant extract, soothing agent, and preservatives. There are some other interesting water-binding ingredients, but they come well after the preservatives, which makes them useless. Other than that, this is a good lightweight moisturizer for the eye area.

☹ **Visible Energie Complete Day Creme for Combination Skin** *($50 for 1.7 ounces)* contains several ingredients that could be problematic for combination skin. Other than that, this is just a bunch of waxy thickening agents with a minimal amount of water-binding agents.

☺ **$$$ Visible Energie Complete Day Creme for Dry Skin** *($50 for 1.7 ounces)* contains mostly water, slip agents, thickeners, silicone, plant oil, fragrance, preservatives, vitamins, and a minimal amount of water-binding agents. This is a very ordinary moisturizer for normal to dry skin, but for the price you would expect more.

☹ **Masque Clarte Immediate/Instant Clarifying Masque, for All Skin Types** *($30 for 2.5 ounces)* contains mostly water, glycerin, detergent cleansing agent (one that is known for being very drying and irritating), plant oil, thickeners, film former, and preservatives. The ingredients are rather ordinary and the exotic plants come well after the preservatives, making them totally insignificant.

☺ **$$$ Masque Creme Hydro Actif/Hydro-Active Moisture Masque** *($35 for 1.6 ounces)* contains mostly water, mineral oil, film former, thickeners, plant oil, more thickeners, vitamin E, water-binding agents, and preservatives. This is a good, emollient, though completely ordinary moisturizer/mask for dry skin.

Yves St. Laurent Makeup

☺ **$$$ FOUNDATION: Teint Sur Mesure Duo De Teint** *($65 for 1 ounce)* is two separate products, foundation and concealer, in the same container. The six shades offered are a limited assortment; clearly, Yves St. Laurent doesn't expect women of color to shop at its counters. The notion is to use the concealer over any area on the face that you want to appear lighter—particularly the lines around the mouth, forehead, and eyes—or all over if you wish, before or after applying the foundation. It's a standard technique that can be accomplished with any good concealer and foundation. The texture is surprisingly light and sheer, with a dry, almost matte finish, even though it blends on rather moist and smooth. This is a very good foundation for someone with normal to slightly oily or combination skin. It doesn't settle into lines or streak. **These colors are excellent:** Golden Blond, Savannah Blond, Sandy Beige, Smoky Beige, and Tender Ivory. **This color is too rose for most skin tones:** Pale Pink.

☺ **$$$ Line Smoothing Foundation** *($44)* doesn't smooth lines, but it does have a lovely silky texture. It goes on easily and blends well with the skin, providing medium to slightly heavy coverage. The sales pitch is that it has light-reflecting properties. One salesperson said that meant it would light up the dark areas in my wrinkles. Please! It simply can't do that. Plus, the color choice available is terrible. **Only these colors look like skin: 8, 7, and 10. These colors should be avoided: 1, 2, 4, 5, 6, and 9.**

☺ **$$$ Teint Libre Moisturizing Foundation** *($32.50)* comes in only four shades, but the colors are good, and the texture is very light and smooth, with a dewy moist finish.

☺ **$$$ Teint Mat Oil-Free Foundation SPF 12** *($45)* comes with fancy marketing language that says this product has microparticles that can capture sebum (oil). Well, the ingredients are clay and magnesium—not the least bit fancy or unique. Other than that, it is a good, in-part titanium dioxide–based sunscreen foundation, with a partially matte finish. This one is best for someone with normal to slightly oily skin. **These colors are great: 2, 3, and 4. These colors are should be avoided: 1, 5, 6, 7, and 8.**

☹ **Teint Perfect Powder with Highlighter** *($36)* is a cream-to-powder foundation that comes with a separate shade meant to work as a highlighter. I do appreciate two-in-one products, but for this one the highlighter color, repeated for all the shades of powder, is too peach for most skin tones.

☹ **Premier Teint Matte** *($45)* is supposed to contain self-adapting pigments that even-out skin tone. Each of the four colors is shiny and either white, peach, lavender, or pink. A matte product that contains shine—what were they thinking?

☹ **Teint Spontane** *($31)* is an ultra-sheer face color/moisturizer that rubs very red or orange color over the face with a slight shine.

☹ **CONCEALER: Radiant Touch Eclat** *($32.50)* has changed from being a lightweight, smooth concealer to a shade of pink that is fairly unworkable for most skin tones, at least as a concealer. It may be effective as a highlighter, but a neutral tone would be far better.

☹ **Anti-Cernes** *($21)* is a greasy mess and easily creases into the lines around the eyes. The two colors are also too peach or pink for most skin tones.

☺ **$$$ POWDER: Silk Finish Pressed Powder** *($33.50)* has a wonderful silky texture, and some of the colors are quite good. **These are the best colors: 3 and 6. The other colors are too pink or peach. Silk Finish Loose Powder** *($33)* has a smooth, satiny feel, and all the colors are very good. **Semi Loose Powder** *($55)* comes in a cake form, but the container shaves off the top layer when you twist it, creating a loose powder. It's less messy than a loose powder, but all the colors are shiny, and that eliminates the purpose of a powder: dusting down shine.

☹ **Sunny Complexion Powder** *($35)* has a great silky texture, but is too shiny.

☹ **BLUSH: Variation Blush** *($31)* and **Blushing Powder** *($30)* are way too shiny, even though the textures are quite silky.

☹ **EYESHADOW:** All of the eyeshadows are ultra-shiny or too blue or contrasting. Why would any woman want to wear yellow and blue eyeshadow, or pink and green? What a shame, because the texture is quite nice. **Variation Solo** *($31)* is a strange quad set that is all the same shade, but two of the divisions are shiny. **Eyeshadow Powder Duo** *($31)* are mostly ultra-shiny colors (only 1, 2, and 5 are matte), but with this limited selection and price, why bother? **This is the only good combination of matte colors: 3. Quad Shadows The Mats** *($45)* are actually a group of four matte eyeshadows in one compact, which is great, but most of the color combinations are just too strange for any kind of softly blended look.

☺ **$$$ Perfecting Eyeshadow** *($35)* is a set of three colors; the highlighter shade remains the same for each of the shades, and the other two are matte eyeshadow colors and interesting to consider.

☺ **$$$ EYE AND BROW SHAPER: Eyeliner Moire** *($32)* are extremely iridescent, vivid colors with matching mascara. I'm sure there's a reason for this fashion statement, but I can't figure out what it might be. The small selections of **Eye Pencils** *($16.50)* and **Eye Brow Pencils** *($15)* are ordinary but fine. The Eyebrow Pencil has a dry mascara wand on one end to stroke through the brow after you apply the pencil.

☺ **$$$ LIPSTICK AND LIP PENCIL: Rouge Pur Lipstick** *($24.50)* is a very greasy cream lipstick that tends to feather easily and doesn't stay well, despite the tint. **Rouge Pur Mat** *($24.50)* goes on moist and creamy and isn't matte in the least. **Sheer Conditioning Lipstick** *($22.50)* has a soft, creamy, beautiful texture and feels great. **Quad Set of Lipsticks** *($45)* is a set of four lip colors that are more glossy than creamy. **Lip Lacquer** *($19)* is a fairly sticky, standard lip gloss in a vivid array of colors. **Lip Liner Pencil** *($16)* is a completely standard and completely overpriced lip liner.

☺ **$$$ MASCARA: Conditioning Mascara and Mascara Essentiel** *($20.50)* are both excellent mascaras, especially the Essentiel. They build very long, thick lashes and stay on great all through the day.

Zhen

Zhen is a line of skin-care and makeup products aimed at the Asian woman. Created by two Asian sisters who were frustrated by the lack of colors that suited their skin tones, this line boasts a "unique collection of yellow-toned foundations" appropriate for all skin types, but most specifically the Asian woman. I concur that most skin types are better served by yellow/neutral-based foundations and powders. However, although I agree with the mission statement the two sisters make, their foundations are not in the least bit yellow-based. I would call most of them glaringly pink, peach, and ash. Didn't the Yee sisters look at these colors in the daylight? I was so shocked by the colors I tested them several times, even traveling to different stores just to make sure the testers I was using hadn't turned color. They hadn't. There is nothing about this line that makes it better for Asian skin, or any other skin color for that matter. Lancome, Bobbi Brown, Clinique, Almay, and Maybelline, to name a few, all have more "yellow" or neutral-based foundations and powders than Zhen does.

The skin-care products are an embarrassment, and contain many of the same irritating ingredients found in Noxzema, only Zhen charges five times more. Why does anyone think that skin is benefited by clove, peppermint, lemon, or eucalyptus? These all have exceptionally high toxicity ratings and shouldn't be used by anyone ever. They do nothing beneficial, they are only capable of causing irritation and redness. For more information about Zhen, call (800) 457-8455 or (612) 323-4817.

Zhen Skin Care

☹ **Cleanser for All Skin Types** *($18 for 7 ounces)* contains way too many seriously irritating ingredients, including peppermint, clove, and cinnamon.

☹ **Cleanser for Normal to Dry Skin** *($18 for 8 ounces)* contains glycolic acid, which is a problem in a cleanser, but it also has other irritating ingredients that should not be put on the skin, including lemon, orange, and pine.

☹ **Cleanser for Normal to Oily Skin** *($18 for 8 ounces)* is a standard detergent-based cleanser but one of the cleansing agents is rather strong and not the best.

☹ **Papaya Face Scrub** *($20 for 4 ounces)* contains several thickeners, plant oil, a small amount of papain, and plant extracts. This is a confusing product, with several ingredients that can leave a film on the skin or clog pores as well as irritating ingredients that are best avoided. Papain and papaya don't help skin, they just irritate it.

☹ **Toner for All Skin Types** *($16.50 for 6 ounces)* contains peppermint, clove, and cinnamon, and is absolutely not recommended for any skin type.

☹ **Toner for Normal to Oily Skin** *($16.50 for 6 ounces)* has even more irritating ingredients than the one above, and is not recommended for any skin type.

☹ **Toner for Normal to Dry Skin** *($16.50 for 6 ounces)* doesn't contain as many irritants as the one for All Skin Types, but it does have lemon and orange, and that won't do for dry skin.

☺ **$$$ Eye Creme** *($22 for 0.5 ounce)* is an OK moisturizer for dry skin, and contains mostly thickeners and silicone. It also has a tiny amount of glycolic acid, but not enough for it to be an exfoliant.

☹ **Moisturizer with SPF 15 for All Skin Types** *($19.50 for 2 ounces)* doesn't contain avobenzone, zinc oxide, or titanium dioxide, and is not recommended.

☺ **$$$ Moisturizing Gel for Oily Skin** *($17.50 for 2 ounces)* contains mostly water, water-binding agents, witch hazel, thickeners, a teeny amount of AHA, and preservatives. The witch hazel can cause irritation; without that, this could have been a good lightweight moisturizer for normal to slightly dry skin.

☺ **$$$ Eye Gel** *($22 for 0.75 ounce)* is similar to the one above only slightly more emollient (this one has plant oils and more emollient thickeners). The same problem from the witch hazel exists here too.

☺ **$$$ Liposome Creme** *($25 for 1.25 ounces)* is similar to the one above only more emollient, and the same review applies.

☺ **$$$ Face Creme** *($25 for 1.25 ounces)* is a very good moisturizer for dry skin. It contains mostly water, water-binding agents, thickeners, plant oil, vitamins, and preservatives.

Zhen Makeup

☹ **FOUNDATION: Matte Foundation** *($15.50)* is a decent matte foundation, but the color selection is lacking in range. Only Pale Beige, Porcelain, and Creamy Beige are neutral enough to be considered true skin-tone colors. The rest are either too peach or too ash for most skin tones.

☹ **Light Diffusing Foundation SPF 8** *($22.50)* would be an OK in-part titanium dioxide–based foundation to consider except that the colors are almost all just awful. You can consider Creamy Beige, Sandy Beige, and Hazelnut, but why bother?

☹ **Foundation Stick with SPF 8** *($18)* also comes in colors that just aren't worth recommending, and the SPF 8 is too low.

☺ **$$$ CONCEALER: Concealer** *($10.50)* is a somewhat matte-textured concealer in a tube. It doesn't crease and it smoothes on nicely, but it comes in only two colors. This is a very good concealer for someone with normal to oily skin.

☺ **$$$ POWDER: Dual Activ Powder Foundation** *($20)* has a dry, matte finish and a very good range of colors. There are only three shades, but they are all good, true skin tones.

☹ **Pressed Face Powder** *($20)* has a soft, silky texture; what a shame it has such a strange color selection. Of the four colors, one is pink, another a vivid yellow, another peach, and one is a shiny bronze shade. I'm sure someone somewhere thinks there is a purpose for these, but I've got no idea what that purpose is. **Loose Powder** *($18)* comes in four shades—all shiny! Don't ask me why. I always thought of powder as dusting down shine, not adding to it. This can be used as an all-over shine for evening wear, but I would never recommend it for daytime. It comes in a strange assortment of colors, like the Pressed Face Powder above.

☺ **$$$ Mosaic Perfecting Powder** *($25)* is simply a talc-based powder that comes fragmented in a multicolored pattern of colors. When you place your brush over the colors it still comes out as one color. This doesn't perfect anything and is only suitable for a limited range of skin tones.

☺ $$$ <u>BLUSH:</u> **Pressed Powder Blush-On** *($14.50)* comes in an attractive though small grouping of matte colors. Only Shell is shiny, and it can be used as a highlighter for evening wear.

☺ $$$ <u>EYESHADOW:</u> **Matte Eyeshadow** *($10)* is a very small but pretty array of matte eyeshadows. The line does have a small selection of shiny eyeshadows, but they are clearly delineated as **Satin Finish** or **Pearl Finish Eyeshadow** *($10)*.

☺ $$$ <u>EYE AND BROW SHAPER:</u> **Waterproof Eye Definers** *($11)* are standard eye pencils, with a boring, small color selection, but they work. **Liquid Eye Liner** *($11.50)* is a standard liquid liner that goes on smooth without peeling or chipping as the day goes by. It comes in only three colors: Black, Brown, and Blue. Of course the Blue is out of the question, but the other two shades are fine. **Brow Pencil Shader** *($9.50)* is just a standard brow pencil, with a brush at one end. **Brow Set** *($11)* is simply a clear gel (like hair spray) that helps keep brows in place.

☹ **Brow Compact** *($25)* are just two matte shades of eyeshadow that are more grainy and heavy than most. It works, but this is overpriced at best and the two colors are unnecessary; no one has brown and black brows.

☺ $$$ <u>LIPSTICK AND LIP PENCIL:</u> **Cream Lipstick** *($10)* is a fairly creamy lipstick, bordering on being almost too greasy. **Matte Lipstick** *($10)* is an excellent matte lipstick with a smooth, nondrying finish. This one stays on very well and doesn't feather! **Lip Veil** *($10)* is nothing more than a good lip gloss. **Lip Pencil** *($12)* is as standard as a lip pencil can get. **Lip Quints** *($25)* are a set of five lip colors in one compact. One shade is a gloss, one is matte, and three are creamy. I find compacts of lip colors very inconvenient to use. I much prefer just grabbing a tube of lipstick and getting it on without the bother of a lip brush. This is an option for someone who prefers blending different textures of lip products.

☺ $$$ **Lip Primer** *($10)* is an unnecessary step if you have a lipstick that stays well and doesn't feather. It can help prevent lipstick color from turning, but if that isn't your problem there is no reason to add another layer to your lips.

☺ $$$ <u>MASCARA:</u> **Sensitive Eyes Mascara** *($12)* is an OK mascara, but nothing special. It tends not to smear, but it doesn't build much length or definition.

☺ $$$ <u>BRUSHES:</u> **Brushes** *($55 for nine brushes)* is a good assortment that covers every inch of your face, including a very tiny and very good eyeliner brush, a great blush and powder brush, a very good contour brush, large and small eyeshadow brushes, and more. At $55 for nine brushes, the average price is just $6.10 a brush. The only brush that is a bit of a waste is the lip brush; it isn't retractable, which makes it a bit too large to tote in your bag, as well as messy.

Zia (Skin Care Only)

Zia Wesley Hosford is the founder of Zia Cosmetics. This line of so-called herbal-based products is supposed to be for the educated consumer who wants the real thing in cosmetics, products that do what they say. Ironically, Sleek & Chic for women and Lean & Mean for men are her showcase products. "Their one purpose is to dissolve fat and cellulite. The amazing thing is that they actually do just that." These "purely natural ingredient" products are supposed to help women lose "an average of 4.25 inches on [their] thighs alone!" If you believe any of that, I have some swamp land I'd love to sell you. Clearly, Zia is hoping your education wasn't past grade school. For more information about Zia products call (800) 334-7546.

☹ **Absolutely Pure Aloe & Citrus Wash for All Skin Types** *($3.75 for 4 ounces)* definitely does contain citrus, which can make this cleanser irritating for all skin types.

☺ **$$$ Fresh Cleansing Gel, for Normal, Sensitive, Combination & Oily/ Problem Skin Types** *($15.50 for 8 ounces)* is a mild, detergent-based cleanser that should work well for most skin types.

☹ **$$$ Moisturizing Cleanser, for Normal, Sensitive, Dry & Mature Skin Types** *($15.50 for 8 ounces)* is basically a wipe-off cleanser with thickening agents and plant oils. It can leave a greasy film on the skin, which isn't good for any skin type.

☹ **Fresh Papaya Enzyme Peel Non-Abrasive Exfoliant for All Skin Types** *($20.95 for 1.5 ounces)* contains papaya, which is a skin irritant and not even a decent exfoliant.

☹ **$$$ Sea Tonic Aloe Toner for Normal, Sensitive, Combination & Oily/ Problem Skin Types** *($14.75 for 8 ounces)* is a mostly water and glycerin toner. If you aren't allergic to the plant extracts in this one (ylang ylang and cypress), you shouldn't have a problem with this product.

☹ **$$$ Sea Tonic Rosewater & Aloe Toner for Normal, Dry & Mature Skin Types** *($14.75 for 8 ounces)* could be a good toner of water and water binding agents, as long as you aren't allergic to the rose water and fragrance in this product.

☹ **Citrus Night Time Reversal Alpha Hydroxy Acid Creme for All Skin Types** *($25.95 for 1.5 ounces)* does seem to contain plenty of AHAs but the pH isn't high enough for them to be effective as exfoliants.

☹ **Even Smoother AHA/Papaya Accelerator for All Skin Types** *($29.95 for 2 ounces)* contains lemon, lime, and citrus, which are too irritating for all skin types. Papaya is not a good exfoliant but it is a good irritant.

☹ **$$$ Aromatherapy Treatment Oils for Dry Skin** *($20.95 for 0.3 ounce)* is basically just safflower oil and a little vitamin E. If the lemon oil in here doesn't bother your skin, it's OK, but this is something you could mix up on your own (without the irritating fragrances) for far less cost and it would be better for your skin.

☺ $$$ **Aromatherapy Treatment Oils for Hydration** *($20.95 for 0.3 ounce)* is, with minor fragrance differences, the same as the one above, and the same comments apply.

☺ $$$ **Aromatherapy Treatment Oils for Oil Control** *($20.95 for 0.3 ounce)* is, with minor fragrance differences, the same as the one above, and the same comments apply.

☺ $$$ **Essential Eye Gel** *($19.95 for 0.5 ounce)* contains mostly water, thickeners, anti-irritant, water-binding agents, witch hazel, plant extracts, vitamin E, and preservatives. The witch hazel can be irritating but there isn't very much in here, so this can be good as a moisturizer for slightly dry skin.

☺ $$$ **Everyday Moisturizers, Fragrance Free for Normal, Sensitive, Combination & Dry Skin Types** *($18.95 for 2 ounces)* contains mostly water, plant oils, thickeners, vitamin E, silicone, and preservatives. This would be a very good moisturizer for someone with dry skin, but there are several ingredients in here that would be a definite problem for someone with combination skin.

☺ $$$ **Eye Treatment Oil for All Skin Types** *($16.95 for 0.3 ounce)* contains thickeners, plant oils, vitamins, and preservatives. This would be a very good moisturizer for someone with dry skin, but there is nothing in here appropriate for normal to oily skin, despite the name.

☺ $$$ **Herbal Moisture Gel Oil Free Moisturizer for Normal, Sensitive, Combination & Oily/Problem Skin Types** *($22.95 for 1.5 ounces)* is a very lightweight gel that contains an anti-irritant, thickeners, and fragrance. This won't do much for skin, but if you have a touch of dry skin this could help soothe it.

☺ $$$ **Nourishing Creme Cellular Renewal for Normal, Dry & Mature Skin Types** *($12.75 for 1 ounce)* contains mostly water, plant oils, thickeners, water-binding agents, emollients, fragrance, and preservatives. This is a very good emollient moisturizer for dry skin, but it won't help cell renewal any more than any other emollient moisturizer. If you have sensitive skin, the fragrance here, including lemon oil, can be irritating.

☺ $$$ **Ultimate "C" Serum** *($49.95 for 0.5 ounce)* contains mostly water, anti-irritant, plant oils, water-binding agents, thickener, vitamins, plant extracts, silicone, and preservatives. There isn't that much vitamin C, and the form used here (ascorbic acid) is not considered one of the better ones. This is still a good moisturizer for dry skin.

☺ $$$ **Ultimate Moisture** *($34.95 for 1.5 ounces)* is similar to the one above, only with more water-binding agents and thickeners. It is a very good moisturizer for dry skin if you don't have a problem with the fragrance.

☺ **$$$ White Willow Day Treatment for All Skin Types** *($34.95 for 1 ounce)* isn't much of a day treatment without sunscreen; all it contains is some plant oil, thickeners, and vitamin A. That makes it a good moisturizer but that's about it. There is white willow bark, but that doesn't do much for the skin.

☺ **$$$ Ziasome Restorative Moisture Treatment for Normal, Dry & Mature Skin Types** *($29.95 for 0.3 ounce)* contains mostly water, water-binding agents, plant oils, vitamins, fragrance, and preservatives. This is a good moisturizer for dry skin.

☹ **Daily Moisture Screen SPF 15 for All Skin Types Except Oily/Problem Skin** *($19.95 for 1.5 ounces)* doesn't contain avobenzone, zinc oxide, or titanium dioxide, and is not recommended.

☹ **Oil-Free Face Block SPF 16, for All Skin Types** *($9.95 for 4 ounces)* doesn't contain avobenzone, zinc oxide, or titanium dioxide, and is not recommended.

☺ **Sans Sun Self Tanning Creme for All Skin Types** *($16.95 for 5 ounces)*, like all self-tanning products, uses dihydroxyacetone to turn the skin brown. This one would work as well as any.

☹ **15 Minute Face Lift for All Skin Types Especially Mature** *($19.95 for 4.4 ounces)* contains mostly cornstarch and egg white! If you want to believe that will lift your skin, whatever I have to say won't stop you.

☹ **Camphor Treatment Mask for Combination & Oily/Problem Skin Types** *($19.95 for 5 ounces)* contains mostly alcohol, sulfur, and camphor. Either one would be enough to hurt blemish-prone skin, but together they're skin killers.

☺ **Super Moisturizing Mask for Normal, Sensitive, Dry & Mature Skin Types** *($19.95 for 5 ounces)* is a good emollient moisturizer with lots of plant oils, lanolin, and thickeners. It would feel soothing for dry skin.

CHAPTER FOUR

The Best Products

The following product lists summarize the individual reviews in Chapter Three. Be sure to read those more-detailed product evaluations before making any final decisions. I hope all of these recommendations will make you feel informed and confident when shopping for makeup and skin care.

I know my lists of suggestions can get quite long, and some women have complained that I should reduce the list to my absolute favorites or to a top-ten list. I understand the frustration when looking at the number of products I do like, and although the field is narrowed, you still may wonder where to begin. I'm not quite sure how to get around the fact that the following products are all superior formulations or perform beautifully; there really isn't a hierarchy. I wouldn't even suggest that someone start with my own products (Paula's Choice), as they are just part of the products I find to be excellent. Most of you know I have a preference for superior formulations for the least amount of money, but this list simply concentrates on performance.

In some ways this notion of narrowing down my list even further is a bit funny to me, because often I am criticized for hating the cosmetics industry and not liking anything that's out there. But then on the other hand, women complain that I like too many things and I should shrink my list down even further! Perhaps there is no way to please everyone. The best I can do is tell you what my research and experience have found to be true, and allow you the consumer to pick up from there. I should mention that one of the purposes of my newsletter, *Cosmetics Counter Update,* is to narrow the range of options, in more detail and with more explanation. In the "Dear Paula" section of the newsletter where readers write to me with their particular concerns and needs, I address those in detail, and make specific recommendations depending on the individual situation and history. In this book, the goal is more general information, giving consumers enough room to find what works best for them among all the products with great, reliable formulations.

The only singling out I did do for the listing below is that I was even more finicky about the presence of any irritating ingredients. A product might have gotten a happy face in Chapter Three, but here I chose only those I felt didn't compromise my criteria.

First Beauty Note: Most cosmetics companies recommend skin-care routines for specific skin types. It is my strong suggestion that you ignore their categories and the corresponding product names. A person with dry skin who follows the cosmetics companies' recommendations could end up using too many products that will overgrease the skin and cause buildup, making the skin look dull and possibly causing breakouts (particularly whiteheads). Someone with oily skin will most likely be sold products that contain strong irritants that can make oily and acned skin worse. **Please consider each product individually for its quality and value to your skin, instead of by its placement in a series of products, its promotional ads or brochures, or the sales pitches you are likely to hear.**

Second Beauty Note: Please keep in mind that a cosmetics company's name for a product does not always, if ever, correspond with my recommendations. Just because a product label says it "gets rid of wrinkles" or is recommended for sensitive skin, or says it is a firming or nourishing serum doesn't mean the formulation itself supports that label or claim. **The same is true for eye creams or throat creams. Despite what the cosmetics industry wants you to believe, those products can be used anywhere on the face, and what counts is what skin type they are good for.** Additionally, you will find many selections in the following list of recommended products with names that sound like they should be in the dry-skin group but that I have included in the oily-skin group, and visa versa. What counts is how the product is formulated, not what the companies want you to believe about their products. There are lots of products labeled as being good for someone with oily skin that are best for someone with dry skin and lots of products with names that sound like they are best for dry skin but are really best for someone with slightly dry or oily skin.

Third Beauty Note: Just as a reminder, I consider all moisturizers as being necessary only where the skin is dry. If you do not have dry skin, you do not need to use a moisturizer. Overusing moisturizer can hurt the skin's healing process and hinder cell turnover. That means that I provide no category for oily-skin moisturizers. Even when a product is labeled as being for someone with oily or combination skin, it is only meant to be used over dry areas and not over oily areas. If you have dry skin in areas where you are oily, then you either have a skin disorder such as rosacea, dermatitis, psoriasis, or seborrhea, or you are using skin-care products that are too drying and irritating for your skin. That doesn't require a moisturizer, but a change in how you are taking care of your skin, or an appointment with a dermatologist.

If you have oily skin but have dry areas under the eye or on the cheeks (and you are certain you have no skin disorders and are not using irritating skin-care products) then consider the moisturizers in the slightly dry skin category below.

The exception to this rule is sunscreens, which absolutely must be used all over, every day, 365 days a year! To that end I do divide up my recommendations in skin-care categories. Unfortunately, there are very few options for women with oily skin. It is a search to find products that don't generate breakouts or feel greasy. Because of this I often recommend using a matte foundation with a good SPF and UVA protection, and then using a regular sunscreen for the rest of your body that is exposed to the sun.

Fourth Beauty Note: The order for application for any given skin-care regime is describe at length in my book *The Beauty Bible*. As a general rule the following is a safe guideline, depending on the products your skin needs:

Cleanser; scrub; eye-makeup remover if needed—by using an eye-makeup remover after the cleanser to get the last traces of eye or face makeup off, you prevent excessive pulling; **toner; topical disinfectant; AHA, BHA, topical retinoid, Azelaic acid, Differin, Metrogel or Metrocream; sunscreen** during the day; and at night a **moisturizer.** If you are using a **skin-lightening** product, it comes before the sunscreen or moisturizer.

Best Cleansers

Perhaps I was too emphatic years ago when I began nagging about the need for water-soluble cleansers, because now there are more water-soluble cleansers than I ever thought possible. When I wrote my first version of this book back in 1985, the only products available to clean the face were wipe-off cleansers and bar soaps (which were all drying, regardless of the claims on the packaging). Today, there are lots of options for the kinds of cleansers I would like most all women to use because of their gentle, effective, nonclogging cleansing action. Unfortunately, lots of water-soluble cleansers are too drying, irritating, or greasy—but happily, there are many that are very gentle on the skin, remove all the makeup without causing irritation or dryness, don't burn the eyes, and leave no greasy residue. It is also essential that a water-soluble cleanser can be removed easily by splashing and not by being wiped off with a damp washcloth. Using a washcloth might prevent the water from dripping all around the sink after you're done splashing, but washcloths can cause irritation (they aren't the gentlest surface I can think of), and that's not great for the skin.

There is one exception to this rule about washcloths, and it has to do with the new ultra-matte foundations on the market. These ultra-matte foundations, like Revlon's ColorStay or Lauder's Double Wear are incredible for oily skin, but they are also very difficult to wash off. If you are wearing this type of foundation, the best option is to use a water-soluble cleanser along with a washcloth to be sure you are getting everything off at night. One reader of my newsletter suggested another alternative I'd like to pass along. She takes an eye-makeup remover and dabs it all over the face, without pulling. Then she splashes her face with water and then follows with a water-soluble cleanser. She says that works great without pulling and without using a washcloth (which she found too irritating). This process actually works well with some foundations and is worth a try.

One thing most water-soluble cleansers have in common, regardless of price, is the basic ingredient list: detergent cleansing agents, foaming agents, and thickeners. Often water-soluble cleansers designed for dry skin can contain oils and can leave a greasy residue, and that's not great for the skin. When any cleanser leaves a film on the skin and then you follow up with an emollient moisturizer, that can cause a buildup of emollients on the skin, preventing cell turnover, and resulting in dull or even drier-looking skin.

Cleansers designed for normal to oily skin can also contain detergent cleansing agents that can dry out the skin and potentially cause irritation. Using a drying cleanser on oily skin doesn't get rid of any extra oil, it just irritates the skin and causes flaking. Inevitably that can mean the need of a moisturizer, and moisturizers used on a regular basis all over the face are almost always a problem for someone with oily or combination skin. Besides, this cycle of drying out oily or combination skin and then following up with a moisturizer is the fastest way I know to cause more skin problems.

Most of the cleansers listed below are for normal to oily/combination skin types. Many cleansers are made for drier skin types, but they are almost all greasy and require being wiped off. For drier skin types, I have found only a handful that would work well, are not drying, and that rinse off completely without leaving any residue.

FOR NORMAL TO OILY/COMBINATION AND/OR BLEMISH-PRONE SKIN TYPES, THE BEST WATER-SOLUBLE CLEANSERS ARE: **Adrien Arpel** Adult Oily Skin Sea Foam Gel Cleanser ($19 for 4 ounces), and Aromafleur Petal Daily Cleanser ($21 for 4.5 ounces); **Alpha Hydrox** Foaming Face Wash, for All Skin types ($5.57 for 6 ounces); **Amway** Clarifying Cleansing Gel for Normal to Oily Skin ($15.60 for 4.2 ounces); **Aveda** All Sensitive Cleanser ($19 for 5.5 ounces), and Purifying Gel Cleanser ($18 for 5.5 ounces); **Avon** Purifying Facial Cleansing Gel ($7.50 for 6.7 ounces); **Basis** Comfortably Clean Face Wash ($4.09 for 6 ounces); **Bath & Body Works** Foaming Face Wash Normal to Combination Skin ($8 for 6 ounces); **Beauty Without Cruelty** 3% Alpha Hydroxy Facial Cleanser Normal/Oily Skin Types ($7.49 for 8.5 ounces); **Biore** Foaming Cleanser ($5.99 for 5 ounces); **BioTherm** BioPur Pure Cleansing Gel ($15 for 150 ml); **Black Opal** Oil Free Cleansing Gel ($4.51 for 6 ounces); **The Body Shop** Balancing Cleansing Gel for Normal to Oily Skin ($9 for 6.76 ounces), Passion Fruit Cleansing Gel for Normal to Oily Skin ($8.15 for 8.4 ounces), Tea Tree Oil Facial Wash ($3 for 2 ounces), and Balancing Cleansing Gel for Normal to Oily Skin ($9 for 6.76 ounces); **Cetaphil** Oily Skin

Cleanser ($5.50 for 2 ounces); **Christian Dior** Equite Purifying Facewash ($27.50 for 6.8 ounces), and Equite Wash-off Cleansing Foam ($27.50 for 6.8 ounces); **Clarins** Oil-Control Cleansing Gel Oily Skin with Breakout Tendencies ($18 for 4.4 ounces); **Clean & Clear** Sensitive Skin Foaming Facial Cleanser ($3.79 for 8 ounces); **Elizabeth Arden** Modern Skin Care 2-in-1 Cleanser ($17.50 for 4.2 ounces); **Exact** Face Wash, Medicated Antibacterial Cleanser (Triclosan) ($4.61 for 6 ounces); **Fashion Fair** Botanical Cleansing Gel ($12 for 6.7 ounces), and Gentle Facial Shampoo Mild for Dry Sensitive Skin ($10 for 2.1 ounces); **Face Stockholm** Foaming Facial Cleanser Normal to Oily Skin ($12 for 4 ounces); **Flori Roberts** Optima Gel Cleanser Gold Oil-Free ($15 for 6 ounces); **Guerlain** Evolution Purifying Foaming Gel ($32 for 5.4 ounces), and Les Gestes Purete Foaming Gel and Refreshing for the Face ($29 for 6.8 ounces); **H₂O Plus** Marine Cleansing Gel (Oil-Free) ($16.50 for 5.7 ounces); **H+ Beauty System** Purifying Foaming Cleanser ($24 for 6.76 ounces); **Lancome** Clarifiance Oil-Free Gel Cleanser ($21.50 for 6.4 ounces); **Dr. Mary Lupo** Gentle Purifying Cleanser ($22 for 7 ounces); **Neutrogena** Fresh Foaming Cleanser Soap-Free Cleanser for Combination Skin ($6 for 5.5 ounces); **Nivea Visage** Visage Hydro-Cleansing Gel ($5.07 for 5.5 ounces); **Dr. Obagi** Nu-Derm, Cleanser I ($24 for 8 ounces); **Orlane** Normalane Foam Cleansing Gel for Mixed and Oily Skins ($25 for 4.2 ounces); **Paula's Choice** One Step Face Cleanser for Normal to Oily/Combination Skin ($9.95 for 8 ounces); **Pond's** Foaming Cleanser & Toner in One for Normal to Oily Skin ($4.39 for 4 ounces); **Purpose** Gentle Cleansing Wash ($4.95 for 6 ounces); **St. Ives** pH-Neutral Extra Gentle Facial Cleansing Liquid ($3.34 for 12 ounces); **Sea Breeze** Foaming Face Wash for Sensitive Skin ($3.78 for 6 ounces); **Shaklee** Enfuselle Purifying Cleansing Gel ($16.50 for 6 ounces); **Trish McEvoy** Essential Cleanser ($37 for 8 ounces); and **Yves Rocher** Bio-Calmille Gel Cleanser ($9.95 for 3.4 ounces).

<u>FOR NORMAL TO DRY AND/OR SENSITIVE SKIN, THE BEST WATER-SOLUBLE CLEANSERS ARE:</u> **Beauty Without Cruelty** Herbal Cream Facial Cleanser Normal/Dry Skin ($7.49 for 8.5 ounces); **BeneFit** All Types Skin Wash ($14 for 4 ounces); **Biogime** Essential Cleansing Milk ($22.50 for 8 ounces); **Biore** Cleansing Gel, Non-Foaming ($5.99 for 5 ounces); **The Body Shop** Foaming Cleansing Cream for Normal to Dry Skin ($9 for 6.7 ounces); **Borghese** Puro Fresco Gentle Fresh Cleanser ($25 for 6.76 ounces); **Cetaphil** Gentle Skin Cleanser ($8.31 for 16 ounces); **Donna Karan New York** Formula for Clean Skin ($25 for 5 ounces); **Estee Lauder** Instant Action Rinse-Off Cleanser ($17.50 for 6 ounces); **Gale Hayman** Total Eye Make-up & Facial Cleanser ($18.50 for 6.76 ounces); **Garden Botanika** Cucumber Cleansing Gel, ($10 for 8 ounces); **H+ Beauty System** Skin Purifying Cleanser ($24 for 6.78 ounces); **Hydron** Best Defense Gentle Cleansing Creme

($16.50 for 6 ounces); **Kiehl's** Gentle Foaming Facial Cleanser for Dry to Normal Skin Types ($13.50 for 8 ounces); **Marcelle** Aquarelle Oil-Free Purifying Cleansing Gel for Oily Skin ($10.58 for 170 ml); **Matrix Essentials** Gentle Cleansing Wash, for Normal, Dry, or Sensitive Skin ($18 for 5.3 ounces); **M.D. Formulations** Facial Cleanser Basic ($16 for 8 ounces); **Neutrogena** Extra Gentle Cleanser ($6.06 for 6.7 ounces); **Le Mirador** Dual Action Facial Cleanser ($19 for 6 ounces); **Oil of Olay** Foaming Face Wash ($3.87 for 6.78 ounces), and Sensitive Skin Foaming Face Wash ($3.87 for 6.78 ounces); **Organic Essentials** Clarifying Facial Cleanser ($15 for 4.2 ounces); **Paula's Choice** One Step Face Cleanser for Normal to Dry Skin ($9.95 for 8 ounces); **Renee Guinot** Purifiant Biologique Gentle Wash and Cleansing Cream All Skin Types ($26.50 for 5 ounces); **ROC** Rinse-off Facial Cleanser ($14.50 for 125 ml); and **Zia** Fresh Cleansing Gel, for Normal, Sensitive, Combination & Oily/Problem Skin Types ($15.50 for 8 ounces).

Best Eye-Makeup Removers

It is definitely not best to wipe off eye makeup or face makeup, because pulling at the skin encourages sagging. However, water-resistant makeup, stubborn makeup, and ultra-matte foundations need more help being removed than most gentle cleansers can provide, especially water-resistant eye makeup. All eye-makeup removers, regardless of price, are created equal, so I have not included a best list for this product type. The formulations are so amazingly similar it is almost shocking. Regardless of the eye-makeup remover you choose, my strong recommendation is to get as much of your makeup off as possible by washing first with a water-soluble cleanser. Any traces of makeup left behind can then gently be removed with minimal pulling by using an eye-makeup remover. (Ultra-matte foundations can be removed with the aid of a washcloth and a water-soluble cleanser, but be gentle, and then you can go over those areas of the face with the eye-makeup remover too if you choose, or with a toner.) I prefer nonoily eye-makeup removers (meaning those with no plant oils or mineral oil) because they leave the least residue on the skin, but mineral oil and plant oils can work just fine in removing makeup.

Best Toners

I have been preaching for years about the need to use only nonirritating, alcohol-free toners, and I am pleased to say that the cosmetics industry has plenty of them to offer these days. But keep in mind that alcohol-free does not mean irritant-free. Unfortunately, many cosmetics lines stick other irritating ingredients in their toners.

Toners and all the products that fall into this category (refining lotions, clarifying lotions, soothing tonics, stimulating lotions, fresheners, and astringents) are an extra cleansing step, and sometimes they can be soothing and slightly moisturizing. I evaluated these products strictly on how soothing or moisturizing and clean they felt on the face without drying the skin or leaving a greasy residue. **I expected a toner for normal to oily skin to leave the face soft and clean but not dry, and a toner for normal to dry skin to leave water-binding agents on the skin to help a moisturizer perform better. For oily skin, a good toner can be the only moisturizer that is needed.**

Does it make sense to spend a lot of money on a toner if it doesn't contain irritating ingredients? No. I found excellent toners that had very gentle ingredients and were relatively inexpensive. Many women enjoy using these products, and because of the soothing, fresh feeling many irritant-free toners can provide, I feel they can be beneficial for many skin types.

Note: If you have slightly dry skin or combination skin, the toners listed for dry skin can be the only moisturizer your skin needs.

FOR NORMAL TO OILY/COMBINATION SKIN, THE BEST TONERS ARE: Avon Moisturizing Alcohol-Free Toner ($7.50 for 6.7 ounces); Bioelements

Equalizer Rebalances Your Skin ($17.50 for 6 ounces); **Biogime** Protective Toner ($19.95 for 6 ounces); **Black Opal** Purifying Astringent ($3.99 for 6 ounces); **Borghese** Hydra-Puro Moisture Renewing Oil-Free Fluide ($35 for 1.7 ounces); **Clarins** Toning Lotion for Dry to Normal Skin ($21 for 8.4 ounces); **Estee Lauder** Verite Soothing Spray Toner ($22.50 for 6.7 ounces); **Forever Spring** Ambrosia Skin Refresher ($14.50 for 4 ounces); **Gale Hayman** Total Skin Toner Freshener & Firmer ($18 for 6.76 ounces); **H$_2$O Plus** Marine Moisture Mist (Hydrate) ($11 for 6 ounces); **Hydron** Best Defense Botanical Toner ($14.50 for 6.5 ounces); **La Prairie** Cellular Refining Lotion ($55 for 8.2 ounces); **Lancome** Eau de Bienfait Cleanser Water with Vitamins for Face and Eyes ($23.50 for 6.8 ounces), and Tonique Douceur Non-Alcoholic Freshener for Dry/Sensitive Skin ($27.50 for 13.5 ounces); **Marcelle** Hydractive Reviving Toner, Dehydrated and Normal to Dry Skin ($11.25 for 180 ml); **Natura Bisse** Sensitive Toner for All Skin Types ($22.50 for 6.5 ounces); **Neutrogena** Alcohol-Free Toner ($6 for 8 ounces); **Paula's Choice** Final Touch Toner for Normal to Oily/Combination Skin ($8.95 for 8 ounces); **Nu Skin** NaPCA Moisture Mist ($19.80 for 8.4 ounces); **Renee Guinot** Lotion Tonique Hydra-Douceur Hydra Soft Toning Lotion Dry and Sensitive Skin, Alcohol-Free ($19.50 for 6.7 ounces), and Lotion Tonique Rafraichissant Fresh Toning Lotion All Skin Types Alcohol-Free ($19.50 for 6.7 ounces); **ROC** Skin Toner Refreshing and Soothing, Dry Skin ($14.50 for 200 ml); and **Shiseido** Benefiance Balancing Softener ($34 for 5 ounces), and Pureness Cleansing Water ($15 for 5 ounces).

FOR NORMAL TO DRY SKIN AND/OR SENSITIVE SKIN, THE BEST TONERS ARE: Alexandra de Markoff Luxury Skin Toner, with Aloe Vera and Comfrey ($28.50 for 6 ounces), and Soothing Lotion, Alcohol Free, for Dry or Sensitive Skins ($48 for 4 ounces); **Aloette** Alcohol-Free Toner ($11 for 8 ounces); **Amway** Moisture Rich Toner for Normal to Dry Skin ($16.60 for 8.1 ounces); **Aveda** All Sensitive Toner ($18 for 5.5 ounces), and Skin Firming/Toning Agent ($18 for 5.5 ounces); **The Body Shop** Hydrating Freshener for Normal to Dry & Dry Skin ($8 for 6.76 ounces); **Borghese** Puro Tonico Comforting Spray Toner ($23 for 6.76 ounces), and Effetto Immediato Spa-Soothing Tonic for Sensitive Skin ($26.50 for 8.4 ounces); **Cellex-C** Firming Freshener ($32.50 for 6.8 ounces); **Charles of the Ritz** Revenescence Softening Lotion 100% Alcohol Free for Dry or Sensitive Skin ($18.50 for 8 ounces); **Christian Dior** Equite Alcohol-Free Softening Toner ($27.50 for 6.8 ounces); **Clarins** Extra-Comfort Toning Lotion Very Dry or Sensitized Skin ($25 for 8.8 ounces); **Erno Laszlo** HydrapHel Skin Supplement Freshener for Extremely Dry and Dry Skin ($30 for 6.8 ounces); **Givenchy** Balancing Mist ($30 for 5 ounces), and Gentle Toning Lotion ($28 for 6.7 ounces); **Jafra** Skin Freshener for Dry Skin ($13 for 8.4 ounces), and Soothing Results Calming Toner for Sensitive Skin ($13 for 8.4 ounces); **M.A.C.** PA-3 Phyto-Astringent Purifying Toner For Dry Skin ($15 for 4 ounces); **Merle Norman** Luxiva Collagen Clarifier ($14.50 for 6 ounces); **Nivea Visage** Alcohol Free Moisturizing Facial Toner ($5.49 for 6 ounces); **Origins** Sprinkler System ($13.50 for 6.7 ounces); **Orlane** B21 Bio-Energic Lotion Vivifiante Preparation for Face Care ($40 for 6.8 ounces), B21 Bio-Energic Vivifying Lotion for All Skins ($40 for 6.8 ounces), and Blue Line Soothing Lotion Alcohol-Free for Dry or Sensitive Skin ($29 for 6.8 ounces); **Paula's Choice** Final Touch Toner for Normal to Dry Skin ($8.95 for 8 ounces); **Physicians Formula** Gentle Refreshing Toner for Dry to Very Dry Skin ($6.95 for 8 ounces); **Rachel Perry** Violet Rose Skin Toner ($9.50 for 8 ounces); **Revlon** Moon Drops Softening Toner Normal to Dry ($5.99 for 8 ounces); **Shiseido** Vital Perfection Balancing Softener ($30 for 5 ounces); **Vichy** Demaquillant Integral One-Step Cleanser for Face and Eyes ($13.50 for 200 ml); **Victoria Jackson** Toning Mist ($9.75, $14.50 for 4 ounces); and **Yves Rocher** Bionutritive Essential Toning Lotion ($9.95 for 6.7 ounces), Hydra Advance Hydrating Toner, for Dehydrated Skins ($9.95 for 6.7 ounces), and Riche Creme Alcohol-Free Toner, with Floral and Herbal Extracts ($14 for 6.7 ounces).

Best Topical Disinfectants

The toner step for someone who struggles with blemishes needs to be a topical disinfectant. I discuss this step at length in my book *The Beauty Bible* and to a lesser extent in Chapter Two of this book. All the recommendations are for over-the-counter products that include benzoyl peroxide with no other irritating ingredients. A range of prescription-strength topical antibiotics are available from dermatologists.

FOR BLEMISH-PRONE SKIN FOR ALL SKIN TYPES, THE BEST TOPI-CAL DISINFECTANTS ARE: **Clean & Clear** Extra Strength Persa-Gel 5% Benzoyl Peroxide Dr. Prescribed Acne Medication Combination Skin Formulation ($3.92 for 1 ounce), and Maximum Strength Persa-Gel 10% Benzoyl Peroxide Dr. Prescribed Acne Medication ($4.99 for 1 ounce); **Mary Kay** Acne Treatment Gel ($6 for 1.25 ounces); **M.D. Formulations** Benzoyl Peroxide 5% for Extremely Oily and Acne-Prone Skin ($25 for 4 ounces), and Benzoyl Peroxide 10% for Extremely Oily and Acne-Prone Skin ($25 for 4 ounces); **Oxy Balance** Deep Action Night Formula ($4.52 for 4 ounces), Oxy Balance Emergency Spot Treatment Sensitive Skin Formula ($4.52 for 1 ounce), and Oxy Balance Emergency Spot Treatment Invisible Formula ($4.52 for 1 ounce); **Paula's Choice** Blemish/Acne Fighting Solution for All Skin Types ($12.95 for 6 ounces); **ProActiv** Repairing Lotion ($22.95 for 2 ounces); and **Serious Skin Care** Clearz-It with 5% Benzoyl Peroxide ($19.95 for 4 ounces).

Best Exfoliants (AHA, BHA, and Topical Scrubs)

Exfoliating the skin (getting rid of unwanted, dead, or built-up layers of sun-damaged skin cells and improving skin-cell turnover), is a procedure that's not easy to discuss accurately. Despite the fact that most beauty experts, as well as dermatologists and plastic surgeons, agree that exfoliating the skin is a wonderful way to take care of both oily and dry skin, *how* to exfoliate is a bone of contention.

A few years back, before Retin-A, there weren't many options when it came to improving cell turnover. During most of the '70s and '80s, the only choices were topical, mechanical scrubs with ingredients such as honey and almond pits, cleansers with scrub particles, facial masks, and irritating toners. Most of these options took a toll on the face, and irritation or dry patches of skin with redness were typical problems. (Then and now my favorite recommendation for a topical scrub, as I've mentioned repeatedly throughout this book, is mixing Cetaphil Gentle Skin Cleanser with baking soda to create an effective, gentle, and inexpensive mechanical scrub. Other scrubs, with their detergent cleansing agents and wax bases, just can't compare and are far more expensive than mixing baking soda and Cetaphil Gentle Skin Cleanser.)

But now, with the addition of alpha hydroxy acids (AHAs), salicylic acid (BHA), and prescription retinoids such as Retin-A and Renova, the topic has become complicated. AHAs and BHA exfoliate the skin chemically instead of mechanically via abrasion. (Prescription retinoids actually alter skin-cell production, changing abnormally produced skin cells back to some level of normal. However, retinoids are not exfoliants as such. Though their net effect is perceived as being the same as an exfoliant, the actual change is radically different.) For AHA and BHA products, the recommendations below all meet my criteria of low pH and appropriate concentration.

If you decide to use an AHA or BHA product, particularly one from my list of recommendations, the question is, Do you still need to use a physical scrub? The answer isn't all that easy, and you will have to judge that for yourself. Most women with normal to dry/sensitive skin should probably use only the AHA product and no other exfoliant (except maybe once in awhile). Someone with normal to oily skin should use a good BHA product and only use a mechanical scrub over breakouts once in awhile (say once or twice a week). Whatever you choose, always listen closely to your skin and remember irritation is never the goal.

What about the products that contain both BHA and AHA, sometimes referred to as polyhydroxy acids? Because I feel strongly that AHAs are best for dry or sun-damaged skin and BHAs for blemish-prone or oily skin, I think mixed-acid products are unwise.

Note: The lack of recommendations for scrubs is due to the fact that most scrubs are extremely abrasive, contain irritants, or have unnecessary waxy thickening agents that would be a problem for oily or blemish-prone skin types.

FOR NORMAL TO OILY/COMBINATION AND/OR BLEMISH-PRONE SKIN, THE BEST SCRUBS ARE:
I still feel strongly that Cetaphil Gentle Skin Cleanser ($8.31 for 16 ounces) mixed with baking soda, or just plain baking soda by itself, is the best topical scrub for this skin type.

FOR NORMAL TO DRY, AND/OR SENSITIVE SKIN, THE BEST SCRUBS ARE:
Cetaphil Gentle Skin Cleanser ($8.31 for 16 ounces) mixed with baking soda; **Guerlain** Evolution Exfoliating Creme for the Face ($29 for 1.7 ounces); **Hydron** Best Defense Micro-Exfoliating Creme ($16.75 for 3.6 ounces); **La Prairie** Essential Exfoliator ($50 for 7 ounces); and **Organic Essentials from Linda Chae** Herbal Exfoliating Scrub ($22.50 for 2.5 ounces).

FOR NORMAL TO OILY/COMBINATION AND/OR BLEMISH-PRONE SKIN, THE BEST ALPHA HYDROXY ACID PRODUCTS ARE:
Alpha Hydrox Extra Strength AHA Oil-Free Formula, 10% AHA Facial Treatment ($10.95 for 1.7 ounces); **Amway** Alpha Hydroxy Serum Plus ($40.20 for 1 ounce); **La Prairie** Age Management Intensified Serum ($140 for 1 ounce), and Age Management Line Inhibitor ($100 for 0.5 ounce); **Dr. Mary Lupo** AHA Renewel Gel I ($25 for 3.5 ounces), and AHA Renewal Gel II ($25 for 3.5 ounces); **M.D. Formulations** Vit-A-Plus with Vitamin A ($35 for 1 ounce), and Vit-A-Plus2 with Alpha Retinyl Complex

($62.50 for 0.4 ounce); **Paula's Choice** 8% Alpha Hydroxy Acid Solution ($10.95 for 4 ounces); **ProActiv** Revitalizing Toner ($16 for 4 ounces); **Serious Skin Care** Glycolic Renewal Gel ($20 for 4 ounces), and Mini Facial Peel Program ($28 for six towelettes); and **Trish McEvoy** Glycolic Lotion ($37 for 2 ounces).

<u>FOR NORMAL TO DRY, AND/OR SENSITIVE SKIN, THE BEST ALPHA HYDROXY ACID PRODUCTS ARE:</u> **Adrien Arpel** Bio Cellular Night Cream with AHA ($35 for 1.25 ounces), and Bio-Cellular Anti Serum with Alpha Hydroxy Complex ($52.50 for ten 0.23-ounce vials); **Alpha Hydrox** AHA Creme, 8% AHA Facial Treatment for Normal Skin ($7.64 for 2 ounces), AHA Enhanced Creme 10% AHA Facial Treatment, for Dry to Normal Skin ($9.50 for 2 ounces), AHA Lotion 8% AHA Facial Treatment, for Dry Skin ($8.64 for 6 ounces), and AHA Sensitive Skin Creme 5% AHA Facial Treatment ($7.89 for 2 ounces); **AlphaMax** Daily Renewal Lotion with AHA and SPF 15 ($29.97 for 2 ounces); **Aqua Glycolic** Face Cream Advanced Smoothing Therapy 10% Glycolic Compound ($11.29 for 2 ounces); **Avon** Stress Shield Serum ($12.50 for 1 ounce); **BeautiControl** Regeneration Face and Neck Complex ($31 for 2 ounces), Regeneration Face and Neck Complex 2 ($31 for 2 ounces), Regeneration Face and Neck Complex 3 ($31 for 2 ounces), Regeneration for Oily Skin ($31 for 2 ounces), Regeneration 2 for Oily Skin ($31 for 2 ounces), Regeneration for Oily Skin 3 ($31 for 2 ounces), Regeneration Extreme Repair ($30 for 4 ounces), and Regeneration Gold ($55 for 1.8 ounces); **Black Opal** Skin Retexturizing Complex with Alpha-Hydroxy Acids ($9.95 for 1 ounce); **Bobbi Brown Essentials** Face Lotion ($38 for 2 ounces); **Color Me Beautiful** Visible Results Glycolic Skin Conditioner for All Skin Types I ($18.50 for 1 ounce), and Visible Results Glycolic Skin Conditioner for All Skin Types II ($18.50 for 1 ounce); **Dr. Obagi** Nu-Derm Exfoderm ($60 for 2 ounces); **Exuviance by Neostrata** Evening Restorative Complex ($27.50 for 1.75 ounces); **Janet Sartin** Revitalizing Cream with Plant Extracts ($44 for 1.7 ounces), Revitalizing Lotion with Plant Extracts ($32 for 1 ounce), and Revitalizing Lotion Advance Strength with Plant Extracts ($35 for 1 ounce); **La Prairie** Age Management Night Cream ($125 for 1 ounce), and Age Management Serum ($125 for 1 ounce); **Dr. Mary Lupo** AHA Renewal Lotion I ($25 for 3.5 ounces), and AHA Renewal Lotion II ($25 for 3.5 ounces); **M.D. Formulations** Facial Lotion with 12% Glycolic Compound ($55 for 2 ounces), Facial Cream with 14% Glycolic Compound ($75 for 2 ounces), Vit-A-Plus Night Recovery Complex ($56.25 for 1 ounce), Vit-A-Plus Revitalizing Eye Cream ($61.25 for 0.5 ounce), Smoothing Complex with 10% Glycolic Compound ($35 for 0.5 ounce), Forte I Facial Lotion with 15% Glycolic Compound ($45 for 2 ounces), Night Cream with 14% Glycolic Compound ($60 for 2 ounces), and Forte I Facial Cream with 15% Glycolic Compound ($32 for 1 ounce); **Murad** Intensive

Formula ($48 for 3.3 ounces), and Murasome Night Reform ($52.50 for 1.4 ounces); **Neostrata** Skin Smoothing Lotion ($16.95 for 6.8 ounces), Polyhydroxy AHA Eye Cream ($22.95 for 0.5 ounce), Polyhydroxy AHA Ultra Moisturizing Face Cream ($22.95 for 1.75 ounces), Skin Smoothing Cream ($12.95 for 1.75 ounces), and Sensitive Skin AHA Face Cream ($17.50 for 1.75 ounces); **Neutrogena** Healthy Skin Face Lotion ($10 for 2.5 ounces); **Pond's** Age Defying Complex With Alpha Nutrium ($10.99 for 2 ounces), Age Defying Complex for Delicate Skin ($11.59 for 2 ounces), Age Defying Lotion With Alpha Nutrium ($10.99 for 3 ounces), and Age Defying Lotion for Delicate Skin With Alpha Nutrium ($12.49 for 3 ounces); **Principal Secret** AHA Booster Complex ($45 for 1 ounce); **Trish McEvoy** Glycolic Face Cream ($37 for 1 ounce); and **Yves St. Laurent** Fruit Jeunesse/Firming Renewal Complex Glucohydroxy Acid ($50 for 1.6 ounces).

FOR NORMAL TO OILY/COMBINATION AND/OR BLEMISH-PRONE SKIN, THE BEST BETA HYDROXY ACID PRODUCTS ARE: **Clinique** Mild Clarifying Lotion ($15.50 for 12 ounces); **Garden Botanika** Skin Correcting Purifying Toning Lotion ($10 for 8 ounces); **Paula's Choice** 1% Beta Hydroxy Acid Solution ($12.95 for 4 ounces); and **Serious Skin Care** Clarifying Treatment with 2% Salicylic Acid ($19.95 for 4 ounces).

FOR NORMAL TO DRY AND/OR SENSITIVE SKIN, THE BEST BETA HYDROXY ACID PRODUCTS ARE: **Clean & Clear** Sensitive Skin Balancing Moisturizer ($3.79 for 4 ounces), Skin Balancing Moisturizer ($3.79 for 4 ounces), and Dual Action Moisturizer ($3.79 for 4 ounces); and **Oil of Olay** Daily Renewal Cream Age Defying Series Beta Hydroxy Complex ($8.91 for 2 ounces).

THE BEST SUNSCREENS WITH ALPHA HYDROXY ACID ARE: **Decleor Paris** Day Alpha Hydrating Cream with Plant Extracts and Alpha-Hydroxy Acids, SPF 12, for All Skin Types ($42 for 1.69 ounces); and **Exuviance by Neostrata** Essential Multi-Defense Day Creme SPF 15 ($25 for 1.75 ounces), Essential Multi-Defense Day Fluid SPF 15 ($22.50 for 2 ounces), Fundamental Multi-Protective Day Creme SPF 15 Sensitive Formula ($25 for 1.75 ounces), and Fundamental Multi-Protective Day Fluid SPF 15 Sensitive Formula ($22.50 for 2 ounces).

Best Moisturizers

One of the most frequently asked questions I receive is from women asking me which moisturizer is the best or which product will really do something about wrinkles. Wrinkle creams are a fairy tale (except for sunscreens); none of them erase or change wrinkling. What isn't a fantasy is the fact that there are a lot of great moisturizers to be found that can help soothe the skin and eliminate dryness (at least while you wear them—the effect is gone once you wash you face), and help make wrinkles look less pronounced. Stop using the product, whatever the exotic name, promise, or claim happens to be and the wrinkles are back the next day or two. Another damning aspect of the moisturizer craze and the belief that one can somehow slow down or stop the wrinkling process is that a lot of women end up using moisturizers who shouldn't be, with the result that there are a lot of women who overmoisturize, and that can hurt the skin's healing process.

Regardless of the label, wrinkle creams, day creams, replenishers, liposome creams, eye creams, throat creams, lotions, serums, gels, and nourishing creams—and all the other creatively named moisturizers—were lumped together in this category. All these concoctions and combinations do the same thing—moisturize the skin—and, for the most part, they do an excellent job. What is offensive is that none of these formulations warrant the outlandish claims, ridiculous prices, or your belief that you've finally found the fountain of youth (because a new antiwrinkle product launch is waiting just a month or so down the road and yet we're still wrinkling!).

Surprisingly enough, when I ignored the claims and price tags, I liked most of the moisturizers I reviewed, which is why the following list is so long. Only a handful contain ingredients that I thought were potentially harmful to the skin or would dry it out and cause irritation.

This listing will prove disheartening to the women who wanted a more narrow range to choose from, but it would be like preferring one type of aspirin or antacid over another; they all work, it just depends what you like best. I can't adjust for an individual's personal preferences when it comes to texture or fragrance (though it would be best if all products were fragrance-free because fragrances—and these include essential oils—can cause irritation.

The problem for most women is finding a moisturizer that is right for their skin type. Some moisturizers contain extremely rich ingredients such as lanolin, vegetable oil, mineral oil, petrolatum, shea butter, cocoa butter, or protein that are best only for women with very dry skin. Lighter-weight moisturizers that contain only one or two oils further down on the ingredient list and a selection of water-binding agents are best for skin that is normal to dry. Someone with combination skin should only be using moisturizer over the areas that are dry, and someone with oily skin should not be using a moisturizer at all. Finding the appropriate type of moisturizer for your skin will be easier if you turn to the specific products as they are described in Chapter Three and review how you think they will suit your skin.

When it comes to day moisturizers versus night moisturizers, the only difference should be whether or not the day moisturizer contains a sunscreen (most sunscreen formulations have a moisturizing base). If your skin is extremely dry, products rich in oils, emollients, and water-binding agents may be necessary for your skin day and night, but the daytime moisturizer must have an SPF of 15, and one of the active ingredients for UVA protection (avobenzone, zinc oxide, or titanium dioxide) must be included. If your skin is dry, but not excessively so, you may want to use a light moisturizing lotion that contains one or two oils and an SPF of 15 with UVA protecting ingredients for daytime and a more emollient moisturizer at night. If you have slightly dry skin, a lightweight moisturizer or a moisturizing gel should be perfect for both morning and night, but you must absolutely use a product with a good SPF during the day. For oily/combination skin a foundation with SPF 15 and UVA protecting ingredients is best for daytime, and at night a moisturizer only over those areas that are dry.

The moisturizer you use on your face will always work around your eyes, throat, chest, or wherever. Try to disregard the scare tactics at the cosmetics counters and the brochures that carry on about special formulations designed exclusively for the eye, throat, or chest area. These claims are not substantiated by the ingredients in the products, which are identical to products supposedly designed just for the face.

Women with oily skin should not get sucked into believing that all skin types, even oily-skin types, require a moisturizer to prevent the skin from wrinkling or to combat surface dehydration. Unless we are talking about a sunscreen with an SPF of 15, or dealing with isolated areas of dryness, **someone with oily skin should not being using a moisturizer. Remember that the words "oil-free" don't mean a product won't feel slick, greasy, or oily on the skin. Many ingredients that don't sound like "oil" have a very slick, oily texture.** The product recommendations for more oily skin types refer to lighter-weight, less emollient formulas, but they should still only be used over dry areas of the face.

So, does it really make sense to spend a lot of money on moisturizers? Does a woman who spends between $50 to $200 really get a much better product than one who spends $10? (and when you break out the per-ounce cost, the difference in price grows even bigger). Those of you who have read this whole book already know the answer. Those of you who didn't read the first half of the book and skipped ahead to this section needn't wait in suspense. The best moisturizers for dry skin can be found in almost every skin-care line. Yes, that's right, almost every line has its share of good moisturizers, so spending a lot of money does not make sense. As you read the following suggestions, understand that when I say best, I mean *best*. "Best" moisturizers by Almay or Avon are the equivalent of "best" moisturizers by Chanel or Borghese. Get used to reading skin-care ingredients, and ignore words like "lift," "firm," "energizing," or "antiwrinkle."

Warning: None of these products are recommended for daytime because they don't contain a sunscreen. Choose from the sunscreen product list for a daytime moisturizer or sun-protection product. And oily skin types should not be using a moisturizer.

FOR NORMAL TO COMBINATION SKIN (COMBINATION MEANS SOME AREAS OF THE FACE ARE DRY WHILE OTHERS ARE OILY, MOISTURIZER SHOULD ONLY BE WORN OVER DRY AREAS), THE BEST MOISTURIZERS ARE: Almay Stress Eye Gel ($8.29 for 0.5 ounce), Time-Off Age Smoothing Moisture Lotion ($11.49 for 2 ounces), and Time-Off Age Smoothing Eye Cream ($8.49 for 0.5 ounce); bare escentuals bare aloe vera ($8 for 2 ounces); Beauty Without Cruelty Green Tea Nourishing Eye Gel ($14.49 for 1 ounce); Bioelements Jet Travel Moisture Boost for Low Humidity ($31.50 for 1 ounce), and Urban Detox Pollution Fighting for City Skin ($31.50 for 1 ounce); BioTherm Bioregard Bi-Active Eye Contour Treatment Gel ($32 for 15 ml), and Symbiose Daily Aging Treatment Liposome Gel ($45 for 50 ml); Black Opal Oil Free Moisturizing Lotion ($3.99 for 1.75 ounces); The Body Shop Eye Supplement for All Skin Types ($12 for 0.5 ounce), Light Moisture Lotion for Normal to Oily Skin ($16 for 3.38 ounces), and Tea Tree Oil Moisturizing Gel, for Oily or Blemished Skin ($13.50 for 8.4 ounces); Cellex-C Hydra 5 B-Complex Moisture Enhancing Gel for All Skin Types ($55 for 1 ounce); Christian Dior Capture Eyes Contour Gel ($45 for 0.5 ounce); Clarins After Sun Gel Ultra Soothing ($20 for 5.3 ounces); Decleor Paris Eye Contour Gel with Plant Extracts, for All Skin Types ($27 for 0.5 ounce); Estee Lauder Diminish Retinol Treatment ($47.50 for 1 ounce), and Clear Difference Oil-Control Hydrator for Oily Normal/Oily and Blemish-Prone Skin ($27 for 1.7 ounces); Gale Hayman Eyelift Gel ($25 for 0.5 ounce); H$_2$O Plus After Sun Refresher Gel (Oil-Free) ($10 for 4 ounces); Jafra Skin Firming Complex ($31 for 1 ounce); Lancome Clarifiance Oil-Free Hydrating Fluide ($35 for 2.5 ounces); Dr. Mary Lupo Vivifying Serum C ($39.95 for 1 ounce); Nu Skin Enhancer Skin Conditioning Gel ($9.15 for 2.5 ounces), and HPX Hydrating Gel ($49.95 for 1.5 ounces); Paula's Choice Completely Non-Greasy Moisturizing Lotion ($9.95 for 4 ounces); philosophy between the lines topical vitamin A ($20 for 0.5 ounce); Principal Secret Eye Relief ($30 for 0.5 ounce); Prescriptives Retinol LSW ($50 for 1 ounce); Rachel Perry Immediately Visible Eye Renewal Gel-Cream with Liposomes ($22.50 for 0.5 ounce); Serious Skin Care A Force Vitamin A Serum ($25 for 1 ounce), and Super Hydrate ($19.95 for 4 ounces); Ultima II Interactives Booster Shot Antioxidant Firming System ($28.50 for 1.7 ounces); Victoria Jackson Eye Repair Gel ($12.50, $19.50 for 0.5 ounce); Yves Rocher Riche Creme Line Smoothing Serum, with Plant Extracts ($14 for 0.3 ounce); and Zia Herbal Moisture Gel Oil Free Moisturizer for Normal, Sensitive and Combination & Oily/Problem Skin Types ($22.95 for 1.5 ounces).

FOR NORMAL TO SOMEWHAT DRY AND DRY SKIN, THE BEST MOISTURIZERS ARE: **Alexandra de Markoff** Skin Tight Firming Eye Cream ($50 for 0.4 ounce); **Almay** Moisture Balance Eye Cream for Normal Skin ($6.79 for 0.5 ounce), Moisture Renew Cream for Dry Skin ($7.99 for 2 ounces), Moisture Renew Eye Cream for Dry Skin ($6.79 for 0.5 ounce), Moisture Renew Moisture Lotion for Dry Skin ($9.99 for 4 ounces), Moisture Renew Night Cream for Dry Skin ($7 for 2 ounces), Perfect Moisture ($5.68 for 4 ounces), Sensitive Care Cream for Super Sensitive Skin ($6.78 for 2 ounces), Time-Off Age Smoothing Night Cream ($9.69 for 2 ounces), Time-Off Wrinkle Defense Capsules with Micro-Fillers ($12.49 for 0.29 ounce), Time-Off Wrinkle Defense Cream with Micro-Fillers ($12.49 for 2 ounces), and Vitalizing Moisture Night Cream ($7.29 for 2 ounces); **Amway** Eye Balm ($14.20 for 0.5 ounce), Revitalizing Night Treatment ($33 for 2.5 ounces), and Progressive Emollient ($33 for 2.5 ounces); **Arbonne** Rejuvenating Cream for All Skin Types ($30 for 2 ounces); **Aubrey Organics** Rosa Mosqueta Rose Hip Moisturizing Cream Normal to Dry Skin ($14.35 for 4 ounces); **Aveda** Firming Fluid ($32 for 1 ounce); **Avon** Anew Instant Eye Smoother ($16 for 0.5 ounce), Anew Retinol Recovery Complex P.M. Treatment ($17.50 for 1 ounce), Anew Moisture Supply Day Cream ($16 for 1.7 ounces), Anew Moisture Supply Night Cream ($16 for 1.7 ounces), Calming Effects Sensitive Skin Lotion ($10.50 for 1.7 ounces), Dramatic Firming Cream for Face and Throat ($12 for 1.5 ounces), Hydrofirming Eye Treatment ($9.50 for 0.5 ounce), Maximum Moisture Super Hydrating Gel ($10.50 for 2.5 ounces), and Lighten Up ($14.50 for 0.5 ounce); **bare escentuals** Rose & Royal Jelly Anti-Oxidant Moisturizer Normal to Dry Skin ($32 for 2 ounces); **Basis** All Night Face Cream ($6.55 for 2 ounces); **BeautiControl** Essential Moisture Lotion ($15.50 for 4.5 ounces), Balancing Moisturizer ($15.50 for 4.5 ounces), Microderm Oxygenating Nighttime Line Control ($26 for 0.81 ounce), and Microderm Oxygenating Firming Gel ($29.50 for 2 ounces); **Beauty Without Cruelty** All Day Moisturizer Normal/Dry Skin ($12.49 for 2 ounces); **BeneFit** Very Aloe Creme For Combo Skin ($25 for 2 ounces); **Bioelements** Absolute Moisture Balances Combination Skin ($29.50 for 2.5 ounces), and Crucial Moisture Fortifies Your Skin with Emollients ($29.50 for 2.5 ounces); **Biogime** Natural Conditioner ($22.45 for 6 ounces), Skin Perfection with Retinol Palmitate and Lipsosomes ($34.95 for 4 ounces), Ultimate Conditioner ($23.45 for 6 ounces), and Retinol Palmitate ($34.95 for 4 ounces); **BioTherm** Bionutrition Comfort Treatment for Dry Skin ($34 for 50 ml), Bionutrition Force II ($34 for 50 ml), Biosensitive Yeux Calming Eye Cream ($35 for 15 g), Fluide Biojeunesse Skin Refining Day Fluid ($35 for 50 ml), Bionuit Overnight Visibly Effective Skin Treatment ($35 for 50 ml), Hydra-Detox Lotion ($35 for 50 ml), Hydra-Detox Cream ($35 for 50 ml), and Face Repair Soothing Balm ($16 for 50 ml); **Bobbi Brown Essentials** Eye Cream ($32.50 for

0.65 ounce), and Hydrating Face Cream ($38 for 1.7 ounces); **Borghese** Effetto Immediato Spa Lift for Eyes ($43 for 1 ounce), Energia Skin Recovery Fluid Oil-Free ($47.50 for 1.7 ounces), Energia Skin Recovery Creme ($47.50 for 1.7 ounces), Fluido Protettivo Advanced Spa Lift for Eyes ($45 for 1 ounce), and Spa Energia Skin Energy Source ($40 for 1.5 ounces); **Cellex-C** Bio-Botanical Cream for Normal to Oily Skin ($45 for 2 ounces), Fruitaplex Line Smoother ($48 for 1 ounce), G.L.A. Dry Skin Cream for Dry Skin ($48 for 2 ounces), G.L.A. Eye Balm for Dry Skin ($44 for 1 ounce), Seline-E Cream, for Normal Skin ($48 for 2 ounces), and Salicea Gel for All Skin Types ($45 for 1 ounce); **Chanel** Complexe Intensif Night Lift Cream ($31 for 1 ounce), Creme No. 1 Skin Recovery Cream ($95 for 1 ounce), Creme No. 1 Skin Recovery Eye Cream ($70 for 0.5 ounce), Dual Benefit Complex Anti-Dryness/Anti-Wrinkle ($65 for 1.7 ounces), Firming Eye Cream ($50 for 0.5 ounce), Lift Serum Extreme Advanced Corrective Complex ($56 for 1 ounce), and Source Extreme ($65 for 1.7 ounces); **Chantal Ethocyn** Ethocyn Hydrating Complex Moisturizer ($40 for 2 ounces), and Ethocyn Essence Vials ($50 for 0.23 ounce); **Charles of the Ritz** Any Age Self Protection for Eyes ($30 for 0.4 ounce), Revenescence Brightening Face and Eye Hydrating Cream ($20 for 1 ounce), Timeless Difference Night Recovery Cream ($35 for 1.7 ounces), and Timeless Difference Eye Recovery Cream ($25 for 0.5 ounce); **Christian Dior** Capture Lift Firming Night Treatment for the Face ($58 for 1 ounce), Capture Rides Wrinkle Creme for Eyes ($45 for 0.5 ounce), Hydra-Star Moisture Creme for Dry Skin ($46 for 1.7 ounces), Hydra-Star Night Treatment Creme for Dry Skin ($56 for 1.7 ounces), Hydra-Star Moisture Creme Emulsion for Dry Skin ($46 for 1.7 ounces), Hydra-Star Moisture Emulsion for Dry Skin ($46 for 1.7 ounces), Hydra-Star Night Treatment Creme, for Normal to Combination Skin ($56 for 1.7 ounces), and Icone Principe Regulateur for All Types of Dryness ($70 for 1.7 ounce); **Circle of Beauty** Lighten It Eye Cream ($8.50 for 0.6 ounce); **Clarins** Extra-Firming Day Cream All Skin Types ($50 for 1.7 ounces), Extra-Firming Night Cream All Skin Types ($60 for 1.7 ounces), Face Treatment Plant Cream "Blue Orchid" for Dehydrated Skin ($29 for 1.7 ounces), Hydration-Plus Moisture Lotion for All Skin Types ($30 for 1.7 ounces), Multi-Active Night Lotion for All Skin Types ($50 for 1.7 ounces), Multi-Active Night Lotion Very Dry Skin ($50 for 1.7 ounces), Revitalizing Moisture Cream with Plant Marine "Cell Extract" ($50 for 1.7 ounces), Revitalizing Moisture Base with Plant Marine "Cell Extract" for All Skin Types ($30 for 1.1 ounces), and Eye Contour Balm "Special" for Very Dry Skin ($30 for 0.7 ounce); **Clientele** Nourishing Night Oils ($100 for ten vials), Preventative Age Treatment ($50 for 2 ounces), Time Therapy ($75 for 1.1 ounces), Wrinkle Treatment ($75 for 1.1 ounces), Elastology Firming Target Treatment Roll-On ($40 for 0.35 ounce), and Elastology Oil-Free Firming Night Cream for Normal/Oily Skin ($95 for 1.1 ounce); **Clinique** Advanced Cream Self

Repair System ($32.50 for 1 ounce), All About Eyes ($25 for 0.5 ounce), Daily Eye Benefits ($25 for 0.5 ounce), Daily Eye Saver ($25 for 0.5 ounce), Dramatically Different Moisturizing Lotion ($10.50 for 2 ounces, $19.50 for 4 ounces), Moisture On-Call ($30 for 1.6 ounces), Moisture On Line ($30 for 1.7 ounces), Moisture Surge Treatment Formula ($32.50 for 2 ounces), and Skin Texture Lotion Oil Free Formula ($19.50 for 1.25 ounces); **Color Me Beautiful** Triple Action Eye Cream, All Skin Types ($18.50 for 0.5 ounce); **Coppertone** After Sun Aloe & Vitamin E Moisturizing Lotion ($4.79 for 16 ounces); **Decleor Paris** Contour Firming Serum for the Eyes with Plant Extracts, for All Skin Types ($36 for 0.5 ounce), Day Hydrating Cream with Plant Extracts ($56 for 1.69 ounces), Instant Beauty Booster, with Plant Extracts for All Skin Types ($42 for 1.69 ounces), Moisturizing Face Cream with Plant Extracts and Essential Wax for Normal Skins ($50 for 1.69 ounces), Moisturizing Face Cream with Plant Extracts and Essential Waxes, for Dry Skins ($50 for 1.69 ounces), Moisturizer Day Cream with Plant Extracts, for Normal Skins ($29 for 1.69 ounces), Soothing Anti Redness Day Cream, with Plant Extracts and Essential Oils ($58 for 1.69 ounces), Soothing Night Cream with Plant Extracts and Essential Oils, for Normal Skins ($35 for 1.69 ounces), Soothing Serum with Plant Extracts and Essential Oils ($69 for 1 ounce), Vitalite Nourishing and Firming Face Cream with Plant Extracts and Essential Oils ($56 for 1.69 ounces), Vitarome Cream with Plant Extracts and Essential Oils, for Dry Skins ($39 for 1 ounce), Corrective Care with Plant Extracts for Sensitive Skins ($19 for 0.5 ounce), and Eye and Lip Precious Contour Balm with Plant Extracts for Mature Skins ($34 for 0.5 ounce); **Dermalogica** Active Moist ($38.50 for 3.5 ounces), Intensive Eye Repair ($35 for 0.5 ounce), Intensive Moisture Balance ($31 for 1.75 ounces), Intensive Moisture Concentrate ($45 for 1 ounce), and Skin Smoothing Cream ($42 for 3.5 ounces); **DHC USA** Rich Moisture for Normal to Drier Skin ($24 for 3.3 ounces), Light Moisture for Normal to Oilier Skin ($24 for 3.3 ounces), Oil-Free Hydrator for Oilier Skin ($22 for 3.3 ounces), Extra Nighttime Moisture ($30 for 1.5 ounces), and Hydrating Nighttime Moisture ($28 for 1 ounce); **Elizabeth Arden** Visible Difference Eyecare Concentrate ($30 for 0.5 ounce), Visible Difference Perpetual Moisture ($38 for 1 ounce), Ceramide Firm Lift Intensive Lotion for Face and Throat ($45 for 1 ounce), Ceramide Night Intensive Repair Creme ($45 for 1 ounce), Eight Hour Cream ($20 for 4 ounces), and Micro 2000 Stressed-Skin Concentrate ($42.50 for 0.85 ounce); **Erno Laszlo** Antioxidant Moisture Complex Cream for Extremely Dry to Normal Skin ($65 for 2 ounces), HydrapHel Complex PM Moisturizer for Extremely Dry and Dry Skin ($55 for 2 ounces), Moisture-Firming Throat Cream for All Skin Types ($23 for 2 ounces), pHelityl Cream PM Moisturizer for Normal Skin ($55 for 2 ounces), pHelityl Lotion AM Moisturizer for Slightly Dry to Slightly Oily Skin ($45 for 3 ounces), and Total Skin Revitalizer Facial Hydration Enhancer for All Skin Types ($54 for 1 ounce); **Estee Lauder** Advanced Night Repair Protective Recovery Complex ($70 for 1.7 ounces), Re-nutriv Firming Eye Creme ($47.50 for 0.5 ounce), Re-nutriv Firming Throat Creme ($53 for 1.7 ounces), Resilience Eye Creme ($42.50 for 0.5 ounce, Skin Perfecting Creme Firming Nourisher ($35 for 1.75 ounces), Swiss Performing Extract Moisturizer ($37.50 for 3.2 ounces), Time Zone Eyes Ultra-Hydrating Complex ($40 for 0.5 ounce), Time Zone Moisture Recharging Complex ($55 for 1.7 ounces), Verite Moisture Relief Creme ($50 for 1.75 ounces), Verite Calming Fluid ($60 for 1.7 ounces), Re-nutriv Intensive Lifting Creme ($150 for 1.7 ounces), Re-nutriv Replenishing Creme ($78 for 1.7 ounces), Nutritious Bio Protein ($45 for 1.7 ounces), and 100% Time Release Moisturizer ($32.50 for 2 ounces); **Exuviance by Neostrata** Hydrating Lift Eye Complex ($22.50 for 0.5 ounce); **Face Stockholm** Aloe Vera Moisture Cream All Skin Types ($24 for 2 ounces), Aloe Vera Facial Lotion All Skin Types ($14 for 4 ounces), Orchid Oil Moisturizer All Skin Types ($24 for 2 ounces), and Vitamin Cream All Skin ($24 for 2 ounces); **Flori Roberts** My Everything Creme ($25 for 3.25 ounces), and My Everything Treatment Oil Control Serum Normal to Oily Skin ($14 for 1 ounce); **Forever Spring** Bio Eye and Throat Intensive Lubrication Complex ($15 for 1 ounce), Collagen Skin Quencher ($22.75 for 4 ounces), Ginseng and Vitamin C Intensive Complex with Vitamins E, A, C, and Lipolic Acid ($31.50 for 2 ounces), Ginseng Facial Feed ($21.25 for 4 ounces), and Petal Soft Eye Cream ($14 for 0.5 ounce); **Freeman Beautiful Skin** Apricot & Vitamin E Ultra Nourishing Lotion ($2.88 for 18 ounces), Skin Control Facial Gel Moisturizer ($2.85 for 4 ounces), and Skin + Vitamin C Complex Eye Cream ($7.99 for 0.5 ounce); **Gayle Hayman** Youth Lift Firming Night Treatment ($55 for 1 ounce), and Youth Lift Total Moisturizer ($35 for 2 ounces); **Garden Botanika** Calendula Moisture Cream for Dry Skin ($10 for 2 ounces), Hydrating Cream with Aloe ($10 for 2 ounces), Nutrient Night Creme ($10 for 2 ounces), Ivy and Yarrow Moisture Creme ($9.50 for 2 ounces), Meadow Sweet Night Cream ($10 for 2 ounces), Nourishing Eye Creme ($9.50 for 1 ounce), and Vitalizing Night Creme ($11 for 2 ounces); **Givenchy** Nutritive Care ($54 for 1.7 ounces); **Guerlain** Evolution Sublicreme No. 1 Light Day and Night Care ($52 for 1.7 ounces), Evolution Sublicreme No. 2 Rich Day and Night Care ($52 for 1.7 ounces), Evolution Sublifluide Day and Night Care ($50 for 1.7 ounces), Evolution Specific Eye Contour Care Emulsion ($37 for 0.5 ounce), Issima Intenserum Beauty Treatment ($175 for ten 0.08-ounce ampoules), Odelys Perfect Care #1 Day and Night (Light) ($52 for 1.7 ounces), Odelys Perfect Care #2 Day and Night (Rich) ($52 for 1.7 ounces), Odelys Stabilizing Serum ($56 for 1 ounce), Odelys Perfect Eye Contour Care ($35 for 0.7 ounce), Hydrobella Creme Souple #1 Light Creme ($50 for 1.7 ounce), and Hydrobella Creme Onctueuse #2 Rich Creme ($50 for 1.7 ounce); **H₂O Plus** Green Tea Antioxidant Face Complex ($30 for 2 ounces), Hydro

Essential Eye Treatment (Hydrate) ($20 for 0.5 ounce), Marine Daily Hydrator (Oil-Free) ($18.50 for 4 ounces), Marine Daily Moisture Cream (Moisturize) ($20 for 2 ounces), and Post-Sun Hydrator ($10.50 for 6 ounces); **H+ Beauty System** Nyaluronic Beauty Serum ($44 for 1.1 ounces), Firming Eye Gel ($38 for 1.1 ounces), Liposomal Beauty Serum ($44 for 1.1 ounces), and Extra Rich Night Cream ($44 for 1.69 ounces); **Hydron** Best Defense Line Smoothing Complex ($37.75 for 0.5 ounce), and Best Defense Moisture Balance Restorative Overnight Liposome Complex ($36 for 2 ounces); **Jafra** Night Cream for Dry Skin ($15 for 1.7 ounces), Night Cream Moisturizer for Dry to Normal Skin ($15 for 1.7 ounces), Night Lotion ($15 for 4.2 ounces), Eye Revitalizing Concentrate ($17 for 0.75 ounce), Royal Jelly Milk Balm Moisture Lotion Dry and Normal to Dry ($60 for 1 ounce), Royal Jelly Milk Balm Moisture Lotion Normal to Oily and Oily ($60 for 1 ounce), Best Defense Fragile Eye Moisturizer, Wrinkle Fighting Complex ($26 for 0.5 ounce), and Time Corrector Firming Moisture Cream ($38 for 1.7 ounces); **Janet Sartin** Continual Action Cream Age Protection with Kalaya Oil ($45 for 1.7 ounces), Eye Care for Sensitive Eyes, Enriched with Kalaya Oil ($45 for 1 ounce), and Hydrating Lotion Advanced Skin Conditioning ($38 for 1.75 ounces); **Jurlique** Day Care Face Cream ($23.59 for 1.4 ounces), Day Care Face Lotion ($24.69 for 1 ounce), Eye Gel ($43.09 for 0.53 ounce), Herbal Extract Recovery Gel ($33.89 for 1 ounce), Moisturizer Cream ($19.19 for 1.4 ounces), and Wrinkle Softener Beauty Cream for Face, Eye Area and Decollete ($18.49 for 0.2 ounce); **Kiehl's** Original Formula Eye Cream, Ultra Nourishing ($10.50 for 0.5 ounce), Panthenol Protein Moisturizing Face Cream ($22.50 for 4 ounces), Light Nourishing Eye Cream ($15.95 for 0.5 ounce), and Moisturizing Eye Balm with Pure Vitamins A & E ($14.50 for 0.5 ounce); **La Prairie** Age Management Stimulus Complex PM (Delicate) ($150 for 1 ounce), Age Management Stimulus Complex PM (Normal) ($150 for 1 ounce), Cellular Balancing Complex ($65 for 1.7 ounces), Cellular Defense Shield Vitamin C Cream ($125 for 1 ounce), Cellular Eye Contour Creme ($80 for 0.5 ounce), Cellular Neck Cream ($105 for 1 ounce), Cellular Night Cream ($105 for 1 ounce), Cellular Skin Conditioner ($70 for 4 ounces), Cellular Wrinkle Cream ($105 for 1 ounce), Essence of Skin Caviar Cellular Eye Complex with Caviar Extract ($85 for 0.5 ounce), and Extrait of Skin Caviar Cellular Face Complex with Caviar Extract ($85 for 1 ounce); **Lac-Hydrin** Five ($9.12 for 7 ounces) or Twelve ($9.12 for 7 ounces); **Lancome** Expressive Eye Contour Age Treatment Fluide ($42.50 for 0.5 ounce), Nutriforce Double Nutrition Fortifying Nourishing Creme ($40 for 1.7 ounces), Primordiale Nuit ($75 for 2.5 ounces), Primordiale Yeux Visibly Revitalizing Eye Treatment ($42.50 for 0.5 ounce), Progres Counter des Yeux Eye Creme ($37.50 for 1.5 ounces), Renergie Double Performance Treatment ($72.50 for 2.5 ounces), Renergie Serum Instant Lift Concentrate ($75 for 1.7 ounce), Trans-Hydrix Multi-Action Hydrating

Creme ($36.50 for 1.9 ounces), and Vitabolic Deep Radiance Booster ($45 for 1 ounce); **Le Mirador** Revitalizing Eye Cream ($22 for 0.5 ounce); **Lorac by Carol Shaw** Moisturizer ($37.50 for 2 ounces); **L'Oreal** Plenitude Advanced Overnight Replenisher ($9.92 for 1.7 ounces), Plenitude Hydra Renewal Daily Dry Skin Cream with Pro-Vitamin B5 ($5.99 for 1.7 ounces), Eye Defense with Liposomes ($9.99 for 0.5 ounce), Wrinkle Defense ($10.44 for 1.4 ounces), Overnight Defense ($11.99 for 1.7 ounces), Revitalift Eye Anti-Wrinkle and Firming Cream ($9.99 for 0.5 ounce), Plenitude Revitalift Anti-Wrinkle Firming Cream ($9.99 for 1.7 ounces), and Revitalift Night Anti-Fatigue + Recovery Complex ($9.99 for 1 ounce); **Lubriderm** Dry Skin Care Lotion Fragrance Free ($6.59 for 10 ounces), Dry Skin Care Lotion Original Fragrance ($6.59 for 10 ounces), Moisture Recovery Gel Creme ($4.29 for 4 ounces), Seriously Sensitive Lotion for Extra Sensitive Skin ($6.59 for 10 ounces), and Seriously Sensitive Lotion for Extra Sensitive Dry Skin ($6.59 for 10 ounces); **M.A.C.** CR-1 Night Emulsion Cellular Recovery for Normal to Oily Skin Types ($28 for 2 ounces), Night Emulsion CR-2 Cellular Recovery for Normal to Dry Skin Types ($28 for 2 ounces), CR-S Night Emulsion Cellular Recovery for Sensitive Skin Types ($28 for 2 ounces), EP-1 Environmental Protective Day Emulsion for Oily Skin ($24 for 1.6 ounces), EP-2 Environmental Protective Day Emulsion for Normal Skin ($24 for 1.6 ounces), EP-3 Environmental Protective Day Emulsion ($24 for 1.6 ounces), EP-S Environmental Protective Day Emulsion for Sensitive Skin Types ($24 for 1.6 ounces), EP-T Environmental Protective Day Emulsion for All Skin Types ($24 for 1.6 ounces), EZR Day/Night Emulsion for All Skin Types ($28 for 1 ounce), and NMF-Natural Moisturizing Factors for All Skin Types ($18 for 4 ounces); **Marcelle** Hydractive Eye Contour Gel ($11.95 for 15 ml), Hydractive Hydra-Repair Night Treatment for All Skin Types ($17.95 for 60 ml), Hydractive Hydra-Replenishing Cream ($15.25 for 40 ml), Moisture Cream ($8.58 for 40 ml, $11.98 for 60 ml), Moisture Lotion ($9.88 for 90 ml, $12.58 for 120 ml), Night Cream ($8.58 for 40 ml), Anti-Aging Cream ($11.95 for 40 ml), Eye Care Cream, and Ultra-Light ($7.68 for 15 ml), and After Sun Lotion, All Skin Types ($7.95 for 120 ml); **Mariana Chicet** Maximum Moisturizing Complex ($38 for 1 ounce), Moisturizing Mist Complex ($8.50 for 4 ounces), Bone Marrow Cream ($29 for 1.35 ounces), Revitalizing Cream ($30.50 for 2 ounces), Ideal Moisturizer ($25.50 for 2 ounces), Revitalizing Lotion Concentrate ($28.50 for 2 ounces), and Oil-Free Moisturizer ($25 for 2 ounces); **Marilyn Miglin** Perfect Balance Oxygen 600 ($37.50 for 4 ounces), Restore ($40 for 4 ounces), Perfect C Firming Creme ($30 for 2 ounces), and Perfect C Serum ($35 for 0.85 ounce); **Mary Kay** Balancing Moisturizer ($16 for 4 ounces), Enriched Moisturizer ($16 for 4 ounces), Extra Emollient Moisturizer ($16 for 4 ounces), Oil-Control Lotion ($16 for 4 ounces), Advanced Moisture Renewal Treatment Cream ($19 for 2.5 ounces), and Instant Action Eye Cream

($15 for 0.65 ounce); **Matrix Essentials** Daily Moisture Lotion for Normal, Dry, and Sensitive Skin ($22 for 2 ounces), and Nourishing Night Cream ($30 for 1 ounce); **M.D. Formulations** Forte Advanced Hydrating Complex Cream Formula ($45 for 1.7 ounces), and Vit-A-Gel with Vitamin A Propionate ($40 for 1 ounce); **Merle Norman** Luxiva Collagen Support ($20 for 2 ounces), Luxiva Night Creme with HC-12 ($37.50 for 2 ounces), Luxiva Day Creme with HC-12 ($21.50 for 2 ounces), Luxiva Energizing Concentrate ($37.50 for 1 ounce), Luxiva Eye Cream ($20 for 0.5 ounce), Luxiva Protein Cream ($39.50 for 4 ounces), and Luxiva Hydrosome Complex Advanced Hydrator ($31.50 for 1 ounce); **Mon Amie** Intensive Eye Serum ($39.95 for 0.5 ounce); **Murad** Cellular Eye Gel ($29 for 0.5 ounce), Murasome Cellular Serum for All Skin Types ($42 for 1.4 ounces), Perfecting Night Cream ($31 for 2.25 ounces), Perfecting Serum ($52 for 1 ounce), and Skin Perfecting Lotion ($27 for 2 ounces), **Natura Bisse** Hydroprotective Concentrate for Dry Skin ($78 for 1.2 ounces), Rose Mosqueta Oil for Dry Aged Skin ($32 for 1 ounce), Sensitive Concentrate Calming Concentrate for All Sensitive Skin Types ($108 for 1.2 ounces), Sensitive Eye Gel Calming Gel for the Eyes ($52 for 0.8 ounce), Sensitive Gel Cream Soothing Gel Cream for All Skin Types ($48 for 2.5 ounces), and Sensitive Night Cream Soothing Night Cream for All Skin Types ($58 for 2.5 ounces); **Neutrogena** Healthy Skin Eye Cream ($9.46 for 0.5 ounce), Healthy Skin Anti-Wrinkle Cream with Retinol ($10.89 for 1.4 ounces), Intensified Eye Moisture 12-Hour Hydration ($7.57 for 0.5 ounce), Light Night Cream Won't Clog Pores ($10.50 for 2.25 ounces), and Moisture Non-Comedogenic Facial Moisturizer for Sensitive Skin ($9.50 for 2 ounces); **Nivea Visage** Eye Contour Gel with Liposomes ($7.97 for 0.5 ounce); **Noevir** 95 Herbal Skin Cream ($40 for 1 ounce), Eye Treatment Stick ($30 for 0.19 ounce), and Eye Treatment Gel ($65 for 0.52 ounce); **Nu Skin** Celltrex Skin Hydrating Fluid ($26.75 for 0.5 ounce), NaPCA Moisturizer ($19.80 for 2.5 ounces), Rejuvenating Cream ($28.45 for 2.5 ounces), and Ideal Eyes Vitamins C&A Eye Refining Creme ($28.60 for 0.5 ounce), Sunright Prime Pre and Post Sun Moisturizer ($16.10 for 5 ounces), and Interim MHA Diminishing Gel ($18.40 for 1 ounce); **Dr. Obagi** Nu-Derm Action ($30 for 2 ounces), Nu-Derm Action Plus ($30 for 2 ounces), and Nu-Derm Eye Cream ($50 for 1 ounce); **Oil of Olay** Moisture Replenishing Cream Daily Care Series ($5.76 for 2 ounces), Night of Olay Night Care Cream ($5.76 for 2 ounces), Oil-Free Beauty Fluid Daily Care Series ($7.99 for 6 ounces), Oil-Free Replenishing Cream, Daily Care Series ($5.76 for 2 ounces), Original Beauty Fluid, Moisture Replenishment Lotion ($7.99 for 4 ounces), Sensitive Skin Beauty Fluid ($6.58 for 4 ounces), and Sensitive Skin Replenishing Cream Daily Care Series ($5.76 for 2 ounces); **Organic Essentials from Linda Chae** Sheer Moisture Lotion ($31 for 1.7 ounces), and Rich Moisture Cream ($35.50 for 1.7 ounces); **Origins** Line Chaser Stop Sign for Lines

($25 for 0.5 ounce), Night-A-Mins ($27.50 for 1.7 ounces), Steady Drencher If Your Skin Acts Dry ($22 for 1.7 ounces), Time Mender ($22 for 1.7 ounces), and Urgent Moisture ($25 for 1.7 ounces); **Orlane** Anagenese Eye Contour Cream Total Time Fighting Care for All Skins ($40 for 0.5 ounce), Anagenese Total Time Fighting Serum ($52.50 for 1.7 ounces), B21 Bio-Energic Absolute Skin Recovery Care ($130 for 1.7 ounces), B21 Absolute Skin Recovery Care Eye Contour ($75 for 0.5 ounce), B21 Bio-Energic Anti-Fatigue Recovery Care ($130 for 1.7 ounces), B21 Bio-Energic Anti-Fatigue Recovery Care Eye Contour ($75 for 0.5 ounce), B21 Bio-Energic Intensive Nurturing Care Nightly Concentrate for Dry and Very Dry Skin ($110 for 1.7 ounces), B21 Bio-Energic Morning Recovery Concentrate ($60 for 1 ounce), B21 Bio-Energic Points Vulnerable Creme for All Skins ($70 for 1 ounce), B21 Bio-Energic Protective and Moisturizing Base ($75 for 1.7 ounces), B21 Bio-Energic Protective Oxytoning System for All Skin Types ($300 for 0.7 ounce), B21 Bio-Energic Ultra-Light Cream for the Day ($75 for 1.7 ounces), B21 Bio-Energic Super Moisturizing Concentrate Day and Night ($95 for 1.7 ounces), B21 Oligo Gentle Soothing Cream for Sensitive Fragile & Allergic Skin Types ($63 for 1.7 ounces), B21 Oligo Light Smoothing Cream ($63 for 1.7 ounces), B21 Oligo Vit-A-Min Vitalizing Lotion for Dry and Sensitive Skin Types ($32.50 for 8.4 ounces), Extrait Vital Biological Cream for Dry and Very Dry Skins ($60 for 1.7 ounces), Extrait Vital Biological Emulsion ($45 for 1.3 ounces), Extrait Vital Eye Contour Serum ($42 for 0.33 ounce), Hydralane Eye Contour Moisture Care ($35 for 0.5 ounce), Hydro-Climat Moisture Shell Multiprotective Fluid ($48 for 1.7 ounces), and After Sun Creme for Face ($30 for 1.7 ounce); **Parthena** Anhydrous Extreme ($24.95 for 4 ounces), Longevity Daily Line Smoothing Fluid ($24.50 for 1 ounce), Longevity Resource Cream ($37.50 for 4 ounces), Eye Power Lift ($19.95 for 2 ounces), and Metamorphosis ($37.50 for four ampoules, total of 1 ounce); **Paula's Choice** Completely Emollient Moisturizer ($9.95 for 4 ounces); **philosophy** dark shadows eye brightener ($25 for 0.5 ounce), eye believe ($25 for 0.5 ounce), the present oil-free moisturizer sensitive skin ($20 for 2 ounces), and thin skin ($24 for 2 ounces); **Physicians Formula** Oil Free Nourishing Eye Gel for Normal to Oily Skin ($5.95 for 0.5 ounce), Extra Rich Rehydrating Moisturizer for Normal to Dry Skin ($8.50 for 4 ounces), Elastin Collagen Moisture Lotion for Normal to Dry Skin ($8.50 for 4 ounces), Collagen Cream Concentrate for Dry to Very Dry Skin ($8.95 for 2 ounces), Intensive Therapy Moisture Cream for Dry to Very Dry Skin ($8 for 2 ounces), and Luxury Eye Cream All Skin Types ($5.95 for 0.5 ounce); **Pond's** Dry Skin Cream, Extra Rich Skin Cream ($4.39 for 3.9 ounces), Nourishing Moisturizer Cream ($5.99 for 2 ounces), Nourishing Moisturizer Lotion ($5.99 for 4 ounces), Overnight Nourishing Complex Cream ($6.29 for 2 ounces), Revitalizing Eye Capsules With Nutrium, Delicate Eye Area ($10.99 for 0.13 ounce), and Skin Smoothing

Capsules with Nutrium ($10.99 for 26 capsules); **Prescriptives** Px Comfort Lotion ($30 for 1.7 ounces), Px Comfort Cream 24 Hour Care for Sensitive Skin ($37.50 for 1.7 ounces), Px Uplift Active Firming Cream ($45 for 1 ounce), Px Uplift Firming Eye Cream ($35 for 0.5 ounce), and Line Preventor 3 ($45 for 1 ounce); **Principal Secret** Extra Nurturing Cream ($40 for 2 ounces); **Purpose** Dry Skin Cream ($5.61 for 3 ounces); **Rachel Perry** Bee Pollen-Jojoba Maximum Moisture Cream ($12.50 for 2 ounces), Ginseng and Collagen Wrinkle Treatment ($14.50 for 2 ounces), and Hi Potency "E" Special Treatment Line Control ($14.50 for 2 ounces); **Ralph Lauren Polo Sport** Water Basics Post Shave Relief Balm ($25 for 4.2 ounces); **Renee Guinot** Base Hydratante, Continue Day Long Moisturizer with Essential Oils, Dry/Dehydrated Skin ($34.50 for 1.7 ounces), Hydrallergic, Day/Night Desensitizing Care, Ultra-Sensitive Skin ($40 for 1.6 ounces), Hydrazone Moisturizing Face Cream, Dry Skin ($67 for 1.6 ounces), Liftosome, Day/Night Cream, All Skin Types ($72 for 1.6 ounces), LongueVie Cellulaire, Vital Face Care, Day/Night Cream, Triple Action Formula ($67 for 1.6 ounces), Surgenerant Profond, Skin Revitalizing Concentrate, Day/Night ($85 for 1 ounce), Surtenseur Cou, Firming Neck Serum Cream, Tightening, Anti-Wrinkle ($40 for 1 ounce), Anti-Rides Yeux, Cream for the Eyes, Wrinkles, Crow's Feet ($34 for 0.5 ounce), Creme Anti-Rides 888, Regenerate, Anti-Wrinkle Night Cream 888, with Cell Vitalizers, and Devitalized Skin ($48.50 for 1.7 ounces); **Renew** Vitamin Enriched Natural Moisture Factor (0.5 ounce); **Revlon** Eterna '27' All Day Moisture Lotion ($11.99 for 2 ounces), and Eterna '27' All Day Moisture Cream ($11.99 for 1 ounce); **ROC** Amino Moisturizing Cream, Dry Skin ($20.50 for 50 ml), Melibiose Anti-Aging Action Enriched Texture ($30 for 40 ml), Melibiose Anti-Ageing Action Light Texture ($30 for 40 ml), Melibiose Anti-Ageing Action Eye Contour ($23 for 15 ml), Revitalizing Night Cream ($28.75 for 40 ml), Retinol Actif Pur Eye and Lip Contour ($28.75 for 15 ml), Retinol Actif Pur Moisturizing Anti-Wrinkle Day Cream ($32.75 for 30 ml), Retinol Actif Pur Night Treatment Cream ($35.75 for 30 ml); **St. Ives** Extra Relief Collagen Elastin Dry Skin Lotion ($3.19 for 18 ounces), Swiss Formula Collagen Elastin Essential Moisturizer ($3.47 for 12 ounces), Swiss Formula Instant Relief Collagen Elastin Dry Skin Lotion (3.19 for 18 ounces), Swiss Formula Peaches and Cream Moisturizing Beauty Lotion ($2.32 for 6 ounces), Swiss Formula Sunflower & Silk Moisture Lotion with Antioxidant Vitamins A&C ($3.19 for 18 ounces), and Swiss Formula Swiss Vanilla Cream Lotion with Soothing Milk Protein ($3.19 for 18 ounces); **Dr. Semel** Collagen Stimulator ($85 for 1 ounce), DNA Repair Aspire ($45 for 2 ounces), Triple Moisture ($45 for 1 ounce), and Tightener ($45 for 1 ounce); **Serious Skin Care** Emu & Aloe Soothing Cream ($24.50 for 2 ounces), Eye Help ($19.95 for 0.05 ounce), and Mega Mins ($28 for 1 ounce); **Shaklee** Balancing Moisturizer ($19.95 for 2 ounces), Enfuselle Eye Treatment ($19.95 for 0.5 ounce), and Enfuselle Hydrating Moisturizer ($19.95

for 1.7 ounces); **Shiseido** Benefiance Revitalizing Cream ($40 for 1.3 ounces), Benefiance Revitalizing Emulsion ($40 for 2.5 ounces), Benefiance Revitalizing Eye Cream ($40 for 0.51 ounce), Benefiance Firming Massage Mask, Vital Perfection Daily Eye Primer ($30 for 0.5 ounce), and Bio-Performance Advanced Super Revitalizer Cream ($60 for 1.7 ounces); **Shu Uemura** Moisture Lotion ($35 for 8.4 ounces), Moisture Fluid ($40 for 1.6 ounces), Refreshing Lotion ($35 for 8.4 ounces), Absolute Cream ($40 for 1.05 ounces), Eye Care Jell ($27 for 0.7 ounce), Aid Oil ($39 for 0.8 ounce), and Principe 21 Bio-Energizing Concentrate ($60 for 1 ounce); **Sothys Paris** Active PhytoContour Anti-Wrinkles, Anti-Circles Eye Serum ($47 for 0.5 ounce), Creme de Nuit, Night Creme for Dry Skins ($39 for 1.7 ounces), Creme de Nuit, Night Creme for Sensitive Skins ($39 for 1.7 ounces), Creme de Nuit, Night Creme to Firm Normal to Dry Skins ($39 for 1.7 ounces), Creme de Nuit, Night Creme to Oxygenate All Skin Types ($39 for 1.7 ounces), Immuniscience Cream for Sensitive Skin ($36 for 1.7 ounces), Immuniscience Fluid for Ultra-Sensitive Skin ($36 for 1.7 ounces), and Serum Nourissant, Nourishing Serum for Dry Skins ($50 for 1 ounce); **Sudden Youth** Moisture Lotion ($15.75 for 8 ounces), Sleeping Beauty Cream ($24.95 for 2 ounces), Elastin Elegance ($42.50 for 2 ounces), and Eye Cream ($24.95); **Tova** Cactine CelRenual ($41 for 1 ounce), Cactine EyeRenual Treatment ($31 for 0.5 ounce), and Cactine Moisture Rich Cream ($26.50 for 1 ounce); **Trish McEvoy** Dry Skin Normalizer, Extra-Rich Improvement Cream ($40 for 1 ounce), Enriched Moisturizer ($37 for 2 ounces), Extra-Light Moisturizer ($37 for 2 ounces), Light Moisturizer ($37 for 2 ounces), and Line Refiner ($25 for 0.18 ounce); **Tyra** Phase III, Premiere Moisturizer ($36 for 4 ounces), and Plus IV Deep Moisturizer ($44 for 4 ounces); **Ultima II** Brighten Up, Tighten Up Eye Cream ($20 for 0.5 ounce), CHR Extraordinary Cream ($68.50 for 1.13 ounces), CHR Extraordinary Lotion ($68.50 for 2 ounces), CHR Lotion Concentrate ($32.50 for 3 ounces), Interactives Balanced State Antioxidant Skin Control Hydrator ($20 for 1.75 ounces), and Smart Move ($25 for 1.7 ounces); **Vaseline Intensive Care** Aloe Vera Triple Action Formula ($3.29 for 10 ounces), Dermasil Dry Skin Treatment Cream ($7.79 for 4 ounces), Dermasil Dry Skin Treatment Lotion ($7.79 for 8 ounces), Dermatology Formula ($2.29 for 11 ounces), and Dry Skin Triple Action Formula ($3.29 for 10 ounces); **Vichy** Adaptive Skin Balancing System, for Combination Skin ($21.50 for 40 ml), Nutritive 1 Balanced Nutrient Cream for Dry Skin ($26 for 40 ml), Optalia Restructuring Eye Gel ($28.50 for 15 ml), Regenium Night Renewal Cream ($31 for 40 ml), Thermal S1: Long Lasting Hydration ($21.50 for 50 ml), Thermal S2: Long Lasting Hydration for Very Dehydrated Skin ($21.50 for 50 ml), Thermal S2 Lotion: Long Lasting Hydration ($21.50 for 50 ml), and Heliocalm Calming Reparative Gel For Face and Body ($15.50 for 100 ml); **Victoria Jackson** Moisturizer ($13.75, $20.50 for 2 ounces), Nourishing Skin Revitalizer

($12.95, $19.95 for 1 ounce), and Skin Renewal System ($30.95, $39.95 for 0.14 ounce of Extra-Intensive Eye Cream and 1.25 ounces of Extra-Intensive Night Cream); **Yves Rocher** A.D.N. Revitalizing Resource Energizing Mask, for Devitalized Skin ($16 for 1.7 ounces), Bio-Calmille Long-Lasting Day Cream ($11.95 for 1.7 ounces), Bio-Calmille Soothing Night Cream ($15.95 for 1.7 ounces), Bionutritive Enrichment Day Cream ($11.95 for 1.35 ounces), Bionutritive Nourishing Night Cream ($17.95 for 1.35 ounces), Hydra Advance Maximum Moisture Renewal Gel for Dehydrated Skins ($19.95 for 1.35 ounces), Response Nature Time Defense Eye Contour Treatment ($19 for 0.5 ounce), Response Nature Time Defense Night Recovery Treatment ($24 for 1.35 ounces), Riche Creme Smoothing Throat Cream, with Botanical Extracts ($24 for 1 ounce), and Riche Creme Wrinkle Smoothing Day Cream, with 10 Botanical Oils ($19 for 1.7 ounces); **Yves St. Laurent** Creme de Nuit Revitalisante/Nighttime Revitalizer, for Combination to Dry Skin ($55 for 1 ounce), Creme de Nuit Revitalisante Peaux Seches a Tres Seches/Intensive Nighttime Revitalizer, for Dry to Very Dry Skin ($55 for 1 ounce), Hydratant Absolu/Absolute Hydration ($57 for 1 ounce), Precurseur Anti-Temps/Time Interceptor Fortifying Complex ($65 for 1 ounce), Prevention + /Time Prevention Day Creme ($65 for 1.7 ounces), and Soin Beaute Instantanee/Instant Firming Gel ($60 for 1 ounce); **Zhen** Face Creme ($25 for 1.25 ounces); and **Zia** Essential Eye Gel ($19.95 for 0.5 ounce), Everyday Moisturizers, Fragrance Free for Normal, Sensitive, Combination & Dry Skin Types ($18.95 for 2 ounces), Eye Treatment Oil for All Skin Types ($16.95 for 0.3 ounce), Nourishing Creme Cellular Renewal for Normal, Dry & Mature Skin Types ($12.75 for 1 ounce), Ultimate "C" Serum ($49.95 for 0.5 ounce), Ultimate Moisture ($34.95 for 1.5 ounces), and Ziasome Restorative Moisture Treatment for Normal, Dry & Mature Skin Types ($29.95 for 0.3 ounce).

FOR DRY TO VERY DRY SKIN, THE BEST MOISTURIZERS ARE: **Adrien Arpel** Moisturizing Blotting Lotion ($23.50 for 2 ounces), Swiss Formula Day Cream #12 with Collagen ($50 for 1 ounce), Swiss Formula Day Eye Creme, with Vitamin A Palmitate and Collagen ($27.50 for 0.5 ounce), and Vital Velvet Moisturizer ($23.50 for 2 ounces); **Alexandra de Markoff** Compensation Skin Serum ($65 for 2 ounces), and Skin Tight Firming Eye Cream ($50 for 0.4 ounce); **Aloette** Night Creme ($14 for 2 ounces); **Amway** Delicate Care Hydrating Fluid for Sensitive Skin Types ($21.15 for 2.3 ounces), and Advanced Daily Eye Creme ($20.30 for 0.5 ounce); **Arbonne** Moisture Cream for Normal to Dry Skin ($18.50 for 2 ounces), Night Cream for Normal to Dry Skin ($20.50 for 2 ounces), Skin Conditioning Oil ($16 for 1 ounce), Bio Hydria Night Energizing Cream ($58 for 2 ounces), and Bio Hydria Eye Cream ($24.50 for 0.75 ounce); **Aveda** Night Nutrients ($38 for 1 ounce), Pure Vital Moisture Eye Creme ($26 for 0.5 ounce), Balancing Infusion for Dry Skin ($18 for 0.33

ounce), and Balancing Infusion for Sensitive Skin ($18 for 0.33 ounce); **Avon** Basics Perfect Day Moisture Cream ($4.99 for 3.4 ounces), Basics Vita Moist Face Cream ($4.99 for 3.4 ounces), Calming Effects Sensitive Skin Creme ($10.50 for 1.7 ounces), and Hydrofirming Cream Night Treatment ($11 for 1.7 ounces); **Beauty Without Cruelty** Maximum Moisture Cream Benefits Dry/Mature Skin ($14.49 for 2 ounces); **BeneFit** Eye Lift ($25 for 1 ounce), Hyaluronic Creme ($22 for 2 ounces), and Vita Hydrating Creme, for Sensitive/Dry Skin ($22 for 2 ounces); **BioTherm** Biosensitive Calming Regulating Daily Cream ($27 for 50 ml), Biosensitive Extra Comfort Cream Calming Regulating ($27 for 50 ml), Hydrologic Moisture Generator ($34 for 50 ml), Reducteur Rides Anti-Wrinkle and Firming Cream, for Very Dry Skin ($37 for 50 ml), Reducteur Rides Anti-Wrinkle and Firming Eye Creme ($30 for 15 g), Intensive Soothing After Sun Balm For Face ($16 for 50 ml), and Soothing Repair Lotion ($17 for 240 ml); **The Body Shop** Carrot Oil for Normal to Dry Skin ($4.95 for 1 ounce), Evening Primrose Oil for Dry Skin ($4.95 for 1 ounce), Sweet Almond Oil for All Skin Types ($4.95 for 1 ounce), Wheat Germ Oil for All Skin Types ($4.95 for 1 ounce), Aloe Vera Moisture Cream ($9.50 for 1.8 ounces), Carrot Moisture Cream ($9.50 for 1.8 ounces), Hydrating Moisture Lotion for Normal to Dry Skin ($16 for 3.38 ounces), Jojoba Moisture Cream ($9.50 for 1.6 ounces), Rich Moisture Cream for Dry Skin ($16 for 3.52 ounces), Rich Night Cream with Vitamin E ($9.50 for 1.4 ounces), and Vitamin E Moisture Cream ($9.50 for 1.8 ounces); **Borghese** Hydra-Puro Intensivo Moisture Renewing Creme ($40 for 1.7 ounces); Puro Protettivo Protective Eye Creme ($32 for 0.5 ounce), Crema Correttivo Firming Eye Cream ($35 for 0.5 ounce), and Dolce Notte ReEnergizing Night Creme ($50 for 1.85 ounces); **Cellex-C** G.L.A. Extra Moist Cream for Excessively Dry Skin ($55 for 2 ounces); **Cetaphil** Moisturizing Lotion ($7.49 for 16 ounces); **Charles of the Ritz** Moisture Balancing Day Care Skin Soother ($18.50 for 2 ounces), Revenescence Cream ($42.50 for 4.4 ounces), and Special Formula Emollient ($28.50 for 4 ounces); **Circle of Beauty** Overnight Eye Treatment ($15 for 0.6 ounce); **Clarins** Extra-Firming Day Cream for Dry Skin ($50 for 1.7 ounces), Face Treatment Cream for Dry or Reddened Skin ($29 for 1.7 ounces), Face Treatment Plant Cream "Santal" for Dry or Extra Dry Skin ($29 for 1.7 ounces), Gentle Night Cream for Sensitive Skin ($49 for 1.7 ounces), After Sun Skin Conditioner with Plant Extracts ($22.50 for 1.4), and After Sun Moisturizer ($20 for 5.3 ounces); **Clientele** Elastology Firming Night Cream for Normal/Dry, Sensitive Skin ($95 for 1.1 ounce); **DHC USA** Collagen Eye Stick ($29 for 0.12 ounce), Pure Squalane ($25 for 1 ounce), Advanced Collagen Treatment ($40 for 1 ounce), and Skin Conditioning Oil ($30 for 1 ounce); **Elizabeth Arden** Millennium Day Renewal Emulsion ($54.50 for 2.6 ounces), Visible Difference Refining Moisturizer Creme Complex ($47.50 for 2.5 ounces), Skin Basics Beauty Sleep ($32.50 for 2.5 ounces), Millennium Eye Renewal

Cream ($39.50 for 0.5 ounce), Millennium Night Renewal Creme ($82 for 1.7 ounces), and Skin Basics Velva Moisture Film ($38.50 for 6.7 ounces); **Estee Lauder** Age Controlling Creme ($60 for 1.7 ounces), Estoderme Creme ($25 for 4 ounces), Estoderme Emulsion ($25 for 4 ounces), Re-nutriv Creme ($75 for 1.75 ounce), and Enriched Under-Makeup Creme ($25 for 4 ounces); **Erno Laszlo** Active pHelityl Cream PM Moisturizer for Slightly Dry Skin ($32 for 2 ounces), Antioxidant Concentrate for Eyes, Intensive Therapy for the Eye Area ($48 for 0.5 ounce), HydrapHel Emulsion AM Moisturizer for Extremely Dry and Dry Skin ($45 for 2 ounces), pHelitone Replenishing Eye Cream for All Skin Types ($42 for 0.5 ounce), and Total Skin Revitalizer for Eyes Hydration Enhancer for the Eye Area ($45 for 0.5 ounce); **Eucerin** Original Moisturizing Creme ($4.19 for 2 ounces), Light Moisture Restorative Creme ($6.99 for 4 ounces), and Light Moisture Restorative Lotion ($6.99 for 8 ounces); **Fashion Fair** Dry Skin Emollient for Excessively Dry Skin ($21 for 2 ounces), Moisturizing Creme with Aloe Vera for Dry Skin ($18.50 for 4 ounces), and Special Beauty Creme with Collagen ($19.50 for 2 ounces); **Forever Spring** Super Rich Emollience ($24.50 for 4 ounces); **Iman** PM Renewal Cream ($20 for 1.8 ounces); **Jafra** Extra Care Cream ($8 for 0.5 ounce), and Royal Jelly Milk Balm Moisture Lotion, Unscented ($60 for 1 ounce); **Janet Sartin** Active Skin Replenishing Cream, Super Rich Nourishing Cream ($39 for 1.85 ounces), Highly Active Collagen Cream ($44 for 1.85 ounces), Nutri Performance Cream, Soothing Emollient to Help Nourish Dry Skin ($39 for 1.85 ounces), Nutri Performance Eye Care Cream ($35 for 0.5 ounce), Superfatted Cream, and Rich Nourishing Cream for Dry Skin ($70 for 4 ounces); **Jergens** Aloe Enriched Lotion, for Very Dry Skin ($2.99 for 6 ounces), Ultra Healing Cream, for Extra Dry Skin ($4.99 for 8 ounces), Ultra Healing Lotion, for Extra Dry Skin ($2.99 for 6 ounces), Ultra Healing Lotion, Fragrance Free, for Extra Dry Skin ($3.49 for 10 ounces), and Vitamin E Enriched Lotion, for Very Dry Skin ($2.99 for 6 ounces); **Kiehl's** Creme d'Elegance Repairateur Superb Tissue Repairateur Creme ($25.50 for 2 ounces); **Lancome** Hydrative Continuous Hydrating Resource ($42.50 for 1.75 ounces), Hydrix Hydrating Creme ($36.50 for 1.9 ounces), Nutrix Soothing Treatment Creme ($32 for 1.9 ounces), Nutribel Nourishing Hydrating Emulsion ($38 for 2.5 ounces), and Renergie Yeux ($40 for 0.5 ounce); **Lubriderm** Skin Therapy Moisturizing Lotion for Normal to Dry Skin ($6.99 for 16 ounces), Skin Therapy Moisturizing Lotion Fragrance-Free, for Normal to Dry Skin ($6.99 for 16 ounces), and Advanced Therapy Gel Cream for Rough and Dry Skin ($5.23 for 7.5 ounces); **Marcelle** Dry Skin Lubricating Cream ($9.95 for 120 ml), and Eye Cream Ultra Rich ($6.78 for 15 ml); **Mariana Chicet** Rich Moisturizer ($27.50 for 2 ounces); **Mary Kay** Extra Emollient Night Cream ($11 for 2.5 ounces); **Merle Norman** Intensive Moisturizer ($15 for 1.25 ounces), and Aqua Lube ($12 for 2 ounces); **Natura Bisse** Elastin Refirming Night

Cream for Deeply Dry Skin ($56 for 2.5 ounces), and Essential Shock Night Cream for Dry Aged Skin ($74 for 2.5 ounces); **Noevir** Special Night Cream ($35 for 0.7 ounce); **Paula's Choice** Extra Emollient Moisturizer for Extra Dry Skin ($11.95 for 4 ounces); **Physicians Formula** Nourishing Night Cream for Dry to Very Dry Skin ($5.95 for 1 ounce), Deep Moisture Cream Normal to Dry ($6.89 for 4 ounces), Emollient Oil for Dry to Very Dry Skin ($5.25 for 2 ounces), and Enriched Dry Skin Concentrate for Dry to Very Dry Skin ($4.79 for 4 ounces); **ROC** Moisturizing Cream, Normal to Combination Skin ($20.50 for 50 ml); **Sudden Youth** Essential Beauty Oils ($15.95 for 1 ounce); **Tova** Cactine Emollient ($23.50 for 1 ounce); **Ultima II** CHR Cream Concentrate ($32.50 for 2 ounces), CHR Double Action Night Cream ($42.50 for 2 ounces), CHR Double Action Eye Cream ($22.50 for 0.5 ounce), Under Makeup Moisture Cream ($22 for 2 ounces), and Under Makeup Moisture Lotion ($27.50 for 4 ounces); **Vichy** Nutritive 2 Reinforced Nutrient Cream for Very Dry Skin ($26 for 40 ml); and **Yves Rocher** Cel Defense Age-Defying Day Cream ($17.50 for 1.35 ounces), Cel Defense Age-Defying Night Cream ($19.50 for 1.35 ounces), Hydra Advance Replenishing Moisture Base for Dehydrated Skins ($15.95 for 1.35 ounces), Hydra Advance Solaire Moisture Replenishing Lotion After-Sun ($11.95 for 5 ounces), Riche Creme Wrinkle Fighting Concentrate ($26 for 1 ounce), Riche Creme Wrinkle Smoothing Night Cream with 10 Botanical Oils ($24 for 1.7 ounces), and Riche Creme Wrinkle Smoothing Eye Cream, with Floral Extracts ($24 for 0.5 ounce).

Best Sunscreens

I've discussed at length why sunscreens are essential for skin care (they are the only true antiwrinkle products), why UVA-protecting ingredients (either avobenzone, zinc oxide, or titanium dioxide) are so crucial, and why I prefer SPF 15 to other numbers, but the bottom line is that sun protection is essential for everyone at any age and every day of the year. If you want to select a sunscreen with a lower rating that's up to you, but my strong advice is not to venture out with anything less than SPF 10, though SPF 15 or greater is by far preferred.

The only thing left to explain is why the lists below are so disproportionate, with vastly more sunscreens for normal to dry skin than for normal to oily. The answer is not reassuring, at least not to those with oily skin or skin prone to breakouts. Sunscreen agents work better in an emollient emulsion than in a matte base or liquid. When a lightweight liquid is available, often the base includes alcohol, and that is just hard on skin due to irritation. Plus, the UVA-protecting ingredients of zinc oxide and titanium dioxide can clog pores! As I mentioned before, from the chin up, someone with oily skin may prefer using a foundation with a good SPF and from the neck down any other good sunscreen formulation. Sadly, as this book goes to print there are no foundations with avobenzone as one of the sunscreen agents; those that have UVA protection usually use titanium dioxide. Either way, this is one area of skin care that is difficult for someone with oily skin, and it takes experimentation to find what works well for you.

All of the following sunscreens are an SPF 15 or greater and contain either avobenzone, titanium dioxide, or zinc oxide.

FOR NORMAL TO OILY/COMBINATION SKIN, THE BEST SUN-SCREENS (KEEPING IN MIND THAT FOUNDATIONS WITH SUNSCREENS WORK GREAT FOR OILY AND COMBINATION SKIN TYPES) ARE: **Estee Lauder** Advanced Suncare Sun Block Lotion Spray No Chemical Sunscreen SPF 15 ($18.50 for 4.25 ounces); **Lancome** SPF 15 Face and Body Lotion with Pure Vitamin E ($21 for 5 ounces), and SPF 25 Face and Body Lotion with Pure Vitamin E ($21 for 5 ounces); **Le Mirador** Triple Action Revitalizing Moisturizer SPF 15 ($21.71 for 2 ounces); **Paula's Choice** Essential Nongreasy Sunscreen SPF 15 ($10.95 for 6 ounces), and All Day Cover Non-Greasy Sunscreen SPF 30+ with Antioxidants Waterproof ($11.95 for 6 ounces); and **Yves St. Laurent** Hydra Fluide/Hydro-Light Day Lotion Oil-Free with SPF 15 ($35 for 1.3 ounces).

FOR NORMAL TO DRY, EXTRA DRY, AND/OR SENSITIVE SKIN, THE BEST SUNSCREENS ARE: **Almay** Time-Off Lasting Moisture SPF 25 ($14.99 for 3.8 ounces), and SPF 30 Waterproof Sunblock Sensitive Skin Formula ($5.40 for 4 ounces); **Aveda** Daily Light Guard SPF 15 ($16.50 for 5 ounces); **Avon** Age Block Daytime Defense Cream SPF 15 UVA/UVB Protection ($12.50 for 1.7 ounces), Sun Age-Fighting Protective Sun Cream SPF 15 Waterproof ($10 for 4.2 ounces), and Sun Age-Fighting Protective Sun Cream SPF 30 Waterproof ($10 for 4.2 ounces); **Bain de Soleil** UV Sense SPF 50 ($9.89 for 3.12 ounces), Mademoiselle Sunblock SPF 15 ($6.99 for 4 ounces), Le Sport Sunblock SPF 15 ($6.99 for 4 ounces), Le Sport Sunblock SPF 30 ($8.99 for 4 ounces), and Kids Sunblock SPF 30 ($8.99 for 4 ounces), Bebe Block SPF 50 ($9.89 for 3.12 ounces), All Day Extended Protection Sunscreen, SPF 30 ($9.19 for 4 ounces), All Day Extended Protection Sunblock, SPF 15 ($6.99 for 4 ounces), and Gentle Block Sunblock, SPF 30 ($8.99 for 4 ounces); **Basis** Face the Day Lotion SPF 15 ($6.55 for 4 ounces), and One Step Face Cream SPF 15 ($6.55 for 1.5 ounces); **Beauty Without Cruelty** SPF 12 Daily Facial Lotion ($9.49 for 4 ounces); **Bioelements** Sun Diffusing Protector SPF 15 Natural Sunblock ($29.50 for 6 ounces); **Biogime** Essential Protector SPF 15 ($30 for 2 ounces), and Sun Protector SPF 15 ($17.95 for 4 ounces); **BioTherm** Maximum Protection Lotion SPF 15 ($15 for 150 ml), Protective Lotion SPF 15 ($18 for 150 ml), Protective Lotion SPF 15 ($18 for 150 ml), Special Wrinkle Sun Block SPF 15 ($19.50 for 50 ml), Sun Block Lotion SPF 25 ($19.50 for 150 ml), Total Intolerance Sun Block SPF 30 ($19.50 for 50 ml), and Total Sun Block SPF 25 ($19.50 for 50 ml); **Bobbi Brown Essentials** SPF 15 Face Lotion ($38 for 1.7 ounces); **The Body Shop** Facial Sun Stick SPF 30 ($6.50 for 0.6 ounce); **Charles of the Ritz** Any Age Self Protection for Face SPF 15 ($25 for 1.8 ounces), and Biochange Replacement Therapy Serum for Changing Skin ($30 for 1.9 ounces); **Clarins** Hydration-Plus Moisture Lotion SPF 15 for All Skin Types ($30 for 1.7 ounces), Sun Block SPF 25 Ultra Protection for Face/Sensitive Areas ($19.50 for 2.7 ounces), Sun Block Stick SPF 19 Sensitive Areas ($16.50 for 0.17 ounce), Sun Care Cream SPF 15 ($18.50 for 4.4 ounces), and Sun Care Milk SPF 19 ($18.50 for 2.7 ounces); **Clientele** Preventative Age Solar Block SPF 25 ($42 for 4 ounces), **Clinique** Weather Everything SPF 15 ($37.50 for 1.7 ounces), City Block Oil-Free Daily Protector SPF 15 ($13.50 for 1.4 ounces), and Special Defense Sun Block SPF 25 ($13.50 for 3 ounces); **Coppertone** Shade UVA Guard SPF 15 ($9.99 for 4 ounces), and Shade UVA Guard SPF 30 ($9.99 for 4 ounces); **DHC USA** Dual Defense SPF 25 ($24 for 3.5 ounces); **Estee Lauder** Advanced Suncare Baby Block Lotion for Children SPF 25 ($19.50 for 4.25 ounces), Advanced Suncare Sun Block for Face SPF 25 ($19.50 for 1.7 ounces), Advanced Suncare Sun Block for Face SPF 15 ($19.50 for 1.7 ounces), and Day Wear Super Anti-Oxidant Complex SPF 15 ($37.50 for 1.7 ounces); **Eucerin** Facial Moisturizing Lotion, SPF 25 ($8 for 4 ounces); **Guerlain** Odelys Perfect Care No. 3 Super Rich, Day and Night ($52 for 1.7 ounce), and Hydrobella Creme Grand Comfort #3 Ultra Rich Creme ($50 for 1.7 ounce); **Janet Sartin** SPF 15 Sunblock Face Cream with Plant Extracts ($39 for 1.85 ounces), Sunblock SPF 15 Waterproof Lotion with Plant Extracts ($18 for 4 ounces), and Sunblock SPF 25 Waterproof Lotion with Plant Extracts ($18 for 4 ounces); **Jurlique** Moist Face Sun Lotion, SPF 15+ Broadband UV Sunscreen ($24.69 for 1 ounce); **Kiehl's** Heidegger's All-Sport Water-Resistant Skin Protector with SPF 30 ($17.95 for 4 ounces), and Sun Shield Sunblock with SPF 15 ($23.50 for 8 ounces); **La Prairie** Soleil Suisse Cellular Anti-Wrinkle Sun Cream SPF 15 ($100 for 1.7 ounces); **Lancome** SPF 15 Water-Light Spray ($21 for 5 ounces), and SPF 30 Face Creme with Pure Vitamin E ($23 for 1.7 ounces); **Marcelle** Protective Block No Chemical Sunscreen Cream SPF 25 ($12.95 for 50 ml), Protective Block No Chemical Sunscreen Lotion SPF 25 ($12.95 for 120 ml), and Protective Block No Chemical Sunscreen Spray SPF 15 ($12.95 for 120 ml); **Dr. Mary Lupo** Daily Age Management Oil Free Moisturizer SPF 15 ($23 for 2 ounces); **Mon Amie** Daytime Moisturizer Replenishment Complex SPF 15 ($24.95 for 1.75 ounces); **Murad** Murasun Daily Sunblock with Antioxidants SPF 15 ($16.50 for 4.2 ounces), and Murasun Waterproof Sunblock with Antioxidants SPF 30 ($19 for 4.2 ounces); **Natura Bisse** Sun Protector SPF 30 Hydrating Sun Block for All

Skin Types ($53 for 4.2 ounces); **Neutrogena** Sensitive Skin Sunblock SPF 17 No Irritating Chemical Sunscreen Ingredients ($7.20 for 4 ounces); **Noevir** Sun Defense SPF 15 ($24 for 4.2 ounces); **Nu Skin** Sunright 15 Maximum Protection Sunscreen ($17.15 for 3.4 ounces), Sunright 23 Face and Hands Ultimate Sunscreen Protection ($13.85 for 4 ounces), and Sunright 28 Ultimate Sunscreen Protection ($17.45 for 3.4 ounces); **Ombrelle** Sunscreen Lotion SPF 15 ($10 for 4 ounces), and Ombrelle Sunscreen Lotion SPF 30 ($10 for 4 ounces); **Origins** Silent Treatment Instant UV Face Protector SPF 15 ($15 for 1.7 ounces); **Orlane** Creme Solaire Total Block Sun Cream For the Face 30+ UVA 11 ($30 for 1.7 ounces), Creme Solaire Vulnerable Points Sun Cream 30 Ultra Protection ($19.50 for 1.7 ounces), and Safe Tanning Cream SPF 18 Ultra Sun Protection for Delicate Skin ($20 for 4.2 ounces); **Paula's Choice** Essential Moisturizing Sunscreen SPF 15 ($10.95 for 6 ounces), and All Day Cover Moisturizing Sunscreen SPF 30+ with Antioxidants Waterproof ($11.95 for 6 ounces); **Physicians Formula** Sun Shield Sensitive Skin Formula Chemical Free Sunscreen SPF 25 ($8.50 for 4 ounces), Sun Shield For Faces Sensitive Skin Formula SPF 15 for All Skin Types ($8 for 2 ounces), and Vital Defense Sun Stick For Faces SPF 30 for All Skin Types ($6.95 for 0.55 ounce); **Pond's** Nourishing Moisture Lotion with SPF 15 ($5.99 for 2.5 ounces); **Prescriptives** Px Insulation Anti-Oxidant Vitamin Cream with SPF 15 ($40 for 1.7 ounces), and Any Wear SPF 15 ($19.50 for 1 ounce); **Principal Secret** Sun Block SPF 20 ($17 for 4 ounces); **Purpose** Dual Treatment Moisturizer with SPF 15 Protection ($7.89 for 4 ounces); **Dr. Semel** UVA/UVB SPF 19 ($50 for 4 ounces), and Licorice Lightning DNA Repair—UVA/UVB SPF 19 ($50 for 4 ounces); **Shiseido** Gentle Sun Block Cream SPF 22 ($20 for 3.8 ounces), Sun Block Face Cream SPF 35 ($22 for 1.7 ounces), and Ultra Light Sun Block Lotion SPF 30 ($25 for 3.3 ounces); **Trish McEvoy** Natural Sunscreen SPF 17 Waterproof ($19 for 5 ounces), and Protective Shield Moisturizer SPF 15 ($37 for 2 ounces); **Vichy** Capital Soleil Protective Gel-Cream SPF 15 ($15.50 for 120 ml), Capital Soleil Protective Lotion SPF 15 ($15.50 for 120 ml), Capital Soleil Sunblock Cream for the Face SPF 25 ($15.50 for 50 ml), Capital Soleil Sunblock Lotion SPF 25 ($15.50 for 120 ml), Capital Soleil Sunblock Lotion for Children SPF 25 ($15.50 for 120 ml), Capital Soleil Total Sunblock Lotion SPF 30 ($15.50 for 120 ml), and Capital Soleil Total Sunblock Cream SPF 45 ($15.50 for 50 ml); **Yves Rocher** Hydra Advance Solaire Moisturizing Sun Block SPF 25 ($17.95 for 5 ounces); and **Yves St. Laurent** Hydra Fluide/Hydro-Light Day Lotion, SPF 15 ($50 for 1.3 ounces).

FOR NORMAL TO DRY, SENSITIVE SKIN THE BEST TINTED SUN-SCREENS ARE: **Bobbi Brown Essentials** Tinted Moisturizer SPF 15 ($35); **Lancome** Immanance SPF 15 ($27), and Lancome Immanance Mat SPF 15 ($27); **Origins** Let the Sunshine SPF 14 ($13.50 for 5 ounces); **philosophy** the naked truth nonchemical sunscreen SPF 15 tinted moisturizer ($16 for 4 ounces); and **Shiseido** Vital Perfection Protective Tinted Moisturizer SPF 10 ($26).

FOR NORMAL TO DRY, SENSITIVE SKIN THE BEST FOUNDATIONS WITH SUNSCREEN ARE: **Almay** Amazing Lasting Sheer Makeup SPF 12 ($8.37); **Clinique** Almost Makeup SPF 15 ($25), City Base Compact Foundation SPF 15 ($20), and Sensitive Skin Foundation SPF 15 ($18.50); **Dermablend** Active Cover Creme Foundation SPF 15 ($18.50); **Elizabeth Arden** Flawless Finish Hydro Light Foundation SPF 10 ($30), Flawless Finish Every Day Makeup SPF 10 ($25), and Flawless Finish Complete Control Matte Makeup SPF 10 ($25); **Erno Laszlo** Multi-pHase Light Diffusing Foundation SPF 15 ($28); **Estee Lauder** Enlighten Skin-Enhancing Makeup with SPF 10 ($27.50); **Maybelline Natural** Defense Makeup with SPF 15 ($5.26); **Physicians Formula** Le Velvet SPF 15 Foundation ($5.50), Le Velvet Liquid Cream Makeup SPF 15 ($5.95), and Sun Shield Foundation SPF 15 ($5.50); **Prescriptives** Matchstick Foundation SPF 15 ($35); **Revlon** Age Defying Extra Cover Creme Makeup SPF 12 ($9.34), New Complexion One-Step Makeup SPF 15 ($8.78), and Age Defying Makeup with SPF 10 ($9.34); and **Ultima II** Beautiful Nutrient Nourishing Makeup SPF 15 ($24).

FOR SOMEONE WITH OILY/COMBINATION AND/OR BLEMISH-PRONE SKIN, THE BEST FOUNDATIONS WITH SUNSCREEN ARE: **BeautiControl** Color Freeze Liquid Makeup SPF 12 ($19.50); **The Body Shop** All-in-One Face Treat SPF 15 ($15); **Elizabeth Arden** Flawless Finish Complete Control Matte SPF 10 ($27); **Erno Laszlo** Multi-pHase Oil-Free Foundation SPF 15 ($28); **Estee Lauder** Double Wear Makeup SPF 10 ($27.50); **Prescriptives** Photochrome Compact Makeup SPF 15 ($35); **Revlon** ColorStay Lite SPF 15 ($8.95); **Shiseido** Liquid Compact Foundation SPF 15 ($35); and **Yves St. Laurent** Teint Mat Oil-Free Foundation SPF 12 ($45).

THE BEST SUNSCREEN MOISTURIZERS WITH ALPHA HYDROXY ACIDS ARE: **Decleor Paris** Day Alpha Hydrating Cream with Plant Extracts and Alpha-Hydroxy Acids, SPF 12, for All Skin Types ($42 for 1.69 ounces); **Exuviance by Neostrata** Essential Multi-Defense Day Creme SPF 15 ($25 for 1.75 ounces), Essential Multi-Defense Day Fluid SPF 15 ($22.50 for 2 ounces), Fundamental Multi-Protective Day Creme SPF 15 Sensitive Formula ($25 for 1.75 ounces), and Fundamental Multi-Protective Day Fluid SPF 15 Sensitive Formula ($22.50 for 2 ounces).

Best Facial Masks

Although I am rarely a woman of few words, I'm not one to get too excited about facial masks. First, I feel quite comfortable stating that there are not many exciting, interesting, or particularly helpful facial masks to choose from. Many facial masks use clay as their main ingredient and then add thickening agents, water-binding agents, or plants (so you think you're getting something special), which isn't necessarily bad for skin, but isn't necessarily helpful either. What is most disturbing are the number of facial masks that add a host of irritating ingredients to the mix so the skin tingles and you feel that is doing something for the face—but all it's doing is causing damage. There are also an array of masks that use a plasticizing agent that is then pulled or peeled off the skin. These do impart a temporary soft feeling on the skin by pulling off a layer of skin, but that is hardly beneficial or lasting. Facial masks can be a pampering interval for women, but for good skin care, what you do daily is vastly more important than what you do once a week or once a month.

FOR NORMAL TO OILY/COMBINATION AND/OR BLEMISH-PRONE SKIN, THE BEST MASKS ARE: Beauty Without Cruelty Purifying Facial Mask ($8.49 for 4 ounces); Circle of Beauty Pore Purge Clay Mask ($10.50 for 8 ounces); Freeman Beautiful Skin Avocado & Oatmeal Mineral Mud Mask ($2.85 for 6 ounces); Forever Spring Baby Soft Facial Clay ($15 for 4 ounces); Garden Botanika Desert Mud Mask ($7.50 for 2 ounces); Murad Purifying Clay Masque ($22.50 for 2.25 ounces); Paula's Choice Oil Absorbing Face Mask ($9.95 for 6 ounces); philosophy never let them see you shine oil absorbing serum ($12 for 1 ounce), and stuck in the mud ($18 for 2 ounces); and Vichy Purifying Thermal Mask ($18 for 50 ml).

FOR NORMAL TO DRY AND/OR SENSITIVE SKIN, THE BEST MASKS ARE: Amway Hydrating Masque ($17.10 for 2.6 ounces); Arbonne Mild Masque ($17 for 5 ounces); Avon Avon Intensive Hydrating Facial Mask ($8.50 for 3.4 ounces), and Soothing Hydrating Mask Rose & Apple Blossom ($4.99 for 3 ounces); BeneFit Seaweed Mud Mask ($19 for 2 ounces); Bioelements Cremetherapy Very Emollient Mask ($23 for 2.5 ounces), and Restorative Clay Active Treatment Mask ($21.50 for 2.5 ounces); BioTherm Hydro-Cure Soothing and Moisturizing Mask ($20 for 75 ml); Chanel Natural Exfoliating Mask ($42 for 2.5 ounces); Charles of the Ritz Moisture Intensive Facial ($20 for 4 ounces); Clarins Purifying Plant Facial Mask ($23.50 for 1.7 ounces), and Revitalizing Moisture Mask with Plant Marine "Cell Extract" for All Skin Types ($28 for 1.7 ounces); Clinique Skin Calming Moisture Mask ($18.50 for 3.4 ounces); Decleor Paris Moisturizing Creamy Face Mask with Plant Extracts for All Skin Types ($32 for 1.69 ounces), Regulating Face Mask with Plant Extracts and Natural Aromatic Essences for Combination Skins ($26 for 1.69 ounces), and Timecare Mask with Plant Extracts and Aromatic Essences ($34 for 1.69 ounces); Dermalogica Intensive Moisture Masque ($32.50 for 2 ounces), and Skin Hydrating Masque ($28.50 for 2.5 ounces); Estee Lauder Quick Lift 4-Minute

Mask N/D ($18.50 for 3.4 ounces), Soothing Creme Facial ($18.50 for 3.4 ounces), and Triple Creme Hydrating Mask ($27.50 for 2.5 ounces); **Face Stockholm** Sage and Aloe Mask All Skin Types ($18 for 2 ounces); **Garden Botanika** Chamomile Moisture Mask ($8.50 for 2 ounces); **Givenchy** Hydra-Tricellia Mask ($40 for 2.8 ounces), and Hydrating Cream Mask ($40 for 1.7 ounces); **Guerlain** Evolution Fresh Complexion Mask ($37 for 1.7 ounces), Issima Revitalizing Moisturizing Mask ($65 for 2.5 ounces), and Odelys Moisturizing Creme Mask ($33 for 2.6 ounces); **Jafra** Refreshing Moisture Mask for Dry and Dry to Normal Skin ($12.50 for 2.5 ounces), and Soothing Results Cooling Yogurt and Honey Mask, for Sensitive Skin ($12.50 for 2.6 ounces); **Janet Sartin** Triple Performance Moisture Mask with Kalaya Oil ($25 for 1.7 ounces), and Moisture Mask for Dry Skin ($22 for 2.2 ounces); **Jurlique** Deep Penetrating Cream Mask ($28.75 for 1.7 ounces); **Kiehl's** Moisturizing Masque ($35 for 2 ounces), and Soothing and Cleansing Algae Masque for Balancing Skin Types ($39.95 for 4.5 ounces); **La Prairie** Cellular Moisture Mask ($65 for 1 ounce); **Marcelle** Gentle Purifying Mask ($10.25 for 50 ml); **Mary Kay** Moisture Rich Mask ($12 for 4 ounces); **Origins** Drink Up 10 Minute Moisture Mask ($17.50 for 3.4 ounces); **Orlane** B21 Bio-Energic Hydro-Energizing Masque for All Skins ($55 for 1.7 ounces); **Renee Guinot** Masque Anti-Rides Defatigant, Instant Relaxing Anti-Wrinkle Mask with Cell Vitalizers, Devitalized Skin ($31 for 1.7 ounces); **Shu Uemura** Balancing Mask ($33 for 2.2 ounces); **Sothys Paris** Beauty Mask for Normal to Combination Skin ($31 for 1.7 ounces); **Yves Rocher** Bio-Calmille Relaxing Soothing Mask ($11.95 for 1.7 ounces); **Yves St. Laurent** Masque Creme Hydro Actif/Hydro-Active Moisture Masque ($35 for 1.6 ounces); and **Zia** Super Moisturizing Mask for Normal, Sensitive, Dry & Mature Skin Types ($19.95 for 5 ounces).

Best Skin-Lightening Products

Only a small group of products fit into this category of effective skin-lightening products. The preponderance of evidence indicates that the best ingredient for effectively inhibiting melanin production is hydroquinone. Over-the-counter hydroquinone products are available in strengths of 1% to 2%, and higher concentrations are available from dermatologists and plastic surgeons. Some formulations include kojic acid to boost the effectiveness of the hydroquinone, and others include some amount of AHA and BHA to increase cell turnover, and that is just fine—both of those are good additions to improve the color of sun-damaged skin. Skin-lightening properties are often attributed to other ingredients, such as plants or vitamins, but there is no evidence that these have any effect on the skin. **Keep in mind that no skin-lightening product will work if an effective sunscreen is not used on a daily basis.**

<u>FOR ALL SKIN TYPES THE BEST SKIN-LIGHTENING PRODUCTS</u> <u>ARE:</u> **Avon** Banishing Cream Skin Lightening Treatment ($8.50 for 2.5 ounces); **Bioelements** Pigment Discourager ($18.50 for 0.5 ounce); **Black Opal** Advanced Dual Complex Fade Gel ($11.95 for 0.75 ounce); **Color Me Beautiful** Fade Away for All Skin Types ($15 for 1.9 ounces); **Fashion Fair** Vantex Skin Bleaching Creme with Sunscreens ($14 for 2 ounces); **M.D. Formulations** Skin Bleaching Lotion ($30 for 1.5 ounces), and Forte Skin Bleaching Gel with 2% Hydroquinone in a Base Containing 10% Glycolic Compound ($30 for 1.5 ounces); **Paula's Choice** Remarkable Skin Lightening Lotion for All Skin Types ($12.95 for 4 ounces); and **philosophy** when lightening strikes ($45 for 4 ounces).

Best Self-Tanners

Because all self-tanners use the exact same ingredient, dihydroxyacetone, to turn the skin brown, there is no way to differentiate one from the other: they all perform essentially the same. Where self-tanners do differ is in the amount of dihydroxyacetone used; however, there is no way for me to determine how much each product contains. Even if I could find out how much dihydroxyacetone was in a given formula, because skin interaction with the amount of the active ingredient varies so widely, there isn't a hierarchy of too much or too little being either a positive or a negative. It all depends on your skin, and even more primarily on your application technique.

Best Foundations

Perhaps no area of makeup is more treacherous and just plain hard to get exactly right than finding the perfect foundation. The problems are many, but the most difficult to overcome are hopes for flawless looking skin, color choice, and texture. Women want a foundation that fits like a second, secret skin but still provides coverage and camouflage, erases wrinkles, hides blemishes, and reflects a radiant look. That is no short order. Foundations have their limitations, and some women find that hard to accept and keep looking endlessly for the right one. For instance, some women make a personal quest of finding an oil-free foundation that will last through the evening. If you have oily skin, that just isn't possible without intermittent touchups during the day. Plus, selecting oil as the only nefarious ingredient for oily skin is irrationally narrow. There are lots of ingredients that aren't an oil or oily but that are still notorious for clogging pores. Light reflecting or diffusing foundations promise to diminish the appearance of wrinkles, and those claims are equally bogus. All it takes is one application to check out how impossible that is too achieve with a foundation. Indeed, there are lots of great foundations, but only some (certainly not all) of your high hopes can be fulfilled.

Choosing the right foundation color is not only time-consuming, it is exceedingly frustrating. **The only way to discover what fits is to apply the foundation on your skin, perhaps two different colors on either side of your face, and then to check it in the daylight. If the color isn't an exact match, you have to go back in and try again.**

The last hurdle is finding a pleasing texture, one that feels soft and silky but doesn't streak, cake, or look thick, and that takes experimentation too. Now tell me that isn't a challenge!

If you can splurge on only one product, foundation is it. This is the one area where spending a little bit more is the best option, not because expensive means better, but because it's just way too risky to buy a foundation you can't try on first.

Beauty Note: I feel strongly that pressed-powder-style foundations are best for normal to slightly dry or slightly oily skin. Because this is a unique group of products to use as a foundation, and one which involves personal preference more than skin type, I've included those in a separate category. *needs a "SPF" in formula*

<u>FOR VERY OILY SKIN, THE BEST FOUNDATIONS ARE:</u> **Almay** Amazing Lasting Makeup ($7.35); **BeautiControl** Color Freeze Liquid Makeup SPF 12 ($19.50); **BeneFit** Matte Tint Liquid Foundation ($20); **Estee Lauder** Double Wear Makeup SPF 10 ($27.50); **Lancome** MaquiControle ($30), Teint Idole ($32.50), and Eau de Teint ($25); **Maybelline** Great Wear Makeup ($4.72); **Revlon** ColorStay ($8.22), and ColorStay Lite SPF 15 ($8.95); and **Smash Box** Anti-Shine Foundation ($32). *— Avon —*

<u>FOR NORMAL TO OILY/COMBINATION SKIN, THE BEST FOUN-DATIONS ARE:</u> **Almay** Amazing Lasting Sheer Makeup SPF 12 ($8.37); **Amway** Oil-Free Foundation ($18.90); **Aveda** Base Plus Balance ($20.50); **Avon** Calming Effects Illuminating Foundation ($8.95), and Perfect Match Self Adjusting Foundation ($5.50); **Black Opal** True Color Liquid Foundation Oil-free ($5.95); **Bobbi Brown Essentials** Oil-Free Foundation ($35); **Bonne Bell** No Shine Oil Control Makeup ($2.09); **Borghese** Cura Naturale Time Defying Makeup Oil-Free SPF 8 ($28.50); **Clinique** Stay True Oil-Free ($14.50); **Elizabeth Arden** Flawless Finish Complete Control Matte Makeup SPF 10 ($25); **Erno Laszlo** Multi-pHase Oil-Free Foundation SPF 15 ($28); **Fashion Fair** Oil-Free Liquid ($17.50); **Flori Roberts** Maximum Matte Souffle Oil-Free Makeup ($20); **Lancome** Teint Idole ($32.50), and Eau de Teint ($25); **Laura Mercier Classique** Oil-Free Foundation ($35); **Mary Kay** Day Radiance Formula III Oil-Free for Oily and Combination Skin ($11);

Maybelline Great Wear Makeup ($4.72); Origins Some Coverage ($14.50), More Coverage ($14.50), and Most Coverage ($14.50); and Yves St. Laurent Teint Sur Mesure Duo De Teint ($65 for 1 ounce).

FOR NORMAL TO DRY SKIN, THE BEST FOUNDATIONS ARE: Bobbi Brown Essentials Moisturizing Foundation ($35); The Body Shop Every Day Foundation ($8.50); Borghese Cura Naturale Time Defying Makeup Normal to Dry Skin SPF 8 ($28.50); Chanel Teint Extreme Lumiere with Non-Chemical SPF 8 ($50), Teint Caresse Naturel ($42), and Teint Lumiere Creme with Non-Chemical SPF 8 ($55); Charles of the Ritz Superior Moisture Foundation for Normal to Dry Skin ($20), and Moistureful Line Defying Makeup SPF 20 ($26.50); Christian Dior Teint Dior Eclat Satin ($42.50); Clinique Balanced Makeup Base ($13.50), Soft Finish Makeup ($18.50), and Almost Makeup SPF 15 ($16.50); Club Monaco Oil-Free Foundation ($18), and Liquid Makeup ($18); Color Me Beautiful Liquid Foundation ($18), and Illusion Age Defying Foundation SPF 15 ($20); Cover Girl ContinuousWear Natural Makeup ($6.29); Elizabeth Arden Flawless Finish Hydro Light Foundation SPF 10 ($30), and Flawless Finish Every Day Makeup SPF 10 ($25), Erno Laszlo Multi-pHase Light Diffusing Foundation SPF 15 ($28); Estee Lauder Minute Makeup SPF 15 ($27.50), Enlighten Skin-Enhancing Makeup with SPF 10 ($27.50), and Lucidity Light Diffusing Makeup SPF 8 ($27.50); Face Stockholm Matte Foundation ($21); Fashion Fair Liquid Sheer Foundation ($12.50); Gayle Hayman Light Coverage Treatment Makeup ($15); Guerlain Perfect Light SPF 8 Foundation ($44); Lancome MaquiVelour Hydrating Foundation ($30); Laura Mercier Classique Moisturizing Foundation ($35); M.A.C. Matte Finish ($20), Satin Finish ($18), and EP-T Day Emulsion Moisturizer ($28); Make Up For Ever— Paris Soft Modeling Film ($24); Mary Kay Day Radiance Formula II for Normal to Dry Skin SPF 8 ($11); Maybelline Natural Defense Makeup with SPF 15 ($5.26); Mon Amie The Foundation ($19.95); Nars Balanced Foundation ($37), and Oil Free Foundation ($37); Orlane Satilane ($35); philosophy our foundation ($25); Prescriptives Makeup ($30), Matchstick Foundation SPF 15 ($35), and Custom Blended Foundation Oil Free ($55); Revlon Age Defying Makeup with SPF 10 ($9.34); Shiseido Stick Foundation ($29), and Fluid Foundation ($29); Smash Box Liquid Foundation ($28); Stila Oil Free Liquid Makeup ($30); Trish McEvoy Cream Powder Makeup ($40); and Ultima II Beautiful Nutrient Nourishing Makeup SPF 15 ($24), and Beautiful Nutrient Nourishing Compact Makeup ($24).

FOR EXTRA DRY SKIN, THE BEST FOUNDATIONS ARE: Alexandra de Markoff Countess Isserlyn Creme Makeup ($45), and Countess Isserlyn Soft Velvet Makeup Oil-Free ($42.50); Amway Liquid Foundation ($17.05); Avon Face Lifting Moisture Firm Foundation Liquid ($8.95), and Face Lifting Moisture Firm Foundation Cream ($8.95); **Borghese** Cura Naturale Time Defying Makeup SPF 8 Creme for Very Dry Skin ($35); **Christian Dior** Teint Dior Actuel ($42.50); **Clinique** Extra Help ($18.50); **Elizabeth Arden** Flawless Finish Sponge-On Cream Makeup ($25); **Guerlain** Issima Foundation ($53); **Mary Kay** Day Radiance Formula I Foundation for Dry Skin SPF 8 ($11 for refill, $8 for compact); **Merle Norman** Luxiva Ultra Foundation with HC-12 ($22); **Prescriptives** Custom Blended Foundation Moisturizing Formula ($55); **Revlon** Age Defying Extra Cover Creme Makeup SPF 12 ($9.34); and **Stila** Complete Coverage Foundation ($40).

FOR MAXIMUM COVERAGE REGARDLESS OF SKIN TYPE, THE BEST FOUNDATIONS ARE: **Almay** Amazing Lasting Makeup ($7.35); **Clinique** Continuous Coverage Makeup SPF 11 (nonchemical) ($14.50); **Dermablend** Active Cover Creme Foundation SPF 15 ($18.50), The Cover Creme Foundation ($18), and Leg & Body Cover ($13.50); **Estee Lauder** Maximum Coverage with Non-Chemical SPF 12 ($25); **Maybelline** Great Wear Foundation ($4.72); and **Revlon** ColorStay ($9.34).

BEST PRESSED-POWDER FOUNDATIONS (GENERALLY BEST FOR NORMAL TO SLIGHTLY DRY OR SLIGHTLY OILY SKIN AND BEST USED AS POWDER NOT FOUNDATION) ARE: **Amway** Versatile Matte Pressed Powder Foundation ($18.20); **Aveda** Dual Base Minus Oil ($19.50); **BeautiControl** Perfecting Wet/Dry Finish Foundation ($19.50); **BeneFit** Sheer genius ($26); **The Body Shop** All-in-One Face Base ($15); **Borghese** Cura Naturale Time Defying Makeup Dual Effetto SPF 8 ($28.50); **Chanel** Double Perfection Makeup ($42); **Christian Dior** Teint Dior Dual Poudre Foundation ($42.50); **Clarins** Compact Powder Foundation ($29.50); **Clinique** Super Powder Double Face Powder Foundation ($15.50); **Color Me Beautiful** Perfection Microfine Powder Foundation ($20); **Elizabeth Arden** Flawless Finish Dual Perfection Makeup ($25), and Flawless Finish Control Matte Powder Makeup ($25); **Estee Lauder** Compact Finish Double Performance Makeup ($27.50); **Face Stockholm** Powder Foundation ($24); **Garden Botanika** Natural Color Powder Plus ($12.50); **Guerlain** Treatment Powder Foundation ($47); **Lancome** Dual Finish Powder ($27.50); **L'Oreal** Dualite Powder ($7.45); **M.A.C.** Studio Fix Pressed Powder Foundation ($19); **Shiseido** Dual Compact Powdery Foundation ($30); **Trish McEvoy** Dual Powder ($28); and **Youngblood** Natural Mineral Cosmetics ($29.95) (this is a loose powder foundation).

BEST CREAM-TO-POWDER OR LIQUID-TO-POWDER FOUNDATIONS (GENERALLY BEST FOR NORMAL TO SLIGHTLY DRY OR SLIGHTLY OILY SKIN) ARE: **The Body Shop** All-in-One Face Treat SPF 15 ($15); **Borghese** Molto Bella Liquid Powder Makeup ($35); **Chanel** Teint Perfecting

Compact Makeup ($40); **Clinique** City Base Compact Foundation SPF 15 ($20); **Lancome** Cool Finish Foundation ($46 for the foundation insert and $2.50 for the compact); **Mary Kay** Cream-to-Powder Foundation ($11 for refill, $8 for compact); **Prescriptives** Photochrome Compact Makeup SPF 15 ($35); **Revlon** New Complexion One-Step Makeup SPF 15 ($8.78); and **Shiseido** Advanced Performance Compact Foundation SPF 10 ($30), and Liquid Compact Foundation SPF 15 ($35).

Best Concealers

Finding a good under-eye concealer is a task that has become a great deal easier since the last edition of this book. A concealer shouldn't be too dry or too creamy, should definitely not crease into the lines under the eye (this requirement cannot be ignored, particularly by those of us with an increasing number of under-eye lines), and should provide good, even coverage. I found some great concealers in all price categories. I also found a lot of concealers that are still too thick, too greasy, too peach, too pink, too dark, or too expensive.

THE BEST CONCEALERS FOR ALL SKIN TYPES ARE: **Almay** Cover-Up Stick ($3.43), Extra Moisturizing Undereye Cover Cream ($6.50), Time-Off Age Smoothing Concealer ($6.18), Amazing Lasting Concealer ($6.19), and Sensitive Care Concealer ($5.95); **Aveda** Conceal Plus Protect ($13.50); **Chanel** Quick Cover Concealer ($32.50); **Christian Dior Hydrating Concealer** ($19.50); **Circle of Beauty** No Flaw Maximum Cover Concealer ($7); **Clinique** Quick Corrector ($9.50), and Soft Concealer Corrector ($10.50); **Club Monaco** Concealer ($10); **Cover Girl** Invisible Concealer ($3.69); **Dermablend** Quick Fix (cover stick) ($15); **Erno Laszlo** Anti Cerne Concealer ($25); **Estee Lauder** Smoothing Creme Concealer with SPF 8 ($16); **Jafra** White Souffle ($9); **Lancome** Effacernes Waterproof Anti-Cernes Waterproof Protective Undereye Concealer ($17.50), and MaquiComplet ($17.50); **Laura Mercier** Secret Concealer ($18); **L'Oreal** Mattique Conceal Oil-Free Cover-Up ($4.73), and Feel Perfecte Concealer ($5.89); **M.A.C.** Concealer ($10); **Maybelline** Great Wear Concealer ($4.19); **Revlon** New Complexion Concealer ($6.75), and ColorStay Concealer ($7.29); **Stila** Face Concealer ($16), and Eye Concealer ($16); **Ultima** II WonderWear Concealer ($14.50); and **Zhen** Concealer ($10.50).

Best Powders

It doesn't make sense to spend a lot of money on a finishing powder because there is so little difference between products. Most all pressed and loose powders are talc-based, and when talc is excluded the other minerals still perform similarly. I am often asked about the risk of talc as a cosmetic ingredient. While it is true that prolonged inhalation of talc can cause lung problems because it is similar in chemical composition to asbestos (asbestos is a known lung irritant and cancer-causing agent), that is only true for those working in the manufacture of talc or talc-related products. But that kind of exposure is radically different than exposure to the tiny amounts of talc found in makeup application.

The rest of the ingredients vary only slightly, although the companies make absurd claims about light-reflecting properties and micro-encapsulated color, all of which are nonsense. When I think of the number of pressed powders priced between $16 and $30, I just shake my head at the audacity of the cosmetics companies. Unfortunately, after recommending that you go inexpensive for this product group, I can't muster much enthusiasm for the finishing powders available at the drugstore. Not that many of these aren't superior products, but more often than not there is no way to test the color. In regard to drugstore finishing powders, I made my suggestions based on what I think are the safest choices for the products with the best texture, but if you are inexperienced or haven't had luck finding the best color, trying on a powder is generally the best way to make a decision.

Note: The recommendations for skin type that follow are more interchangeable than you might think. Choosing a powder truly has more to do with your preference (what kind of finish you like), how much of the product you use, and what kind of foundation you wear.

THE BEST FINISHING POWDERS (BOTH LOOSE AND PRESSED) FOR NORMAL TO OILY/COMBINATION SKIN, ARE: Amway Loose Powder ($17.50); **Arbonne** Translucent Pressed Powder ($16); **Aveda** Pressed Powder Plus Antioxidants ($17.50), and Pure Finish Loose Powder ($18.50); **bare escentuals** bareMinerals mineral veil ($22), and pressed mineral veil ($24); **BeautiControl** Oil-Free Translucent Pressed Powder ($10.50); **BeneFit** Powder tint ($22); **Black Opal** Oil Absorbing Pressed Powder ($6.82); **Christian Dior** Pressed Powder ($35), Loose Powder ($42.50), and Dior Light Oil-Free Pressed Powder ($35); **Clinique** Soft Finish Pressed Powder ($15.50), Stay Matte Sheer Pressed Powder ($15.50), Blended Face Powder with Brush ($15.50); **Club Monaco** Loose Powder ($18); **Color Me Beautiful** Translucent Loose Powder ($13.50); **Dermablend** Setting Loose Powder ($15), and Setting Pressed Powder ($15); **Estee Lauder** Double-Matte Oil-Free Loose Powder ($18.50), and Double-Matte Oil-Free Pressed Powder ($20); **Face Stockholm** Loose Powder ($18); **Jane** Staying Powder Loose Powder ($2.99); **Gale Hayman** Semi Translucent Face Powder ($17); **Iman** Luxury Pressed Powder Oil-Controlling ($15); **Laura Mercier Classique** Pressed Powder ($25), and Loose Powder ($28); **Lorac** Face Powder ($22.50), and ($32); **M.A.C.** Blot Powder ($12); **Mary Kay** Powder

Perfect Loose Powder ($12.50), and Powder Perfect Pressed Powder ($7.50); **Maybelline** Shine-Free Oil-Control Translucent Pressed Powder ($3.35); **Mon Amie** Pressed/Translucent Powder ($19.95); **Physicians Formula** Shine Away Neutral Oil Control Pressed Powder ($5.95); **Prestige** Pressed Powders ($4.51); **Stila** The Loose Powder ($27), and Pressed Powder ($32); and **Zhen** Dual Activ Powder Foundation ($20).

THE BEST FINISHING POWDERS (BOTH LOOSE AND PRESSED) FOR DRY SKIN, ARE: **Almay** Luxury Finish Loose Powder ($7.79); **BeautiControl** Loose Perfecting Powder ($10.50); **Borghese** Powder Milano ($30); **Club Monaco** Pressed Powder ($16); **Estee Lauder** Lucidity Translucent Loose Powder ($26), Lucidity Translucent Pressed Powder ($20), and Enlighten Powder ($20); **Guerlain** Pressed Powder ($38); **La Prairie** Translucent Pressed Powder ($36), and Foundation Finish Loose Powder ($40); **Lancome** Poudre Majeur Pressed Powder ($26.50); **M.A.C.** Pressed Powder ($18), and Loose Powder ($14); **Make Up For Ever—Paris** Poudre Libre ($27), and Compact Powder ($27); **Maybelline** Finish Matte Pressed Powder ($3.29); **Nars** Pressed Powder ($24); **Origins** Original Skin Pressed Powder ($13.50 for the powder refill and $4 for the compact); **Orlane** Translucent Powder ($35); **Prescriptives** All Skins Pressed Powder ($22.50), and All Skins Loose Powder ($24.50); **Shiseido** Natural Pressed Powder ($23); **Victoria Jackson** Pressed Powder ($11.95, $17.95); and **Wet 'n' Wild** Pressed Powder ($2.49).

THE BEST BRONZING PRODUCTS ARE: **Bobbi Brown Essentials** Bronzing Stick ($25), and Bronzing Powder ($26); **Bonne Bell** Gel Bronze Face and Body Bronzer ($2.09), and Cream Bronze Face Bronze ($2.09); **The Body Shop** Twist & Bronze ($11); **Clarins** Bronzing Duo ($24); and **Club Monaco** Bronzers Pressed Powder ($16).

Best Blushes

Blush is probably one of the easiest cosmetics to get right because it is hard to buy a bad blush. Not that there aren't some real losers out there, but there are far more winners. The problem with blush is usually application, and that is where good brushes come into play. Using the proper brushes is essential for getting blushes to go on correctly.

Blushes received high marks if most of the colors were matte, had a soft, nongrainy texture, blended on smoothly, did not fade or dissipate with time, and came in a good selection of colors. There are plenty that qualify, so don't spend a lot of money on blush unless you need to test the color first. Many drugstore blushes are of a superior quality and provide the same results as those at the department store.

THE BEST POWDER BLUSHES ARE FROM THE FOLLOWING COMPANIES: Alexandra de Markoff; Almay; Arbonne; Aveda; bare escentuals; Black Opal; BeautiControl; Bobbi Brown Essentials; The Body Shop; Bonne Bell; Borghese; Charles of the Ritz; Christian Dior; Circle of Beauty; Clarins; Clinique; Elizabeth Arden; Estee Lauder; Face Stockholm; Fashion Fair; Garden Botanika; Guerlain; Il Makiage; Iman; Jafra; Jane; Janet Sartin; Lancome; Laura Mercier Classique; Lorac; M.A.C.; Make Up For Ever–Paris; Maybelline; Maybelline Shades of You; Merle Norman; M Professional; Origins; philosophy; Physicians Formula; Prescriptives; Prestige; Color Principal; Revlon; R Pro; Shiseido; Shu Uemura; Stila; Trish McEvoy; Ultima II; Victoria Jackson; Wet 'n' Wild; and Zhen.

THE BEST CREAM OR GEL BLUSHES ARE FROM THE FOLLOWING COMPANIES: Bobbi Brown Essentials; Clinique; Club Monaco; Estee Lauder; Lancome; M Professional; Mon Amie; and Origins.

Best Eyeshadows

By now many of you know my opinions about shiny eyeshadows as well as blue, green, or any brightly colored eyeshadow. It still is my goal to find the best matte shades available, and I am thrilled to say that the cosmetics industry does deliver. There are more than enough matte shades available in all price ranges. You can shop both the drugstore and cosmetics counters and find wonderful textures and colors. You still have lots of shiny products to wade through, or to choose, if that's your preference.

Be aware that almost all of the lines listed below have some shiny eyeshadows mixed in with their matte colors.

THE BEST MATTE EYESHADOWS CAN BE FOUND IN THE FOLLOWING LINES: Almay; Arbonne; Aveda; Black Opal; Bobbi Brown Essentials; Borghese; Charles of the Ritz; Club Monaco; Elizabeth Arden; Estee Lauder; Face Stockholm; Garden Botanika; Guerlain; Iman; Jane; Lancome; Laura Mercier Classique; Lorac; L'Oreal; M Professional; M.A.C.; Make Up For Ever—Paris; Merle Norman; Mon Amie; Nars; Natural Glow from Naturistics; Origins; philosophy; Physicians Formula; Prescriptives; Prestige; Color Principal; Revlon; R Pro; Shiseido; Shu Uemura; Stila; Trish McEvoy; Ultima II; Yves St. Laurent; and Zhen.

Best Eye and Brow Shapers

Some cosmetics companies sell two different eye pencils, one for the brow and the other for lining the eye. Other cosmetics companies are more straightforward and sell only one that does both jobs. That is the practical and honest approach.

There is usually little to no difference between eye and brow pencils. The contrasts mainly involve color choice. When there is a difference, the brow pencil often has a drier consistency. That can make drawing on a brow difficult, though it does tend to look less greasy.

An eye pencil with a dry texture makes it difficult to line the eyelid after you've applied your eyeshadows; if the pencil is on the greasy side, it will line the lid more easily, but it is also more likely to smear under the lower lashes in a very short time. **I have always preferred (and still do) to line the eyes with regular eyeshadow powder and a small, thin eyeliner brush.** I usually line my lower lashes with a soft brown eyeshadow and my eyelid with a black or dark brown eyeshadow. You can also wet the brush and apply the eyeshadow as you would a liquid liner in a more vivid line. In fact, even when I line my eyes with a pencil, I go over it with an eyeshadow to make sure it has a better chance of staying all day. The difference in the look and in how long it lasts compared with using a pencil alone, is amazing—particularly if you have oily or combination skin. If, however, the technique of lining your eyes with an eyeshadow and a tiny brush has eluded you and you prefer pencils, there are still many good ones. You can shop the more expensive lines, but it is a waste of money, because, regardless of the price, almost all the pencils I tested in all price ranges had more similarities than differences.

Eyebrow pencil has long been the standard method for making eyebrows appear thicker or more defined (and it still is), but greasy pencils look overly made-up and dry ones are not that easy to apply and can still look thick and heavy. It is my strong recommendation that you fill in the brow with a powder, either an eyeshadow or a specific eyebrow powder.

Several companies sell colored eyebrow gels as a way to fill, lift, and define the brow. There are also a few companies that make a clear brow gel that isn't much different than using hair spray on a toothbrush and brushing it through the brow. For the most part, the natural-colored brow gels are great. I strongly recommend them as another way to make eyebrows look fuller but not artificial. If you can learn how to use the eyebrow gels, they can be a great alternative to pencils.

Most every line has its share of extremely standard but very good pencils, so the preference for texture is up to you. Just be aware that liquid liners, brow powders, and brow gels do differ.

THE BEST LIQUID LINERS ARE: **Almay** Eye Defining Liquid Liner ($4.79), and I-Liner ($6.50); **Amway** Fine Liner ($13.45); **Jafra** Liquid Eyeliner ($8); **Lancome** Maquiglace Liquid Liner ($18.50), and Precision Point Artliner Automatic Eye Lining Felt Pen ($23.50); **L'Oreal** Lineur Intense ($5.47), and Super Liner ($5.68); **Lord & Berry** Ink Well ($3.37); **M.A.C.** Creme Liner ($9.50); **Nat Robbins** Perfect

Liquid Eyeliner ($2.49); **Revlon** Jetliner Intense ($4.84); **R Pro** Liquid Eyeliner ($5.99); **Ultima II** WonderWear Liquid Eye Definer ($12); and **Zhen** Liquid Eye Liner ($11.50).

THE BEST EYEBROW POWDERS (BUT ALSO REFER TO THE LIST OF MATTE EYESHADOWS AS DEFINITE OPTIONS FOR BROW POW- DERS) ARE: Circle of Beauty Color Up Brow Cake ($8); **Clinique** Brow Shaper ($12); **Elizabeth Arden** Great Color Brow Makeup ($15); **Face Stockholm** Brow Shadow ($16); **Lancome** Le Kohl Poudre ($14), and Le Crayon Poudre for the Brows ($16.50); **M Professional** Eyebrow Powder and Blush ($2.25); **Maybelline** Ultra-Brow Brush-On Brow Color ($3.42); **Merle Norman** Only Natural ($9.50); **R Pro** Liquid Eyeliner ($5.99); and **Physicians Formula** Eyeliner Palette Multi-Colored Cake Liner ($10.20).

THE BEST BROW GELS ARE: **Borghese** Milano ($20); **Chanel** Brow Shaper ($28.50); **Face Stockholm** Brow Fix ($12); **Max Factor** Brow Tamer ($4.99); **Ori- gins** Just Browsing ($11); **Merle Norman** Tinted Brow Sealer ($10.50); and **Revlon** ColorStay Brow Color ($6.94).

Best Lipsticks and Lip Pencils

By now we are all over the search for lipsticks that will last all day, right? We also know that the greasier or glossier the lipstick, the less likely it is to last, and the more matte the lipstick, the longer it is likely to stick around, although if it is too matte it may be too drying. If you don't have a problem with dry lips and you want to try a matte look, mattes and ultra-mattes are certainly an option. It is very difficult to make lipstick suggestions. There are great discussions on the Web about the best lipstick and lip pencil, but this is one area where preference plays a bigger role than any other issue. One woman who wrote me summed it up quite well by saying, "You seem not to like glossy lipsticks because they don't stay on well, but I love lipsticks that are glossy and don't mind reapplying frequently to get the look I want." I agree, some women just prefer glossy lipsticks and others creamy or matte. I still prefer a soft matte finish, but the options out there are incredible and there really isn't a "best."

If you do want to use a lip gloss or a sheer glossy lipstick during the day it would be best if the lipstick contained a good SPF with UVA protection.

All the lines have great lipsticks and lip glosses, depending on your preference. Rather than listing all of those, I am only including a list of specialty lipstick products that are relatively unique. Just keep in mind that price has nothing to do with how well a lipstick performs.

THE BEST MATTE LIPSTICKS ARE FROM: **Aveda** Lip Matte Plus Fresh Essence ($14); **Color Me Beautiful** More Than Matte Lipstick ($9.50); **Face Stockholm** Matte Lipstick ($15); **M Professional** Matte Lipstick SPF 15 ($2.99); **M.A.C.** Matte Lipstick ($13.50); **Make Up For Ever—Paris** Matte Lipstick ($16); **Nars** Matte Lipstick ($19); **Prestige** Lasting Lip Color ($3.89); and **Zhen** Matte Lipstick ($10).

THE BEST ULTRA-MATTE LIPSTICKS ARE FROM: **Almay** Amazing Lasting Lipstick ($7.95); **Cover Girl** Marathon ($4.32); **Charles of the Ritz** LipSTICK ($14); **Coty** Lip Writer Stayput Lipstick ($4.50); **Estee Lauder** Indelible ($16); **Jafra** Always Color Stay On Lipstick ($9); **Lancome** Rouge Idole ($16.50); **L'Oreal** Endure Stay-On Lip Colour ($6.39); **Lord & Berry** Kiss Proof Lipstick ($3.37); **Maybelline** Budgeproof Lipstick ($4.72), and Shades of You Lasting Finish Long-Wearing Matte Lipstick ($4.72); **Nat Robbins** Stay-Put Lipcolor ($2.99); **Shu Uemura** Powder Lipstick ($27); and **Ultima II** Lip Sexxxy ($12.50).

THE BEST LIPSTICKS OR LIP PRODUCTS WITH A HIGH SPF AND UVA PROTECTION ARE FROM: **Black Opal** Simply Sheer Lipstick with SPF 15 ($4.05); **Clinique** Lip Block SPF 15 ($7.50); **L'Oreal** Sheer Colour Riche SPF 15 ($6.28); **M Professional** Matte Lipstick SPF 15 ($2.99); **Nu Skin** Sunright Lip Balm 15 ($5.65); **Paula's Choice** Total Protection Lip Care SPF 15 ($6.95); and **Physicians Formula** Bare Radiance Protective Lip Shine SPF 15 ($4.49).

THE BEST PRODUCTS TO PREVENT LIPSTICK FROM BLEEDING ARE: **BeautiControl** Lip Control Creme ($7); **The BodyShop** No Wander ($6.50); **Coty** Stop It Anti-Feathering Stick for Lips ($3.57), and Hold It Wear Extending Base for Lips ($4.16); and **Revlon** Moon Drops Color Lock Anti-Feathering Lip Base ($6.20).

THE BEST LIPSTAINS ARE: **The Body Shop** Lipstain ($7.50), and **Lip Ink** ($15).

THE BEST PRODUCTS TO PREVENT CHAPPED AND DRY LIPS ARE: **Adrien Arpel** Freeze-Dried Protein Lip Peel and Salve ($39.50); **BeautiControl** Lip Apeel ($16.50 for 1.25 ounces); and **Paula's Choice** Exfoliating Lip Treatment ($7.95 for 0.5 ounce).

There is no reason to spend more than a few dollars on lip pencils. I can say without any hesitation that lip pencils priced over $6 are a waste of money. There is little to no difference between a higher-priced pencil and a less-expensive one. You can spend $22 on Estee Lauder's very attractive retractable lip pencil in the metallic blue case or you can spend $4 or $5 on Almay's or Revlon's lip pencils and get the same look. The decision is up to you. The only real difference is that a few are greasier than others, but that has nothing to do with price. Rather than listing every cosmetics line I've reviewed, I will just say that all of them have great lip liners; some have more color choices than others, but that's about the only difference.

The only real pitfall is believing that expensive lipsticks or lip pencils are somehow superior. Nothing could be further from the truth. Some of my favorite lipsticks are from M Professional (I love their mattes), Aveda, Zhen, Coty, and L'Oreal. When it comes to pencils, the $4 versions are identical to the $20 ones. Choosing not to see this is the way lots of women stay loyal to cosmetics companies regardless of the benefit to themselves.

Best Mascaras

I am still surprised by how many good mascaras there are at both drugstores and department stores. In fact, I think they've improved all around. All price ranges include excellent mascaras. Obviously, it is foolish to buy the most expensive mascara when reasonably priced ones are equally good. Given that this is one product you can't readily test at the counters, try a few of the inexpensive ones I suggest and see what works for you. It really is the most sensible and beautiful decision.

THE BEST MASCARAS ARE: **Alexandra de Markoff** Professional Secrets Mascara ($20); **Almay** One Coat Mascara ($4.95), Mascara Plus ($4.95), and Triple Thick Mascara ($4.99); **Amway** Smudgeproof Mascara ($14.20); **Borghese** Maximum Mascara for Sensitive Eyes ($17), and Superiore State of the Art Mascara ($16); **Chanel** Instant Lash Mascara ($20), and Instant Waterproof Mascara ($20); **Charles of the Ritz** Perfect Finish Lash ($12); **Christian Dior** Fascination Mascara ($19), Lengthening Mascara with Cashmere ($19), and Mascara Parfait ($18); **Clarins** Volumizing Mascara ($15.50); **Clinique** Naturally Glossy Mascara ($11), Full Potential Mascara ($11), Super Mascara ($11), and Gentle Waterproof Mascara ($11.50); **Color Me Beautiful** Lush Lash ($9.50); **Color Principal** Double Duty Mascara ($19); **Cover Girl** Long 'N Lush ($3.87), Curved Brush Professional Advanced Mascara ($3.05), Straight Brush Professional Advanced Mascara ($3.05), Super Thick Lash ($4.76), and Natural Lash Darkener ($3.95); **Elizabeth Arden** Twice as Thick Two Brush Mascara ($15), Two Brush Mascara Regular ($15), Defining Mascara ($15), and Two Brush Waterproof Mascara ($17); **Erno Laszlo** MultipHase Mascara ($19); **Estee Lauder** More Than Mascara ($15); **Givenchy** Mascara ($19); **Jane** Flashes Ultra Rich Mascara ($2.29); **Lancome** Definicils, Intencils, and Keracils ($16.50), Eternicils (waterproof) ($17), and Aquacils (waterproof) ($17); **Lorac by Carol Shaw** Mascara ($16); **Lord & Berry** Dramatic Eyes Waterproof Mascara ($3.37); **L'Oreal** Lash Out Extending Mascara ($5.39), Le Grand Curl ($5.39), Voluminous Mascara

($4.99, and Voluminous Waterproof ($5.39); **M Professional** Mascara ($2.82); **Make Up For Ever—Paris** Mascara ($16); **Max Factor** 2000 Calorie Mascara ($4.95), and S-T-R-E-T-C-H Mascara ($4.95); **Maybelline** Great Lash Pro Vitamin ($4.72), Illegal Lengths Mascara ($4.55), Volum' Express ($4.16), Extremely Gentle Mascara ($3.99), Volum' Express Waterproof Mascara ($4.16), Illegal Lengths Waterproof Mascara ($4.55), and Great Lash Waterproof Mascara ($3.99); **Natural Glow from Naturistics** Soft and Full Thickening Mascara ($2.81); **Origins** Fringe Benefits Mascara ($11); **Revlon** Lengthwise Mascara ($5.48), Lashfull Mascara ($5.48), and Lashful Mascara Curvaceous ($5.48); **Shiseido** Waterproof Mascara ($18); **Trish McEvoy** Mascara ($16); **Ultima II** Flutters Lengthening Mascara ($13), and WonderWear Mascara ($13); and **Yves St. Laurent** Conditioning Mascara ($20.50), and Mascara Essentiel ($20.50).

Best Brushes

More than ever before, professional-sized brushes are available in all price ranges. Keep in mind that the texture of the brush is more important than the source of the bristles. While many cosmetics companies love bragging about the type of animal hair used, you are not buying a mink coat. What counts is softness and firmness, no matter where it came from.

THE BEST ASSORTMENTS OF BRUSHES ARE FROM THE FOLLOW-ING COMPANIES: Aveda; bare escentuals; BeneFit; Bobbi Brown Essentials; Borghese; Chanel; Club Monaco; Estee Lauder Classique; Expressions Brushes; Face Stockholm; Janet Sartin; Joan Simmons Brushes; Laura Mercier; Lorac by Carol Shaw; M.A.C.; Maybelline; Nars; Origins; philosophy; Prescriptives; Prestige; R Pro; Shu Uemura; Stila; Trish McEvoy; and Zhen.

Best Specialty Products

This is a list of miscellaneous products that have interesting effects that just don't fit in the above categories.

Borghese Spa Mani Moisture Restoring Gloves ($38.50) are special gloves lined with silicone that can help keep moisture in the skin.

Rejuveness ($39.50 to $295, depending on the size ordered) are pliable sheets of silicone, used as a way to reduce the appearance of thick or raised scarring.

philosophy the coloring book ($160) is a great group of ten eyeshadows, four blushes, five lip colors, two liner pencils and a decent set of makeup brushes in one convenient kit.

Shiseido Pureness Oil-Blotting Paper ($10 for 100 sheets) are small sheets coated with a light layer of clay to be pressed against the skin to absorb oil.

Stila's Face Planner ($35 to $45 for the case/$12 to $14 for the pages) is a very clever way to assemble a makeup bag.

Appendix

WEB Sites for the Companies Reviewed

Adrien Arpel: *www.adrienarpel.com*

Aloette: *www.aloette cosmetiques.qc.ca/ menuen.html*

Alpha Hydrox: *www.alpha-hydrox.com*

Amway: *www.amway-usa.com/usa*

Arbonne: *www.arbonne.com*

Aubrey Organics: *www.aubrey-organics.com*

Aveda: *www.aveda.com*

Aveeno: *www.scjohnsonwax.com/aveeno.html*

Avon: *www.avon.com*

bare escentuals: *www.bareescentuals.com*

BeautiContol: *wwwbeauti.com/index.html*

Biogime: *www.biogime.com*

Biore: *www.jergens.com*

Bobbi Brown Essentials: *www.bobbibrown cosmetics.com*

The Body Shop: *www.the-body-shop.com*

Cetaphil: *www.cetaphil.com*

Clearasil: *www.clearasil.com*

Clinique: *www.clinique.com*

Cover Girl: *www.covergirl.com*

Dermablend: *www.sheen.com/derma/ dblend.htm*

Dermalogica: *www.dermalogica.com*

Exuviance by Neostrata: *www.neostrata.com/ consumer.html*

Fashion Fair: *www.ebonymag.com/ff/ ffmain.html*

Flori Roberts: *www.sheen.com/flori/flori.htm*

Freeman Beautiful Skin: *www.freeman cosmetics.com/index2.html*

Galderma: *www.galderma.com/products/usa*

Gale Hayman: *www.galehayman.com/ welcome.htm*

Guerlain: *www.guerlain.com*

H₂0 Plus: *www.h2oplus.com*

Hard Candy: *www.hardcandy.com*

IGIA: *www.igia.net*

Iman: *www.sheen.com/iman/iman.htm*

Janet Sartin: *www.sartin.com*

Jurlique: *www.jurlique.com*

L'Oreal: *www.lorealcosmetics.com*

La Prairie: *www.laprairie.com*

Lancome: *www.lancome.com*

Le Mirador: *www.themarshallplan.com/ lmrsp01.shtml*

Lip Ink: *www.lipink.com*

Lubriderm: *www.skinhelp.com*

M Professional: *www.mprofessional.com*

Mary Kay: *www.marykay.com*

Murad: *www.murad.com*

Neostrata: *www.neostrata.com/index.html*

Neutrogena: *www.neutrogena.com*

Nivea Visage: *www.nivea.com*

Noevir: *www.noevirusa.com*

Nu Skin: *www.nuskin.com*

Dr. Obagi: *www.rdgi.com/obagi/index.htm*

Ombrelle: *www.ombrelle.com*

Parthena: *www.parthenacosmetics.com*

Paula's Choice: *www.cosmeticscop.com*

philosophy: *www.philosophy.com*

Posner: *www.sheen.com/posner/posner.htm*

PropapH: *www.propaph.com*

Rachel Perry: *www.rachelperry.net*

Rejuveness: *www.rejuveness.com*

Revlon: *www.revlon.com*

Dr. Semel: *www.drsemel.com/index.html*

St. Ives: *www.stives.com*

Sea Breeze: *www.seabreezezone.com/home.html*

Shaklee Enfuselle: *www.enfuselle.com*

Shiseido: *www.shiseido.co.jp/e/index.htm*

Shu Uemura: *www.shu-uemura.co.jp*

Smash Box: *www.smashbox.com*

TheraCel: *www.theracel.com*

Urban Decay: *www.urbandecay.com*

Victoria Jackson: *www.vmakeup.com*

Yves Rocher: *www.yvesrocher.com*

Zhen: *www.dgi.net/zhen*

Animal Testing and Cosmetics

Companies that do not use animal testing:

Acne-Statin
Adrien Arpel
Alexandra de Markoff
Almay
Aloette
Alpha Max
Amway
Arbonne
Aubrey Organics
Aveda
Avon
bare escentuals and bareMinerals
Basis
Bath & Body Works
BeautiControl
Beauty Without Cruelty
BeneFit
Bioelements
Biogime
Biore
BioTherm
Black Opal
Blistex
Bobbi Brown Essentials
The Body Shop
Bonne Bell
Borghese
Cellex-C
Chanel
Chantal Ethocyn
Charles of the Ritz
Christian Dior
Clarins
Clear LogiX
Clientele
Clinique
Color Me Beautiful
Decleor Paris
Dermablend
Donna Karan New York

eb5
Estee Lauder
Exuviance by Neostrata
Fashion Fair
Flori Roberts
Forever Spring
Freeman Beautiful Skin
Garden Botanika
Guerlain
H_2O Plus
Il Makiage
Iman
Jafra
Jane
Janet Sartin
Jergens
Jurlique
Kiehl's
L'Oreal
La Prairie
Lancome
Lord & Berry
Marilyn Miglin
Mary Kay
Matrix Essentials
Maybelline
Merle Norman
Mon Amie
Murad
Neostrata
Neutrogena
Nivea Visage
Noevir
Nu Skin
Dr. Obagi
Origins
Orlane
Paula's Choice
philosophy
Physician's Formula
Posner
Prescriptives
Prestige Cosmetics

Principal Secret
PropapH
Rachel Perry
Ralph Lauren Polo Sport
Rejuveness
Renee Guinot
Revlon
St. Ives
Serious Skin Care
Shu Uemura
Smash Box
TheraCel
Tova
Trish McEvoy
Ultima II
Urban Decay
Victoria Jackson
Wet 'n' Wild
Youngblood
Yves Rocher
Yves St. Laurent
Zhen
Zia

Companies continuing to use animal testing:

Aapri
Aveeno
Bain de Soleil
Cetaphil (Galderma)
Clean & Clear
Clearasil
Coppertone
Coty
Cover Girl
Dove
Elizabeth Arden
Erno Laszlo
Johnson & Johnson
Max Factor
Noxzema
Oil of Olay
Oxy Balance

Purpose
Sea Breeze
Shiseido
Suave
Vaseline Intensive Care

Companies with unknown animal-testing status:

Aqua Glycolic
Dermalogica
Exact
Givenchy
Hard Candy
Hydron
Lac-Hydrin

Laura Mercier Classique
Le Mirador
Lip Ink
Lorac by Carol Shaw
Lubriderm
M Professional
M.D. Formulations
Make Up Forever—Paris
Marcelle
Mariana Chicet
Dr. Mary Lupo
Moisturel
Nars
Nat Robbins
Natura Bisse

Nature's Cure
Ombrelle
Organic Essentials from
    Linda Chae
Pan Oxyl
Parthena
pHisoDerm
ProActive
Dr. Semel
Sisley
Stila
Stridex
Sudden Youth
Tyra

Information Sources

Cosmetic, Toiletry, and Fragrance Association (CTFA)
1101 17th Street N.W., Suite 300
Washington, DC 20036-4702
Tel: (202) 331-1770

Cosmetic, Toiletry, and Fragrance Association (CTFA) Scientific/Regulatory Reference Guide, 1997 Edition
1101 17th Street N.W., Suite 300
Washington, DC 20036-4702
Tel: (202) 331-1770

Cosmetic Ingredient Review Board
1101 17th Street N.W., Suite 310
Washington D.C. 20036-4702
Tel: (202) 331-0651

Household & Personal Products Industry (HAPPI) (magazine)
Rodman Publishing
17 South Franklin Turnpike
Ramsey, NJ 07446
Tel: (201) 825-2552

Cosmetics & Toiletries® magazine
Allured Publishing Corp.
362 S. Schmale Road
Carol Stream, IL 60188-2787
Tel: (630) 653-2155

Drug & Cosmetics Industry (DCI) (magazine)
Advanstar Communications
P.O. Box 5045
Pittsfield, MA 01203-9683
Tel: (888) 527-7008

Encyclopedia of Common Natural Ingredients, 2nd Edition
by Albert Y. Leung and Steven Foster
John Wiley & Sons, Inc.
605 Third Avenue
New York, NY 10158-0012
Tel: (212) 850-6000

The Food and Drug Law Journal
1000 Vermont Ave. N.W., Suite 200
Washington, DC 20005-4903
Tel: (202) 371-1420

Personal Care Formulas
Allured Publishing Corp.
362 S. Schmale Road
Carol Stream, IL 60188
Tel: (630) 653-2155

Cosmeceuticals, Active Skin Treatment
Allured Publishing Corp.
362 S. Schmale Road
Carol Stream, IL 60188-2787
Tel: (630) 653-2155

**The Chemistry and Manufacture
of Cosmetics**
Allured Publishing Corp.
362 S. Schmale Road
Carol Stream, IL 60188-2787
Tel: (630) 653-2155

*Personal Care for People Who Care,
9th Edition*
National Anti-Vivisection Society
53 W. Jackson Blvd.
Chicago, IL 60604
Tel: (800) 888-6287

F-D-C Reports— "The Rose Sheet"
5500 Friendship Blvd., Suite One
Chevy Chase, MD 20815-7278
Tel: (800) 844-8974

Cosmetic Dermatology (journal)
Quadrant HealthCom Inc.
26 Main Street
Chatham NJ, 07928-2402
Tel: (973) 701-8900

*The Journal of the American
Medical Association*
Subscriber Services Center
P.O. Box 10945
Chicago, IL 60610
Fax: (312) 464-5831

www.ncbi.nlm.nih.gov/pubmed
(Web site for the National Library
of Medicine)

The New England Journal of Medicine
Massachusetts Medical Society
10 Shattuck Street
Boston, MA 02115-6094
Tel: (617) 734-9800

www.lancet.com
(medical journal on-line)

www.FDA.gov
(Web site for the U.S. Food and Drug
Administration)

www.Medscape.com
(medical journal on-line)

*www.matrix.ucdavis.edu/DO/desk/
desk.html*
(Dermatology Online Journal)

www.AAD.org
(on-line information from the American
Academy of Dermatology)